First Principles of Gastroenterology

Gastroenterology

The Basis of Disease and an Approach to Management

FOURTH EDITION

First Principles of Gastroenterology

Gastroenterology

The Basis of Disease and an Approach to Management

A.B.R. THOMSON and E.A. SHAFFER,
editors

FOURTH EDITION

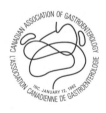

Endorsed by

Supported by an education grant from   AstraZeneca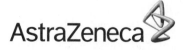

The publication of this book was endorsed by the Canadian Association of Gastroenterology and the Canadian Association for the Study of the Liver and supported by an education grant from AstraZeneca Canada Inc.

Publishers:

Co-editors
Dr. A.B.R. Thomson
University of Alberta
519 Newton Research Building
11315-87 Ave.
Edmonton, AB T6G 2C2

and

Dr. E.A. Shaffer
University of Calgary, Foothills Hospital
1403-29 St. NW, Room C210
Calgary, AB T2N 2T9

AstraZeneca Canada Inc.
1004 Middlegate Road
Mississauga, ON
L4Y 1M4

Canadian Cataloguing in Publication Data

Main entry under title:

First principles of gastroenterology : the basis of disease and an approach to management
4th ed.
Issued also in French under title: Principes fondamentaux de gastro-entérologie
Endorsed by: Canadian Association of Gastroenterology and Canadian Association for the Study of the Liver.
Includes bibliographical references and index.
ISBN 0-920163-20-3 (bound) ISBN 0-920163-18-1 (pbk.)

1.   Gastroenterology.
I.   Thomson, A.B.R. (Alan Bryan Robert), 1943 -   .
II.   Shaffer, E.A. (Eldon A.), 1941 -   .
III.   Canadian Association of Gastroenterology.
IV.   Canadian Association for the Study of the Liver.
V.   AstraZeneca Canada Inc.

RC801.F57 2000   616.3'3   C00–932020-2

Great care has been taken to ensure the accuracy of the contents of this publication. However, the publishers cannot be responsible for errors or any consequences arising from the information published herein.

Project Management: MacLean Communications Inc., Milton, ON
                     Tel: (905) 878-9752 or e-mail: kathy@macleancomm.com
Copy Editor: Cy Strom, Toronto, ON Tel.: (416) 214-0183 ext. 12

Printed on recycled paper and bound in Canada.

We invite you to visit our website based upon the 3rd edition of this textbook at www.gastroresource.com

Dedication

Without the caring support from our families for our academic work, the meaning of our accomplishments would disappear. We acknowledge and express our sincere thanks for the encouragement and love of Jeannette, James, Matthew, Jessica and Benjamin Thomson, and of Beryl, Andrea, Emily and Alexandra Shaffer.

A.B.R. Thomson
E.A. Shaffer

Contents

Preface

It was almost 10 years ago that Alan Thomson and Eldon Shaffer conceived the idea that there was a need for the type of introductory textbook useful to students, residents, family physicians and specialists alike. This book would need to cover the pathophysiological basis of gastrointestinal and hepatobiliary disease, and would also need to list learning objectives and contain abundant illustrations, be well indexed, and provide a logical and practical approach to patient management. It was recognized that such a book was not intended to replace the standard encyclopedic tomes or excellent in-depth reviews, but would instead provide a complementary first step to the vast and exciting field of gastroenterology, including processes and diseases of the hepatobiliary and pancreatic systems and nutrition. The editors also recognized that there was a place for consideration of important topics such as ethical issues, the clinical trials that form the basis of much of our modern practice, and of course, the crucial new area of molecular biology as it applies to clinical practice and patient care.

It was only when this idea for *"First Principles"* was taken to Mr. Peter Dixon that the possibility of success became real. Mr. Dixon had a vision of the importance of such a tribute to Canadian gastroenterology, the insight that such a book must be made available in both Canadian official languages, English and French, and the understanding that it was essential to bring out such a textbook in a timely manner and at a modest cost. It was through his energetic and enthusiastic support of this concept that it was possible to obtain the generous arm's-length sponsorship of AstraZeneca Canada Inc. The book is of the very highest quality in both content and presentation, and for this we are most thankful to MacLean Communications Inc. and in particular Ms. Kathy Dixon and Mr. Cy Strom for the careful copy editing and proofreading.

The editors then turned their efforts to making the textbook available to all members of the medical community worldwide. This led, again with the generous support of AstraZeneca Canada Inc., to the successful achievement of a CD-ROM and the establishment of a website containing the Gastro Resource Centre and the text of *First Principles of Gastroenterology:* www.gastroresource.com.

Now this textbook is available to all students, residents and practitioners throughout the world. Video tapes of endoscopic procedures have been provided through the generous and enthusiastic support of Dr. Norm Marcon and his colleagues at the Wellesley Hospital, Toronto, Ontario. The text has been enriched with photomicrographs of important pathological examples supplied by Dr. Lawrence Jewell. The Internet version of the textbook will be updated regularly, providing the framework for evidence-based practice of gastroenterology and an important role for Canadian physicians in maintaining the very best knowledge basis while providing compassionate and competent patient care.

We appreciate the continued endorsement of the Canadian Association of Gastroenterology and the Canadian Association for the Study of the Liver. To our readers, we welcome your suggestions and comments – this textbook is at the forefront of medical knowledge and we are eager to use modern teaching and communications methods to help you remain at the forefront.

To all our chapter captains and contributors, thank you most sincerely for the excellent job which you have done in writing this material. It is a pleasure working with you and we look forward to many future years of successful collaboration.

Alan B.R. Thomson
Eldon A. Shaffer

Endorsement

The Canadian Association of Gastroenterology and its members are proud sponsors of the fourth edition of *First Principles of Gastroenterology*. This highly successful endeavor is written for the undergraduate and graduate student of gastrointestinal and liver disease, and for the practicing clinician providing gastrointestinal and liver health care to patients. The discipline of gastroenterology and hepatology, like all of medicine, is undergoing enormous change, and our understanding of physiology and pathophysiology is taking quantum leaps forward. This textbook addresses the discipline, ranging from the domains of molecular genetics and cell biology to population health and wellness. The Canadian Association of Gastroenterology hopes that you find it informative and stimulating.

Richard N Fedorak, MD
President, Canadian Association of Gastroenterology

On behalf of the Canadian Association for the Study of the Liver (CASL), I am pleased to endorse this fourth edition of *First Principles of Gastroenterology*. I believe that it has assumed a place amongst the standard textbooks in gastroenterology and hepatology. It is detailed enough for everyday clinical use, but also concise enough to be read cover-to-cover. Many CASL members contributed to the sections dealing with the liver, and it has been gratifying to see the continuing growth and diffusion of this Canadian text. Congratulations to the editors and contributors for making this book a success.

Samuel S. Lee, MD, FRCPC
President, Canadian Association for the Study of the Liver

First Principles of Gastroenterology

The Basis of Disease and an Approach to Management

FOURTH EDITION

1
Common Symptoms and Signs in Gastroenterology

R.R. Gillies, W.G. Thompson, M.C. Champion,
S. Grégoire, J.M. Watters, D.G. Patel, L.J. Scully,
A.S.C. Sekar, R.F. Bursey, J.M. Fardy and
D.G. MacIntosh

1. INTRODUCTION / W.G. Thompson

The key to accurate diagnosis and effective management of gastrointestinal problems is flawless history-taking. Since up to 50% of gastrointestinal disorders are associated with no anatomical change, no physical findings and no positive test result, diagnosis and therapy must often be based on the medical interview. The gastrointestinal history must include an accurate description of the symptom itself, a past history of gastrointestinal disorders, treatment or surgery and a meticulous search for symptoms that might suggest organic disease. Finally, the physician should assess the patient's psychosocial state, with particular attention directed toward traumatic events or concerns associated with the onset of his or her complaints.

The physician should determine the time of onset of the symptom, its occurrence in the past, its periodicity, its location and radiation if appropriate, its aggravating and relieving factors, and its relationship to other symptoms. A review of past history should include not only any previous gastrointestinal surgery or diseases, but also systemic illnesses (such as diabetes or severe cardiovascular disease) that might affect the gut. One should pay particular attention to "alarm" symptoms such as gastrointestinal hemorrhage, profound weight loss, voluminous diarrhea or episodes of extreme abdominal pain, which might indicate organic disease. Similarly, such phenomena as anemia, fever or incapacity to work may indicate a more serious gastrointestinal disorder demanding investigation, treatment and follow-up. A family history of inflammatory bowel disease or bowel cancer may indicate a more careful investigation as well.

When considering a gastrointestinal complaint, the astute physician cannot ignore the patient's psyche. Many studies establish that those who bring gastrointestinal complaints to a physician, even if they are organic in nature, frequently have psychosocial disabilities. Failure to identify and manage the patient's reaction to his or her psychosocial environment (whether it be hostility toward a spouse, an abnormal fear of cancer or a profound loss) may lead to an unsatisfactory therapeutic outcome.

The following is a synopsis of the common gastrointestinal symptoms. These notes include a description of the symptom itself, a word about how the symptom is generated, the important historical features and associated physical findings, and a brief approach to diagnosis and management. These serve as introductory comments; greater detail can be found throughout the text in discussions of specific diseases. The final section of this chapter presents a sequential approach to the examination of the abdomen.

2. GLOBUS / W.G. Thompson

2.1 Synonyms
Globus hystericus; lump in the throat.

2.2 Description
Globus is a lump in the throat or a perceived inability to swallow unassociated with meals. Nearly one out of every two persons experiences this symptom, often at the time of an intense emotional experience.

2.3 Mechanism
Globus is a "functional" disorder since no pathologic or pathophysiologic abnormality has been clearly identified. Many believe that globus is due to a dysmotility of the upper esophageal sphincter.

2.4 Important Historical Features
Generally speaking, patients with globus can swallow meals normally but feel an inability to swallow their saliva between meals. The tendency of globus to occur when the patient is experiencing intense emotion has led in the past to the use of the epithet "globus hystericus." Since one-half of the population experiences this symptom, the term *hystericus* hardly seems justified. Patients may have psychogenic features such as anxiety, but are not overt in displaying other conversion features. There are no physical findings.

2.5 Differential Diagnosis
Globus is easily distinguished from true dysphagia by its occurrence between meals and by the lack of difficulty in swallowing such items as bread and meat. The sensation may be continuous.

2.6 Management

There is no treatment beyond reassurance. No diagnostic tests are indicated. If deep-seated emotional features exist, they may warrant a psychiatric opinion.

3. HEARTBURN / W.G. Thompson

3.1 Synonyms

Pyrosis.

3.2 Description

Heartburn is a burning sensation experienced behind the sternum. It characteristically occurs or is worsened when the subject is bending over, straining or lying down, especially after a meal. It is aggravated by certain foods (acidic drinks, chocolate, coffee), obesity or anxiety. Unlike angina, it is not usually worsened by exercise or exertion.

3.3 Related Symptoms

Heartburn may be associated with a sensation of reflux into the gullet, or even actual regurgitation into the mouth (with the risk of aspiration). It should be distinguished from *rumination*, in which the subject regurgitates meals routinely and then swallows them again, usually with no consequence beyond disgust in the observer.

3.4 Mechanism

Heartburn is associated with reflux of gastric contents (usually acidic) into the esophagus. The mechanism is complex. Decreased tone or inappropriate relaxation of the lower esophageal sphincter favors reflux. Anatomic disturbances such as obesity or hiatus hernia may also be important. In diseases in which peristalsis of the esophagus is disturbed (e.g., scleroderma) any acid that does reflux into the esophagus will not be adequately cleared.

Contrary to popular opinion, the presence of a hiatus hernia has a minor role in the genesis of heartburn (Figure 1). Both hiatus hernia and heartburn occur in approximately one-third of subjects (not necessarily the same third). Thus, individual cases may have heartburn without hiatus hernia and vice versa.

The mechanism of heartburn is obscure. There appear to be no nerve endings for pain in the esophageal mucosa. Severe esophagitis may exist in the absence of heartburn or indeed of any symptoms. Conversely, individuals with heartburn may have an apparently normal esophagus. This gives rise to the suspicion that gastroesophageal reflux may be associated with a disturbance in esophageal motility that is responsible for the sensation of heartburn.

GASTROESOPHAGEAL REFLUX

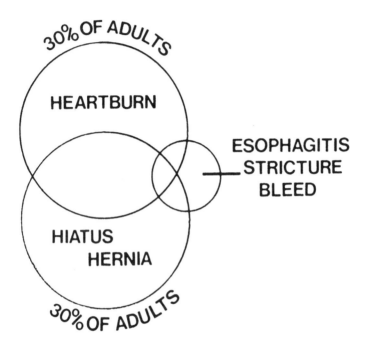

FIGURE 1. Heartburn and hiatus hernia each occurs in about 30% of adults, so some overlap is inevitable; a causal relationship has not been established. Complicated GERD may occur with heartburn, hiatus hernia, both or neither.

3.5 History and Physical

When heartburn is suspected, one should determine the effect of position, food, stress and exercise on the discomfort. The interviewer should carefully exclude such symptoms as dysphagia, odynophagia, weight loss, bleeding and anemia, which indicate complications of reflux or more serious esophageal disease.

There are no physical findings that can be associated with heartburn. The presence of substernal or costochondral tenderness suggests a musculoskeletal origin for the symptom.

3.6 Differential Diagnosis

The presence of heartburn implies that the individual has gastroesophageal reflux disease (GERD). If the burning retrosternal sensation is aggravated by bending and relieved by antacids, then no further investigation is necessary. Some, however, have a retrosternal sensation that cannot be distinguished from that of angina pectoris, particularly if it is in some way related to effort, relieved by nitroglycerin and associated with other features of heart disease. As discussed in the chapter on the esophagus, esophageal spasm may be responsible for chest pain. However, it is often difficult to prove this relationship even with sophisticated motility equipment. Musculoskeletal disturbances such as costochondritis may be responsible for chest pain; costochondritis is characterized by tenderness of one or more costochondral joints.

3.7 Approach to Investigation and Management

One-third of adults have experienced heartburn and one in ten suffer heartburn at least once per week. If the heartburn is not incapacitating and is unaccompanied by dysphagia or anemia, then a trial of therapy is a reasonable first approach. Foods that delay gastric emptying (e.g., fat) or that weaken the lower esophageal sphincter (e.g., chocolate, onions) should be avoided. Antacids or alginate compounds such as Gaviscon® are usually successful in relieving the symptoms or even preventing them. Having small meals, fasting before bedtime, elevating the head of the bed and avoiding bending or exertion on a full stomach may be beneficial as well.

In the event that such simple management fails to relieve heartburn, or that dysphagia, anemia or bleeding occurs, then some investigation is necessary. An endoscopy provides the most information, since it allows the degree of inflammation of the esophagus to be assessed. This permits the physician to plan treatment on the basis of its severity. Generally speaking, mild esophagitis may be successfully managed with an H_2 blocker, while severe (grade 3 or 4) esophagitis will require a proton-pump inhibitor. In either case, long-term treatment is usually required. If a stricture is present, it should be biopsied. If the stricture proves to be nonmalignant, dilation may be carried out. A more detailed discussion of pharmacologic therapy for gastroesophageal reflux disease is found in Chapter 5, "The Esophagus."

4. WATERBRASH / W.G. Thompson

4.1 Description

Waterbrash is the spontaneous flooding of the mouth with a clear, slightly salty fluid, which may be of sufficient quantity to require expectoration.

4.2 Mechanism

The source of the fluid appears to be the salivary glands. It is believed to result from a vagal cholinergic reflex, with afferents originating in the upper gastrointestinal tract and efferents destined for the salivary glands.

4.3 Important Historical Points
The fluid, with a neutral or somewhat salty taste, is quite distinct from the acidic or bitter contents that are refluxed from the stomach. The symptom commonly accompanies upper gastrointestinal distress such as heartburn, peptic ulcer disease and even acute gastroenteritis. By itself, it has no pathologic significance.

4.4 Differential Diagnosis
Waterbrash must be distinguished from gastroesophageal reflux disease and rumination. Diagnosis and management depend upon the underlying upper gastrointestinal disorder.

5. DYSPHAGIA / A.S.C. Sekar

5.1 Description
Dysphagia means difficulty in swallowing. Some patients describe food sticking in the throat or retrosternally.

5.2 Important Historical Points and Differential Diagnosis
A careful history is important. Mechanical narrowing is a common cause; an inflammatory stricture must be distinguished from a carcinoma. If the dysphagia is relatively short in duration (e.g., only a few months) and is worsening, this suggests a progressive mechanical narrowing of the lumen such as may occur with an esophageal carcinoma. With benign disease, symptoms are often present for a longer period of time than with carcinoma. A previous history of heartburn or acid regurgitation in a patient with progressive dysphagia might point to an esophageal stricture secondary to gastroesophageal reflux disease. Not all patients with a benign esophageal stricture have a clear history of preceding heartburn or acid regurgitation. This is particularly true in the elderly patient. A history of ingestion of caustic agents such as lye suggests an esophageal stricture secondary to severe chemical esophagitis.

Infections of the esophagus can also cause difficult swallowing. Infections, usually due to Candida albicans or herpes virus, are often accompanied by significant pain on swallowing, termed *odynophagia*. Often the odynophagia is so severe that the patient even has difficulty swallowing his or her saliva. Although herpes esophagitis can occur in relatively healthy patients, Candida esophagitis is associated with diabetes, an underlying malignancy or immunosuppression.

The patient may point to the site of obstruction, but this is not always reliable. A stricture of the lower esophagus may be experienced at the xiphoid area or as high as the throat. Upper esophageal obstruction is experienced high in the throat region, not low in the chest.

Dysphagia can also occur with motor disorders of the esophagus. These conditions include esophageal spasm and achalasia. With motor disorders of the esophagus, the dysphagia may be for both solids and liquids. The dysphagia is intermittent and may have a long history. Sometimes with esophageal spasm the dysphagia may be accompanied by pain (odynophagia), especially with extremely cold or hot liquids. These patients are usually able to wash down impacted particles of food, whereas patients with a mechanical cause (such as a stricture) may need to regurgitate impacted particles of food to obtain relief.

A common cause of intermittent dysphagia is a mucosal ring at the gastroesophageal junction (lower esophageal or Schatzki's ring). On occasion when a relatively large bolus of food is swallowed the ring can cause mechanical obstruction, producing a dramatic onset of acute dysphagia (sometimes associated with pain). Often such patients will have to leave the table and regurgitate. Patients with a Schatzki's ring usually have symptoms for many years before they seek medical attention.

A rare cause of upper esophageal dysphagia is the Paterson-Kelly syndrome or Plummer-Vinson syndrome. Here, a chronic iron deficiency anemia is associated with narrowing of the upper esophagus due to a web.

Cricopharyngeal dysphagia may be due to a cricopharyngeal or Zenker's diverticulum, which develops from an abnormality of the cricopharyngeal sphincter. Patients with a diverticulum often complain of regurgitating food that they swallowed a day or so earlier.

There are non-esophageal causes of dysphagia. Underlying neuromuscular disease may cause cricopharyngeal dysphagia, where patients have difficulty initiating a swallow. A large goiter or mediastinal tumor can cause extrinsic compression of the upper esophagus.

5.3 Approach to Diagnosis and Management

A barium swallow is the most important initial investigation in the diagnosis of dysphagia. It might reveal a Zenker's diverticulum, an esophageal stricture (benign or malignant) or a Schatzki's ring. If inflammation of the esophagus is suspected, endoscopy with biopsies is indicated. If a stricture is identified on a barium swallow, endoscopy with biopsies is necessary to determine whether this stricture is benign or malignant. Also, benign strictures can be dilated following the endoscopic diagnosis. A barium swallow may help diagnose motility disturbances such as esophageal spasm and achalasia.

Esophageal manometry is often required to confirm such motility distur-bances.

Once a cause of dysphagia has been established, management will depend on the cause. Strictures secondary to gastroesophageal reflux disease are man-aged with periodic esophageal dilations and long-term proton pump inhibitors (e.g., omeprazole). Esophageal strictures can be dilated following endoscopy. Esophageal carcinoma requires either surgery, radiation or palliative insertion of prosthesis. Esophageal motility disturbances can sometimes be managed medically with nitroglycerin or calcium channel blocking agents. Achalasia and esophageal spasm sometimes require surgical myotomy or pneumatic dilation.

6. DYSPEPSIA / W.G. Thompson

6.1 Synonyms
Indigestion.

6.2 Description
Dyspepsia is an imprecise term. It is best described as a chronic (over three months), recurrent, often meal-related epigastric discomfort, pain or fullness. The location of the pain and the relationship to meals resemble the classic description of peptic ulcer disease, so the physician must consider the possi-bility that a dyspeptic patient has a peptic ulcer. Dyspepsia is usually a daily experience, yet is seldom disabling.

6.3 Mechanism
The mechanism of dyspepsia is uncertain. Even in those dyspeptic patients who have a peptic ulcer, the cause of the pain is uncertain. It is disputed whether the discomfort is related to (1) impaired gastric emptying, (2) a disor-der of the basic electrical rhythm of the stomach, (3) pyloroduodenal dys-motility or (4) gut hypersensitivity. None are proven.

Although many patients believe that specific foods are responsible for dys-pepsia, only fat appears to be a consistent offender. Fat may induce dyspepsia by slowing gastric emptying or by releasing cholecystokinin, which is known to affect the smooth muscle of the upper gastrointestinal tract.

Other upper gastrointestinal symptoms relate to dyspepsia. These include nausea, vomiting (rarely), belching and a feeling of gaseous distention. Terms such as gallbladder dyspepsia, pancreatic dyspepsia, appendiceal dyspepsia and gaseous dyspepsia are misleading and serve no useful purpose. There should be no confusion between the episodic nature and severity of pain due to biliary colic or pancreatic disease and the more predictable and regular occurrence of dyspepsia. Indeed, dyspeptic symptoms are equally common in those who have and in those who do not have gallstones.

It is important as well to distinguish dyspepsia from the recumbency-aggravated retrosternal burning that we call "heartburn." Heartburn results from gastroesophageal reflux and has different diagnostic and therapeutic approaches than dyspepsia.

6.4 Important Historical Points

In an individual case it is almost impossible to distinguish ulcer from non-ulcer dyspepsia. Large studies have shown that, statistically, epigastric pain occurring at night and relieved with antacids is more likely to be associated with peptic ulcer disease. The pain of dyspepsia is not incapacitating. Of course, evidence of complications such as bleeding, weight loss or vomiting would not be expected in nonulcer dyspepsia. The pain or discomfort of the irritable bowel syndrome may occur in the epigastrium. This is generally distinguished from discomfort originating in the upper gastrointestinal tract by its association with defecation and a coexistent alteration in bowel habit.

On physical examination epigastric tenderness will not distinguish between ulcer and nonulcer dyspepsia. In the latter there should be no complications suggestive of peptic ulcer disease, such as peritoneal signs, a succussion splash or the presence of an epigastric mass.

6.5 Approach to Diagnosis and Management

Dyspepsia occurs in about 10% of the population, many of whom do not seek medical help. Of those who do, approximately one-third will not have a peptic ulcer. There is little evidence that those who have nonulcer dyspepsia will eventually develop an ulcer. Yet the symptoms usually persist for long periods in the patient's life. Since peptic ulcer is now curable, the proportion of dyspeptics with ulcer is steadily declining.

Thus, investigation and management will depend upon the establishment of a clear diagnosis at the outset, the cost of investigation and the cost of treatment. Since anti-ulcer medication is very effective and seemingly safe, one attitude would be to treat all such individuals without investigation. In the United States, where x-ray and endoscopy are very expensive and the cost must be borne by the individual, indiscriminate therapy has achieved some currency. In such countries as Canada, where drug costs are similar but procedural costs are much less and are not borne by the individual, it seems more efficacious to establish the diagnosis at the outset before committing the patient to drug therapy. Now that we know that most non–NSAID-induced ulcers are due to the presence of Helicobacter pylori and are cured once these gastric bacteria are killed, other approaches are proposed. The current recommendation is that those who have both an ulcer and H. pylori should be given appropriate antibiotics. Those without an ulcer will not benefit from eradication of the organism, but once the organism has been found it is difficult not to treat. New strategies suggest testing dyspeptics for H. pylori and endoscoping only those who test positive. Others would treat indiscriminately. Cost and outcome analysis has not established which is the best approach. More details on this fast-evolving issue are found in Chapter 6, "The Stomach and Duodenum."

Although a carefully conducted upper gastrointestinal series will discover most ulcers, endoscopy is more accurate and will detect mucosal lesions as well. The advantage of early diagnosis is that if no ulcer is found then the futile use of expensive, systemic drugs can be avoided in those with nonulcer dyspepsia. Further, the uncertainty factor in failing to establish a diagnosis compounds inappropriate therapy and aggravates patient unease.

7. NAUSEA AND VOMITING / M.C. Champion

7.1 Synonyms
Barf, upchuck, bring up.

7.2 Description
Nausea is a psychic as well as physical experience and defies precise definition. Vomiting is evacuation of the stomach contents through the mouth. Nausea normally precedes vomiting. There can be associated tachycardia, hypersalivation, waterbrash and excessive perspiration.

7.3 Mechanism (Figure 2)
A variety of stimuli may produce nausea (labyrinthine stimulation, pain, unpleasant memories). The neural pathways mediating nausea are not known, but evidence suggests that they are the same pathways that mediate vomiting. During nausea, gastric tone and peristalsis are reduced. The tone of the duodenum and proximal jejunum tends to be increased, with frequent reflux of duodenal contents into the stomach.

Vomiting occurs as the gastric contents are forcefully brought up to and out of the mouth. This occurs by forceful sustained contraction of the abdominal muscles at a time when the cardia of the stomach is raised and open and the pylorus is contracted. Elevation of the cardia eliminates the intra-abdominal portion of the esophagus and relaxes the lower esophageal sphincter. This allows the stomach contents to enter the esophagus. The act of vomiting is completed with rapid upward displacement of the diaphragm and reversal of thoracic pressure from negative to positive. The glottis closes, the soft palate rises, the mouth opens and the stomach contents are expelled. The control of

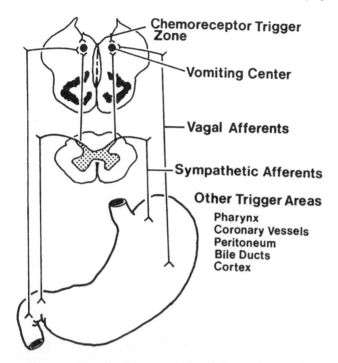

Chemoreceptor Trigger Zone

Vomiting Center

Vagal Afferents

Sympathetic Afferents

Other Trigger Areas
Pharynx
Coronary Vessels
Peritoneum
Bile Ducts
Cortex

FIGURE 2.   The vomiting center and chemoreceptor trigger zone control vomiting. Peripheral trigger areas send visceral afferent impulses, which excite the vomiting center into action.

vomiting consists of two anatomically and functionally separate units, a vomiting center and a chemoreceptor trigger zone. The vomiting center is in the reticular formation of the medulla and is excited directly by visceral afferent impulses (sympathetic and vagal) arising from the gastrointestinal tract and other peripheral trigger areas. These trigger areas are found in the pharynx, cardiac vessels, peritoneum, bile ducts, cortex and stomach. The chemoreceptor trigger zone is on the floor of the fourth ventricle, on the blood side of the blood–brain barrier. The chemoreceptor trigger zone is unable to cause vomiting without an intact vomiting center.

7.4 History and Physical
Patients may complain of nausea and hypersalivation. With gastrointestinal causes of the nausea (and vomiting) there may be associated symptoms of heartburn or epigastric pain. Prior to vomiting, patients may retch (spasmodic, abortive respiratory movements with the glottis closed).

History-taking should probe for precipitating factors, other symptoms that suggest the underlying cause, drug use and dietary habits. The history should also explore psychological trauma or disturbances of body image suggestive of anorexia nervosa.

Physical examination is often normal. An abdominal mass may point to an underlying cause (e.g., gastric carcinoma). Prolonged vomiting may cause dehydration.

7.5 Differential Diagnosis

Prolonged nausea, by itself, rarely has an organic origin. There are many causes of nausea and vomiting, including intracerebral problems (e.g., hydrocephalus, brain tumor), stimulation of the peripheral trigger areas (e.g., severe chest pain, pain from kidney stones), systemic disease (malignancy), medications and pregnancy. Upper gastrointestinal diseases (esophagitis, peptic ulcer disease, gastric carcinoma) are common. Early morning nausea and vomiting suggest pregnancy, gastroesophageal reflux disease, alcohol withdrawal, a metabolic cause (e.g., uremia) or a psychogenic origin.

7.6 Approach to Diagnosis and Management

In approaching a patient with nausea and vomiting, one should look for and correct any underlying causes. Prolonged vomiting may cause dehydration and the patient may need to be rehydrated intravenously. Medications should be discontinued.

There are many drugs that have anti-emetic actions. Antihistamines act on the vestibular apparatus as well as on the chemoreceptor trigger zone. Phenothiazines also exert their action on the chemoreceptor trigger zone. Metoclopramide and domperidone are both anti-emetics and gastric prokinetics (which stimulate the stomach to empty). Domperidone exerts its action on the chemoreceptor trigger zone, whereas metoclopramide also crosses the blood–brain barrier and affects the vomiting center. Cisapride, a newer gastric prokinetic, has no effect on the chemoreceptor trigger zone or vomiting center. Like the other prokinetic agents, it may improve nausea and vomiting if they are due to gastric stasis or gastroparesis.

8. ANOREXIA / M.C. Champion

8.1 Description

Anorexia is the lack (or loss) of appetite. Anorexia is a common and important, but nonspecific, symptom. It can be a presenting feature in patients with organic or psychological disease. Anorexia and weight loss may be the early signs of malignancy.

8.2 Mechanism

The hypothalamus plays a major role in regulating the intake of food. At one time it was generally held that a "satiety center" and a "feeding center" in the hypothalamus exerted the fundamental control over food intake. Stimulation of the satiety center was believed to inhibit the feeding center and gastric hunger contractions. The feeding center was considered to be an integrative station that coordinates complex reflexes associated with food intake. However, it is now believed that control of appetite is best considered as multiple neuropharmaco-logic interactions in the hypothalamus rather than the effect of a distinct satiety center and feeding center.

8.3 History and Physical

The history should detect other symptoms that may suggest underlying organ-ic or psychological disease. A calorie count is also helpful to assess the actual intake of food. The amount and duration of weight loss should also be docu-mented.

Physical examination may be normal except for evidence of weight loss. It may point to the underlying organic problem, such as cardiac failure or malig-nancy.

8.4 Differential Diagnosis

Many (and perhaps most) illnesses feature a loss of appetite. These range from gastrointestinal disease to malignancy, chronic renal failure, congestive heart failure and many psychiatric diseases, such as depression and anorexia nervosa.

8.5 Approach to Investigation and Management

Investigation should exclude organic disease. The approach depends upon the patient's symptoms and signs. If no physical ailment is discovered, careful screening may be necessary to exclude psychiatric disease.

9. GAS AND BLOATING / W.G. Thompson

9.1 Synonyms and Related Terms

Burbulence, flatulence, burp, belch, borborygmi, gaseous distention, wind, flatus, fart.

Gas and bloating embrace three unrelated phenomena. *Farting* is a physio-logic phenomenon due to the production of gas by colon bacteria. Excessive belching or burping is associated with *aerophagia* (air swallowing). This is also partly physiological, but it may become exaggerated through habit. The mechanism of *bloating* is obscure. These phenomena are unrelated, yet they often occur together.

9.2 Farting, Gas, Wind, Flatus

9.2.1 *MECHANISM*

Farting is a physiologic excretory process. Normally, the gut contains 100 to 200 mL of gas. An average person on a normal diet emits about 1 L per day. We pass 50 to 500 mL a mean of 13.6 times per day, although there is great variation from person to person and from time to time. Those prone to produce greater amounts of gas or who are unduly sensitive may suffer socially. Most emitted gas originates in the colon. Some carbohydrates such as cellulose, glycoproteins and other ingested materials, not assimilated in the small intestine, arrive intact in the colon where resident bacteria digest them to produce hydrogen, carbon dioxide, methane and trace gases.

Intestinal floras differ from person to person. Some bacteria produce hydrogen, while others consume it. In one person out of three, an organism called Methanobrevibacter smithii converts hydrogen to methane. The presence of this organism and the methane-producing trait are a result of early environment. Spouses do not share the trait with one another. Another product of fermentation, carbon dioxide, is also released when hydrochloric acid reacts with bicarbonate in the intestines. However, this gas is quickly absorbed. Hydrogen, carbon dioxide, methane and swallowed nitrogen comprise 99% of colon gas. The remaining 1% consists of trace gases that compensate for their small quantities by their strong odors. Smelly gases include hydrogen sulfide ammonia, skatole, indole and volatile fatty acids.

Borborygmi is the name given to the noises generated as air and fluid gurgle through the gut. Bloating is not due to excessive gas.

9.3 Aerophagia

9.3.1 *MECHANISM*

During inspiration, the normally negative intraesophageal pressure draws in ambient air. Forced inspiration against a closed glottis (intentionally closed windpipe) draws in even more air. The air may be forced out again as intraesophageal pressure increases with expiration. Adolescents love to shock their elders with voluntary belching. As a practical application, those who have lost their larynx because of cancer put this learnable skill to use in generating esophageal speech. More commonly, aerophagia is an unwanted but learned habit in those who repeatedly belch in response to other gut symptoms.

Some air is ingested with each swallow, perhaps more with food. Nervous patients undergoing abdominal x-rays accumulate more intestinal gas than those who are relaxed. Other mechanisms of aerophagia include thumb sucking, gum chewing, drinking carbonated drinks, rapid eating and wearing poor dentures. Stomach gas has the same composition as the atmosphere.

In achalasia, where the lower esophageal sphincter cannot relax, the stomach is gasless. In bowel obstruction or a gastrocolic fistula colon gases reach the stomach. Sometimes gastric stasis permits bacteria to grow and produce hydrogen in the stomach. Normally, gastric gas is swallowed air.

9.3.2 CLINICAL MANIFESTATIONS OF AEROPHAGIA

Belching is to bring forth wind noisily from the stomach. The word *burp* means to "cause to belch," as one would burp a baby, but colloquially, the terms are used interchangeably. A belch after a large meal is a physiologic venting of air from the stomach. A meal stretching the muscle of the stomach, which can stretch to accommodate food, causes distress with little increase in intragastric pressure. A satisfying belch eases the discomfort. Some individuals seem unduly sensitive to intragastric pressure. People with gastroenteritis, heartburn or ulcers swallow more frequently. If release of gas transiently relieves the distended feeling, a cycle of air swallowing and belching may be established. The swallow-belch cycle may continue long after the original discomfort is forgotten.

Of course, venting gas is important, as those unable to do so will attest. When the lower esophageal sphincter is reinforced by antireflux surgery, belching may be impossible. Bedridden patients such as those recovering from surgery may trap air in the stomach. In the supine position gastric contents seal the gastroesophageal junction so that air cannot escape until the subject assumes the prone position.

While a patient may insist that his or her stomach is producing prodigious amounts of gas, in reality air is drawn into the esophagus and released. A little may even reach the stomach. Some can belch on command, and the inspiration against a closed glottis is demonstrable. Most sufferers are relieved to have their habit pointed out, but some are incredulous. Quitting the habit is often difficult. Repeated and intractable belching is termed *eructio nervosa*.

9.4 Functional Abdominal Bloating

9.4.1 MECHANISM

Those complaining of bloating and distention are often convinced that it is due to exess intestinal gas. Although the sensation may induce aerophagia, it seldom results from it. Farting may temporarily relieve bloating, but intestinal gas production does not cause it. Research has demonstrated that gas volume in bloaters is not abnormal. Despite visible distention, x-rays and computerized tomography (CT) show no large collections of intestinal gas. The distention disappears with sleep and general anesthesia.

Gut hypersensitivity may explain the sensation of abdominal bloating. The hypersensitive gut feels full at lower than normal filling, and abdominal muscles relax to accommodate the perceived distention. The stomach is and feels distended with normal amounts of air.

Abdominal girth of female irritable bowel syndrome (IBS) patients complaining of distention may increase 3 to 4 cm over an eight-hour day. CT has demonstrated the change in profile despite unchanged gas content or distribution. There were no corresponding changes in control subjects. Lumbar lordosis (arching of the spine) is sometimes increased. When women deliberately protrude their abdomens, the configuration is different from when they are bloated, so a conscious mechanism poorly explains increased abdominal girth. Perhaps abdominal muscles are weakened. The reality of the phenomenon is indisputable; the mechanism remains a mystery.

9.4.2 CLINICAL FEATURES

Bloating occurs in 30% of adults and is frequent in 10%. Amongst those with the irritable bowel syndrome and dyspepsia the figures are much higher. It is often the most troublesome feature of these conditions. Typically, the abdomen is flat upon awakening, but distends progressively during the day, only for the distention to disappear with sleep. Women complain of the need to let out their clothing and sometimes volunteer "It's as if I'm six months pregnant." Many report that bloating occurs quickly, in some cases within a minute. It is often aggravated by eating and relieved by lying down. Menstrual periods and stress affect a few cases. Usually, it is most obvious in the lower abdomen, but many report it near the umbilicus or all over the belly.

9.4.3 DIFFERENTIAL DIAGNOSIS

Observable bloating has been called *hysterical nongaseous bloating, pseudotumor* or *pseudocyesis* (false pregnancy). If distention is present at the time of the examination (more likely late in the day) and absent on other occasions, the phenomenon is likely functional. There is no abdominal tympany to suggest gaseous intestines, and sometimes the distended abdomen can be mistaken for ascites or a tumor.

Bloating is often associated with dyspepsia or IBS. On its own, it is not a symptom of organic disease and should prompt no investigation. In intestinal obstruction or postoperative ileus (paralyzed intestines), gas accumulates and distends the gut to cause discomfort and pain. In such a case, there are other symptoms and signs with which to make a diagnosis.

10. **CONSTIPATION** / W.G. Thompson

10.1 **Synonyms**

Costiveness, obstipation.

TABLE 1. Causes of chronic constipation

Functional
Irritable bowel syndrome
Functional constipation

Motility disorders of unknown mechanism
Atonic colon
Failure of defecation
    Obstruction by hyperactive anal sphincter
    Impaired rectoanal reflex

Pharmacologic
Opiates, antidepressants, calcium
Laxative abuse

Organic
Hypothyroidism
Depression
Hirschsprung's disease
Pseudo-obstruction
    Hollow viscera myopathy
    Hollow viscera neuropathy
Obstructing lesions (e.g., carcinoma, diverticulitis)

10.2 Description

Constipation defies accurate definition. What is "normal" frequency? Ninety-five percent or more of the population have between three movements per day and three movements per week. Some people consider that fewer than three movements a week without discomfort or dissatisfaction is normal. The effort needed to pass the stool and the consistency of the stool are probably of greater importance. Most would agree that hard bowel movements that are difficult to pass constitute constipation even if they occur as often as daily. One definition of constipation is the need to strain at stool on more than 25% of occasions. Thus constipation may be defined as persistent symptoms of difficult, infrequent or seemingly incomplete evacuation.

10.3 Mechanism

Some causes of constipation are summarized in Table 1; organic causes are discussed elsewhere in this text. The commonest kind of constipation is that associated with irritable bowel. In this instance, the stool is hard, difficult to pass, and often scybalous (i.e., like rabbit stools or sheep stools). Frequently, passage of such stools is accompanied by abdominal pain and alternates with diarrhea.

Some other functional causes of constipation are difficult to define. In simple atonic constipation, stool in the rectum fails to stimulate the defecation reflex. That is, a full rectum fails to initiate the evacuating response of the internal sphincter. In others, there is no gastrocolonic response to a meal. Still others are part of a generalized motility disorder called chronic idiopathic intestinal pseudo-obstruction. This disorder may be confined to the colon, but often affects other parts of the gastrointestinal tract. In this group must be included problems associated with long-standing use or abuse of laxatives. It is not certain whether the laxative use causes or results from the motility disorder.

10.4 Important Historical Points and Physical Examination Features

The physician's questions should elicit details about the nature of the stool. The presence of hard, pellet-like, difficult-to-pass stools, sometimes with a little bit of blood coating the edge, in an otherwise healthy young person strongly suggests the irritable bowel syndrome. On rectal examination or sigmoidoscopy the rectum is often empty or contains only scybala. This type of constipation is often interspersed with periods of normalcy or diarrhea.

The atonic type of constipation, on the other hand, is relentless and is associated with a full colon and/or rectum. Often, examination of the abdomen reveals distention, and one may palpate large amounts of stool in the more proximal colon.

Various sensory or anorectal dysfunctions may also cause constipation.

Constipation and blood mixed with the stool raise the possibility of an obstructing lesion, such as a carcinoma. Hirschsprung's disease may present in adults, although usually there is a history of childhood constipation. Other possibilities include a spinal lesion, hypothyroidism, hypercalcemia, depression or drug use (e.g., opiates).

10.5 Approach to Diagnosis

Sigmoidoscopic examination using either the rigid or flexible instrument is necessary to rule out local diseases such as fissures, fistulas or distal proctitis. Many cancers are within the range of the sigmoidoscope. One might also detect melanosis coli, a pigment in the rectal mucosa that indicates chronic laxative use.

If the constipated patient is over 40, has blood or pus in the stool, or has had significant weight loss, a barium enema is indicated to rule out polyps, cancer or Crohn's disease of the colon.

A gut transit study may be revealing. Twenty radiopaque markers are ingested and daily plain abdominal x-rays are taken. If 80% of the markers have disappeared in five days, the transit time is said to be normal. In cases of longer transit, the position of the markers may help distinguish colonic inertia from anorectal disorder. More sophisticated studies are then required.

10.6 Approach to Management

Obviously, the best management of constipation is to treat any underlying disease. For the constipation of irritable bowel syndrome, a good response can be expected if sufficient bulk is added to the diet. It is best to avoid the chronic use of stimulant laxatives because of their potential to damage the myenteric plexus in the colon. If overused, laxatives may cause excessive loss of fluids and electrolytes. Colonic inertia or anorectal dysfunction causing severe constipation or obstipation requires specialist care.

11. DIARRHEA / W.G. Thompson

11.1 Synonyms

Lax bowels, the flux.

11.2 Description

Diarrhea is best described as too frequent passage of too loose (unformed) stools. Diarrhea is frequently accompanied by urgency, and occasionally incontinence. When considering a patient with diarrhea the following must be considered: frequency (>3 movements/day), consistency (loose/watery), urgency, volume (>200 g/day) and whether the condition is continuous. Persistent, frequent, loose, urgent, large-volume stools are most likely to have a pathology. Lesser and intermittent symptoms are more likely to be functional.

11.3 Mechanism

Diarrhea is due to one or more of four mechanisms: osmotic attraction of excess water into the lumen of the gut, secretion of excess fluid into the gut (or decreased absorption), exudation of fluid from the inflamed surface of the gut, and rapid gastrointestinal transit.

Osmotic diarrhea results if the osmotic pressure of intestinal contents is higher than that of the serum. This may result from malabsorption of fat (e.g., in celiac disease) or of lactose (e.g., in intestinal lactase deficiency). Certain laxatives, such as lactulose and magnesium hydroxide, exert their cathartic effect largely through osmosis. Certain artificial sweeteners, such as sorbitol and mannitol, have a similar effect. Characteristically, osmotic diarrhea ceases when the patient fasts.

Secretory diarrhea occurs when there is a net secretion of water into the lumen. This may occur with bacterial toxins, such as those produced by E. coli or Vibrio cholerae, or with hormones, such as vasoactive intestinal polypeptide (VIP), which is produced by rare islet cell tumors (pancreatic cholera). These provoke adenylate cyclase activity in the enterocyte (intestinal epithelial cell), increase cyclic AMP and turn on intestinal secretion. A similar effect may occur as a result of excess bile salts in the colon (choleretic enteropathy) and from the cathartic affect of hydroxylated fatty acids resulting from the bacterial action on malabsorbed fat. Such a diarrhea does not diminish with fasting. Osmotic and secretory diarrhea result from abnormalities in the small intestine such that the flow of water through the ileocecal area overcomes the absorptive capacity of the colon.

Exudative diarrhea results from direct damage to the small or large intestinal mucosa. This interferes with the absorption of sodium salts and water and is complicated by exudation of serum proteins, blood and pus. Infectious or inflammatory disorders of the gut cause this kind of diarrhea.

Acceleration of intestinal transit may result in diarrhea (e.g., as a result of hyperthyroidism). The rapid flow-through impairs the ability of the gut to absorb water, resulting in diarrhea.

In most instances of diarrhea two or more of these four mechanisms are at work, so these pathogenetic concepts are seldom of great help in diagnosis.

11.4 Important Historical Points and Physical Examination Features

It is important to establish the frequency of defecation, the duration of the diarrhea, the nature of the stool and its volume. If diarrhea has been present for less than two weeks, it is most likely a result of an infection or toxin. A history of many previous attacks, on the other hand, may indicate a recurrence of inflammatory bowel disease. The frequency of the stool gives some idea of severity; one should establish whether incontinence is also present. To elicit the latter history may require direct questions. Stool from malabsorption is often foul-smelling and contains oil droplets. A history of nutrient deficiency, anemia or weight loss also suggests malabsorption. Watery diarrhea, particularly when large in volume, supports a diagnosis of small bowel disease. However, a large villous adenoma of the distal colon may produce a watery diarrhea. The presence of blood or pus in the stool suggests an exudative diarrhea, a type of diarrhea that is often relatively small in volume and indicative of colitis. Loose bowel movements interspersed with normal or even constipated ones are evidence of the irritable bowel syndrome.

There are many causes of diarrhea, some of which are summarized in Table 2. The presence of profound weight loss and malnutrition in a young person points to a malabsorption syndrome due to small bowel or pancreatic disease or to inflammatory bowel disease. Metabolic conditions such as hyperthyroidism or the overuse of (magnesium-containing) antacids or laxatives might also be responsible for chronic diarrhea.

Travel to tropical countries can be marred by an attack of so-called traveler's diarrhea. The most common cause is toxigenic E. coli (it is known as toxigenic because a toxin is produced). However, a large variety of intestinal

TABLE 2.   Anatomic approach to the causes of chronic diarrhea

Gastric
Dumping syndrome

Small intestine
Celiac disease
Lymphoma
Whipple's disease
Parasitic infection (Giardia lamblia)
Abnormal intestinal tract motility with bacterial overgrowth (scleroderma, amyloidosis, diabetes, hyperthyroidism)

Large bowel
Villous adenoma (adenocarcinoma)
Inflammatory bowel disease (ulcerative colitis, Crohn's disease)
Irritable bowel (diarrhea phase)
Functional diarrhea
AIDS-related infections

Pancreatic
Chronic pancreatitis
Islet cell tumors
    Gastrin secretions
    VIP secretions

Drugs
Antacids
Antibiotics
Alcohol
Antimetabolites
Laxatives
Digitalis
Colchicine
Sorbitol, fructose
Many others

Metabolic
Hyperthyroidism
Hypoparathyroidism
Addison's disease
Diabetes
Carcinoid syndrome

infestations can occur with travel. Pseudomembranous colitis may occur within weeks of the use of antibiotics. Campylobacter or cryptococcosis may be acquired from pets. Contaminated water may result in giardiasis, amebiasis or cryptococcosis. Chronic use of alcohol may damage the small intestinal mucosa. Diabetics frequently have diarrhea because of autonomic neuropathy, perhaps with bacterial overgrowth.

Finally, it is essential to establish if the patient is homosexual. Almost any of the usual gastrointestinal pathogens can be spread by homosexual activity, including lymphogranuloma venereum and gonococcus. In addition to the "gay bowel syndrome," homosexuals are liable to the gastrointestinal complications of AIDS.

11.5 Differential Diagnosis and Management
The recent onset of acute diarrhea requires careful examination of the stool for pus cells and culture for bacterial pathogens, or a study for ova and parasites in the case of suspected protozoa. Viral studies are important in infants, and special studies are required in AIDS.

The differential diagnosis of chronic diarrhea is very complex. A careful history is often the most important diagnostic tool. Patients examined for the first time deserve at least a sigmoidoscopy to rule out local colon disease. If a small intestinal diarrhea is suspected, a three-day collection of stool to determine daily weight and fat content is necessary. If there is steatorrhea, or if stool weight exceeds 500 g per day, there is likely to be small intestinal or pancreatic disease. Smaller volumes, particularly if accompanied by blood, point to inflammation of the colon.

12. MALNUTRITION / D.G. Patel

12.1 Description
Nutrition may be defined as the process by which an organism utilizes food. This complex process involves ingestion, digestion, absorption, transport, utilization and excretion. Any alteration in one or many of these factors can produce malnutrition. Globally, primary malnutrition due to lack of food is the most common cause of malnutrition. Malnutrition in the Western world is mainly due to inadequate intake of nutrients, malabsorption and/or the hypercatabolism accompanying a critical illness. Protein-energy undernutrition is increasingly recognized in eating disorders such as anorexia nervosa.

12.2 Mechanism
The malnutrition associated with gastrointestinal disorders is usually multifactorial and varies with the nature and activity of the disease.

1. Lack of food intake due to anorexia or food-related symptoms such as dysphagia, pain or vomiting.
2. Maldigestion due to pancreatic disease. Deficiency of bile salts due to cholestatic hepatobiliary disease or to ileal disease leads to maldigestion of triglyceride and lipid-soluble vitamins. Steatorrhea (fat malabsorption) produces negative caloric balance and deficiency of fat-soluble vitamins.
3. Malabsorption due to mucosal disease of the small intestine or loss of surface area due to intestinal bypass, fistula or resection.
4. Excessive loss of nutrients, as in protein-losing enteropathy and loss of zinc in diarrheal illness.
5. Therapeutic agents that may selectively affect nutrient utilization – e.g., cholestyramine use for bile acid–induced diarrhea can worsen steatorrhea.
6. Alcoholism – an extremely common cause of malnutrition in the Western world. Social and economic status, behavior problems, isolation and depression cause reduced intake of nutrients. Alcoholics rarely consume a well-balanced diet and depend very heavily on "empty" calories from alcohol. Protein and vitamin deficiencies, particularly of the B-complex group, are extremely common. Alcohol is a toxic agent that even in the presence of adequate nutritional intake can produce damage to the pancreas, liver and small bowel mucosa, aggravating malnutrition.

12.3 Signs of Malnutrition

1. Weight loss in the absence of edema is a good indicator of energy deficiency.
2. Muscle wasting, particularly in the temporal area and dorsum of the hand between thumb and index finger, suggests protein-calorie deficiency.
3. Dry, scaly skin with pigmentation results from vitamin and trace metal deficiency.
4. Angular mouth fissure (cheilosis) is due to riboflavin deficiency.
5. Glossitis and depapillation of the tongue are due to B_{12}, folate or iron deficiency.
6. Hepatomegaly may be due to fatty liver, a common finding in protein malnutrition or alcoholism.
7. Peripheral neuropathy (decreased position sense), decreased vibration sense or ataxia may result from B_{12} deficiency.
8. Weakness and paresthesia of the legs are signs of nutritional polyneuropathy, especially in alcoholics (due to thiamine or pyridoxine deficiency).
9. Anemia due to iron, folate or B_{12} deficiency or chronic disorders.
10. Peripheral edema.
11. Hypoalbuminemia.

13. ACUTE ABDOMEN / J.M. Watters

13.1 Description

The term *acute abdomen* describes abdominal pain and related symptoms and signs that are sufficiently severe as to suggest a serious intra-abdominal condition. Pain has usually been present for 72 hours or less and sometimes for only a few hours. Since some patients with an acute abdomen require resuscitation and early surgical treatment, it is important to assess the patient and establish a plan of management as soon as possible.

13.2 Mechanism

Acute abdominal pain may be referred to the abdominal wall from intra-abdominal organs (visceral pain) or may involve direct stimulation of the somatic nerves in the abdominal wall (somatic pain). The nerve supply to the viscera is bilateral, and visceral pain is not usually lateralized. Foregut pain is typically epigastric in location, midgut pain is central, and hindgut pain is felt in the lower abdomen. Organs that are bilateral give rise to pain that is predominantly felt on one or the other side of the body. Somatic pain is more precise in location than visceral pain and corresponds more directly to the anatomic site of the underlying pathology. Rarely, pain may be referred to the abdomen from extra-abdominal sites. Unusually, acute abdominal pain is a feature of systemic disease.

Visceral pain arises from tension in the bowel wall (e.g., distension or vigorous contraction), mesenteric traction, or irritation of the mucosa or serosa of the bowel (e.g., chemical irritation, bacterial contamination, ischemia). Somatic pain occurs with stimulation of pain receptors in the parietal peritoneum and abdominal wall.

13.3 History

The initial location and character of acute abdominal pain and their evolution often give useful clues to the site and nature of the underlying pathology. A history of pain with movement – e.g., riding in a car or walking – suggests the presence of peritonitis if it is not otherwise obvious. Steady, severe pain is more ominous than colicky pain. Severe pain of sudden onset suggests a catastrophic event – e.g., perforation of an ulcer, embolism or thrombosis of a mesenteric artery, or rupture of aortic aneurysm. Colicky pain corresponds to peristaltic waves and eases or disappears between waves. Examples are the intermittent, central abdominal pain of uncomplicated small bowel obstruction, and the intermittent flank pain radiating anteriorly to the groin accompanying ureteric obstruction. However, when the viability of obstructed small bowel is compromised, for example, the now-ischemic segment of bowel causes unremitting pain that is localized to the area of the involved loop.

Biliary "colic" is a misnomer in that the pain is typically steady. It is usually epigastric and relatively diffuse, becoming more localized in the right upper quadrant if the process evolves into acute cholecystitis.

Radiation of pain may provide important clues to diagnosis. Irritation of the diaphragm, from blood in the peritoneal cavity, for example, may cause shoulder tip pain. Biliary tract pain may radiate to the right scapular region. Pain arising from retroperitoneal structures may be perceived in the back – e.g., pancreatitis, symptomatic abdominal aortic aneurysm.

13.4 Associated Symptoms

Anorexia, nausea and vomiting are nonspecific but are more common in diseases of the gastrointestinal tract than elsewhere. Abdominal distention and obstipation accompanying acute abdominal pain suggest intestinal obstruction. In a patient with colonic obstruction and/or perforation, a recent change in bowel habit or blood in the stool (prior to the onset of pain) suggests the possibility of a colon cancer. Bloody diarrhea may arise from severely inflamed, ulcerated or infarcted bowel. In women an accurate menstrual history aids the diagnosis of ovarian disease, ectopic pregnancy and pelvic inflammatory disease.

13.5 Physical Examination

Examination is carried out with the patient supine. Analgesia may impair the sensitivity of physical examination when signs are subtle, but should be given promptly when pain is severe, once assessment has been completed or when assessment is unavoidably delayed.

Inspection should note any abdominal distention or masses. The patient with peritonitis typically lies immobile, since any movement increases peritoneal irritation and pain. With ureteral colic, the patient may appear restless, seeking a more comfortable position.

Auscultation may reveal a range of bowel sounds, from the silent abdomen of peritonitis to the hyperactive sounds of bowel obstruction. Bruits suggest vascular disease, but an epigastric bruit may also be found normally.

Gentleness is the key to palpation. Palpation detects and localizes tenderness, muscle guarding, rigidity and masses. *Guarding* refers to the involuntary contraction of initially relaxed muscles of the abdominal wall in response to the pain stimulated or exacerbated by palpation. In some instances (e.g., classically perforated duodenal ulcer), the muscles are in a state of continuous contraction and are rigid or "board-like" even without palpation. Guarding may be localized (e.g., uncomplicated appendicitis) or generalized throughout the abdomen (e.g., perforated diverticulitis with diffuse contamination of the peritoneal cavity).

In more subtle situations, peritonitis is suggested by the triggering of pain in the area of suspected pathology (e.g., appendicitis) through palpation elsewhere on the abdominal wall, by having the patient cough or by gently shaking the pelvis. Gentle percussion is also a very useful way to assess peritoneal irritation, as well as to assess the nature of abdominal distention. Testing for "rebound" tenderness by deeply palpating the area of concern and then suddenly releasing the abdominal wall is very distressing to the patient with peritonitis, may be misleading in the patient without peritonitis, and does not contribute to diagnosis.

Rectal examination should be carried out and recorded by at least one examiner. Tenderness above the peritoneal reflection indicates pelvic peritonitis (e.g., appendicitis or diverticulitis). The sites of inguinal and femoral hernias should be specifically examined. Femoral pulses should be palpated. A careful physical examination will identify pertinent extra-abdominal findings (e.g., jaundice, lymphadenopathy) and systemic effects of an acute abdominal condition (e.g., hypotension, tachycardia, tachypnea).

13.6 Differential Diagnosis

Intra-abdominal conditions requiring laparotomy are the most common causes of an acute abdomen. Some conditions require immediate surgery (e.g., ruptured abdominal aneurysm). They must always be included in the differential diagnosis, therefore, and confirmed or excluded promptly. In some instances, the specific diagnosis and the need for surgery may take some time to establish. The relative likelihood of specific diagnoses varies to an extent with the age of the patient. Clinical presentations are more likely to be atypical in the elderly and in patients with coexisting conditions (such as diabetes or stroke). Particular care must be taken not to overlook an important intra-abdominal process in such patients.

One must always consider in the differential diagnosis (1) intra-abdominal conditions for which surgery is not indicated (e.g., acute pancreatitis, primary bacterial peritonitis) and (2) extra-abdominal (e.g., pneumonia) or systemic conditions (e.g., diabetic ketoacidosis) that can be accompanied by acute abdominal pain.

13.7 Approach to Diagnosis

In many instances, a careful history and physical examination provide the clinical diagnosis. Complete blood count (CBC) and urinalysis are routine. Other bloodwork is obtained as indicated. Serum amylase or lipase, electrolytes, creatinine and glucose are frequently obtained. Chest x-ray and views of the abdomen are obtained routinely unless the diagnosis is clear – e.g., with appendicitis.

More sophisticated diagnostic imaging may be necessary. Ultrasound is very useful in the diagnosis of biliary tract and gynecologic disease and is often used in suspected appendicitis. A contrast enema may be obtained to show the level of a large bowel obstruction and to exclude pseudo-obstruction. Intravenous pyelography can demonstrate kidney nonfunction or hydroureter in suspected renal pain. An opaque calculus may be seen on plain abdominal x-rays. In suspected bowel ischemia, mesenteric angiography is used to confirm the diagnosis and assess therapeutic options. In suspected diverticulitis, ultrasound and CT scanning will demonstrate thickening of the wall of the sigmoid colon and evaluate the presence of an associated abscess or gross perforation. A water-soluble enema can also be helpful in confirming the diagnosis and assessing perforation. Increasingly, abdominal CT scanning is being used for diagnosis of the acute abdomen. The choice of investigation should be discussed with a radiologist.

13.8 Approach to Management
An early, specific diagnosis based on history and examination can often be established in the patient with an acute abdomen and is the ideal basis for further management. In some instances (e.g., possible appendicitis), careful observation with repeated examination and selected imaging studies (e.g., ultrasound) allow a diagnosis to be reached. Many acute abdominal pains of mild to moderate severity resolve, at least in the short term, without a confirmed diagnosis.

In patients with more serious conditions, intravenous fluid administration, other supportive measures and monitoring must be instituted following rapid initial assessment and before a specific diagnosis is made. Diagnostic and therapeutic maneuvers proceed in a coordinated manner. Occasionally patients with an acute abdomen require urgent laparotomy without a definitive preoperative diagnosis.

14. CHRONIC ABDOMEN / W.G. Thompson

14.1 Synonyms
Recurrent abdominal pain; recurrent abdominal pain in children.

14.2 Description
Ten percent of children suffer recurrent abdominal pain and approximately 20% of adults have abdominal pain at least six times per year unrelated to menstruation. The pain is chronic when it is continuous and has been present for six months or more, unrelated to gastrointestinal functions such as eating and defecation. It is often a feature of dyspepsia or the irritable bowel syndrome. Characteristically, the pain has no relationship to bodily functions, and no gastrointestinal, hepatobiliary, genital or renal cause for the pain can be found.

14.3 Causes and Mechanism
The mechanisms of abdominal pain are discussed above, in Section 13 ("Acute Abdomen"). Of course, chronic abdominal pain may be caused by many organic diseases. *Peptic ulcer* generally produces pain after meals or on

an empty stomach and is relieved by food or antacid. Abdominal pain awakening the patient at night is a particularly discriminating feature. Peptic ulcers are now more common in the elderly, especially women on NSAIDs. In them the pain may be atypical.

Biliary colic may be due to cystic or common bile duct obstruction by a stone. Characteristically this pain is significant enough to awaken the patient at night or require a visit to the emergency room for analgesia. It lasts from 1 hour to 12 hours; beyond that time consider acute cholecystitis or pancreatitis. Attacks are sporadic and at intervals, not continuous. Biliary pain is located in the epigastrium, the right upper quadrant and/or the right scapula. It leaves the patient shaken but well. Should the gallbladder become inflamed, cholecystitis results. Obstruction of the common bile duct with a stone results in pain, jaundice and sometimes fever (cholangitis).

Pancreatitis is a devastating illness, with steady epigastric pain radiating to the back and sometimes accompanied by shock. It almost always requires admission to hospital.

Ischemic bowel disease, subacute bowel obstruction caused by Crohn's disease, *neoplasm* or *volvulus* may present with recurrent bouts of abdominal pain, often related to eating. These conditions are usually progressive and accompanied by physical signs.

In a patient with *diverticular disease*, a peridiverticular abscess may develop, causing recurrent bouts of severe left lower quadrant abdominal pain and fever. Usually, diverticula are asymptomatic and symptoms that do occur are those of coincident irritable bowel syndrome.

Renal colic due to a stone in the ureter is rarely chronic but may be recurrent. It consists of severe flank pain radiating to the groin and testicle, and may be accompanied by hematuria. Typically, a patient smitten with renal colic is unable to lie still.

Gynecologic conditions ranging from mittelschmerz (ruptured ovarian cyst) to pelvic inflammatory disease may account for recurrent abdominal pain. Menstruation-related pain in a young woman suggests endometriosis. Chronic pelvic pain often relates to the irritable bowel syndrome.

Chronic appendicitis probably does not exist.

The chronic abdomen is seldom explained by the above mechanisms. *Functional abdominal pain* may originate in any part of the gastrointestinal tract or biliary tree. It is unrelated to bodily function and may be continuous. The commonest cause of recurrent abdominal pain is the irritable bowel syndrome, in which there is a relationship to disordered defecation. It is uncertain whether such pain is due to a normal perception of abnormal gut motility or an abnormal perception of normal motility, or indeed if it is due to the gut at all; there are frequently accompanying psychosocial difficulties.

14.4 Important Historical Points and Physical Examination Features

Pain, when related to a bodily function – defecation, eating, micturition or menstruation – should focus the investigation upon the involved system. Certain physical findings (such as an abdominal mass, or blood or mass upon rectal examination) point to specific organic diseases. Fever, weight loss, rectal bleeding and/or anemia indicate further tests. These features are absent in chronic functional abdominal pain.

14.5 Differential Diagnosis, Diagnosis and Management

Management of the organic causes of the chronic abdomen can be directed at the underlying disease process. In many instances, however, there is no organic basis. Here, the physician's responsibility is to reassure the patient that no serious disease exists, and help the patient coexist with the symptoms in the light of the patient's social background. One might improve digestion through regular and better eating habits, and treat bowel dysfunction, particularly constipation, with increased dietary bulk.

14.6 Pain and Emotion

There are patients who have severe recurrent abdominal pain unrelated to bodily function or organic disease. Such patients see many doctors without satisfaction; the genesis of the symptom is thought to be psychogenic. This pain is often given such descriptors as "illness behavior" and "pain proneness." Some have hypochondriasis and do not improve when organic disease has been disproved. An extreme example is the Münchausen syndrome, where the patient deliberately relates a tall tale of medical duress in order to precipitate treatment, perhaps even surgery.

Functional pain is frequent in those who have recent conflicts, have experienced a death in the family, or have become overly concerned with fatal illness. Depression and anxiety are frequent. Here, it is important not to carry out extensive investigation in a fruitless search for an elusive cause. This only reinforces the patient's belief that something is wrong and undermines the patient's confidence in the benign diagnosis.

Such pain may be an emotional expression, in which case regular visits are necessary to allow the patient to vent his or her problems. Drugs, especially narcotics, should be used with restraint, and the physician should strive to develop a strong doctor–patient relationship while dealing with the patient's depression, anxiety, frustration and often hostility. Some individuals benefit from low-dose antidepressants, as in other chronic pain syndromes. These patients test our skill in the art rather than the science of medicine.

15. JAUNDICE / L.J. Scully

15.1 Definition

A state characterized by increased serum bilirubin levels and a yellow appearance due to deposition of bile pigment in the skin and mucus membranes.

15.2 Mechanism

Bilirubin is a waste product of hemoglobin metabolism. Interruption of the breakdown pathway at any of a number of steps, or a marked increase in load due to red cell destruction, results in an increase in serum bilirubin and (if high enough) clinical jaundice.

Under normal circumstances senescent red blood cells are taken up and destroyed in the reticuloendothelial system. Through a number of steps the heme molecule of hemoglobin is converted to bilirubin and, tightly bound to albumin, is transported in the plasma to the liver cells. Hepatocytes take up bilirubin, conjugate it to glucuronide and excrete the bilirubin diglucuronide in bile into the duodenum. In the bowel, bacteria break down bilirubin to urobilinogen, 80% of which is excreted in the feces, contributing to the normal stool color. The remaining 20% is reabsorbed and excreted in bile and urine (enterohepatic circulation of urobilinogen).

Functional or anatomic obstruction at almost any level in this pathway (from hemoglobin breakdown to uptake by the hepatocellular membrane to excretion into the biliary system) will result in jaundice, with an increase in serum bilirubin. A large increase in the breakdown products of hemoglobin alone (e.g., hemolytic anemia) will cause an increase in serum unconjugated bilirubin. If the problem lies after the uptake and conjugation step, the increase is in serum conjugated bilirubin. Causes of jaundice are usually classified as (1) hemolysis, (2) genetic defects in bilirubin handling, (3) hepatocellular disease and (4) obstruction.

15.3 Clinical Presentation

Clinical jaundice is detected when the serum bilirubin level reaches 2–4 mg/dL (40–80 μmol/L). It is usually preceded by a few days of pale stools (as excretion of bilirubin into the intestine is decreased) and dark urine (due to increased glomerular filtration of conjugated bilirubin). Jaundice is usually first detected in the sclera, although the bilirubin is actually deposited in the overlying conjunctival membranes. Yellow skin without scleral icterus should suggest carotenemia or the ingestion of such drugs as quinacrine.

Most patients with jaundice, excluding those in whom it is secondary to hemolysis, have nausea, anorexia and discomfort over the liver. There may be hepatomegaly, masses in the epigastrium or pancreas or a dilated gallbladder.

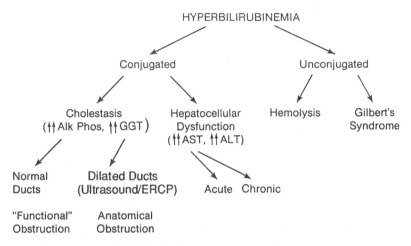

FIGURE 3. Causes of hyperbilirubinemia.

Signs of chronic liver disease such as spider nevi or palmar erythema are important. Pruritus may result, presumably from the deposition of bile salts (or a retained pruritogen normally excreted in bile) in the skin.

Several genetic defects in the conjugation or excretion of bilirubin may cause long-standing unconjugated or conjugated hyperbilirubinemia.

15.4 Approach to Diagnosis
Initially the most important information is whether the jaundice is due to conjugated or unconjugated hyperbilirubinemia (Figure 3). Serum bilirubin can be fractionated from "total" into conjugated and unconjugated, but the presence of bile in the urine determined by a test strip at the bedside confirms that the bilirubin rise is predominantly in the conjugated form. If the bilirubin is unconjugated, hemolysis or genetic defects are implicated. If the bilirubin is conjugated, "liver biochemical tests" (AST, ALT, GGT and alkaline phosphatase) will help determine if the jaundice is primarily due to obstruction/ cholestasis (high GGT and alkaline phosphatase) or hepatocellular damage (high AST and ALT). Cholestatic jaundice requires ultrasound as the best, first test to detect biliary tract disease. If the jaundice is cholestatic, then an ultrasound of the abdomen is required to determine if there is obstruction of the ducts or intrahepatic bile duct dilation.

15.5 Management
The management of obstructive jaundice is directed toward the cause where possible (e.g., removal of obstructing gallstone). Jaundice secondary to hepato-

cellular disease, such as viral hepatitis, does not require any specific treatment. Jaundice due to alcohol, toxin or drug requires withdrawal of the offending agent.

16. ASCITES IN CHRONIC LIVER DISEASE / L.J. Scully

16.1 Definition
Ascites is the accumulation of nonsanguinous fluid in the peritoneal cavity.

16.2 Mechanisms
With significant liver disease, albumin synthesis is reduced. Low serum albumin results in a decrease in intravascular osmotic pressure. This causes renal blood flow changes, resulting in sodium and water retention. Increased aldosterone levels, possibly due to decreased catabolism of this hormone by the liver, also contribute. There is a generalized salt and water retention, but the fluid accumulation may be confined to the peritoneal cavity or may be associated with peripheral edema. Ascites develops because of increased portal pressure and the transudation of fluid from the capillaries in the portal system to the peritoneal cavity. Hepatic lymph production also increases and extravasates directly into the peritoneal cavity.

16.3 Signs and Symptoms
Ascites most commonly presents with increasing abdominal girth, often associated with an uncomfortable feeling of distention, and sometimes nausea and anorexia. Shortness of breath may develop, resulting from either elevation of the diaphragm or pleural effusion. Ankle edema may accompany ascites.

Clinical examination reveals flank fullness on inspection. "Shifting dullness" or a "fluid thrill" may be elicited. Smaller amounts of fluid may be detected on ultrasound when clinical signs are absent. One should look for other signs of portal hypertension, such as dilated abdominal wall veins or an enlarged spleen.

16.4 Differential Diagnosis
Newly developed ascites must have a diagnostic aspiration to determine the albumin level, cell count and cytology. The fluid should be clear and straw-colored. Occasionally, lymph can accumulate in the peritoneal cavity, causing "chylous ascites," which requires different management. Ascitic fluid may become infected, in which case the white blood cell count will be elevated in the fluid. If the fluid is sanguinous, other causes – such as infection or malignancy – must be sought. The serum ascites albumin gradient is the best way

TABLE 3. The important causes of upper GI bleeding

Duodenal ulcer
Gastric ulcer
Gastric erosions
Ulcerative esophagitis
Esophagogastric varices
Mallory-Weiss tear
Carcinoma, lymphoma
Angiodysplasia

of confirming if the ascitic fluid is secondary to portal hypertension. In this situation the gradient is high – i.e., >11 g/L – whereas it is low if the ascites is due to peritoneal carcinomatosis. This is far more accurate than our previous assessment of transudative versus exudative ascites.

16.5 Approach to Management
Management initially includes bed rest and salt restriction. Most cases also require adding a diuretic such as spironolactone. Careful aspiration of large quantities (up to 8 L) of ascitic fluid may be necessary in some resistant cases; this can be safely performed, and if the serum albumin level is very low an intravenous infusion of albumin is given before the paracentesis.

17. GASTROINTESTINAL BLEEDING / R.R. Gillies

17.1 Description
Blood issuing from the GI tract is a cause for alarm, and justifiably so! The visible evidence is described as hematemesis, hematochezia and/or melena.

Hematemesis – vomited blood, either red (fresh) or dark brown (altered by reaction with HCl) – comes from a source proximal to the duodenojejunal junction.

Hematochezia – blood in the stool – comes from the left colon, or even above if the volume of blood is large and the transit rapid.

Melena – black, tarry, smelly stool, looser and larger with larger hemorrhages – comes from the upper GI tract, in which case bacterial action has longer to break down the blood. It may even come from the lower tract when transit is delayed. The important causes of upper gastrointestinal bleeding are shown in Table 3, and of lower gastrointestinal bleeding in Table 4.

TABLE 4.   The important causes of lower GI bleeding

Hemorrhoids, anal fissure
Carcinoma, adenomatous polyps
Angiodysplasia
Ulcerative colitis
Crohn's disease
Diverticular disease
Ischemic colitis
Certain bacterial infections
Amebic colitis
Meckel's diverticulum

17.2 Important Historical Points and Physical Examination Features

Vomiting blood usually signifies a major hemorrhage. In a briskly bleeding duodenal ulcer, rapid transit may result in passage of red blood and clots per rectum without vomiting. Even before being passed per rectum, a large hemorrhage into the upper tract will announce itself by hyperactive bowel sounds. It is obvious that such a large-volume blood loss will have major cardiovascular effects compared to a rectal lesion causing passage of red blood and clots.

The symptoms associated with blood loss may occur before any blood appears externally (e.g., the features of an acute anemia – weakness, faintness, sweating, pallor, thirst and collapse). While the first clues as to the site of bleeding are gathered, we need to know more about how the patient is tolerating the blood loss. A rapid, thready pulse; hypotension; cold, sweaty skin; and pallor tell us that emergency restoration of blood volume is needed to keep the patient alive. Vital signs may be normal while the patient is recumbent, but a blood pressure fall of 15 mm Hg when the patient sits up indicates a significant blood loss. Cardiovascular compensation may be perfect – for the moment! A large-diameter IV line (at least 18 gauge) must be inserted. The patient should be given first saline or plasma and then, as soon as it is available, blood as indicated by any features of hypovolemia.

Once resuscitation is under way, one can assess the site and etiology of the bleeding. First, take a detailed history, particularly noting upper and lower GI symptoms, previous episodes of bleeding, previous GI surgery, ASA or NSAID intake, ethanol abuse, and diseases or treatments that could cause clotting defects. Ulcer pain often stops as bleeding starts; ulcer pain does not precede ulcer bleeding in 20–25% of cases.

Next, do a thorough physical examination, with attention to vascular lesions of the skin and mucosa, ecchymoses, the liver, peripheral signs of cir-

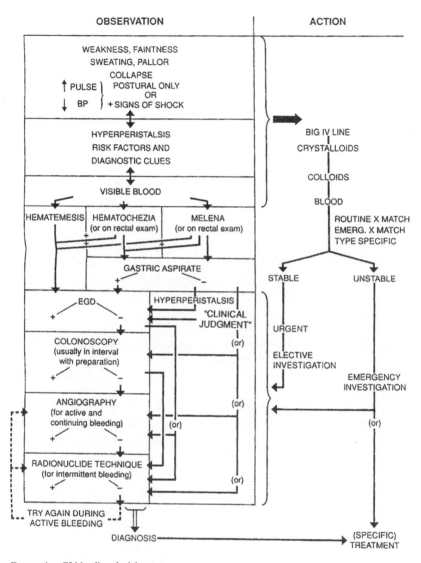

FIGURE 4. GI bleeding decision tree.

rhosis, splenomegaly and prominent superficial abdominal veins. Inspection of the nares and oropharynx avoids the embarrassment of missing epistaxis as a source of swallowed blood. Rectal examination allows stool examination.

17.3 **Approach to Diagnosis** (Figure 4)

When the passage of blood from either end of the GI tract has been reported but not observed, or when hematochezia or melena without hematemesis has been observed, the passage of a nasogastric tube for a single aspiration will help determine if bleeding is proximal or distal to the pylorus. Providing the patient's response to IV volume replacement is satisfactory, one can make a decision as to the timing and type of investigation needed to identify the cause of bleeding. Upper GI endoscopy is the most reliable technique to detect lesions proximal to the duodenojejunal junction. Sometimes perendoscopic injection, heater probe application or snare-cautery polypectomy may be employed to stop bleeding from identified lesions. Whether endoscopy is emergent, urgent or elective depends on the status of the patient. Remember that the status may rapidly deteriorate. One must be prepared to change the plan just as rapidly.

Bleeding lower GI tract lesions may be identified and treated endoscopically. Usually this is feasible only later, after proper bowel preparation removes the accumulated blood. When active bleeding continues from the small or large bowel, mesenteric angiography is the best choice to discover the bleeding site. If the bleeding is less brisk and is intermittent, radionuclide imaging may point to the site. Bleeding must occur during either test to make it useful.

When all else fails, total enteroscopy – endoscopy of the entire small bowel – should be done. Usually this is more efficient at laparotomy where the surgeon can assist by manipulating the loops of bowel over the advancing scope.

17.4 **Approach to Management**

Remember that the objective is a live patient. Continued, careful assessment of the patient's cardiovascular response to blood loss and replacement will guide interventions, including surgical. Specific treatment depends upon the underlying disease and will be dealt with in subsequent sections.

18. **ABDOMINAL MASS / S. Grégoire**

18.1 **Description**

When an abdominal mass is discovered on physical examination, one must define its nature. Using a systematic approach often permits the identification of the mass before the use of sophisticated tests.

18.2 **Important Points in History and Physical Examination**

Important clues in the history and general physical examination may help to identify the enlarged viscus. For example, in a young patient presenting with diarrhea, weight loss and abdominal pain, finding a right lower quadrant mass would suggest inflammatory bowel disease. However, an abdominal mass may be discovered during physical examination of an asymptomatic individual. Certain observations made during the abdominal examination may be helpful. (See also Section 20.)

18.2.1 INSPECTION
Where is the mass located? A practical approach is to divide the abdomen into four quadrants (see Section 20.1). Starting from the principle that an abdominal mass originates from an organ, surface anatomy may suggest which one is enlarged. A mass seen in the left lower quadrant, for example, could be of colonic or ovarian origin but, unless there is situs inversus, one would not consider an appendiceal abscess!

Does the mass move with respiration? In the upper abdomen a mobile intra-abdominal mass will move downward with inspiration, while a more fixed organ (e.g., aorta, pancreas) or an abdominal wall mass (e.g., hematoma of rectus muscle) will not.

Is there visible peristalsis?

18.2.2 AUSCULTATION
Careful auscultation for bowel sounds, bruit or rub over an abdominal mass is part of the systematic approach.

18.2.3 DEFINING THE CONTOUR AND SURFACE OF THE MASS
This is achieved by inspection, percussion and palpation. Is the organ air-filled (e.g., stomach) or fluid-filled? Is it a well-defined mass (e.g., liver, spleen) or are its borders difficult to define (matted loops of small bowel)? Is the surface regular? An enlarged liver due to fatty infiltration may have a smooth surface, while a cirrhotic organ is usually irregular and nodular. What is the consistency of the mass? Firm? Hard or soft? Is it pulsatile? In the absence of ascites, ballottement of an organ situated in either upper quadrant more likely identifies an enlarged kidney (more posterior structure) than hepatomegaly or splenomegaly.

18.3 Differential Diagnosis
The following suggests an approach to the differential diagnosis of an abdominal mass located in each quadrant:

18.3.1 RIGHT UPPER QUADRANT
This location suggests liver, right kidney, gallbladder and, less commonly, a colon or gastroduodenal mass. A pancreatic mass is rarely palpable.

18.3.1.1 *Liver*

As a subdiaphragmatic organ, the liver moves downward with inspiration. This anterior organ has an easily palpable lower border, which permits assessment of its consistency. A bruit or venous hum can be heard in certain conditions. An enlarged left lobe can usually be felt in the epigastric area.

18.3.1.2 *Right kidney*

The kidney may protrude anteriorly when enlarged and be difficult to differentiate from a Riedel's lobe of the liver. It may be balloted.

18.3.1.3 *Gallbladder*

This oval-shaped organ moves downward with inspiration and is usually smooth and regular.

18.3.1.4 *Colon*

Colon masses are deep and ill-defined, and do not move with respiration. High-pitched bowel sounds suggest obstruction.

18.3.2 *LEFT UPPER QUADRANT*

Location in the left upper quadrant suggests spleen or left kidney. Less commonly, a colonic (splenic flexure) or gastric mass can be felt. A pancreatic mass is rarely palpable.

18.3.2.1 *Spleen*

This anterior organ moves downward with inspiration. Since it has an oblique longitudinal axis, it extends toward the right lower quadrant when enlarged. It has a medial notch and the edge is sharp.

18.3.2.2 *Left kidney*

Its more posterior position and the presence of ballottement helps distinguish the left kidney from the spleen.

18.3.2.3 *Colon, pancreas, stomach*

It is practically impossible to differentiate masses in these organs by physical examination. The history helps but often one must resort to radiology or endoscopy.

18.3.3 *RIGHT LOWER QUADRANT*

A mass in this area has its origin either in the lower GI tract (colon, distal small bowel, appendix) or in a pelvic structure (ovary, uterus, fallopian tube).

18.3.3.1 *Lower GI tract*
These deeper organs are usually ill-defined. Clinical context is important. Inflammatory bowel disease usually would be associated with pain on palpation but carcinoma of the cecum would be painless.

18.3.3.2 *Pelvic organs*
Bimanual palpation is the preferred method.

18.3.4 *LEFT LOWER QUADRANT*
As with a right lower quadrant mass, the differential diagnosis here is between lower GI (in this quadrant the sigmoid colon) and pelvic origin. The shape of the organ and pelvic examination should help differentiate the two.

18.4 Approach to Diagnosis
To complete the assessment of an abdominal mass, one may choose among several different investigational tools. The use of specific tests depends on availability and on the organ studied.

Generally, ultrasound is useful. This noninvasive, safe, cheap and widely available method identifies the mass and provides information on its origin and nature. Ultrasound may also be used to direct a biopsy. Other noninvasive modalities are nuclear imaging and CT scan. Hollow organs may be demonstrated radiographically through the use of contrast media (e.g., barium enema, GI series, ultrasound, intravenous pyelogram, endoscopic retrograde cholangiopancreatography, etc.). Sometimes, laparotomy or laparoscopy will be necessary to make the diagnosis.

19. PROCTALGIA FUGAX / W.G. Thompson

19.1 Description
Proctalgia fugax is a sudden severe pain in the anus lasting several seconds or minutes and then disappearing completely.

19.2 Mechanism
The pathophysiology of proctalgia fugax is uncertain. Although some observations (under obviously fortuitous circumstances) suggest a rectal motility disorder, the symptom appears more likely to result from spasm of the skeletal muscle of the pelvic floor (specifically, the puborectalis).

19.3 History and Physical Examination
Proctalgia fugax occurs in about 14% of adults and is somewhat more common in females than males. The pain may be excruciating, but since it is so short-lived patients seldom report it to their physician. In 90% of instances it lasts less than five minutes and in many cases less than a minute. About one-

third of patients suffer attacks following defecation. A small minority report attacks following sexual activity. There are no physical signs.

19.4 Differential Diagnosis

Perianal disease may cause pain but it usually accompanies, rather than follows, defecation. One should be particularly careful to exclude the presence of an anal fissure, which may be difficult to see on anal inspection. Pain originating from the coccyx may be accompanied by coccygeal tenderness both externally and from within the rectum. An acute attack of anal pain lasting several hours may indicate a thrombosed hemorrhoid. However, constant pain for many months or years is not likely to be proctalgia fugax or to have an organic explanation.

19.5 Management

Beyond reassurance there is no treatment.

20. EXAMINATION OF THE ABDOMEN / R.F. Bursey, J.M. Fardy and D.G. MacIntosh

Examination of the abdomen is an important component of the clinical assessment of anyone presenting with suspected disease of the gastrointestinal tract. As in all other parts of the examination, care must be taken to show respect and concern for the patient while ensuring an appropriate and thorough examination.

While performing the examination it is useful to keep in mind the concepts of sensitivity and specificity. How confident can we be that a suspected physical finding is in fact present and has clinical significance? For example, how sensitive and specific is our bedside examination for hepatomegaly? What is the clinical significance of an epigastric bruit heard in a thin 20-year-old female versus a 55-year-old hypertensive, obese male?

In the following sections we will describe an appropriate sequential examination of the abdomen and highlight some of the potential pitfalls of this process.

20.1 Inspection

Ensure that the abdomen is exposed from the costal margin to symphysis pubis. When describing the location of an abnormality it is useful to divide the abdomen into four quadrants with a perpendicular line through the umbilicus from the xiphoid process to the symphysis pubis. A horizontal line through the umbilicus then allows the abdomen to be divided into 4 areas: the left upper, right upper, left lower and right lower quadrants (Figure 5). On occasion it may be helpful to divide the abdomen into 9 regions with the spaces marked by vertical lines through the left and right mid-clavicular lines and horizontal

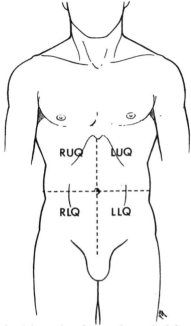

FIGURE 5. Division of the abdomen into four quadrants: the left upper quadrant, right upper quadrant, left lower quadrant and right lower quadrant.

lines passing through the subcostal margins and anterior iliac crests (Figure 6). The overall appearance such as scaphoid, protruberant, or obese should be described, and the location of any surgical scars noted. One should look for any abnormal surface markings, including cutaneous lesions as well as vascular markings. A comment should also be made about the apparent ease of movement of the abdominal wall with respiration and change in body position. Occasionally organomegaly or a mass will be visible. It is helpful to look at the abdomen from the foot of the bed as well.

20.2 Auscultation
It is useful to auscultate the abdomen prior to palpation or percussion, as bowel sounds induced by further examination may mask vascular bruits or pleural rubs. When listening for vascular bruits it is useful to keep in mind the surface markings. The aorta enters the abdomen at or just to the left of the xiphoid process and bifurcates to the left and right common iliac arteries at the level of the umbilicus. The renal arteries are found approximately one-half the distance between the xiphoid process and the umbilicus, and auscultation

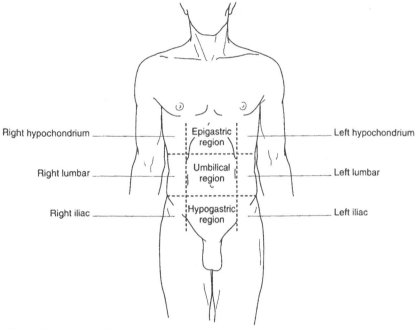

Right hypochondrium

Right lumbar

Right iliac

Epigastric region

Umbilical region

Hypogastric region

Left hypochondrium

Left lumbar

Left iliac

FIGURE 6.   Division of the abdomen into nine regions.

is best performed within 2 cm of the midline. Bruits are often best heard at the bifurcation of major vessels; therefore it is also appropriate to listen at the bifurcation of the common iliacs into the internal and external iliacs, approximately halfway between the umbilicus and the inguinal ligament. One should listen over the inguinal ligament for femoral bruits as well.

A venous hum is best heard overlying the portal vein, which is found in an area approximated by an elliptical shape between the umbilicus and the midclavicular line where it crosses the right subcostal margin. Arterial bruits are usually heard only during systole and best heard with the diaphragm of the stethoscope, as they are high pitched. A venous hum is more likely to be continuous and best heard with the bell of the stethoscope, as this is a low-pitched sound. There are, however, no studies to suggest these findings are helpful or reliable in routine examination. Venous hum can occur in portal venous hypertension of any cause. Undifferentiated liver patients in one study had a prevalence of bruits reported as less than 3%. The ability of clinicians to distinguish hepatic arterial bruits from other arterial bruits such as a renal artery bruit has not been studied.

Friction rubs may occur overlying the liver or spleen and are always abnormal, though rare. Even with careful auscultation of patients with known liver tumors, fewer than 10% are found to have a rub.

20.2.1 *BOWEL SOUNDS*

Auscultation for bowel sounds is a rather controversial subject. Bowel sounds should be listened for prior to palpation or percussion, but the yield of this examination is low. The diaphragm of the stethoscope should be placed on the abdomen, as least initially in the right lower quadrant near the ileocecal valve. The particular characteristics of the bowel sounds or even absence of them is not diagnostic of a particular condition, perhaps except for the very high pitched noises of acute small bowel obstruction. In fact, it is probably more helpful in this regard to observe how the bowel sounds change over a period of several hours.

20.3 Palpation

Palpation of the abdomen should be done in an orderly sequence with the patient in the supine position. Light palpation should be done first in all four quadrants assessing for areas of potential tenderness. Light palpation is a one-handed technique. If no areas of obvious tenderness are elicited, then deep palpation is performed, again in all four quadrants using a two-handed technique. Pressure is applied with one hand over the other hand, which is placed on the abdominal wall, as it is thought that deep palpation with one hand may lead to the inadvertent nonrecognition of suble fullness or mass if the hand applying deep pressure is also responsible for detecting the abnormality. The accuracy of this is untested. It is stated that if a patient has difficulty relaxing the abdominal wall musculature, then placing the soles of the patient's feet on the bed with hips and knees flexed will aid relaxation; in all likelihood, however, a calm, organized approach with verbal reassurance by the examiner will be just as effective.

The techniques of palpation of liver and spleen are discussed in Sections 20.5 and 20.6.

20.4 Percussion

Percussion of the abdomen will detect the presence of bowel gas. The technique as it relates to defining organomegaly and the presence of fluid is discussed in later sections.

20.5 Examination of the Liver

Examination of the liver consists mainly of palpation for the lower edge of the liver and percussion to determine the span. This examination is performed after inspection for right upper quadrant swelling and extrahepatic signs of liver disease. To palpate the lower edge of the liver the examiner starts with gentle pressure in the right lower quadrant of the abdomen. The patient is asked to breathe gently and slowly, in order to bring the liver edge down to the examining fingertips of the right hand. The examiner moves the right hand in a cephalad direction about 2 cm with each breath. If the edge is not felt, no further examination is required. If liver disease is suspected the lower liver edge can be located by percussion.

If the edge is located, mark the lower border in the mid-clavicular line. Percuss for the upper border starting in the third intercostal space with a finger that is held flat and lies within the space. Move down one interspace at a time until the percussion note changes from resonant to dull. To confirm the change of percussion note strike the third and fourth fingers laid in adjacent interspaces. The note on the top finger should be resonant and on the lower dull. Measure the distance between the upper and lower percussion edges in the mid-clavicular line. Determination of the liver span can be done with firm or gentle percussion to locate the lower border. Gentle percussion is the recommended technique, as this method appears to better estimate liver span as judged by ultrasound. Remember that the upper edge of the liver is dome shaped and not straight across.

The scratch test has been used to find the lower liver margin. The diaphragm of the stethoscope is placed at the right costal margin in the mid-clavicular line. A finger moves up the abdomen in the mid-clavicular line, scratching gently and with consistent pressure. When the liver edge is reached, there is a sudden increase in the scratching sound heard through the stethoscope. In one comparative study the scratch test was not felt to offer any advantage over the techniques of palpation and percussion.

When the liver edge is palpable, trace the edge working laterally to medially. Try to determine the characteristics of its surface – for example, soft, firm or nodular. These characteristics may help in the assessment of patients with liver disease; however, agreement about the characteristics is poor, even among experts. Auscultation is rarely helpful. An attempt should be made to assess the left lobe in the epigastrium using these techniques.

What is the significance of a palpable liver edge? A recent review suggested that a palpable liver is not necessarily enlarged or diseased. When clinical examination is compared to nuclear medicine scanning, about one-half of palpable livers are not enlarged. The inability to feel a liver edge does not rule out hepatomegaly, but does reduce its likelihood.

What is the normal percussion span? Only one study has been done to establish the normal span. Castell examined 116 healthy subjects using firm percussion. The mean span in the mid-clavicular line was 7 cm in women and 10.5 cm in men. The following nomograms were developed to predict estimated liver dullness in a normal population using firm percussion technique: Male liver dullness equals (0.032 × weight in pounds) + (0.183 × height in inches) − 7.86. The female liver dullness equals (0.027 × weight in pounds) + (0.22 × height in inches) − 10.75. The 95% confidence intervals were ±2.64 cm. Therefore a 5 ft. 10 in., 175 lb. male would have an estimated liver span of 10.2 cm (range 7.6–12.8) and a 5 ft. 5 in., 130 lb. female would have an estimated liver span of 7.1 cm (4.5–9.7 cm) by this formula.

20.6 Examination of the Spleen

The normal spleen is a curved, wedge-shaped organ located beneath the rib cage in the upper left quadrant. The spleen lies beneath the left tenth rib and normally weighs about 150 g, measuring approximately 12 cm in length, 7 cm in width and 3 cm in thickness. The normal spleen usually cannot be palpated, but as it enlarges it descends below the rib cage, across the abdomen toward the right lower quadrant. An enlarged spleen may have a palpable notch along its medial edge.

Examination of the spleen should begin with observation of the left upper quadrant for an obvious mass, though such a mass is quite uncommon. The examiner should then proceed with percussion over the area of the spleen to look for evidence of dullness, implying splenetic enlargement. The two most useful methods are percussion over Traube's space and Castell's sign.

The surface markings for Traube's space are the left sixth rib, the left mid-axillary line and the left costal margin. An enlarged spleen may cause dullness over Traube's space. Percussion should be carried out at one or more levels of Traube's space from medial to lateral. This maneuver has a sensitivity and specificity between 60 and 70% for splenetic enlargement; however, the sensitivity and specificity increases to approximately 80% in non-obese patients who are fasting.

Castell's method involves percussion in the lowest intercostal space in the left anterior axillary line. In normal individuals this area is resonant on percussion and remains resonant on inspiration. In patients with mild splenic enlargement this area will be resonant on percussion and become dull on maximal inspiration. This method has a sensitivity and specificity of approximately 80% for detection of splenic enlargement and would seem particularly suited for detection of a minimally enlarged spleen that may not be palpable.

Palpation of the spleen should begin in the right lower quadrant and proceed toward the left upper quadrant in order to follow the path of splenic enlargement. Palpation should initially be carried out in the supine position with a bimanual technique using the left hand to gently lift the lowermost portion of the left rib cage anteriorly. The fingertips of the right hand are used to palpate gently for the spleen tip on inspiration. The hand is moved from the right lower quadrant, advancing toward the left upper quadrant. If the spleen is not palpated in the supine position the patient should be moved into the right lateral decubitus position and again with bimanual technique the spleen tip should be sought using the fingertips of the right hand on inspiration. This technique has a sensitivity of about 70% and specificity of 90% for splenic enlargement.

20.7 Examination for Suspected Ascites

The presence of ascites – free fluid within the abdominal cavity – is always due to an underlying pathological process. Most often the underlying etiology is cirrhosis of any type. Other potential causes include severe right-sided heart failure, lymphatic obstruction, primary intra-abdominal malignancy and peritoneal metastases. It is easy to identify large-volume ascites clinically, but the sensitivity of the examination techniques falls with lower volumes of fluid. Ultrasound, which can detect as little as 100 mL of free fluid, is the gold standard against which the clinical diagnostic maneuvers are compared.

An approach involves inspection for bulging flanks, followed by palpation for the presence or absence of fluid waves combined with percussion to demonstrate flank dullness as well as shifting dullness. One has to be aware that adipose tissue in the flanks may be occasionally mistaken for free fluid. To demonstrate a fluid wave it is necessary to enlist the aid of the patient or another individual. With the patient in the supine position, place one hand on the patient's flank. With the other hand briskly tap the other flank. A third hand is placed in the mid-abdomen with sufficient pressure applied to dampen any wave that may pass through adipose tissue in the anterior abdominal wall. If fluid is present a shock wave will be felt with the palpating hand. The sensitivity of this technique is approximately 50% but it has a specificity of greater than 80%.

When percussing for free fluid one should place the finger parallel to the expected edge and percuss from resonance in the mid-abdomen to dullness in the flanks. This area is then marked and the patient rolled to the opposite side. For example, if flank dullness is demonstrated on the left then the patient should be rolled onto the right side. One should allow approximately 30 seconds for the fluid to move between the mesentery and loops of bowel into the inferior portion of the abdomen. The previous area of dullness in the left flank should now be resonant. It does not matter which side one chooses to start with. In three separate studies shifting dullness had a sensitivity that ranged from 60–88% and a specificity that ranged from 56–90%.

In one study involving six gastroenterologists and 50 hospitalized alcoholic patients, the overall agreement was 75% for the presence or absence of ascites and reached 95% among senior physicians.

Interestingly, symptoms are often as useful as physical examination techniques for the clinical diagnosis of ascites. The most useful findings to make a diagnosis of ascites are a positive fluid wave, shifting dullness or peripheral edema. The absence of these findings is useful in ruling out ascites, as is a negative history of ankle swelling or increasing abdominal girth.

SUGGESTED READING LIST

Section 20 Examination of the Abdomen

Castell DO, O'Brien KD, Muench H, Chalmers TC. Estimation of liver size by percussion in normal individuals. Ann Intern Med 1969; 70(6):1183–1189.

Grover SA, Barkun AN, Sackett DL. Does this patient have splenomegaly? JAMA 1993; 270:2218–2221.

Naylor CD. Physical examination of the liver. JAMA 1994; 271:1859–1865.

Sapira JD. The art and science of bedside teaching. In: Urban & Schwarzenberg 1990.

Williams JW, Jr, Simel DL. Does this patient have ascites? How to divine fluid in the abdomen. JAMA 1992; 267:2645–2648.

2
Nutrition in Gastrointestinal Disease
J.S. Whittaker, U.P. Steinbrecher, M. Lemoyne and H.J. Freeman

1. INTRODUCTION

Food assimilation is the major function of the gastrointestinal tract, and important manifestations of many gastrointestinal diseases are their nutritional effects. Digestion and absorption of nutrients are discussed elsewhere. This chapter reviews physiologic considerations that are essential for planning proper nutritional management. The focus will be on the role of the liver in regulating the supply of carbohydrate and lipid fuels as well as ensuring the availability of essential substrates to peripheral tissues. The clinical features of malnutrition and specific effects of malnutrition on the gastrointestinal tract and liver will be discussed along with diet therapy in gastrointestinal disease. Finally, an approach to clinical nutrition will be presented, including nutritional assessment and the rational use of enteral and parenteral nutritional support.

2. ESSENTIAL PHYSIOLOGIC CONCEPTS IN NUTRITION

To maintain a continuous supply of nutrients in the bloodstream in the face of intermittent dietary intake, a complex set of regulatory mechanisms have evolved. These allow the storage of nutrients during feeding, and their release from storage pools during the interdigestive period so as to maintain nutrient levels in the bloodstream within remarkably narrow limits. Short-term regulation between the fed state and the interdigestive state is mediated principally by (1) the concentration of several key substrates and (2) a set of regulatory hormones, which include insulin, glucagon, catecholamines and corticosteroids (Table 1).

Taken together, the actions of glucagon, catecholamines and corticosteroids work to increase plasma glucose and free fatty acid levels in direct opposition

TABLE 1.   Hormonal regulation of nutrient metabolism

Hormone	Principal metabolic actions
Insulin	Increases glucose uptake in peripheral tissues Stimulates protein synthesis Inhibits lipolysis and glycolysis Increases amino acid uptake into muscle (particularly important post-exercise)
Glucagon	Increases cyclic AMP levels in the liver and adipose tissue, with stimulation of fatty acid mobilization, glycogenolysis, glycolysis and gluconeogenesis, thereby increasing plasma glucose
Catecholamines	Increase cyclic AMP levels in the liver, skeletal muscle and adipose tissue, with release of glucose, free fatty acids and lactate
Corticosteroids	Increase gluconeogenesis Increase amino acid mobilization from the periphery (chiefly skeletal muscle) Increase fatty acid release from extremities Decrease glucose utilization by peripheral tissues by increasing post-receptor insulin resistance Increase glucagon release

to insulin. Therefore, the release of these hormones, which occurs in response to low glucose levels and/or stress, leads to insulin resistance.

The fate of glucose in the fed and the fasting states is detailed in Figure 1. Glucose is rapidly absorbed following ingestion as starch, disaccharides or monosaccharides. The glucose is transported via the portal system to the liver, which extracts a considerable fraction of portal venous glucose. The remainder enters the systemic circulation and causes pancreatic secretion of insulin. The high portal vein insulin and glucose concentrations lead to hepatic glucose uptake with conversion to glycogen and fatty acids. The peripheral rise in insulin, which occurs in association with the rise in plasma glucose concentration, causes a large peripheral uptake of glucose, first by muscle cells, and second by adipocytes. Glucose is the essential substrate for brain, renal medulla and red cell metabolism; other organs mainly use fatty acids for energy. The rise in plasma insulin also leads to amino acid uptake by muscle and has an antiproteolytic effect. These effects on muscle protein have led to the designation of insulin as an "anabolic hormone." In the postabsorptive or interdigestive state, plasma glucose is low, with low plasma insulin levels. The low plasma insulin influences the metabolism of all three macronutrients (i.e., carbohydrates, fat and protein). Glycogenolysis occurs in the liver to maintain plasma glucose levels. The low plasma insulin also allows lipolysis to take place, such that fatty acids can be utilized as the major energy substrate. Finally, the low plasma insulin leads to proteolysis,

A. Fed state

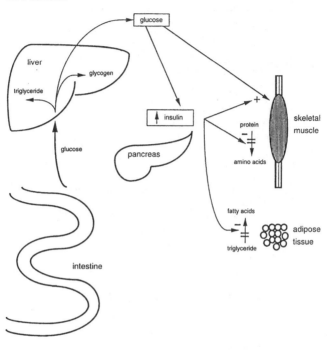

B. Interdigestive state

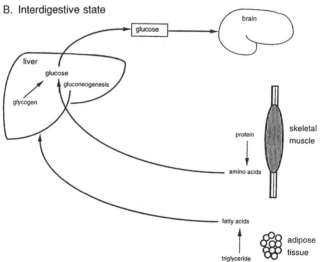

FIGURE 1.   Carbohydrate, fat and protein metabolism.

particularly of muscle protein, which leads to release of alanine and gluta-mine, which can be used for gluconeogenesis in the liver. This gluconeogen-esis occurs in concert with glycogenolysis to assure an ongoing supply of glucose for the body.

Other hormones, such as glucagon, catecholamines and growth hormone, play less important roles in macronutrient metabolism, but in general have been termed the "stress hormones," since they are released during times of stress and have anti-insulin effects. In particular, if for any reason there is a low blood sugar, all these hormones are released and will promote an eleva-tion in plasma glucose.

The flux of lipid nutrients in the fed and the interdigestive states is contrasted in Figure 2. In the fed state, fat enters the circulation from the intestine as chy-lomicrons, which are large droplets of triglyceride emulsified by a surface mono-layer of phospholipid and apolipoproteins. Additional apolipoproteins are trans-ferred onto the chylomicrons from HDL. The artificial fat emulsions used for parenteral nutrition are very similar to chylomicrons in that they contain a core of triglyceride with a surface monolayer of phospholipid. They initially contain no apolipoproteins, but acquire these from HDL very rapidly once they have entered the circulation. One of the apolipoproteins, apolipoprotein C-II, is par-ticularly important in that it is an essential cofactor for the action of lipoprotein lipase. This enzyme is attached to the capillary endothelium in tissues, such as the heart and adipose tissue, that are active in utilizing fatty acids. Chylomicrons bind to the enzyme and the core triglyceride is rapidly hydrolyzed. The released fatty acids are then taken up and utilized in the peripheral tissues. As the chy-lomicron particle shrinks in size, the excess surface material is transferred back to HDL, and ultimately the remnant particles are cleared via a specific receptor in the liver. The process of lipolysis is extremely efficient, and the half-life of chylomicron triglyceride in the circulation is normally less than 15 minutes. The lower panel of Figure 2 depicts the postabsorptive or interdigestive state. Chy-lomicrons are absent, but triglyceride fuels are available in the circulation in the form of VLDL, which are secreted by the liver. The substrates for triglyceride assembly include free fatty acids released from adipose tissue through the action of a hormone-sensitive lipase, and fatty acids synthesized in the liver from acetyl-CoA. The newly secreted VLDL acquire apolipoproteins and cholesterol ester from HDL. Lipolysis of VLDL in peripheral tissues is mediated by lipoprotein lipase. As the particle decreases in size, free cholesterol transfers to HDL, where it is esterified through the action of lecithin-cholesterol acyltransferase (LCAT), and the resultant cholesterol ester is then transferred back to the lipolyzed parti-cle, where it forms part of the core. When lipolysis is completed, what is left behind is termed an LDL particle. This is smaller and more dense than VLDL, has lost all apolipoproteins except apolipoprotein B, and has a core of cholesterol

A. Fed state

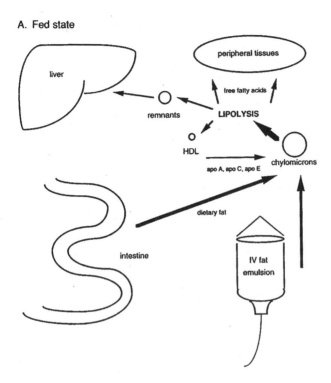

B. Postabsorptive state

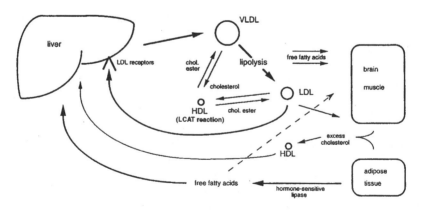

FIGURE 2.   Lipoprotein metabolism.

ester rather than triglyceride. LDL is cleared relatively slowly, with a half-life of several days. The uptake of LDL is mediated by a specific membrane receptor, termed the LDL receptor, whose activity in turn is regulated by intracellular cholesterol levels. The most active tissues (on a weight basis) for LDL clearance are steroidogenic tissues, such as the adrenals, gonads and the liver; because of its size, the liver accounts for over half of total LDL catabolism. As peripheral tissues cannot degrade cholesterol, excess cholesterol is returned to the liver via HDL, where it is used for bile acid synthesis or excreted in the bile.

Starvation leads to a number of adaptive responses. There is a depletion of liver glycogen within 24 to 48 hours, with stimulation of gluconeogenic enzymes to allow the production of glucose from amino acids released through protein breakdown in skeletal muscle. Lipolysis in adipose tissue leads to increased fatty acid levels and activation of enzymes responsible for β-oxidation of fatty acid in the liver (acyl-CoA-carnitine acyltransferase). In addition to acetyl-CoA, fatty acid oxidation generates ketone bodies. One important adaptive response to starvation is the induction of 3-hydroxybutyrate dehydrogenase in the brain, which allows this organ to utilize ketone bodies as a fuel. Decreased dependence on glucose reduces the need for excess gluconeogenesis and spares muscle protein. In a relatively lean 70 kg man with 12% body fat, survival without food can be expected to be about 60 days or longer.

3. CLINICAL AND LABORATORY FEATURES OF PROTEIN-ENERGY MALNUTRITION

Protein-energy malnutrition may result from a number of causes. These are shown in Table 2. Intake or assimilation may be impaired or, alternatively, losses may be increased, as occurs with excessive enteric protein loss in protein-losing enteropathies. In some disorders, multiple causes may be present. Moreover, requirements may be significantly increased in some patients as a result of growth, pregnancy, tissue injury or a superimposed disease process. In some patients with chronic debilitating diseases, multiple factors may be responsible.

Malnutrition has been classically divided into kwashiorkor (protein restricted) and marasmus (protein-calorie restricted). In kwashiorkor, the subject ingests a moderate number of calories, usually as complex carbohydrate (e.g., rice), but very little protein. The carbohydrate is absorbed as glucose, causing rises in plasma glucose and insulin, and leading to decreased lipolysis and proteolysis. The liver is therefore supplied with inadequate amino acids, with little oral intake and little peripheral mobilization from skeletal muscle stores. Transport of triglyceride made from ingested glucose is

TABLE 2. Causes of protein-energy malnutrition

Impaired intake
Insufficient quantity or quality
Impaired intake due to systemic disease (e.g., cerebrovascular accident, chronic infections)
Impaired intake due to localized gastrointestinal disease (e.g., benign or malignant esophageal stricture)

Impaired digestion and/or absorption
Selective enzyme defect (e.g., enteropeptidase deficiency, trypsinogen deficiency)
Generalized enzyme defect (e.g., pancreatic exocrine insufficiency)
Impaired small intestinal assimilation (e.g., celiac disease)

Excessive enteric protein loss
Gastric or intestinal mucosal disease (e.g., Ménétrier's disease, intestinal lymphangiectasia)
Extraintestinal disease with lymphatic blockage (e.g., pericarditis, lymphoma)

Disorders with multiple causes
Advanced malignancy
Chronic renal failure with uremia
Other chronic debilitating diseases

---

impaired since there is inadequate production of apoprotein, which is needed for the formation of VLDL. The liver becomes fatty and enlarged. Furthermore, other proteins, including albumin, are inadequately produced by the liver in kwashiorkor, and serum albumin falls, with resulting peripheral edema. With marasmus the subject takes inadequate amounts of protein and calories. The low caloric intake means that only small amounts of carbohydrate are taken; plasma glucose and insulin are low. Hence, lipolysis and proteolysis occur, with adequate delivery of amino acids from muscle to the liver for protein production. Fatty liver does not occur, and serum albumin levels tend to be normal, with no peripheral edema. Often patients fall between these two extremes of nutritional states, but there are examples of kwashiorkor and marasmus in Western clinical practice. Anorexia nervosa is a classic example of marasmus. Marked muscle wasting and loss of subcutaneous tissue (adipose tissue) occur with normal-sized nonfatty livers and no peripheral edema. In contrast, the intensive care unit patient who has received intravenous dextrose (glucose) without amino acids for a prolonged period will often show a fatty liver and marked hypoalbuminemia and edema. Other changes in the liver that may occur in nutritional disorders are listed in Table 3.

Clinical vitamin deficiencies are listed in Table 4. Except for cheilosis and glossitis, which are seen with multiple vitamin B deficiencies, physical find-

TABLE 3.   Effects of specific nutritional disorders on the liver

Nutritional disorders	Effects on the liver
Common conditions	
Alcoholism	Steatosis, alcoholic hepatitis and cirrhosis
Obesity	Steatosis, steatohepatitis and cholelithiasis
Uncontrolled diabetes	Glycogenosis, steatosis and steatohepatitis
Protein deficiency	Pigment stones
Kwashiorkor	Steatosis and decreased protein synthesis
Fasting	Mild unconjugated hyperbilirubinemia, especially in Gilbert's syndrome
Uncommon conditions	
Jejunoileal bypass	Steatosis and steatohepatitis
Gross dietary iron excess	Bantu siderosis/hemochromatosis
Senecio alkaloids	Veno-occlusive disease
Dietary aflatoxins	Hepatocellular carcinoma (?)
Chronic arsenic ingestion	Noncirrhotic portal hypertension, angiosarcoma and hepatocellular carcinoma
Hypervitaminosis A	Hepatic fibrosis and cirrhosis

ings of vitamin deficiencies are seldom observed in protein-calorie malnourished patients in developed countries. Trace elements are elements that are required in small quantities (mg amounts or less) for normal growth and/or function. Essential trace elements for humans include iron, iodine, zinc, chromium, copper, selenium, cobalt (as vitamin B_{12}), molybdenum, manganese and possibly vanadium. Except for iron deficiency due to blood loss and/or poor intake, deficiency states of trace elements are rare in subjects with some oral intake, since only minute amounts are required.

4. EFFECTS OF MALNUTRITION ON THE GASTROINTESTINAL TRACT AND PANCREAS

Protein-energy malnutrition may produce major structural and functional changes in the gastrointestinal tract and pancreas, which, in turn, may aggravate the underlying poor nutritional condition. In severe protein-energy malnutrition, for example, acinar cell atrophy occurs and exocrine cells have decreased numbers of zymogen granules. Pancreatic secretion may be reduced following stimulation with cholecystokinin and/or secretin. With malnutrition, the activities of enzymes contained in pancreatic juice (i.e., trypsin, chymotrypsin, lipase, amylase) are reduced. With reversal of malnutrition these can return to normal levels, but this may require several weeks.

In addition to pancreatic exocrine changes, the entire wall and mucosal lining of the stomach and intestine may be reduced in thickness. Microscopically, marked changes may develop, including severe "flattening" of the small intestinal mucosa, similar to celiac disease. In contrast to celiac disease, however, reduced numbers of crypt mitoses are seen. Changes may be present throughout the small intestine in an irregular patchy distribution, although the jejunum appears to be most severely affected. Some brush-border enzymes (e.g., disaccharidases) may be reduced; as a result, malabsorption of a variety of substances (e.g., lactose) may be observed. Altered uptake of glucose and D-xylose has also been reported, and steatorrhea may be present with impaired absorption of fat and some fat-soluble vitamins. In addition, there may be increased protein loss from the gut, leading to increased fecal nitrogen loss. Finally, specific nutrients may be deficient and cause alterations in certain tissues. In particular, folic acid and vitamin B_{12} deficiencies may lead to subtotal villous atrophy in association with crypt hypoplasia (Table 5).

Restitution of small bowel mucosa occurs after renutrition. There is growing evidence that mucosal atrophy occurs during total parenteral nutrition with associated increased intestinal permeability, especially in stressed metabolic states, and that atrophy is absent or minimal in patients fed enterally. Therefore, whenever possible, intestinal (i.e., enteral) feeding is preferred to parenteral feeding. When refeeding occurs after a period of malnutrition, however, it should be appreciated that gut function may be impaired, with resultant malabsorption and diarrhea, and that total refeeding via the gut may not initially be achieved. In this circumstance, partial enteral refeeding with parenteral supplementation is usually given, provided there are no contraindications to enteral feeding (e.g., bowel obstruction).

There is increasing evidence that the colonic mucosa uses short-chain fatty acids (especially butyrate) as an energy source. In patients who undergo a colostomy, the bowel that is left distally does not have a fecal stream. The mucosa of this bowel may develop inflammation, called "diversion colitis." This condition can be corrected by administering short-chain fatty acid enemas. A major source of the short-chain fatty acids in the colon is fermented dietary fiber, and thus fiber may be considered a "nutrient."

5. DIETARY THERAPY IN GASTROINTESTINAL DISEASE

5.1 General Principles

A number of specific diets are useful in different gastrointestinal disorders.

TABLE 4. Vitamin deficiency syndromes

Vitamin	Name of deficiency state	Clinical occurrence	Common clinical features
1. Water-soluble			
B₁ (thiamine)	Beriberi: Dry (neurologic) Wet (cardiac)	Refeeding after starvation	Neurologic: Peripheral neuropathy, Wernicke-Korsakoff Cardiac: Heart failure
	Wernicke-Korsakoff syndrome		
B₂ (riboflavin)	—	Rare	B-complex deficiency*
B₆ (pyridoxine)	—	Only with pyridoxine-antagonist drugs (isoniazid, cycloserine, penicillamine)	Neurologic: Convulsions B-complex deficiency* Anemia
B₁₂ (cyanocobalamin)	Pernicious anemia (when secondary to idiopathic gastric atrophy)	Achlorhydria Terminal ileal disease or resection Bacterial overgrowth Diphyllobothrium latum Pancreatic insufficiency	Hematologic: Pancytopenia Neurologic: Subacute combined degeneration Peripheral neuropathy Glossitis
Folic acid	—	Pregnancy Poor intake Malabsorption	Hematologic: Pancytopenia Glossitis
Niacin	Pellagra	Poor diet	Characteristic dermatitis Dementia Diarrhea
Pantothenic acid	—	Rare	—
Biotin	—	Excess egg white ingestion ? TPN	Dermatitis Glossitis Anorexia
C (ascorbic acid)	Scurvy	Infants, the elderly and alcoholics with very poor intake	Purpura Gum disease (when teeth present)

TABLE 4. Vitamin deficiency syndromes (cont'd)

Vitamin	Name of deficiency state	Clinical occurrence	Common clinical features
2. Fat-soluble			
A	—	Third World children Severe low intake	Night blindness, corneal changes, xerophthalmia, xeroderma and hyperkeratosis
D	—	Inadequate sun exposure Inadequate intake Renal disease	Osteomalacia (rickets in children) Hypocalcemia
E	—	Cholestatic liver disease (especially children)	Neurologic: Posterior column degeneration, areflexia
K	—	Warfarin anticoagulant Long-term antibiotics (especially with TPN) Newborn infants	Hemorrhage with prolonged prothrombin time

*B-complex deficiency: cheilosis, angular stomatitis, glossitis.

TABLE 5.   Effects of depletion of specific nutrients on the intestine

Nutrient	Effects
Protein-energy malnutrition (e.g., especially, kwashiorkor)	Total or subtotal villous atrophy and crypt hypoplasia
Folic acid deficiency	Total or subtotal villous atrophy and crypt hypoplasia; macrocytic and/or "megaloblastic" enterocytes
Vitamin B$_{12}$ deficiency	Total or subtotal villous atrophy and crypt hypoplasia; macrocytic and/or "megaloblastic" enterocytes
Vitamin E deficiency	(?) Small intestinal ceroidosis (i.e., "brown bowel syndrome")
Vitamin A deficiency	Reduced numbers of intestinal goblet cells

These may involve diet restriction or supplementation, or alternatively, a change in the consistency or content of specific nutrients. In patients with steatorrhea, for example, luminal fatty acids are present and involved in the pathogenesis of diarrhea. In these patients, reduction in diarrhea can be accomplished, in part, by a reduction in the oral intake of triglycerides; a low-fat diet may be beneficial. In some patients with steatorrhea, supplementation with medium-chain triglycerides may be useful because these are hydrolyzed more rapidly by pancreatic enzymes, do not require bile acid micelles for absorption, and are primarily directed to the portal rather than the lymphatic circulation. Because medium-chain triglycerides undergo ω-oxidation to metabolically nonutilizable dicarboxylic acids, the effective caloric content of medium-chain triglycerides is less than expected. Medium-chain triglycerides in a daily dose of 60 mL will provide approximately 460 calories. Low-fat dietary supplements may be provided in the form of a number of commercially available products prepared as complete nutritional supplements. Fat-soluble vitamins can be replaced using oral water-miscible formulations, if steatorrhea is present. For vitamin K, a water-soluble form is available. Fat-soluble vitamins require bile acid micelles for absorption; thus, if steatorrhea is due to bile acid depletion (as might occur in the short bowel syndrome following surgical resection for extensive Crohn's disease), increased amounts of vitamins may be required.

   Bloating and cramping pain may follow ingestion of lactose-containing foods. This may be due to lactase deficiency (e.g., small bowel disease, "ethnic" lactase deficiency). Dietary lactose restriction may be indicated in patients

TABLE 6.   Dietary guidelines for celiac disease patients

Foods to avoid
Wheat, rye, barley, oat products
Triticale (wheat–rye hybrid)
Millet and sorghum
Malt and hydrolyzed vegetable protein

Acceptable foods
Corn, rice, buckwheat products
Wine and distilled alcoholic beverages
Fruits and vegetables
Meat
Nuts
Dairy products (unless lactose-intolerant)

---

if there is a history of lactose intolerance or a positive lactose tolerance test (i.e., rise in blood sugar less than 20 mg/dL after 50 g of lactose) accompanied by characteristic symptoms. An alternative test involves measurement of breath hydrogen; a rise of more than 20 ppm is consistent with lactose intolerance. Lactose may be found in milk, including buttermilk, even if it has been naturally fermented. Commercial yogurt should also be avoided, since this often has milk or cream added after fermentation to avoid the sour taste produced by fermenting lactose. Ice cream and sherbets have high lactose concentrations and should be avoided. Cheese or desserts made from milk or milk chocolate as well as sauces or stuffings made from milk, cream or cheese should also be avoided. Calcium supplements may be necessary with dairy product restriction, particularly in postmenopausal women. Liquid dairy products may be used to a limited extent by patients who have lactose intolerance; in these patients, a yeast enzyme preparation (i.e., lactase from Kluyveromyces lactis) added to milk at 4°C (15 drops/L) can hydrolyze up to 99% of the lactose in 24 hours. Nonliquid dairy products cannot be treated with enzyme preparations, although lactase tablets may be chewed prior to eating solid food.

5.2 Celiac Disease
Celiac disease, also known as gluten-sensitive enteropathy or celiac sprue, is a malabsorption disorder resulting from ingestion of proteins derived from certain cereal grains of the grass family, Gramineae: wheat, rye, barley and possibly oats. It is believed that the alcohol-soluble gliadin fraction of wheat gluten or similar alcohol-soluble proteins from the other grains (termed *prolamins*) cause the intestinal damage. Consequently, absolute restriction is required for life. Table 6 provides some dietary guidelines for celiac disease

patients. Gluten, however, is a particularly ubiquitous substance and can be found in coffee, catsup, dip, frozen TV dinners, ice cream and even in the capsules of medications! Although wheat, rye, barley and possibly oats are important, corn and rice do not appear to activate celiac disease. Data on other grains are not as clear. Buckwheat is not derived from the grass family and is usually permitted. Millet and sorghum are often allowed, but have not been thoroughly evaluated. Triticale, a hybrid of wheat and rye, should be avoided. Rye whiskey, Scotch whiskey and other cereal-derived alcohols can be consumed, since gluten is not present in distilled spirits. Similarly, brandy and wine made from fruit pose no difficulties. Beer and ale are produced from barley; it is not entirely clear if they can activate disease and would best be avoided. Malt made from barley should be avoided, as well as hydrolyzed vegetable proteins used as flavor enhancers in processed foods, since they may be made from soy, wheat and other cereal proteins.

For both symptomatic and asymptomatic patients with celiac disease, a lifelong gluten-free diet is recommended. Multivitamin supplements are frequently required and specific vitamin, mineral and trace element deficiencies should be corrected. Iron and folate supplementation may be needed and poor absorption of oral iron may sometimes necessitate parenteral administration. Supplements of calcium and vitamin D may be required to prevent mobilization of skeletal calcium, and in some patients magnesium may be needed.

5.3 Inflammatory Bowel Disease

Malnutrition in patients with inflammatory bowel disease, especially Crohn's disease, is a frequent problem. Weight loss may be seen in over 65% of patients and growth retardation may be observed in up to 40% of children. As shown in Table 7, there are multiple causes for malnutrition, especially in patients with Crohn's disease with small bowel involvement. The goal of nutritional management is to ensure adequate nutrient intake with modifications that reduce symptoms. Although only limited studies are available, evidence suggests that energy expenditure in quiescent Crohn's disease and ulcerative colitis is no greater that one would predict for a healthy individual. If the disease is quite active, or is accompanied by fever or sepsis, resting energy expenditure increases. Interestingly, patients even with quiescent Crohn's disease have evidence of increased fat oxidation at rest, similar to findings in starved individuals. There may be increased caloric as well as nutrient requirements, particularly if gastrointestinal losses are substantial and malabsorption is significant. Attention should also be placed on micronutrient deficiencies in these patients, particularly if concomitant malabsorption is present. For example, patients with significant ileal disease or resection require regularly administered parenteral vitamin B_{12}.

TABLE 7. Malnutrition in inflammatory bowel disease

Reduced oral intake
Disease-induced (e.g., postprandial abdominal pain and diarrhea, sitophobia, anorexia, nausea and vomiting)
Iatrogenic (e.g., restrictive diets, "fad" diets)

Malabsorption
Reduced absorptive surface (e.g., shortened small intestine due to prior resection, diseased segments)
Bacterial overgrowth (e.g., associated with strictures and bypassed loops, stasis)
Bile salt deficiency after ileal resection (e.g., impaired micelle formation and steatorrhea)
Lactase deficiency (e.g., associated with small bowel disease)
Drug-induced malabsorption

Increased nutrient loss
Protein-losing enteropathy
Diarrhea losses of electrolytes, minerals and trace elements (e.g., potassium, zinc)
Gastrointestinal blood loss (e.g., iron loss)

Drug-induced malabsorption
Cholestyramine (e.g., bile acids; fat; fat-soluble vitamins, including vitamins D and K)
Sulfasalazine (e.g., folic deficiency associated with reduced absorption and increased requirement related to hemolysis)
Steroids (e.g., calcium absorption and mobilization)

Increased requirements
Chronic inflammatory disease, fever, superimposed infection

Frequently, the diet consistency or form will require modification to permit intake of adequate amounts of various nutrients. In some, symptoms may be improved by a diet with increased fiber. Increased amounts of pectin or guar, for example, may be helpful in patients with increased stool water content, as these fibers tend to have a significant water-retaining capacity.

Lactose intolerance appears to be no more common in ulcerative colitis than in healthy individuals. However, the effect of lactose intolerance in a patient with impaired colonic absorption may be much more profound in terms of diarrhea. There remains ongoing debate as to the prevalence of lactose intolerance in Crohn's disease, but it is likely equal to or slightly higher than that in the general population. Owing to the problems with malnutrition in Crohn's disease, a lactose-restricted diet should not be recommended unless there is clear-cut improvement in diarrhea with lactose restriction.

Specific drugs may also alter nutrient absorption. Cholestyramine is the classic example of an agent that interferes with nutrient (especially cations such as zinc) and drug absorption.

6. DIETARY THERAPY IN LIVER DISEASE

Two important manifestations of chronic liver disease, ascites and porto-systemic encephalopathy, have dietary modification as a cornerstone of treatment. The prime dietary objective in the treatment of ascites is sodium restriction. Some authorities have recommended restriction of dietary sodium intake to as little as 10–20 mmol/day for patients with symptomatic, large-vol ascites. However, it is almost impossible to design a palatable diet or provide sufficient protein to maintain nitrogen balance with such stringent restrictions, and therefore these will not be satisfactory for long-term use. Well-motivated patients can often be maintained on a 40 mmol sodium diet (equivalent to about 1 g of sodium or 2.5 g of sodium chloride).

The treatment of portosystemic encephalopathy includes dietary protein restriction. Management will obviously need to be individualized for patients with fulminant hepatic failure or stage IV coma, but patients with chronic liver disease and mild to moderate encephalopathy should usually have dietary protein intake restricted to 0.5–0.8 g/kg body weight. Even more rigorous restriction may be necessary to control encephalopathy in the short term, but is difficult to maintain for prolonged periods because of limited patient compliance and negative nitrogen balance. It is believed that vegetable protein may be less ammoniagenic than meat, but part of this may relate to decreased efficiency of absorption of vegetable protein. Disproportionately high levels of aromatic amino acids are found in plasma of patients with decompensated cirrhosis. Hence, nutritional supplements rich in branched-chain amino acids have been advocated; however, unequivocal evidence for their efficacy is lacking.

Patients with advanced cirrhosis often have hepatic glycogen depletion. During fasting, glucagon and catecholamines will be released to maintain blood glucose levels. In the absence of hepatic glycogen stores, this requires gluconeogenesis, and the substrate is provided to a significant extent from muscle catabolism. Utilization of the amino acids for gluconeogenesis will lead to ammonia production. It is not known whether dietary manipulations designed to provide a continuous supply of glucose, and therefore to reduce gluconeogenesis, would improve the hyperammonemia in these individuals. Cholestatic liver diseases, including primary biliary cirrhosis (PBC), secondary biliary cirrhosis, sclerosing cholangitis and biliary atresia, may be accompanied by malabsorption of fat-soluble vitamins. Vitamin K deficiency can be easily confirmed with the demonstration of a prolonged prothrombin time that corrects with administration of parenteral vitamin K. Assays for vitamins D,

TABLE 8. Diet therapy for hereditary liver diseases

Disorder	Dietary intervention
Tyrosinemia	Low-phenylalanine diet
Hereditary fructose intolerance	Low-fructose, low-sucrose diet
Galactosemia	Galactose-free diet
Glycogen storage disease	Continuous glucose feeding
Cerebrotendinous xanthomatosis	Deoxycholic acid supplementation
Wilson's disease	Low-copper diet, zinc supplementation (together with chelating agent)
Hemochromatosis	Avoidance of excess dietary iron, selection of foods containing phytates or tannins to reduce iron absorption (together with appropriate phlebotomy treatment)
Cystic fibrosis	Low-fat diet, pancreatic enzyme supplements, fat-soluble vitamin supplements

A and E are generally available only in specialized laboratories. If confirmatory tests are not available and if there are strong clinical grounds for suspecting a deficiency state, appropriate replacement therapy should be initiated. Table 8 lists a number of hereditary liver diseases for which appropriate therapy includes specific dietary interventions.

7. NUTRITION INTERVENTION

7.1 Nitrogen Requirements
In a well-nourished adult in steady state, total nitrogen intake will equal nitrogen output in urine, stool and skin. This is termed (zero) "nitrogen balance." Nitrogen is assimilated almost exclusively as protein, and, on average, 6.25 g protein is equivalent to 1 g nitrogen. The nitrogen is excreted predominantly as urea in the urine, but stool and skin losses account for about 2–3 g daily. If a 70 kg man consumes 1 g protein/kg (= 70 g protein or 11.2 g N), then about 8–9 g of nitrogen can be expected in the urine, assuming nitrogen balance. In the steady state, ingestion of more nitrogen will merely result in excretion of

more nitrogen in the urine, with the excess protein oxidized in the liver and used as an expensive energy source. In growing children or in malnourished adults, the nutritional goal is a positive nitrogen balance, meaning that body tissue is being formed in excess of what is being broken down (i.e., there is net growth). It is less clear that patients with conditions associated with protein loss, such as nephrotic syndrome and protein-losing enteropathy, benefit from extra protein intake. Indeed, there remains concern with nephrotic syndrome that extra protein may contribute to a fall in glomerular filtration rate (GFR), as has been reported in other renal conditions.

Nitrogen balance studies have shown that well-nourished adults can maintain nitrogen balance when given as little as 0.5 g/kg protein intake, if energy requirements are met or exceeded. It is important that the protein supplied be of high quality; it should include all essential amino acids and a balanced mix of nonessential amino acids. Malnourished, septic, injured or burned patients will require more protein, in the order of 1.5–2.0 g/kg daily. Pregnant patients should also be given 1.5 g/kg protein daily. It is less clear that patients with conditions associated with protein loss, such as nephrotic syndrome and protein-losing enteropathy, benefit from extra protein intake.

7.2 Energy Requirements
Basal energy requirements in healthy subjects are accurately predicted by the Harris-Benedict equation:

MALES: Energy (kcal/d) = 66 + (13.75 × W) + (5.00 × H) – (6.78 × A)

FEMALES: Energy (kcal/d) = 655 + (9.56 × W) + (1.85 × H) – (4.68 × A)

where W = weight in kg, H = height in cm and A = age in years.

Basal energy requirements, as predicted by these equations, increase in the presence of fever (13% per °C), sepsis or injury (up to 20–30%), and burns (up to 100%). Modest physical activity usually requires about 30% above basal requirements.

7.3 Types of Nutritional Intervention
The options for refeeding include oral refeeding, tube feeding and total parenteral nutrition. An assessment by a dietitian regarding current food intake and food preferences is essential. It may well be possible by determining food preferences to provide a well-balanced, nutritionally complete diet. In addition, supplements of high-calorie, high-protein foods such as milkshakes or com-

mercially prepared liquid formula diets may allow for adequate intake. If the patient will not or cannot eat, however, nutritional intervention may be indicated. Examples of patients who will not eat include those with anorexia due to tumor or chemotherapy, and those with anorexia nervosa. Such patients generally have a normal or near-normal nonobstructed bowel, and can be fed enterally. Patients who cannot eat because of severe gastrointestinal illness include those with bowel obstruction or ileus. If nutritional intervention is required in these patients, parenteral (intravenous) nutrition will be necessary.

7.3.1 *ENTERAL NUTRITION*
Enteral nutrition generally refers to nutrition provided through a tube that has been inserted into the gastrointestinal tract. Usually the tube is a fine-bore (10 French [3.3 mm] or less) Silastic® or polyurethane tube placed via the nose into the stomach, duodenum or jejunum. When long-term feeding is required, it is often preferable for cosmetic and comfort reasons to perform a gastrostomy radiologically or endoscopically, the latter commonly referred to as a PEG (percutaneous endoscopic gastrostomy). These tubes can be placed through the pylorus to feed into the jejunum with only local anesthetic and mild sedation. If pulmonary aspiration is a potential problem, the tube should be placed into the jejunum.

A multitude of commercial enteral formulas are available for infusion. The formulas have been traditionally divided into polymeric, oligomeric and modular. Polymeric formulas (also called defined formula diets) provide nitrogen as whole protein, often casein, egg white solids or soy protein. Carbohydrate is provided as corn syrup, maltodextrins or glucose oligosaccharides, with sucrose added for sweetness in oral formulas. Fat is usually provided as soy oil, although corn oil and safflower oil may be used. Medium-chain triglycerides (MCT oil) are rarely used. Protein may be provided as milk (usually dry or skim), with lactose as a major carbohydrate. These formulas are contraindicated in patients with lactose intolerance.

Oligomeric formulas (also called elemental diets) provide nitrogen as oligopeptides from partially hydrolyzed whole protein or as crystalline amino acids. Carbohydrate tends to be provided as glucose oligosaccharides or glucose. Fat is usually present in small quantities, enough to meet the requirement for linoleic acid (an essential fatty acid), which is about 2–4% of total calories. MCT oil is added to some formulas. The oligomeric diets were formulated to require minimal digestion by the gastrointestinal tract, with little necessity for bile and pancreatic secretions, and minimal "work" by the enterocyte in terms of brush-border enzyme activity or re-esterification. Hence, these diets have been commercially promoted as ideal for patients with decreased bile output (cholestasis), pancreatic insufficiency and short bowel.

However, there is little evidence that these diets are superior to polymeric diets, except with pancreatic insufficiency. Crohn's disease is another condition in which elemental diets may be superior to polymeric diets, although this too remains controversial. Furthermore, since the diet is "predigested," osmolality is high. Finally, the high cost of these diets (often 5 to 10 times that of polymeric diets) rarely justifies their use except in patients with severe pancreatic disease or possibly Crohn's disease.

Most of these formulas provide enough protein, calories, water, electrolytes, minerals, vitamins and trace elements in 2 L/day for most "nonstressed" patients. In other words, these diets are "complete." Excess requirements may exist in patients with multiple injuries, major infections or burns.

Modular formulas are those that contain or predominantly contain one kind of nutrient. There are commercially available modules for protein, fat, carbohydrates, vitamins, electrolytes and trace elements. These modules are not required for the majority of patients, and are rarely used. However, they may be used if different nitrogen-to-calorie ratios are indicated for a patient. Examples of this might include burns or protein-losing enteropathy, if more protein is to be given, or liver disease, if less protein is to be given. Modular feeding is time-consuming, since solutions must be mixed by the hospital, and are more expensive than "complete" formulas.

Finally, specialized amino acid solutions have been made for use in special circumstances – for example, liver disease, renal disease and "stress," such as trauma and sepsis. For liver disease, these solutions are composed mostly or exclusively of branched-chain amino acids, whereas for renal disease the solutions are predominantly essential amino acids. In general, these solutions are expensive and their efficacy is controversial.

Complications of enteral feeding may be divided into aspiration, mechanical, gastrointestinal and metabolic. In general, enteral feeding is well tolerated, and provided the complications are known, preventive and/or corrective measures may be undertaken to minimize patient risk.

Aspiration of the infused formula, with development of pneumonia, is a potentially lethal complication of tube feeding. Proper positioning of the tube requires radiographic verification. Risk factors for aspiration include patients on a ventilator and those with gastroesophageal reflux, poor or absent gag reflex, and impaired mentation. To minimize aspiration, it is suggested that patients, when possible, be fed with the head of the bed elevated 20–30°. Gastric contents should initially be checked by aspirating the tube every four to six hours, and if residue is present more than two hours following infusion, it should be temporarily stopped. Unfortunately, the small nasoenteric tubes in current use often collapse when aspirated, so small returns do not guarantee that the stomach is not becoming distended with fluid. Hence, examination for epigastric distention and succussion splash should be done. If there is any concern, an upright (if possible) plain film to assess gastric size may be useful. It has also been suggested that the feeding tube be placed into the small bowel well beyond the pylorus to minimize aspiration in those at risk, though studies have failed to confirm this.

Mechanical problems in patients with nasoenteric tubes include problems in the upper respiratory tract, esophagitis with development of esophageal ulceration and stenosis, tracheoesophageal fistula, and gastric outlet and small bowel obstruction. Upper respiratory problems include pharyngeal irritation, nasal erosions and necrosis, sinusitis and otitis media. These mechanical problems can be largely avoided by the use of soft, small-bore nasoenteric tubes.

Gastrointestinal problems related to nasoenteric feeding are common, occurring in 20–30% of patients. The most frequent complaints are nausea, vomiting, abdominal distention and altered bowel habit. Symptoms may be minimized by feeding at a slow rate with dilute solutions, but these symptoms may be just as common as with full-rate, full-strength solutions. Alternatively, a different enteral solution may be tried. If a lactose-containing solution is being used (generally not recommended for tube feeding), changing to a lactose-free solution is indicated. For constipation, fiber-containing solutions may be tried, although they are often unhelpful. Fiber, however, is a potential energy source for the colon, as previously discussed, and may therefore be important for maintenance of the colonic mucosa. At the present time, fiber-containing solutions are not routinely used.

Metabolic complications include overhydration, dehydration, hyperglycemia (including hyperosmolar nonketotic coma) and electrolyte disturbances. Electrolyte problems include hyponatremia, hyper- and hypokalemia, hyper- and hypophosphatemia and hypomagnesemia. In healthy, reasonably nourished individuals with normal cardiac, liver and renal function, these problems are not common. It is recommended that appropriate blood tests be done at intervals over the first few weeks to check for these potential problems.

7.3.2 *TOTAL PARENTERAL NUTRITION*
Total parenteral nutrition (TPN) involves intravenous administration of all known essential nutrients. This form of therapy is as effective as oral or enteral intake in terms of growth and maintaining body nitrogen. Indications include inability to eat for a minimum of 7 to 10 days with a nonfunctional gut. Total parenteral nutrition is also used for "bowel rest," especially in Crohn's disease, intestinal fistulas and pancreatitis, even if adequate absorption is possible. Several studies suggest, however, that bowel rest is not helpful in Crohn's disease. Furthermore, other studies have shown that elemental

diets can be used instead of TPN, except when bowel obstruction is present. In general, if the gut is functional, enteral feeding is preferred since it is safer, cheaper and more physiologic.

7.3.2.1 Solutions

7.3.2.1.1 *Amino acids* "Protein" is supplied as synthetic crystalline, L-amino acid solutions; these are commercially available in 7–10% concentrations. Most available amino acid mixtures are devised for patients without special requirements. Solutions with added branched-chain amino acids are available for hepatic failure, and solutions with essential amino acids are available for renal failure.

7.3.2.1.2 *Fat* There is a human requirement for linoleic acid, which is a precursor of arachidonic acid, which is in turn a precursor of prostaglandins. Linoleic acid, an essential fatty acid, cannot be produced by humans. It has been recommended that this be supplied as 4% or more of total caloric intake. Commercial fat solutions consist of soybean or safflower oil, emulsified with egg phospholipid, and made isotonic at 300 mOsmol/L with added glycerol. Commercially available fat emulsions are available at concentrations of 10% or 20%.

7.3.2.1.3 *Carbohydrate* Glucose is the preferred carbohydrate for intravenous use. Glucose is widely available in concentrations from 5–70%. The osmolality of these solutions may be markedly hyperosmolar up to about 2,500 mOsmol/L.

7.3.2.1.4 *Nonprotein energy source* Once the initial 100 g of glucose is provided for use in the brain, renal medulla and red blood cells, glucose and fat are equally effective in preserving body nitrogen after an equilibration period of four to five days. Glucose is very inexpensive as an energy source, but requires insulin for uptake into cells, and hyperglycemia can be a problem when large amounts of glucose are utilized. The high osmolality of glucose solutions means that only dilute solutions can be used in peripheral veins, and if glucose is used as a major energy source, a large central vein is necessary to prevent thrombosis. Furthermore, glucose has a respiratory quotient (R.Q. = CO_2 produced/O_2 consumed) of 1.0, meaning that large amounts of carbon dioxide may be produced. Finally, glucose infusion leads to catecholamine release and increased metabolic rate, further increasing CO_2 production. These changes may be deleterious for patients being weaned from ventilators, or with borderline respiratory function.

Lipid solutions offer the benefit of being iso-osmolar, containing linoleic acid and having a lower respiratory quotient of 0.7, with less carbon dioxide production. Drawbacks include somewhat higher cost compared to glucose, and poor tolerance in patients with hyperlipidemia.

7.3.2.2 Routes of delivery

7.3.2.2.1 *Central* The most flexible way to deliver total parenteral nutrition is through a large central vein, usually the superior vena cava, via either the internal jugular or subclavian approach. With the large flow through the superior vena cava, solution osmolality is not of great concern, and thrombosis of this vessel is rare.

7.3.2.2.2 *Peripheral* The hypertonicity of parenteral nutritional solutions (10% amino acids approach 1,000 mOsm/L, 50% dextrose are 2,500 mOsm/L, while fat solutions are iso-osmolar to plasma at 300 mOsm/L) makes peripheral nutrition extremely difficult and therefore rarely used. When parenteral nutrition needs to be given peripherally, a typical mixture might consist of 5% amino acid/10% dextrose Y-connected to 1.5 L of 10% lipid. This would provide 50 g "protein," 350 kcal of glucose and 1,650 kcal of lipid, with a final osmolality of over 600 mOsm/L. The peripheral vein site will need to be changed at least every 48 hours, and the lipid dose may lead to marked hypertriglyceridemia. In general, there should be very little indication for this approach.

7.3.2.3 Complications

Complications of total parenteral nutrition may be divided into local and systemic. Local problems relate to the catheter site, and in the case of central lines involve all the complications of central catheters, including inadvertent arterial catheterization with bleeding, pneumothorax, hemothorax and inadvertent infusion of solutions into the pleural cavity. The complication of pneumothorax is much more common with subclavian insertion than with internal jugular insertion, meaning that internal jugular insertion is a safer technique, overall. Air embolism may occur at the time of insertion or any time thereafter with a central line. Catheter embolization may occur, and as mentioned, thrombosis has been reported, particularly with the use of stiff catheters. For long-term use, Silastic® catheters are preferred. It is essential that catheter placement be done by persons with considerable experience to minimize these complications.

Systemic complications include sepsis, metabolic problems and bone disease. Bacteremia or fungemia occurs in 3–7% of patients given total parenteral nutrition, and this appears to arise predominantly from the hub where the catheter joins the intravenous tubing. Catheters are always inserted in a strictly aseptic manner, with personnel fully gowned and gloved. Metabolic problems include hyperglycemia, which can be treated by reducing the amount of glucose given in the solutions, hypertriglyceridemia when excess calories and/or excess lipid is given, and alterations in electrolytes. In particular, total parenteral nutrition causes anabolism with increased intracellular water, so that potassium and phosphate are driven into cells, leading to possible hypokalemia and hypophosphatemia. These complications are very uncommon if adequate amounts of these electrolytes are provided and careful monitoring is performed. Liver disease remains a frustrating complication of total parenteral nutrition and occurs in up to 90% of cases, but in most cases the changes are restricted to enzyme elevations. In general, mild elevations in AST and alkaline phosphatase occur in the second week, with occasional elevations in bilirubin occurring later. Liver biopsy may show mild cholestasis. Overfeeding, particularly with glucose calories, may result in steatosis; this can be treated by reducing total calories and glucose. Rarely, long-term TPN (extending over years) may result in cirrhosis without a well-defined cause.

SUGGESTED READING LIST

Rombeau JL, Caldwell MD (eds.). Clinical nutrition: parenteral nutrition. 2d ed. Philadelphia: WB Saunders, 1994.
Rombeau JL, Rolandelli RH (eds.). Clinical nutrition: enteral and tube feeding. 3d ed. Philadelphia: WB Saunders, 1996.

OBJECTIVES

1. Know the biochemical pathways important to the understanding of carbohydrate, fat and protein metabolism both in the fasting and fed state.
2. Be able to describe the clinical changes important in malnourished states.
3. Understand the role of diet and nutrition in important gastrointestinal diseases, specifically inflammatory bowel disease, celiac disease and liver disease.
4. Be able to give an overview of the types of nutritional intervention currently available.

3
Gastroenterology and Medical Ethics
J.J. Sidorov

Basic moral principles and rules of medical ethics are as old as the medical profession itself. They were succinctly formulated in such codes as the Hippocratic Oath and Maimonides' Prayer, and have served for centuries as an unchanged moral base for medical practice. Major social and moral changes, particularly those of the second half of the 20th century, have challenged many of these classical values and modified others: witness the introduction of new attitudes toward sexuality and developments in transplantation of human tissues and organs, and opposing views on abortion. Promotion of the patient's autonomy and of human rights has led to the firm establishment of the right of the individual patient to be fully informed and consulted on all medical considerations and decisions related to his or her well-being, health and even death. The influence of such professionals as philosophers, ethicists, sociologists, anthropologists and lawyers has altered concepts of the patient–doctor relationship.

The change from a classical paternalistic to a modern participatory patient–doctor relationship has significantly altered the pattern of medical practice. When a patient consults a physician, a contractual arrangement takes place. The patient provides the physician with the personal, intimate information necessary for proper evaluation and rational management. Complete patient care must take into consideration the patient as a total person, including his or her personal moral values.

The rapid expansion of medical knowledge and technology has also introduced a range of expensive, complex, and often aggressive diagnostic and therapeutic procedures. The rising costs of many new, highly skilled, labor-intensive techniques have led to the rationing of our progressively diminishing health-care resources and raised difficult questions of fairness and

TABLE 1. Ethical principles and professional obligations

Ethical principles	Professional obligations
Beneficence	Confidentiality
Nonmaleficence	Fidelity (promise-keeping)
Respect for autonomy	Interest
Justice, fairness	Veracity (truth-telling)

TABLE 2. Hierarchy of ethical pathways

General ethical principle
Specifically applicable ethical value
Competing and/or conflicting values
Mutually exclusive values
Changing moral values

priorities: who gets what and why, at whose expense, and under what circumstances?

Application of current biomedical ethical principles to the changing clinical and social situation has thus become an essential part of the practice of modern medicine (Table 1).

Since ethics is an integral part of the practice of medicine, it is governed by the same forces that shape the intellectual processes of diagnosis, prognosis, treatment and the general management of a patient. Ethical reasoning and the application of ethical principles reflect, therefore, the same trends and changes affecting current clinical practice, such as evidence-based medicine and clinical diagnostic pathways and practice guidelines.

The evidence-based practice of medicine is intimately linked to general ethical principles such as beneficence and nonmaleficence. In order to uphold these principles, physicians must continue to constantly upgrade their professional knowledge and its clinical application. Failure to consider the available confirmed scientific evidence when making a clinical decision, and through it harming a patient, is unethical. As an example, it would be unethical, because of the physician's lack of evidence-based knowledge to the contrary, to give advice against pregnancy to a young woman with inflammatory bowel disease who desires to start a family.

Clinical diagnostic pathways and practice guidelines are interlocked with corresponding ethical pathways and guidelines. In addition to understanding the rationale of clinical pathways and guidelines, it is also essential to be aware of the rationale of the associated ethical pathways and guidelines.

In order to apply ethical reasoning to a clinical situation it is necessary first to identify the general underlying ethical principle (Table 1). This is followed by identification of specific ethical values applicable to each step of a particular pathway (Table 2).

The *general ethical principle* is a basic moral principle in force throughout the entire contact with an individual patient, such as a moral obligation to always act in the patient's best interest (Table 1).

The *specific ethical value* is a moral obligation applicable to a specific clinical situation or action. For example, testing for H. pylori is ethically justified only if there is an intention to act on the result of the test.

Competing and/or conflicting ethical values are at issue when there is conflict or incompatibility between individual and societal moral values. For example, scarcity of resources may be used to argue for restricting an expensive treatment to a select category of patients (e.g., only to the patients who contracted hepatitis C through blood transfusion during a specified time).

Mutually exclusive moral values mark the situation that arises when different moral values are upheld in otherwise identical situations. Often, these are traditional moral values of different cultures. In contrast to diseases, which are transcultural, moral values are often culture-specific. For example, while veracity (truth-telling) is one of the fundamentals of Western medical ethics, some other cultures consider it immoral to tell a terminally ill patient the truth about his or her condition.

Changing moral values are a feature of a changing society. Certain moral norms change as society changes, though at a different pace in different societies (e.g., differences in the moral justification and acceptance of "assisted suicide" and euthanasia in different countries).

Gastroenterologists share common ethical principles with and encounter problems similar to those faced by their colleagues in other medical disciplines. Like other specialists, gastroenterologists must often apply general medical ethical principles to specific areas of their activities. One such area is diagnostic and therapeutic endoscopy. Others include the treatment of patients with new, potent drugs, the active participation of gastroenterologists in drug trial studies, and their relationship with industry.

Transplantation of the liver, intestine and pancreas also raises ethical issues, particularly related to economy of resources. The demands that organ transplantation places on society lead to political rather than purely medical decisions concerning the allocation of resources and assignment of priorities. These decisions are not only based on the principle of individual beneficence, but they also are greatly influenced by social perceptions of justice and fairness. Gastroenterologists are being exposed to escalating pressure to control costs, ration resources and act as gatekeepers for organ transplantation. In addition to purely medical decisions, assessing patient suitability involves ethical issues. Should, for example, an individual with self-induced liver disease from abusing alcohol or other drugs, or from following a particular lifestyle, be accepted for transplantation?

Commerce involving organs or parts of organs is another area of ethical concern. Organ sale elsewhere in the world has been justified in that it is the only way to meet current needs. The issue is clouded by a lack of absolute ethical standards that could be uniformly applied in all parts of the world. Although medicine is generally transcultural, ethics is often culture-specific, as it depends on historical, religious, social and cultural factors. Ethical principles applicable to contemporary Western societies do not apply to parts of the world with completely different cultural and social traditions.

The availability of cadaveric organs is the main limiting factor in adult liver transplantation in Canada. According to a recent study, at least 37 patients died in Canada in 1991 while waiting for a new liver.

The Council on Ethics and Judicial Affairs of the American Medical Association has recommended a system of mandated choice, in which "everyone would be asked whether they consent to organ donation."

The Council of Europe has adopted a policy in 13 countries of "presumed consent" in which the onus is placed on the individual to opt out of cadaveric organ donation.

No such system exists in Canada. Canadian physicians therefore find themselves morally responsible for ensuring that no potentially available organ is wasted. Accordingly, a failure to secure such an organ, either by discouraging a donation as a result of personal bias, or failing through a passive attitude to consider the possibility and appropriateness of timely retrieval of a patient's organs, amounts to withholding a potentially lifesaving treatment from a waiting recipient.

The advent of fiberoptic endoscopy has had a major impact on research and clinical practice in gastroenterology. Ethical issues peculiar to gastrointestinal endoscopy are often not obvious. Gross violations of a code of ethics are easily detected and identified. The difficulty arises, however, when assessing skill, competence and quality control. It is often difficult to draw a clear line between professional competence and the safety of a procedure on one hand, and ethical behavior on the other.

Ethical considerations arising from invasive diagnostic and therapeutic gastroenterological procedures have been recently addressed in Canada by the Canadian Association of Gastroenterology in its consensus report "Consensus in Endoscopy." The patient's informed consent, based on a full understanding of risks and benefits, must be obtained prior to the procedure and sedation. While society's resources should be economically utilized, economic constraints should not adversely influence the quality of the care.

In addition to mandatory training requirements, the physician's technical and cognitive skills must be maintained through strict adherence to specified standards and must be further improved through constant learning.

Performance of endoscopic procedures in excess of diagnostic and therapeutic requirements and beyond the needs of approved research is unethical.

An innovative procedure or a significant modification of a standard procedure cannot be undertaken without prior approval by the institutional review board or the hospital ethics committee, and without the fully informed consent of the patient.

Life-support measures that provide nutrition through a variety of oral, enteral and parenteral routes have become the principal form of treatment of not only critically ill patients, but often also patients who are terminally ill.

Nonetheless, the belief that nutritional support is beneficial to terminally ill patients has been recently questioned.

Recent reports provide increasing evidence that withholding artificial nutrition and hydration is actually devoid of suffering, providing that oral food and liquids are given as requested by the patient and that proper care is taken of mouth and lips. While insufficient to maintain the patient's weight and life, this limited nutrition and hydration keeps the patient comfortable.

Since food and water have a strong emotional connotation as the essence of life, any attempt at withholding these is strongly resisted by care-givers. Furthermore, some physicians may not only try to persuade but may also resort to coercion and force a patient to accept a given form of artificial feeding. Strong ethical arguments are nevertheless being put forward that prolonging the life of a terminally ill patient through artificial nutrition and hydration prolongs suffering and delays the natural process of death. It therefore violates the ethical principle of beneficence and nonmaleficence. When carried out against the patient's expressed wish or through coercion it also violates the principle of autonomy.

Close cooperation between the pharmaceutical industry and the medical profession has greatly contributed to recent progress in research and to educational opportunities. The development of new drugs requires clinical trials. Development of a new drug from the initial invention of a chemical structure until its final approval for general use takes an average of 10 to 15 years and may cost up to $100 million before realizing any financial return. The industry is quite aware that commercial objectives must not override ethical considerations and has developed the guidelines governing the conduct of such studies. By subscribing to such codes, the industry has accepted responsibility for proper monitoring and supervision of sound clinical trials. For their part, those physicians involved in a clinical study must possess adequate knowledge and devote the necessary time to ensure that no breach of ethical principles occurs.

It is unethical to enter a patient into a trial unless the investigator truly believes that the new drug or procedure will provide benefits beyond those already available. The investigator must be free to publish the results regardless of the outcome, unencumbered by the private interests of the sponsor. The principal investigator shares with the sponsor the responsibility for the scientific validity, ethical content and correctness of the clinical evaluation of the product undergoing trial. The investigator may be remunerated for clinical work (such as physical examination, endoscopies and other technical procedures) if charged for at standard rates. It is unethical, however, to derive personal financial benefit as a reward for participating in or conducting the study.

Medical research using human subjects requires careful scrutiny. A recent study by an international group of reviewers found that a significant proportion of studies involving humans, and published in some of the leading gastroenterology journals, failed to meet ethical standards as defined by the reviewers. Approximately 40% would have been rejected by reviewers had they been members of the review boards at the institutions where the work was done. Some 12% of these "rejections" involved perceived danger to participating patients; the remainder involved poor study design or problems of statistical analysis. Between 10 and 15% of medications used were subsequently discovered to be potentially toxic.

There seem to be several places where a potential deficiency may originate. Concern about personal career development and academic pressure to demonstrate research productivity might induce an investigator to disregard what might at first appear to be a trivial issue. Casual supervision and inadequate quality control by senior, experienced and established investigators could be another factor. Poorly conducted research leading to faulty conclusions based on avoidable deficiencies and errors is unethical. Just because a project has received the approval of an institutional review board, there is no guarantee that it will remain ethical throughout. Finally, the system of peer review, the traditional method of ensuring the quality of scientific investigation, is not infallible. Close supervision based on clearly defined institutional publication policies and periodic careful review of the study's progress may eliminate many of these ethical pitfalls. The ethical component must be part of the scientific review.

The complexity of current scientific, technical, philosophical and social developments and other conditions in the contemporary world present a plethora of ethical issues that we need to consider in our daily work – clinical practice, research or teaching. We should always consider the patient not only as a collection of symptoms, signs and pathological processes but also as an individual with emotions, problems and moral standards. Biomedical ethics is an integral part of such care. Familiarity with basic bioethical principles (Table 1) is as essential for the practice of medicine as the knowledge of pathophysiology is for the understanding of the disease process.

SUGGESTED READING LIST

Bailey RJ, Barkun A, Brow J, et al. Consensus in endoscopy. Can J Gastroenterol 1996; 10:237–242.

Bricker BM. Industrial marketing and medical ethics. N Engl J Med 1989; 320:1690–1692.

Canada. Health Protection Branch, Health and Welfare Canada. Code of good monitoring practice for clinical investigators. 1983.

CMA guidelines for drug–company supported CME. CMAJ 1986; 135:384A.

Davies IB, Grind IM, Pottage A, Turner P. Development of new drugs in man: a review. J Roy Soc Med 1986; 79:96–99.

DeDombal PT, Holt PR, Sidorov JJ. Ethics in gastroenterology: proceedings of a workshop meeting of the World Organisation of Gastroenterology held at St. George's House, Windsor Castle, Berkshire, England, 29 April – 2 May 1986. Leeds: University of Leeds Printing Service, 1986:21–24.

Duggan JM. Resource allocation and bioethics. Lancet 1989; 1:772–773.

Engler RL, Covell JW, Friedman PJ, Kitcher PS, Peters RM. Misrepresentation and responsibility in medical research. N Engl J Med 1987; 317:1383–1389.

Gibinski K. Ethics and training in digestive endoscopy. Endoscopy 1989; 21:232–233.

Grad MR. Human experimentation and informed consent. CMAJ 1984; 131:932–935.

Leaf A. The doctor's dilemma — and society's too. N Engl J Med 1984; 310:718–720.

MCann RM, Hall WJ, Groth-Juncker A. Comfort care for terminally ill patients. JAMA 1994; 272:1263–1266.

McGregor M. Pharmaceutical "generosity" and the medical profession. Ann RCPSC 1988; 21:289.

Mullen MA, Kohut N, Sam M, Blendis L, Singer PA. Access to adult liver transplantation in Canada: a survey and ethical analysis. CMAJ 1996; 154:337–342.

Omery A, Caswell D. A nursing perspective on the ethical issues surrounding liver transplantation. Heart and Lung 1988; 17:626–630.

Rawlins MD. Doctors and the drug makers. Lancet 1984; 2:276–278.

Reagan MD. Health care rationing: what does it mean? N Engl J Med 1988; 319:1149–1151.

Reagan MD. Physicians as gatekeepers: a complex challenge. N Engl J Med 1987; 317:1731–1733.

The Royal College of Physicians of London. The relationship between physicians and the pharmaceutical industry: a report of the Royal College of Physicians. J Roy Col Phy of London 1986; 20:235–241.

Sabesin SM, Williams JW, Evans LS. Ethical and economic issues. In: Maddrey WC (ed.), Transplantation of the liver. New York: Elsevier, 1988:331–343.

Sidorov JJ. Ethical dilemmas in gastroenterology. Med North Am 1995; 472–476.

Sidorov JJ. Ethics in gastrointestinal research. Scand J Gastroenterol 1988; 23(Suppl. 144):100–113.

Singer PA, Siegler M, Whitington RF, et al. Ethics of liver transplantation with living donors. N Engl J Med 1989; 321:620–621.

Sircus W. Ethics of diagnostic and therapeutic endoscopic procedures. Scand J Gastroenterol 1988; 23(Suppl. 144):105–106.

Thompson WG. The ethics of physician–pharmaceutical company relationships. CMAJ 1988; 129:835–836.

Williams JR. Human organ sales. Ann RCPSC 1985; 18:401–404.

Younger SJ, Allen M, Bartlet ET, et al. Psychosocial and ethical implications of organ retrieval. N Engl J Med 1985; 313:321–323.

4
Pharmaceutical Research and Clinical Trials: The Basis for New Knowledge

A. Archambault and B.G. Feagan

1. INTRODUCTION

The scientific study of new drugs is an important research activity that requires close cooperation between investigators in industry and in academia. Despite the relatively small size of the Canadian pharmaceutical market (3% of global drug expenditures), Canadian investigators have played a leading role in the development of new drug treatments for both peptic ulcer disease and inflammatory bowel disease. Since the development of a new drug may require 10 to 15 years of investment in research before a product reaches the market, and only one out of 8,000 substances initially tested in animal models can be expected to result in the development of a useful treatment in humans, this activity is both time-consuming and expensive. The goal of this chapter is to familiarize the reader with the activities necessary for the development of new drug treatments.

2. CLINICAL RESEARCH REGULATIONS AND SUPERVISION

Investigators, sponsors and institutional authorities share equal responsibility for producing high-quality data and following ethical recommendations for the conduct of biomedical research involving human subjects. The Declaration of Helsinki – first proposed in Finland in 1964 and most recently revised by the World Medical Assembly in South Africa in 1996 – is a universally accepted ethical code.

In 1987 the Medical Research Council of Canada (MRC) approved guidelines for research involving human subjects. The latest guidelines for good clinical research practices are stipulated in a document entitled *Good Clinical*

Practice: Consolidated Guideline, issued by the International Conference on Harmonisation of Technical Requirements for Registration of Pharmaceuticals for Human Use (ICH). They were officially adopted by the Therapeutic Products Programme (TPP) of the Canadian government in 1997.

In the United States, federal regulations concerning the development of new drugs and their subsequent admissibility for clinical investigation were in place as early as 1938. Following the tragic events surrounding the use of thalidomide in the 1950s, important amendments were adopted: review of preclinical data, the informed consent of patients and the reporting of preclinical findings became mandatory in 1962. In an attempt to standardize compliance with regulatory requirements, good clinical practice (GCP) rules for sponsors (1977) and for investigators (1978) were developed by industry. The investigational new drug (IND) regulation was established in 1987.

A comprehensive set of guidelines for drug trials emerged in October 1990 as a result of a meeting where the tenets of good practice were compared by scientists from the European Community and North America. Uniform standards were subsequently defined.

Although some differences exist among countries in the government regulations governing clinical research in humans, these guidelines are becoming more uniform.

3. CLINICAL RESEARCH DEVELOPMENT

The research process includes both preclinical studies and clinical trials.

3.1 Preclinical Studies

The pharmaceutical industry must identify chemical structures for synthesis and subsequently assess the biological effects of these compounds in laboratory and animal models. Compounds that show promising biological effects are selected for further study.

Preclinical studies are usually conducted in the research laboratory of pharmaceutical companies or in university centers. Once a potential compound has been identified, a pharmacological expert analyzes the main biological effects of the drug, its duration of action and the adverse effects of the compound in various animal species. Pharmacokinetic studies performed in animals define the absorption, volume of distribution, metabolism and excretion of the candidate compound. Toxicological studies are performed to identify any possible mutagenic or teratogenic effects of the drug. Compounds that meet the requirements of these early studies are further assessed to determine the optimal dosage and route of administration. From these studies a drug may be selected for further development. These goals usually can be achieved within two to four years. At this time a submission to the regulatory authorities for authorization to administer the potential new drug (IND: investigational new drug) to humans is applied for. The latter process involves a well-defined procedure that may require an additional few months for approval. During this process the preclinical data are reviewed by an appropriate national regulatory body, such as the U.S. Food and Drug Administration (FDA) or the TPP in Canada. These agencies follow similar procedures, and for this reason multicenter studies are often performed using similar protocols in the two countries.

3.2 Clinical Trials
Four phases of clinical drug development are recognized.

3.2.1 *PHASE I*
These studies are carried out in small numbers of *normal, healthy volunteers.* The primary objective is to test the compound for safety and tolerability. These studies are done initially with a single dose, then with multiple doses. Pharmacokinetic and pharmacodynamic studies in humans must be performed with close medical surveillance and continuous monitoring of patients for adverse effects. During the time that Phase I studies are underway, animal studies for toxicity and potential carcinogenicity are continued.

3.2.2 *PHASE II*
At this phase, pilot studies to evaluate the efficacy and safety of a new drug are performed in *patients with the specific disease of interest.* The studies are usually short-term and may either be placebo-controlled or employ a comparison with a standard therapy. The emphasis in Phase II is on the definition of the most appropriate dose, dosing interval and route of administration. These studies often provide information that is vital for the design of Phase III trials. The latter provide definitive data regarding the efficacy and safety of a new drug.

Animal studies for toxicity and carcinogenicity continue during this phase.

3.2.3 *PHASE III*
These studies, which are usually conducted in a large number of patients, are designed to demonstrate either short- or long-term efficacy and provide further safety data. A Phase III trial usually compares a fixed dose of the new drug to conventional therapy under conditions that approximate those of usual clinical care. The therapeutic profile of the drug is defined by the results of these studies, which determine the final indications, dosage, route of administration, contraindications, adverse effects and possible drug interactions.

The duration of Phases II and III is often in the range of three to five years. Following accumulation of appropriate Phase II and III data, a submission to regulatory authorities is filed (NDS: New Drug Submission). These data are then scrutinized by the appropriate government experts. In Canada it may require up to an additional two years before approval to market the product is received.

3.2.4 PHASE IV

Following approval for general use, the evaluative process continues. Clinical studies are performed with approved or marketed drugs to gather more information on possible adverse events, to compare them with alternative treatments, and to detect interactions with other drugs. Due to the low prevalence of most serious adverse events, Phase IV observational studies (postmarket surveillance) are often the only means of adequately defining the safety profile of new compounds. During this period, new indications, new formulations or effective combinations of the new drug with existing therapies may be explored. The knowledge of a new pharmaceutical grows gradually through the various phases of clinical research, and it is never 100% complete. All relevant findings must be documented and reported, regardless of the time that has passed since the initial approval of the drug for general use.

4. METHODOLOGY IN CLINICAL RESEARCH

The randomized, controlled trial is the benchmark for the evaluation of new drug therapies. Random allocation is a powerful means of controlling for the potential effects of confounders and serves to minimize bias (systematic deviation from the truth) on the part of physicians and patients. Concealing the treatment allocation from the patient and investigator (blinding), which reduces the potential for bias, is also a fundamental component of a rigorously designed clinical trial. Considerable controversy has arisen regarding the use of placebo controls in evaluating new drugs. Some authors have argued against their use on the basis that patients are denied treatment of proven efficacy and thus may experience some degree of morbidity by participation in a placebo-controlled study. However, a placebo comparison allows an evaluation of the new therapy against the alternative of no treatment, and thus is scientifically valid and ethical when the standard therapy has only modest efficacy or causes important adverse effects. In Phase III trials it is vital that investigators choose as a primary measure of response an outcome that is clinically meaningful. In the past there has been an over-reliance on surrogate markers of efficacy such as improvements in laboratory tests. In some instances these have been shown not to correlate with clinically meaningful events. Investigators should consider utilization of quality of life measures as measures of response in addition to the more conventional outcomes of death, occurrence of disease-related complications and clinical activity indices. Once an appropriate outcome has been identified, the planning of a clinical trial requires input from a biostatistician. Careful consideration is given to the number of patients required, which is dependent upon the alpha (false positive) and beta (false negative) error rates selected by the investigator, the size of treatment effect that is considered to be clinically meaningful and the estimated rate of occurrence of the outcome of interest in the placebo (or standard therapy) group. If interim analyses are planned, these must be defined prior to initiation of the study, and appropriate statistical techniques employed to account for the increase in the alpha error rate that results from the use of multiple statistical testing procedures.

5. PLANNING OF CLINICAL TRIALS

5.1 Protocol Design and Implementation

The study protocol should explicitly state the rationale for studying the drug in the disease of interest. The source and chemical nature of the compound, its pharmacology and toxicology, and the data obtained in previous clinical investigations must be present in appropriate detail. All study protocols must be approved by the appropriate regulatory authorities. The objectives of the study must be clearly stated and appropriate methodology employed to ensure that these are met. The study treatment schedule should define the drug administration (dosage, strength, route of administration, the blinding process, packaging and labeling) in sufficient detail.

The inclusion and exclusion criteria, baseline, pre- and post-treatment measurement and evaluation visits and procedures for reporting adverse events and treatment overdoses must be clearly specified.

A study discontinuation procedure is defined in the event of lack of efficacy, intolerable side effects, poor patient compliance or the occurrence of a treatment endpoint.

Detailed definitions of the statistical analysis, data management procedures, administrative structure of the study and insurance and liability requirements are also necessary.

The protocol should contain a description of the background information that is provided to the patient and the informed consent document. For the patient's protection, lay language must be used. Diary forms and informed consent papers must be translated into the patient's primary language.

Once a protocol has been developed, an appropriate study administrative structure should be organized. An executive (steering) committee is constituted, which is responsible for the strategic aspects of conducting the trial. Usually other committees are organized to oversee the operational aspects of the trial, to monitor the safety of participants, and to adjudicate key outcomes.

5.2 Selection of Investigators and Centers

The selection of the investigators for clinical research will depend on the nature of the drug and the phase of the investigation. Experts in clinical pharmacology are selected for Phase I and II studies; experts in medical practice or medical specialties will usually be selected for Phase III and IV studies. The principal investigator in each center is responsible for the study in accordance with the protocol and for the accurate and complete reporting of the results: he or she must sign a formal statement of agreement for the study and its commitments and provide copies for the sponsor and government authorities. Investigators are selected on the basis of several criteria, including their past record in peer-reviewed medical research, their current interest in the proposed study and available time to participate. Appropriate on-site hospital or private clinic facilities with adequate space, equipment, safe drug storage, assistance from a research nurse and access to a certified laboratory are essential prerequisites for participation in clinical trials. The laboratory must be able to conduct the study according to the guidelines of good laboratory practices (GLP) adopted by the FDA in 1978. In addition, the investigators should be able to make an estimate of the number of study subjects available at their centers so a recruitment projection can be derived. The investigators must agree to have their facility and data audited at any time by the sponsor's representatives or by the regulatory authorities (FDA or TPP).

6. INFORMED CONSENT FORM AND ETHICAL ISSUES

The informed consent form is a written description of the nature and purpose of the trial. This document includes an explanation of the nature of randomization and includes a description of the benefits, foreseeable risks, discomforts and potential side effects of participating in the study. The consent form should inform the patient that he or she has the right to withdraw from the study at any time without prejudice, and that alternative treatments are available, should he or she decide not to participate in the study. The consent form is presented to the patient, preferably in the presence of an impartial witness, by the investigator or a qualified delegate; sufficient time must be allowed for the patient to consider the information and to ask questions.

This form is an acknowledgment that specific information has been given; it is never proof that the subject has been fully informed. It does not indicate the degree of comprehension or autonomy of the patient. Even if the informed consent is for the protection of the investigator and the patient, it has no legal power in North America.

7. CLINICAL MONITORING

An essential aspect of the conduct of clinical research is monitoring. All aspects of these investigations must be open and verifiable upon independent audit.

Accountability of the drug dispensed to the patients includes surveillance of the expiry date, lot numbers, stability and storage conditions. Compliance with the study medication requirements should be assessed by direct questioning and/or pill counts. All unused medication should be returned to the investigator.

The patient's condition before, during and after the treatment period, laboratory data, concomitant therapy, and adverse events should be accurately recorded using standardized procedures at specified times. Information that is recorded in the case report form should be consistent with information documented in the patient's medical record. Principles of good clinical practice (GCP) should be followed. The number and extent of audits will vary from study to study, depending upon specific requirements.

At the completion of the study, the final evaluation of data for both efficacy and safety is undertaken by an adjudication committee. This committee ensures the accuracy, completeness and legibility of the data. Finally, the results and conclusion of the study are summarized in a final report which must be reviewed and signed by the investigators. Publication of the data in a peer-reviewed medical journal follows.

8. INSTITUTIONAL REVIEW COMMITTEE (IRC)

No patient can be enrolled in a clinical trial before an institutional review committee has accepted the protocol and the informed consent form.

During this process, the scientific aspects of a trial are evaluated by experienced clinical researchers in each institution where the study is performed. Modifications to the protocol suggested by the IRC should be carefully considered by the investigators.

The committee should comprise at least five sufficiently qualified members: both sexes must be represented and members should be sensitive to local racial and cultural issues. There should be at least one nonscientific member and one member who is not affiliated with the institution. There should be no conflicting interests for any of the committee members.

The elements of the informed consent to be considered by the members of the committee are numerous. These are specifically outlined in the Declaration of Helsinki and in the *Tri-Council Policy Statement: Ethical Conduct for Research Involving Humans* (August 1998), governing research funding in Canada.

Confirmation of acceptance of a study by the IRC must be transmitted with the signed agreement form to the government authorities.

9. CONCLUSION

The efficacy and safety of a drug must be well established by appropriate therapeutic trials before it can be accepted for clinical use. Internationally accepted regulatory standards, scientific principles of clinical trial design and good clinical practice rules have evolved to meet these requirements. This chapter should provide the medical student with some basic information concerning drug development and with a better understanding of this important area of clinical research.

BIBLIOGRAPHY

Canada. Health Protection Branch, Health Canada. Drugs Directorate guidelines.
a. Clinical trial review and approval (March 1997).
b. Preparation of human new drug submissions (1991).
c. Conduct of clinical investigations. Catalogue no. H42-2/14 (July 1989).

Canada. Medical Research Council of Canada. Guidelines on research involving human subjects. Minister of Supply and Services Canada, 1987. Catalogue no. MR 21-5/1987E.

The clinical trial in Canada, USA, in Nordic and EEC countries. 2nd Symposium on drug development sponsored by the Faculty of Pharmacy of the Université de Montréal and the Health Protection Branch, Canada, May 6–7, 1990, Montréal, Québec. Montréal: Université de Montréal, 1990 (binder).

Declaration of Helsinki: Recommendations Guiding Physicians in Biomedical Research Involving Human Subjects.

France. Ministère des affaires sociales et de l'emploi. Ministre chargé de la santé et de la famille. Bulletin officiel. Direction des journaux officiels, 26, rue Desaix, 75105 Paris, France.

Good clinical practice: consolidated guideline. ICH harmonized tripartite guideline, adopted by the Therapeutic Products Directorate of Health Canada. Catalogue no. H42-2/67-11-1997E.

Good Clinical Research Practices Limited. Clinical study monitoring (binder).
Three-day course presented in Mississauga, Ontario, March 1991.
Bolaychuk WP, Ph.D.
Ball GT, C.D., Ph.D.
Kimpton DJ.
European office: Round Windows, Grayshott Road, Headly Down, Hampshire, U.K. GU 358JL.

Guidelines for research and ethical rules from FDA (U.S.A.)

Review articles. Drug Information Journal (January/June 1982):7–96.

5
The Esophagus
W.G. Paterson, S. Mayrand and C.D. Mercer

1. INTRODUCTION

The esophagus is a hollow muscular organ whose primary function is to propel into the stomach the food or fluid bolus that it receives from the pharynx. Symptoms of esophageal disease are among the most commonly encountered in gastroenterology. Fortunately, most symptoms are due to benign disease that can be easily remedied. The physician must be on the lookout, however, for the more serious disorders, which can present with a similar spectrum of symptoms. This chapter will focus on the pathophysiology, diagnosis and management of the more common esophageal disorders. Rare diseases involving the esophagus will be dealt with only briefly.

2. ANATOMY

2.1 Muscular Anatomy
The esophagus is a hollow muscular tube closed proximally by the upper esophageal sphincter (UES) and distally by the lower esophageal sphincter (LES). The UES consists predominantly of the cricopharyngeus and the caudal fibers of the inferior pharyngeal constrictor muscles. The UES forms a transverse slit at the C5–C6 vertebral level due to surrounding bony structures and cartilage. In the proximal one-quarter to one-third of the esophagus, the muscle is striated. There is then a transition zone of variable length where there is a mixture of both smooth and striated muscle. The distal one-half to one-third of the esophageal body and LES are composed of smooth muscle. The LES is located at the junction between the esophagus and stomach, usually localized at or just below the diaphragmatic hiatus. Despite its distinct physiological function, it is not easily distinguished anatomically.

2.2 Innervation

The motor innervation of the esophagus is via the vagus nerves. The cell bodies of the vagal efferent fibers innervating the UES and the proximal striated-muscle esophagus arise in the nucleus ambiguus, whereas fibers destined for the distal smooth-muscle segment and the LES originate in the dorsal motor nucleus. The esophagus and LES also receive sympathetic nerve supply (both motor and sensory) arising from spinal segments T1–T10. Sensory innervation is also carried via the vagus and consists of bipolar nerves that have their cell bodies in the nodose ganglion and project from there to the brainstem.

2.3 Blood Supply

Arterial blood supply to the UES and cervical esophagus is via branches of the inferior thyroid artery. Most of the thoracic esophagus is supplied by paired aortic esophageal arteries or terminal branches of bronchial arteries. The LES and the most distal segment of the esophagus are supplied by the left gastric artery and by a branch of the left phrenic artery. Venous drainage is via an extensive submucosal plexus that drains into the superior vena cava from the proximal esophagus and into the azygous system from the mid-esophagus. In the distal esophagus, collaterals from the left gastric vein (a branch of the portal vein) and the azygos interconnect in the submucosa. This connection between the portal and systemic venous systems is clinically important; when there is hypertension, variceal dilation can occur in this area. These submucosal esophageal varices can be the source of major gastrointestinal hemorrhage.

2.4 Lymphatic Drainage

In the proximal third of the esophagus, lymphatics drain into the deep cervical lymph nodes, whereas in the middle third, drainage is into the superior and posterior mediastinal nodes. The distal-third lymphatics follow the left gastric artery to the gastric and celiac lymph nodes. There is considerable interconnection among these three drainage regions.

2.5 Histology

The wall of the esophagus consists of mucosa, submucosa and muscularis propria. Unlike other areas of the gut, it does not have a distinct serosal covering, but is covered by a thin layer of loose connective tissue. The mucosa consists of stratified squamous epithelium in all regions of the esophagus except the LES, where both squamous and columnar epithelium may coexist. Beneath the epithelium are the lamina propria and the longitudinally oriented muscularis mucosa. The submucosa contains connective tissue as well as lymphocytes, plasma cells and nerve cells (Meissner's plexus). The muscularis propria consists of an inner circular and an outer longitudinal muscle layer. The circular muscle layer provides the sequential peristaltic contraction that propels the food bolus toward the stomach. Between the circular and longitudinal muscle layers lies another nerve plexus called the myenteric or Auerbach's plexus, which mediates much of the intrinsic nervous control of esophageal motor function.

3. PHYSIOLOGY

The major function of the esophagus is to propel swallowed food or fluid into the stomach. This is carried out by sequential or "peristaltic" contraction of the esophageal body in concert with appropriately timed relaxation of the upper and lower esophageal sphincters. The esophagus also clears any refluxed gastric contents back into the stomach and takes part in such reflex activities as vomiting and belching.

3.1 Deglutition: Primary Peristalsis
The act of deglutition is a complex reflex activity. The initial phase is under voluntary control. Food is chewed, mixed with saliva and formed into an appropriately sized bolus before being thrust to the posterior pharynx by the tongue. Once the bolus reaches the posterior pharynx, receptors are activated that initiate the involuntary phase of deglutition. This involves the carefully sequenced contraction of myriad head and neck muscles. The food bolus is rapidly engulfed and pushed toward the esophagus by the pharyngeal constrictor muscles. Simultaneously there is activation of muscles that lift the palate and close off and elevate the larynx in order to prevent misdirection of the bolus. Almost immediately upon activation of this reflex, the UES opens just long enough to allow the food bolus to pass through; it then rapidly shuts to prevent retrograde passage of the bolus. The oropharyngeal phase is thus completed and the esophageal phase takes over. This involves two major phenomena: (1) the sequential contraction of the circular muscle of the esophageal body, which results in a contractile wave that migrates toward the stomach; and (2) the relaxation and opening of the LES, which allows the bolus to pass. The peristaltic sequence and associated UES and LES relaxation induced by swallowing are termed *primary peristalsis*. These can be assessed manometrically using an intraluminal tube to measure pressures. The typical sequence seen during primary peristalsis is depicted in Figure 1. *Secondary peristalsis* refers to a peristaltic sequence that occurs in response to distention of the esophagus. This is a localized peristaltic wave that usually begins just above the area of distention. It is associated with LES relaxation, but not with UES relaxation or deglutition.

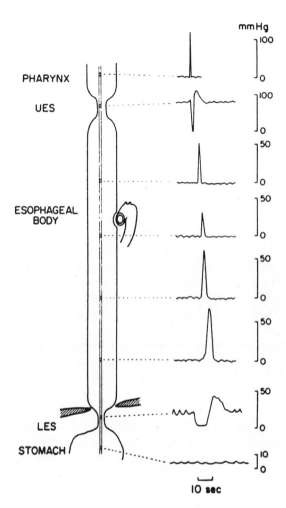

FIGURE 1.   Schematic representation of primary peristalsis as recorded by intraluminal manometry. Swallowing is marked by a rapid pharyngeal contraction coincident with abrupt relaxation of
the UES. This is followed by postrelaxation contraction of the UES and sequential contraction of
the esophageal body, which produces a pressure wave that migrates toward the stomach. A swallowed food bolus is pushed in front of this migrating contraction wave. The LES relaxes within
1 to 2 seconds of the onset of swallowing and remains relaxed until the esophageal pressure wave
has reached the distal esophagus. LES pressure then recovers and is followed by a postrelaxation
contraction, which occurs in continuity with the distal esophageal contraction.
SOURCE: Goyal RK, Paterson WG. Esophageal motility. In: Wood JD (ed.), Handbook of physiology: motility and circulation, vol. 4. Washington DC: American Physiological Society, 1989.
Used with permission.

3.2 Upper Esophageal Sphincter Function

The UES serves as a pressure barrier to prevent retrograde flow of esophageal contents and the entry of air into the esophagus during inspiration. This high-pressure zone is created by tonic contraction of the UES muscles, which is produced by tonic neuronal discharge of vagal lower motor neurons. With deglutition this neuronal discharge ceases temporarily and permits relaxation of the UES. UES opening will not occur with relaxation of the muscles alone; it requires elevation and anterior displacement of the larynx, which is mediated by contraction of the suprahyoid muscles. Relaxation lasts for only one second and is followed by a postrelaxation contraction (Figure 1).

3.3 Esophageal Body Peristalsis

There is a fundamental difference in the control mechanisms of peristalsis between the upper (striated-muscle) esophagus and the lower (smooth-muscle) esophagus. In the striated-muscle segment, peristalsis is produced by sequential firing of vagal lower motor neurons so that upper segments contract first and more aboral segments subsequently. In the smooth-muscle segment, the vagal preganglionic efferent fibers have some role in the aboral sequencing of contraction, but intrinsic neurons are also capable of evoking peristalsis independently of the extrinsic nervous system. Transection of vagal motor fibers to the esophagus in experimental animals will abolish primary peristalsis throughout the esophagus; however, in this setting, distention-induced or secondary peristalsis will be maintained in the smooth-muscle but not in the striated-muscle segment. Furthermore, if vagal efferent fibers are stimulated electrically (Figure 2), a simultaneous contraction will be produced in the striated-muscle esophagus that begins with the onset of the electrical stimulus, lasts throughout the stimulus, and ends abruptly when the stimulus is terminated. In the smooth-muscle esophagus, however, the response to vagal efferent nerve stimulation is quite different, in that onset of contractions is delayed relative to the onset of the stimulus. The latency to onset of the contraction increases in the more distal segments of the esophagus (i.e., the evoked contractions are peristaltic).

This experimental observation indicates that intrinsic neuromuscular mechanisms exist and can mediate peristalsis on their own. Further evidence for this mechanism is found in studies where strips of esophageal circular smooth muscle are stimulated electrically in vitro. The latency to contraction after stimulation is shortest in the strips taken from the proximal smooth-muscle segment and increases progressively in the more distal strips.

This latency gradient of contraction is clearly important in the production of esophageal peristalsis. Although the exact mechanisms are unclear, initial or deglutitive inhibition is important. With primary or secondary peristalsis, a

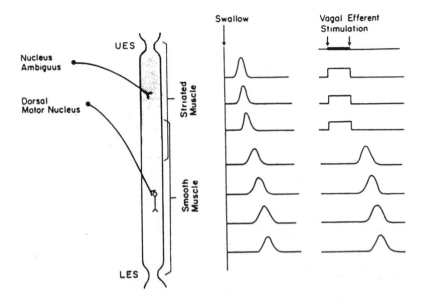

FIGURE 2. Schematic representation of esophageal peristaltic contractions as evoked by swallowing and vagal efferent nerve stimulation. Swallowing evokes sequential esophageal contractions that pass smoothly from the striated- to the smooth-muscle segment. Electrical stimulation of the distal cut end of a vagus nerve, which simultaneously activates all vagal efferent fibers, evokes peristaltic contractions only in the smooth-muscle segment of the esophagus. In the striated-muscle esophagus, vagal stimulation causes simultaneous contractions that occur only during the period of stimulation. This demonstrates that the striated-muscle esophagus is dependent on central neuronal sequencing for its peristaltic contraction, whereas intrinsic neuronal mechanisms are capable of producing a persistaltic sequence in the smooth-muscle segment. SOURCE: Goyal RK, Paterson WG. Esophageal motility. In: Wood JD (ed.), Handbook of physiology: motility and circulation, vol. 4. Washington DC: American Physiological Society, 1989. Used with permission.

wave of neurally mediated inhibition initially spreads rapidly down the esophagus. This is caused by the release of the inhibitory neurotransmitter nitric oxide, which produces hyperpolarization (inhibition) of the circular smooth muscle. It is only after recovery from the initial hyperpolarization that esophageal muscle contraction (which is mediated primarily by cholinergic neurons) can occur. Thus, the duration of this initial inhibition is important with respect to the differential timing of the subsequent contraction. Derangements of the mechanisms behind this latency gradient lead to nonperistaltic contractions and dysphagia. Such derangements could result from problems with either the intrinsic neural mechanisms (enteric nervous system) or the central neuronal sequencing.

3.4 Lower Esophageal Sphincter Function

The LES is an intraluminal high-pressure zone caused by tonic contraction of a region of physiologically distinct circular smooth muscle at the junction of the esophagus and stomach. This results in a pressure barrier that separates the esophagus from the stomach and serves to prevent reflux of gastric contents up into the esophagus. In normal individuals, resting LES pressure averages between 10 and 30 mm Hg above intragastric pressure. Patients with very feeble resting LES pressure are prone to develop gastroesophageal reflux disease (GERD). Unlike that of the UES, the resting tone of the LES is primarily due to myogenic factors that result in tonic contraction of the sphincter. Extrinsic innervation as well as circulating hormones can modify the resting tone; however, the muscle fibers themselves have inherent properties that result in their being tonically contracted.

At the time of deglutition or when the esophagus is distended, the LES promptly relaxes. Swallow-induced LES relaxation is mediated by vagal efferent fibers that synapse on inhibitory neurons of the myenteric plexus. The inhibitory neurotransmitter released from these intrinsic neurons is nitric oxide. LES relaxation usually lasts about five to seven seconds, and is sufficient to abolish the gastroesophageal pressure barrier. This permits the food bolus to pass unimpeded from the esophagus to the stomach. The LES also relaxes to permit belching or vomiting. Inadequate LES relaxation is seen in achalasia and results in dysphagia.

4. SYMPTOMS AND SIGNS OF ESOPHAGEAL DISEASES

4.1 Symptoms

4.1.1 *DYSPHAGIA*

This sensation of food sticking during swallowing is a manifestation of impaired transit of food through the mouth, pharynx or esophagus. It is important to differentiate oropharyngeal ("transfer") dysphagia from esophageal dysphagia. If the patient has problems getting the bolus out of the mouth, then one can be certain of an oropharyngeal cause; if the food sticks retrosternally, an esophageal cause is indicated. Some patients, however, will sense food sticking at the level of the suprasternal notch when the actual obstruction is the distal esophagus. Thus, it can be difficult to determine the site of the problem when patients refer their dysphagia to the suprasternal notch or throat area. With these patients it is important to elicit any ancillary symptoms of oropharyngeal-type dysphagia, such as choking or nasal regurgitation. It may also be helpful to observe the patient swallowing in an attempt to determine the timing of the symptom; with esophageal dysphagia referred to the suprasternal notch, the sensation of dysphagia onsets several seconds after swallowing begins.

The history can also be used to help differentiate structural from functional (i.e., motility disorders) causes of dysphagia. Dysphagia that is episodic and occurs with both liquids and solids from the outset suggests a motor disorder, whereas when the dysphagia is initially for solids such as meat and bread, and then progresses with time to semisolids and liquids, one should suspect a structural cause (e.g., stricture). If such a progression is rapid and associated with significant weight loss, a malignant stricture is suspected.

Associated symptoms help determine the etiology of dysphagia. For instance, a reflux-induced stricture should be suspected if the dysphagia is associated with heartburn or regurgitation, esophageal cancer if there is associated mid-back pain and weight loss, a motor disorder such as diffuse esophageal spasm if there is angina-like chest pain, and a "scleroderma esophagus" if there is arthralgia, skin changes or Raynaud's phenomenon.

4.1.2 ODYNOPHAGIA

This refers to the sensation of pain on swallowing. Local inflammation or neoplasia in the mouth and pharynx can produce such pain. When the pain is retrosternal, one should suspect nonreflux-induced forms of esophagitis, such as infection, radiation or pill-induced (chemical) injury. Less commonly it occurs with esophageal cancer, a deep esophageal ulcer (e.g., Barrett's ulcer) or esophageal motor disorders.

4.1.3 HEARTBURN OR PYROSIS

The sensation here is one of retrosternal burning. Typically it begins in the low retrosternal area and radiates up to the throat. It may be precipitated by bending over or lying down, and usually begins shortly after consuming certain foods or beverages. It is often associated with regurgitation of acidic material into the back of the throat. "Heartburn" with these features indicates gastroesophageal reflux. This very common symptom has been experienced at one time or another by over one-third of the population and therefore does not necessarily indicate serious disease. Many patients will complain of "heartburn," but this should not be taken at face value: this term is used by some patients to describe unrelated symptomatology. It is therefore important to have patients describe exactly what they mean by the term *heartburn*.

4.1.4 REGURGITATION

This refers to the spontaneous appearance of food or fluid in the back of the throat or in the mouth. Some patients describe this symptom as "vomiting"; therefore it is important to determine whether there is associated nausea, retching, etc., when patients present with "vomiting." The taste and consistency of the regurgitated material is an important historical detail. Regurgitation of acidic or bile-stained fluid indicates gastroesophageal reflux. Regurgitation of undigested food or stagnant fluid devoid of an acidic taste indicates an esophageal transport problem (e.g., achalasia). (With achlorhydria, gastric contents also lack acid.) In motor disorders and mechanical obstruction of the esophagus, food may become stuck and then rather quickly will be regurgitated if it does not pass through into the stomach. Some patients regurgitate food back into their mouths after a meal only to chew and swallow it all over again. This is called *rumination* and, although a rarity in humans, it is a normal physiological event in certain animals.

4.1.5 NONHEARTBURN CHEST PAIN

This is also an indication of esophageal disease. Chest pain, and in particular mid-dorsal pain, is seen in advanced esophageal cancer. The most common type of nonheartburn esophageal chest pain, however, is a pain that is qualitatively similar to the pain of ischemic heart disease. This pain can be squeezing or crushing and can radiate into the jaw or arms. Unlike ischemic heart pain, angina-like chest pain of esophageal origin is not predictably elicited by exertion and often occurs spontaneously, in relationship to meals or in the middle of the night. It is associated with other esophageal symptoms. Clearly, patients with this type of pain need to have ischemic heart disease excluded. Once this is done, many will be found to have some form of esophageal motor disorder. In addition, this angina-like pain can be precipitated by gastroesophageal reflux.

4.1.6 WATERBRASH

This sudden appearance of copious amounts of saliva in the mouth must be differentiated from regurgitation of fluid. With waterbrash, acid reflux into the esophagus stimulates hypersalivation via a (cholinergic) neural reflex.

4.1.7 BLEEDING

This may be a symptom of certain esophageal diseases. Mucosal laceration in the region of the gastroesophageal junction (*Mallory-Weiss tear*), as a consequence of retching or vomiting, is a common cause of upper gastrointestinal tract bleeding. Esophageal varices can cause massive hematemesis and melena. Deep esophageal ulcers may also bleed massively, but this is uncommon.

Usually the bleeding from ulcerative lesions of the esophagus or esophageal cancer is occult. When the patient does present with hematemesis or melena from esophagitis, the rate of bleeding is usually slow; therefore, significant hemodynamic compromise is uncommon.

4.1.8 *RESPIRATORY/LARYNGEAL SYMPTOMS*
These may be a manifestation of esophageal disease or oropharyngeal swallowing disorders. Aspiration at the time of swallowing will cause coughing, choking and eventual hoarseness. In addition, patients with motor disorders or gastroesophageal reflux disease (GERD) may regurgitate esophageal or gastric contents up into the larynx and subsequently aspirate. These patients may present with pneumonia, chronic cough, wheezing, hoarseness or laryngitis. Gastroesophageal reflux may also trigger coughing and wheezing via a vaso-vagal reflex.

4.2 Signs
It is uncommon for esophageal disease to be associated with specific physical findings. Signs of weight loss and malnutrition can be found if the esophageal problem is so severe that adequate caloric intake is not maintained. There may be signs of metastatic disease (e.g., hepatomegaly, supraclavicular lymphadenopathy) in esophageal cancer. Patients with GERD rarely have respiratory tract signs such as wheezing, hoarseness or lung consolidation. It is important to look for signs of connective tissue disease (especially scleroderma) in patients with reflux symptoms or dysphagia.

The physical examination is more often helpful in patients with oropharyngeal dysphagia. Careful examination of the head and neck for structural and neurologic abnormalities is mandatory. It is also important to look for more generalized neurologic or connective tissue abnormalities. Observing the patient swallow is also useful when oropharyngeal dysphagia is present.

5. INVESTIGATIONS USED IN THE DIAGNOSIS OF ESOPHAGEAL DISEASE

5.1 Barium X-ray
This most commonly used method of investigating the esophagus evaluates both structural lesions and motor disorders. It is the single most important test in evaluating patients with dysphagia. Proper communication between physician and radiologist is vital. Videotaping the barium swallow allows for playback and slow-motion review. This is very helpful in assessing the rapid events of the oropharyngeal phase of swallowing. Use of marshmallows, barium-coated cookies and different consistencies of barium further assesses swal-

lowing disorders, as delays in transport may not be apparent with simple liquid barium. The disadvantage of barium x-rays is that they are relatively insensitive in detecting mucosal disease, even if air contrast technique is added.

5.2 Endoscopy with Mucosal Biopsy and Brush Cytology

Fiberoptic endoscopy directly visualizes the esophageal mucosa as well as other areas of the upper gastrointestinal tract. Its direct view is superior to barium x-rays for assessing mucosal disease of the esophagus, and the esophagoscope permits assessment of structural lesions that are identified. Furthermore, pinch biopsies and/or brush cytology of specific lesions are easily obtained through the endoscope. Microscopic evidence of esophagitis may be found even when the mucosa looks grossly normal. Endoscopy is the single most useful test in the evaluation of patients with reflux symptoms, as it permits one to establish the presence or absence of esophagitis or Barrett's esophagus (Section 7.3). Endoscopy gives little reliable information regarding esophageal function.

5.3 Bernstein (Acid Perfusion) Test

This tests the sensitivity of the patient's esophagus to acid perfusion. A tube is placed into the distal esophagus and saline, acid and then antacid are infused sequentially, with the patient kept unaware as to what is being administered. The patient is questioned periodically about the presence or absence of symptoms and their quality. This test may be useful in determining whether a patient's atypical chest or epigastric pain is secondary to acid reflux. The test is positive if the patient's presenting pain is reproduced during acid perfusion and relieved by antacid perfusion.

5.4 Esophageal Manometry

This involves recording intraluminal pressures at multiple sites along the esophagus (Figure 1). The most commonly used method involves a perfused multilumen catheter bundle with side holes at 5 cm intervals. Each catheter is connected to a pressure transducer, which in turn is attached to a physiograph. LES pressure and swallow-induced LES relaxation are measured, as are pressure responses to swallowing at several esophageal sites. Pharyngeal peristalsis and UES function can also be measured. Esophageal manometry is the "gold standard" in the assessment of esophageal motor disorders. Motor dysfunction, however, may be intermittent and therefore not detected at the time of the study. Manometry is now commonly combined with provocative tests (acid perfusion, balloon distention and/or pharmacological stimulation of the esophagus with bethanechol or edrophonium) in an attempt to evoke abnormal contractions and reproduce the patient's chest pain (Section 11).

Esophageal pH

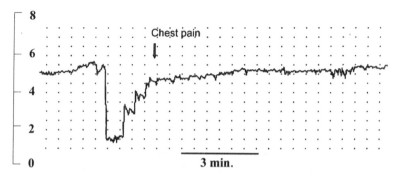

Figure 3.   Extract from an intraesophageal 24-hour pH study in a patient with unexplained chest pain. Note that intraluminal pH abruptly drops, indicating a gastroesophageal acid reflux event. This is followed shortly thereafter by the patient's recording chest pain.

5.5 Ambulatory Esophageal pH Monitoring

This is performed using a pH electrode passed via the nose into the distal esophagus, which continuously records intraluminal pH over a 24-hour period. Acid reflux events can be identified by an abrupt drop in pH to < 4. The results of this test are compared to a healthy control population to determine whether an abnormal degree of gastroesophageal reflux is present. The test is most useful, however, in determining whether atypical symptoms coincide with acid reflux events (Figure 3), and in objectively assessing the response to therapy in patients with refractory symptoms.

5.6 Radionuclide Studies

These assess either gastroesophageal reflux or esophageal transit. In the latter instance, food or fluid labeled with a radioisotope is swallowed and gamma camera scanning is performed over the chest. Computer programs measure transit time in the upper, middle and lower thirds of the esophagus. This has been reported to be a sensitive way of detecting motor dysfunction in patients with dysphagia. It may therefore be a useful screening test, but fails to give reliable information concerning the type of motor disorder present. Gastroesophageal reflux can be quantitated by having the patient ingest the radioisotope and then scanning over the chest and upper abdomen. Binders are placed over the abdomen to increase intra-abdominal pressure; reflux is present if the isotope is seen to travel back up into the esophagus. The role of this test in the assessment of patients with reflux disease remains to be defined, as its sensitivity and specificity are rather poor.

6. ANATOMIC VARIANTS

6.1 Congenital Anomalies

Embryologically the gastrointestinal and respiratory tracts start out as a single tube; however, by the second month of gestation they have completely divided. Problems with this process lead to various congenital anomalies, the most common being tracheoesophageal fistula with esophageal atresia. In 85–90% of cases, the proximal esophagus ends in a blind pouch while the distal esophagus consists of a blind pouch in continuity with the stomach. Neonates with this abnormality develop immediate aspiration with feeding. There is no air in the bowel on x-ray films of the abdomen, contrary to what is observed in those with fistulas involving the distal esophagus. In 1–2% of cases there is an "H-type" fistula with atresia. The patient presents with repeated pulmonary infections and abdominal distention. The latter is caused by air getting into the gastrointestinal tract via the fistula when the infant cries. Because the H-type fistula may be very small, the condition may go unnoticed until adulthood, when it is detected during the investigation of recurrent pulmonary infections. Some of these fistulas may close spontaneously but produce paraesophageal inflammation and ultimately localized esophageal stricture formation.

Treatment of esophageal fistulas (with or without atresia) is surgical. The prognosis is now quite good and mortality is usually related to coexistent congenital malformations. It is important to remember that many of these patients will have gastroesophageal reflux as well as abnormal esophageal peristalsis following surgery, which may cause significant long-term problems.

Congenital esophageal stenosis is a rare anomaly that is also probably related to abnormal differentiation of the gastrointestinal and respiratory tracts, as resected specimens have been found to have pulmonary epithelium and/or bronchial remnants. Sequestered pulmonary remnants with connections to the esophagus but not associated with stenosis have also been described.

6.2 Hiatus Hernia

The majority of hiatus hernias are acquired. Rarely, a hiatus hernia can be caused by a congenitally short esophagus. Hiatus hernias can be divided into two types: (1) sliding and (2) paraesophageal (Figures 4 and 5, respectively). A *sliding hiatus hernia* refers to the condition where a circumferential cuff of cardia and proximal stomach migrates up through the diaphragmatic hiatus and into the thorax. This may reduce and reform spontaneously. These hernias are very common and increase in incidence with advancing age. Generally they are of no clinical significance, despite the fact that many patients and physicians persist in attributing a wide variety of symptoms to them. Large hiatus hernias may be associated with iron deficiency anemia that is presum-

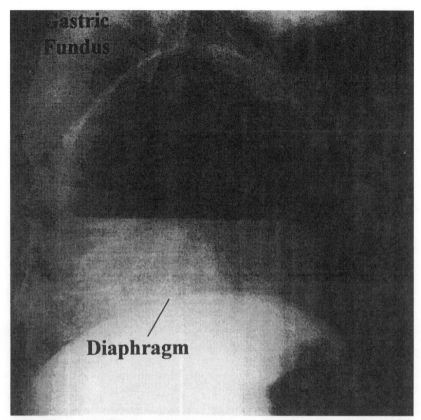

FIGURE 4.   Lateral chest x-ray of a large, sliding-type hiatus hernia. The gastric fundus is seen in the chest, well above the diaphragm. Note the air-fluid level within the herniated stomach.

ably caused by recurrent superficial ulcerations at the site where the diaphragm exerts pressure on the herniated stomach. If no other source of GI blood loss is discovered after thorough investigation, and patients continue to be iron-deficient despite supplementation and antiulcer treatment, surgical correction of the hernia should be performed.

The etiology of the sliding hiatus hernia is obscure. Certainly there is laxity and dilation of the diaphragmatic hiatus and associated laxity of the phrenoesophageal ligament; however, these may well be secondary and not primary pathophysiologic factors. In some cases, persistent gastroesophageal reflux may result in inflammation and consequent esophageal shortening, which in turn leads to the development of a hiatus hernia.

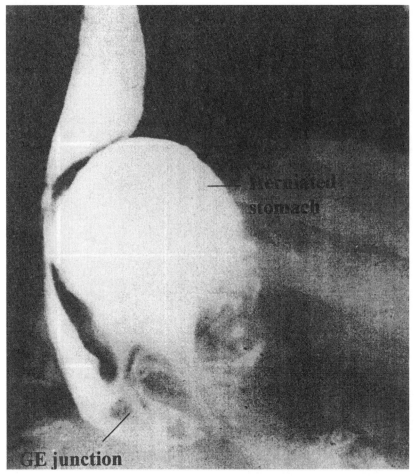

FIGURE 5. Barium contrast study of a paraesophageal-type hiatus hernia. Note that the gastro-esophageal (GE) junction has maintained its normal position at the hiatus, but a large portion of the gastric fundus has migrated up through the hiatus alongside the distal esophagus. The herni-ated portion of the stomach is compressing the distal esophagus.

A sliding hiatus hernia is often seen in association with GERD; the precise role of the hernia in the pathogenesis of the reflux remains uncertain. Certainly the majority of people with hiatus hernias do not have significant reflux disease, and occasionally patients with severe reflux esophagitis will not have a hiatus hernia. It appears that a hiatus hernia may contribute somewhat to gas-troesophageal reflux, but it is most unlikely that this is the prime etiologic factor. A hiatus hernia may contribute to GERD by providing a reservoir of gastric acid that has ready access to the distal esophagus whenever the LES relaxes.

Paraesophageal hiatus hernias are uncommon. These consist of the fundus of the stomach migrating through the hiatus alongside the esophagus without any displacement of the gastroesophageal junction. Although these hernias may be asymptomatic, most surgeons believe that they should be treated surgically when the diagnosis is made because the herniated portion may become strangulated and infarcted. They may also cause dysphagea by compressing the distal esophagus (Figure 5). The treatment consists of reduction of the herniated stomach into the abdomen, elimination of the hernia sac and closure of the herniated defect by reapproximating the crura.

7. GASTROESOPHAGEAL REFLUX DISEASE (GERD)

GERD is the most common condition to affect the esophagus. The disease spectrum ranges from patients with heartburn and other reflux symptoms without morphologic evidence of esophagitis (the so-called acid-sensitive esophagus) to patients with deep ulcer, stricture or Barrett's epithelium. Everyone has some degree of gastroesophageal reflux; it becomes pathological only when associated with troublesome symptoms or complications. Fortunately, the vast majority of patients suffering from GERD have an easily controlled disorder. At the other end of the spectrum, there are patients who develop severe damage to the esophagus. Some will develop Barrett's metaplasia as a consequence of gastroesophageal reflux, which in turn predisposes them to adenocarcinoma.

7.1 Pathophysiology

GERD results from the reflux of gastric contents into the esophageal lumen. Early pathogenesis concepts focused on anatomic factors: reflux was considered a mechanical problem, related to the development of a hiatus hernia. We now know, however, that a hiatus hernia can occur without GERD, and conversely, GERD can occur without a hiatus hernia. Many factors are involved in the pathogenesis of GERD.

7.1.1 BARRIERS TO GASTROESOPHAGEAL REFLUX

By far the most important barrier to gastroesophageal reflux is the LES. Factors such as the intra-abdominal location of the sphincter, extrinsic compression exerted by the diaphragmatic crura and the angle of His (which forms a "mucosal flap valve") may augment this barrier but play a minor role relative to the LES itself. Some patients developing reflux esophagitis have feeble LES tone, but in most, resting LES pressure is nearly normal.

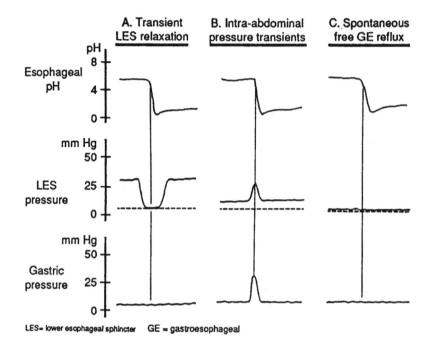

LES= lower esophageal sphincter   GE = gastroesophageal

FIGURE 6.   Schematic representation of three different mechanisms of gastroesophageal (GE) reflux.

A. Transient LES relaxation refers to the sudden occurrence of LES relaxation that causes obliteration of the gastroesophageal pressure barrier and permits gastric contents to reflux up into the esophagus. The reflux event is marked by the sudden drop in esophageal pH. These transient LES relaxations are sometimes related to incomplete or failed peristalsis but may also occur in isolation.

B. Intra-abdominal pressure transients are sudden increases in intragastric pressure caused by coughing, sneezing or deep inspiration. The increased intragastric pressure overcomes the LES pressure and results in reflux.

C. Spontaneous free reflux occurs when there is very low or nonexistent LES pressure, which permits spontaneous reflux across the gastroesophageal junction. In healthy volunteers without GERD, virtually all reflux episodes are due to transient LES relaxation. In patients with reflux esophagitis, approximately two-thirds of the reflux episodes are due to transient LES relaxation. The remaining one-third are caused by either intra-abdominal pressure transients or spontaneous free gastroesophageal reflux.

SOURCE: Dodds WJ, Dent J, Hogan WJ, et al. Mechanisms of gastroesophageal reflux in patients with reflux esophagitis. N Engl J M 1982; 307:1547–1552. Used with permission.

Gastroesophageal reflux occurs by three major mechanisms, as outlined in Figure 6.

7.1.2 ESOPHAGEAL CLEARANCE

Once reflux occurs, the duration of insult to the esophageal mucosa depends on the rapidity with which the esophagus clears this material. Once the initial (primary) peristaltic wave has passed, the bolus (a portion of which frequently remains) is cleared by one or two secondary peristaltic waves. The remaining small adherent acidic residue is then neutralized by saliva, which is carried down by successive swallows. Disorders of salivation or esophageal motor function will impair this clearance mechanism and predispose to the development of GERD.

Patients with severe GERD may have frequent prolonged nighttime reflux episodes because during sleep, peristalsis seldom occurs and salivary flow virtually ceases. Hence the contact time of refluxed material with the esophagus is markedly increased.

7.1.3 GASTRODUODENAL FACTORS

In some patients delayed gastric emptying further predisposes to the development of GERD. Bile salts and pancreatic enzymes, if refluxed back into the stomach, can in turn reflux into the esophagus and may inflict worse damage than when gastric juice is refluxed alone. Such reflux into the stomach and then the esophagus may occur after gastric surgery, when the pylorus is destroyed. Whenever there is increased gastric pressure or an increase in gastric contents, there is greater likelihood that reflux will occur when the sphincter barrier becomes deficient.

7.1.4 MUCOSAL RESISTANCE

The degree of damage to esophageal mucosa depends not only on the composition of the refluxed material and the amount and duration of reflux, but also on defensive factors within the mucosa itself. These include protective secretions from esophageal glands, the integrity of tight junctions between adjacent epithelial cells and esophageal blood flow. Certain patients are more susceptible to the development of actual mucosal damage, for reasons that are not clear.

7.2 Clinical Features

Most patients present with heartburn and acid regurgitation that onset after eating certain foods or following various postural maneuvers (e.g., bending over, lying flat). Frequency varies from once a week or less to daily episodes

TABLE 1. Diagnostic tests in GERD

Tests to determine the presence of reflux
Ambulatory 24-hour pH recording
Barium meal
Radionuclide scintigraphy

Tests to determine whether symptoms are due to reflux
24-hour pH recording
Bernstein (acid perfusion) test

Tests to determine the presence of mucosal damage
Endoscopy
Mucosal biopsy
Barium meal

---

with disruption of sleep. Other presenting symptoms include waterbrash, angina-like chest pain, dysphagia and various respiratory symptoms (hoarseness, cough, wheezing). The dysphagia may be due to the development of a reflux-induced stricture or to abnormal motility induced by the refluxed acid. Odynophagia is rarely a symptom of GERD and should alert the physician to another diagnosis such as infectious esophagitis.

Reflux symptoms are common during pregnancy because of increased intra-abdominal pressures and the LES-relaxant effect of progesterone.

Physical examination in patients with GERD rarely reveals associated physical signs. In severe cases with stricture formation there may be weight loss secondary to decreased caloric intake, or findings of consolidation, bronchospasm or fibrosis on respiratory examination in patients who have GE reflux with aspiration.

7.3 Diagnosis

In the vast majority of patients, GERD can be diagnosed from the history alone and treated without further investigation. Several tests are useful in the assessment of suspected GERD, depending on the information sought: Is there an abnormal degree of reflux? Are symptoms in fact due to reflux? Is there mucosal damage or other complications (Table 1)? Some specialists believe that all patients with symptomatic gastroesophageal reflux should undergo endoscopy. The argument in favor of this approach is that Barrett's esophagus will be found in about 10% of these patients. This identifies those at increased risk for the development of adenocarcinoma (Section 7.5.2). Most physicians, however, feel that in young patients with typical symptoms that are infrequent and relatively mild, empiric therapy should be instituted first

TABLE 2.   Medical therapy of gastroesophageal reflux disease: a pathophysiologic approach

---

Decrease frequency of reflux episodes
Improve LES function (prokinetic drugs; avoid certain drugs and foods, especially alcohol
    and cigarettes)
Elevate head of bed 4–6 inches on blocks
Weight loss

Augment clearing mechanisms; decrease duration of reflux episodes
Prokinetic agents (cisapride, domperidone, metoclopramide)
Agents that stimulate salivation
Gravity (elevate head of bed, avoid bending over)

Decrease irritant quality and volume of gastric juice
Antacids, alginic acid
H_2-receptor antagonists (cimetidine, ranitidine, famotidine, nizatidine)
M_1 antagonists (pirenzepine)
Proton pump inhibitors (omeprazole, lansoprazole, pantoprazole)
Prokinetic agents (cisapride, domperidone, metoclopramide)

Augment esophageal mucosal defenses
? Sucralfate

---

without further investigation. In patients with frequent or more severe symptoms but without symptoms that suggest complications, endoscopy is necessary to rule out other diseases and to document the presence or absence of
mucosal damage or Barrett's metaplasia. Endoscopic biopsy may also detect
microscopic evidence of esophagitis (hyperplasia of the basal zone layer,
elongation of the papillae and inflammatory cell infiltration) when the
esophageal mucosa appears macroscopically normal.

   Many patients will have normal endoscopy and biopsy even though significant GERD is present. In these patients treatment for GERD should be instituted if symptoms are typical. In patients with atypical or multiple symptoms,
a 24-hour pH reflux study may be necessary to establish that the symptom(s)
are in fact due to acid reflux (Figure 3). It is important to first rule out
ischemic heart disease if the presenting symptom is angina-like chest pain.

   All patients who present with symptoms of complicated GERD (i.e., dysphagia, bleeding or respiratory symptoms) need to be fully investigated. If
dysphagia is present, an upper GI endoscopy, with or without initial barium x-
ray study, should be performed. Further investigations will depend on the
results of the initial tests. Esophageal manometry has little role to play in the
routine assessment of patients with GERD. It is useful in the assessment of
patients with atypical symptoms, and can be combined with an acid perfusion

TABLE 3.   Agents known to decrease LES tone

Theophylline
Caffeine
Fatty meal
Chocolate
Peppermint
Smoking
Ethanol
Calcium channel blockers
Morphine
Meperidine
Benzodiazepines
β-adrenergic agonists
Nitrates
Anticholinergics (including tricyclic antidepressants)

(Bernstein) test as well as with other provocative tests. It is important to perform manometry prior to surgical intervention, because patients with significant underlying primary motor disorders of the esophagus (e.g., scleroderma) often develop severe dysphagia following an antireflux procedure.

7.4 Treatment

7.4.1 MEDICAL TREATMENT
The treatment of GERD is directed toward the abnormal pathophysiology (Table 2). In patients with mild or infrequent symptoms, lifestyle modifications, dietary advice, elevation of the head of the bed and p.r.n. antacids are usually all that is required. If possible, the patient should avoid ingestion of various agents that may inhibit LES tone and promote reflux (Table 3). In patients with more severe symptoms or who do not respond to these simple measures, addition of an H_2-receptor antagonist is indicated. Prokinetic agents such as cisapride may also be used alone or in combination with other agents in the treatment of GERD, but are probably best suited to the subgroup of patients who have gastroparesis or coexistent functional, nonulcer dyspepsia (gas-bloat syndrome). Proton pump inhibitors represent the most efficacious therapy currently available for GERD. They should be used in patients with complicated GERD (e.g., frank erosive esophagitis, peptic stricture or Barrett's ulcer) or in patients who have not responded to H_2-receptor antagonists. It is also reasonable to use these agents as initial therapy in all patients.

GERD is a chronic relapsing condition that usually requires long-term treatment. As a general rule the physician should use the simplest, least expensive and least potent therapeutic regime that will keep the patient's symptoms in check.

7.4.2 SURGICAL TREATMENT

Antireflux surgery should be considered in patients with GERD whose symptoms are not controlled with the aforementioned medical regimen and in younger patients who would prefer to avoid long-term pharmacological therapy. Several different operative techniques are used for this condition. The most popular are the Nissen fundoplication, the Belsey Mark IV repair and the Hill posterior gastropexy. Currently, most surgeons are doing antireflux surgery via a laparoscopic approach, which results in the patient returning to full activity much sooner. All procedures, whether performed laparoscopically or open, adhere to the same basic principles: restoration of the LES to an intra-abdominal position, extrinsic bolstering of the LES pressure and repair of the patulous hiatus.

The results of antireflux surgery depend more on the expertise and experience of the surgeon than on the specific operative procedure. In expert hands, surgery will produce a good-to-excellent result in 85–95% of patients; however, in up to 50% of these patients, objective evidence of recurrent pathological reflux will be present five years after surgery, even though symptomatic benefit is maintained. Overall operative mortality for first-time operations is ≤ 0.5%. Between 10 and 20% of patients develop significant problems with dysphagia and/or gas-bloat symptoms after surgery. Inability to belch or vomit may also occur. In most cases these problems resolve with time. Laparoscopic surgical results are similar to those achieved with open surgery. Advanced laparoscopic surgical skills are required by surgeons performing this type of surgery.

7.5 Complicated GERD

7.5.1 PEPTIC STRICTURE

Chronic GERD may lead to peptic stricture formation (Figure 7). This is a fibrous stricture related to collagen deposition that occurs in the course of repair of esophagitis. Patients are usually asymptomatic until the luminal narrowing has reached 12–14 mm. At this point dysphagia to solids occurs. As the stricture progresses, the dysphagia gradually progresses to semisolids and then liquids. Treatment of peptic strictures involves peroral dilation, using either mercury-filled rubber bougies, rigid dilators passed over guidewires, or balloons passed through endoscopes. In close to 50% of patients one or two dilation sessions prove adequate, and no further dilations are required because ongoing medical treatment of the reflux is successful. In others, the stricture recurs and periodic dilations are required to maintain luminal patency. In patients who are otherwise healthy, consideration should be given to antireflux surgery if frequent dilations are required to maintain luminal patency. The success rate of antireflux surgery is lower in such patients with peptic

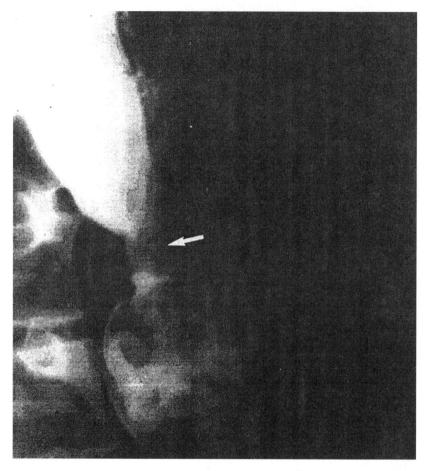

Figure 7.   Barium swallow radiograph in a patient with a tight peptic stricture (arrow). (Radiograph courtesy of Dr. M. Jabbari.)

stricture. Strictures are less likely to recur following dilation if the patient is treated with a proton pump inhibitor. For this reason, long-term treatment with a proton pump inhibitor seems appropriate for patients with peptic stricture.

7.5.2 BARRETT'S ESOPHAGUS

In this condition the squamous epithelium of the distal esophagus is replaced by metaplastic columnar epithelium. Deep ulcers as well as strictures at the new squamocolumnar junction may also develop. Severe hemorrhage may complicate the deep ulcers. This condition occurs in approximately 10% of patients with chronic GERD, although recent prospective studies in which careful biopsies were performed from the region of the gastroesophageal junction suggest that the incidence is actually higher.

Barrett's epithelium is a premalignant condition. At the time of initial presentation, up to 10% of patients found to have Barrett's esophagus will have coexistent adenocarcinoma arising in the Barrett's epithelium. This number gives an exaggerated impression of the magnitude of risk, because Barrett's esophagus patients with cancer are more likely to seek medical attention. The true incidence of adenocarcinoma developing in Barrett's epithelium is only about 1 case for every 200 patient-years of follow-up. This nevertheless represents about a 30- to 40-fold increase over the risk faced by the general population. For this reason patients with Barrett's esophagus should be followed periodically with endoscopy and mucosal biopsy in order to detect early cancer. Most patients will develop severe dysplasia before frank invasive carcinoma occurs. Thus, if patients are found to have severe dysplasia or early mucosal carcinoma, esophageal resection should be considered in order to prevent the development of invasive carcinoma. Recently, photodynamic therapy has been introduced as a less invasive alternative to surgery in patients with severe dysplasia or intramucosal carcinoma complicating Barrett's esophagus. Its exact role remains to be defined. Although there have been case reports of Barrett's esophagus regressing after successful antireflux surgery, it is unlikely that such surgery decreases the risk of cancer in the majority of patients. For this reason, Barrett's esophagus per se should not be an indication for antireflux surgery. Surgery should be performed if the patient has symptoms or complications not readily managed by medical therapy, or in patients unable or unwilling to take lifelong medications.

7.5.3 RESPIRATORY COMPLICATIONS

In some patients the refluxed gastric contents may get past the UES and into the larynx and lungs. This produces recurrent chest infections, chronic cough and laryngitis. In addition, gastroesophageal reflux may trigger bronchospasm or cough via a neural reflex. GERD with aspiration is more commonly seen in the pediatric age group; when present, antireflux surgery should be performed unless there is a well-documented response to medical therapy.

8. NONREFLUX-INDUCED ESOPHAGITIS

8.1 Infectious Esophagitis

Bacteria rarely cause primary esophageal infection, although the esophagus can be involved secondarily by direct extension from the lung. The two most common forms of infectious esophagitis are caused by Candida and herpes viruses. Other viruses (e.g., CMV, HIV) and fungi can also cause esophagitis;

however, this is uncommon and almost invariably associated with immuno-suppression.

8.1.1 *CANDIDA ESOPHAGITIS*

This is by far the most common form of infectious esophagitis. Usually there is a predisposing cause, such as diabetes mellitus, recent antibiotic therapy or some form of immunocompromise. The patient may be asymptomatic. Not all patients will have associated oral thrush. More commonly, however, patients present with odynophagia, retrosternal chest pain and/or dysphagia. Severe cases can be complicated by bleeding, a stricture and sinus tract formation with secondary lung abscess. Barium x-rays reveal an irregular granular or even cobblestone appearance to the esophageal mucosa. Approximately 25% of patients will have a normal barium esophagogram; for this reason, endoscopy with biopsy and brushing are required to make the diagnosis. The typical endoscopic appearance is the presence of small raised whitish plaques. When the plaques are removed the underlying mucosa is seen to be erythematous and friable. Specimens obtained by biopsy or brush cytology should be cultured and examined microscopically for the presence of typical Candida yeast with pseudohyphae formation. Mild cases of Candida esophagitis can be treated with oral nystatin (luminal treatment); however, more extensive disease, especially if the patient is immunocompromised, may require systemic treatment with either ketoconazole or fluconazole. Amphotericin B is required if there is evidence of systemic spread.

8.1.2 *HERPES SIMPLEX ESOPHAGITIS*

Next to Candida, this is the most common form of infectious esophagitis. The clinical presentation is much the same as with Candida esophagitis. There may also be constitutional symptoms of a viral upper respiratory tract infection preceding the esophageal symptoms. Herpetic mouth or skin lesions may also develop. This infection occurs most frequently in immunosuppressed patients, but also develops sporadically in healthy young adults. Endoscopy with biopsy and brush cytology is required to confirm the diagnosis. The pathognomonic finding is the eosinophilic "Cowdry's Type A" intranuclear inclusion body. Herpetic esophagitis is self-limiting in immunocompetent individuals; specific treatment is not indicated. Symptoms of odynophagia often respond to a combination of antacids mixed with viscous Xylocaine®. In severely immunocompromised patients, intravenous acyclovir treatment should be instituted.

8.2 Esophagitis Associated with Immune-Mediated Disease

Rarely, esophagitis can occur in association with Crohn's disease or Behçet's syndrome. The typical lesion is scattered aphthous-type ulcerations, although severe transmural involvement with stricture formation can occur. The esophagus can also be severely involved in pemphigoid, in pemphigus and in epidermolysis bullosa.

Esophagitis occurs in as many as one-third of patients who develop chronic graft-versus-host disease after bone marrow transplantation. The typical lesion is a generalized epithelial desquamation of the upper and middle esophagus. There may be associated ring-like narrowings or strictures due to submucosal fibrosis. A nonspecific esophageal motor disorder may also develop and result in superimposed reflux esophagitis because of poor esophageal clearing. Sarcoidosis and eosinophilic gastroenteritis are two other immune-mediated diseases that (rarely) cause esophageal inflammation.

8.3 Chemical-Induced Esophagitis

8.3.1 CAUSTIC CHEMICAL INGESTION

Strong acids or alkalis ingested accidentally or as a suicide attempt cause marked esophagitis. Alkali tends to be more injurious to the esophageal mucosa than acid and produces liquefaction necrosis as well as thermal burns (due to heat release when the alkali is hydrated by gut secretions). Acids tend to produce superficial coagulation necrosis and eschar formation. Typically the patient develops immediate chest pain and odynophagia. Oral burns also may produce local pain and drooling. There may be respiratory symptoms such as stridor, dyspnea and hoarseness if the airway is contaminated. Symptoms alone do not permit accurate prediction of the presence or absence of esophageal injury; therefore early diagnostic endoscopy should be considered in most patients. Clearly, endoscopy should not be performed if there is evidence of esophageal perforation. In the management of these patients, it is imperative to maintain an adequate airway. Oral intake must be stopped and intravenous fluids administered. Empiric treatment classically has involved antibiotics and corticosteroids, but there is no good evidence documenting the efficacy of this approach. Patients who survive the acute phase of the injury are at risk of developing strictures because of the intense collagen deposition associated with healing. This often requires repeated esophageal dilation to maintain luminal patency.

Lye-induced injury increases the risk of developing squamous cell carcinoma of the esophagus. Typically there is a 30- to 50-year lag time before the development of cancer. For this reason any patient with previous lye injury and new esophageal symptoms should be promptly investigated. The extent of the risk is such that periodic endoscopic surveillance is not indicated.

TABLE 4.   Classification of disorders causing oropharyngeal dysphagia

Central nervous system disease
Cerebrovascular accident (brainstem, pseudobulbar palsy)
Wilson's disease
Multiple sclerosis
Amyotrophic lateral sclerosis
Brainstem neoplasm
Tabes dorsalis

Peripheral nervous system disease
Bulbar poliomyelitis
Miscellaneous peripheral neuropathies
Head and neck neoplasms
Post–radical neck surgery

Muscle disease
Muscular dystrophy
Polymyositis and dermatomyositis
Metabolic myopathy (e.g., hypo- and hyperthyroidism)
Amyloidosis
Systemic lupus erythematosus
Myasthenia gravis

Local disorders
Oropharyngeal inflammation
Oropharyngeal neoplasms
Zenker's diverticulum

Idiopathic conditions
Cricopharyngeal achalasia
Idiopathic oropharyngeal incoordination

8.3.2 PILL-INDUCED ESOPHAGITIS

A large number of oral agents can cause localized esophageal injury. The antibiotic doxycycline and the anticholinergic emepronium bromide are two of the most common culprits. Nonsteroidal anti-inflammatory drugs and slow-release forms of potassium chloride are also frequently implicated. Patients with this type of injury typically take their medication with a small amount of water and then immediately lie down to go to bed. They may then wake up several hours later with severe retrosternal chest pain and odynophagia. Capsules and tablets are notorious for being transported through the esophagus quite poorly unless adequate amounts of fluid are ingested at the same time. This is an important point to remember in counseling all patients who take medicines at bedtime.

Rarely, the medication becomes lodged and causes a deep esophageal ulcer with perforation. More commonly the ulceration is superficial and heals in a few weeks. Late stricture formation may occur. Patients with esophageal motility disorders are particularly prone to this complication.

The bisphosphonate alendronate sodium has also recently been reported to rarely cause esophageal ulceration, but the mechanism of this injury is unclear.

8.4 Radiation-Induced Esophagitis

When included in the field of irradiation the esophagus becomes inflamed in up to 80% of patients receiving therapeutic radiation for cancer. The risk of esophagitis is greater if there is concomitant chemotherapy. The patients typically develop chest pain, dysphagia and odynophagia shortly after the initiation of therapy. This can be a serious problem in such patients, who are often already severely malnourished. Late stricture formation is a well-recognized complication.

9. DISORDERS OF THE OROPHARYNGEAL PHASE OF DEGLUTITION

A variety of structural and functional disorders can disrupt the oropharyngeal phase of deglutition and result in oropharyngeal or "transfer"-type dysphagia (Table 4). In the assessment of these patients it is important to exclude disorders for which specific treatment is available.

The most important investigation is a carefully performed video fluoroscopic study of the swallowing mechanism. In addition to the usual barium studies, it is helpful to observe deglutition when the patient swallows barium-soaked cookies or bread. Not only will this examination identify and characterize disorders of oropharyngeal coordination, it will also help exclude structural lesions. If an inflammatory, neoplastic or other structural lesion is suspected, direct or indirect laryngoscopy is indicated. At present, conventional manometric studies of the pharynx and UES add little to what can be learned from radiologic studies. This is partly because of limitations in recording methods, but also because complex motor events occurring during deglutition (e.g., closure of the nasopharynx, elevation and closure of the larynx – see Section 3, "Physiology") are not amenable to manometric study.

Ideally, treatment of oropharyngeal motor disorders should be directed at the underlying disease. Frequently this is not possible, and nonspecific treatment must be instituted. In some cases reassurance and education are all that is required. Many patients will be able to control their symptoms simply by eating slowly and carefully in a relaxed atmosphere. In patients in whom aspiration develops because of inadequate clearing of the hypopharynx after the

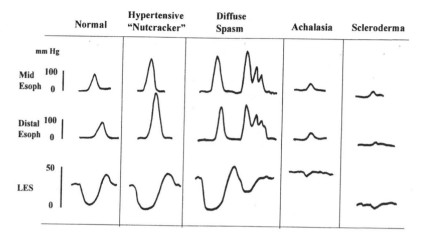

Figure 8. Schematic representation of manometric features of the major esophageal motor disorders. A *normal* tracing is on the left and depicts sequential "peristaltic" contractions in the esophageal body with full LES relaxation. *Hypertensive peristalsis* or *"nutcracker" esophagus* is characterized by normal peristalsis and LES relaxation, but the amplitude of contraction in the distal esophagus is abnormally high (> 180 mm Hg). In *diffuse esophageal spasm*, normal peristaltic waves are interspersed with high-pressure, nonpropulsive (simultaneous) contraction waves and are often repetitive. The resting LES pressure may be abnormally high, but swallow-induced LES relaxation is normal. In *achalasia* there is complete absence of normal peristalsis in the smooth-muscle esophagus (simultaneous contractions only) and swallow-induced LES relaxation is either absent or incomplete. Note also that resting intraesophageal pressures are elevated. *Scleroderma* is characterized by the presence of weak, nonperistaltic esophageal contractions and a markedly hypotensive LES that relaxes normally with swallowing.

initial swallow, it is beneficial to have the patient immediately follow a "bolus" swallow with a second, "dry" swallow. Correcting denture problems and avoiding foods of certain consistency may also help. Most speech pathologists have special expertise as swallowing therapists and can be very helpful in the management of these patients.

For patients in whom these simple measures are not helpful and whose symptoms are such that respiratory and nutritional complications are developing, cricopharyngeal myotomy is often performed. This helps patients with true cricopharyngeal achalasia or Zenker's diverticulum (Section 13). Unfortunately, the response to myotomy is inconsistent in most other patients with oropharyngeal dysphagia, because inadequate opening of the UES is rarely due to dysfunction of the cricopharyngeal muscle alone. More often there is associated weakness of the suprahyoid muscles, which actually open the sphincter, and/or associated problems with pharyngeal peristalsis. Cricopharyngeal myotomy does little to improve such altered physiology. Once cricopharyngeal myotomy has been performed, the patient has lost an important defense mechanism against the aspiration of refluxed material. The patient should therefore be instructed to elevate the head of his or her bed on blocks in order to minimize this risk. For this same reason patients with gross GERD should not undergo cricopharyngeal myotomy unless the reflux can be controlled.

When all other measures fail and nutritional and respiratory complications develop, a gastrostomy feeding tube should be placed.

10. MOTOR DISORDERS OF THE ESOPHAGUS AND LOWER ESOPHAGEAL SPHINCTER

Esophageal motor disorders can be classified as either primary or secondary. Primary disorders refer to those that usually affect the esophagus alone and have no known etiology. Secondary disorders are motility derangements caused by some other systemic or local condition. Examples of secondary disorders include acid-reflux–induced dysmotility, dysmotility related to the neuropathy associated with diabetes or alcoholism, and motor dysfunction secondary to esophageal involvement in scleroderma or other connective tissue disorders. The well-defined primary motor disorders include the hypertensive peristaltic or "nutcracker" esophagus, diffuse esophageal spasm and achalasia (Figure 8). Many cases of primary motility disorders are actually "nonspecific," having a variety of abnormalities that do not fulfill criteria established for the well-defined esophageal motor disorders.

Patients with primary motor disorders typically present with dysphagia and/or chest pain. The pain is often qualitatively similar to angina pectoris and has been classically attributed to smooth-muscle spasm. However, recent studies have suggested that the pain is more often secondary to a lowered sensory threshold to esophageal stimuli such as distention or acid. Some patients with motor disorders will have secondary GERD because of poor clearing or poor LES function. Here, heartburn and regurgitation may be prominent symptoms.

The diagnosis of a motor disorder can be made on the basis of history and barium swallow x-ray. If there is dysphagia referred to the retrosternal area and no evidence of a structural lesion on x-ray, then by exclusion the patient's dysphagia is related to a motor disorder. As mentioned previously, the quality of the dysphagia (e.g., sporadic, unpredictable dysphagia to both liquids and solids) is also helpful in differentiating motor disorders from structural causes of dysphagia. During fluoroscopy, the radiologist is usually able to detect abnormalities of motor function as the barium is swallowed. The use of a solid bolus, such as a piece of bread soaked in barium, may be helpful in diagnosing esophageal rings or webs. Endoscopy primarily rules out secondary causes of the disorder (i.e., ulcerative esophagitis and neoplasm). In order to define specifically the type of motor disorder present, however, esophageal motility studies are required. The manometric features of the important esophageal motor disorders are depicted schematically in Figure 8.

10.1 "Nutcracker" Esophagus

This motility disorder is characterized by normally propagated but high-amplitude peristaltic waves in the distal esophagus. The duration of the contraction wave is also often prolonged. LES relaxation is normal, although in many patients the resting LES pressure is elevated. Patients often present with angina-like chest pain and usually do not complain of dysphagia. Nutcracker esophagus is the most frequent abnormal manometric finding in patients referred for evaluation of noncardiac angina-like chest pain. The etiology is unknown. Rarely, this disorder progresses to diffuse esophageal spasm or even vigorous achalasia. Reassurance that the pain is not cardiac but is secondary to a benign esophageal condition is the most important part of treatment. Nitrates and calcium channel blockers (to relax smooth muscle) have been used extensively, but have no proven benefit. In some patients with nutcracker esophagus, pain is actually triggered by acid reflux; these patients often respond dramatically to appropriate antireflux therapy.

10.2 Diffuse Esophageal Spasm

This is characterized by normal peristalsis interspersed with frequent high-pressure nonpropagated or "tertiary" waves and multipeaked waves. Patients often present with dysphagia and chest pain. In advanced diffuse esophageal spasm, the x-ray will show a corkscrew pattern as different segments of the esophagus vigorously and simultaneously contract. The etiology is obscure, but may relate to degenerative changes in the intrinsic and extrinsic esophageal nerves. Management involves reassurance and the use of nitrates or calcium channel blocking agents. Patients with severe disease unresponsive to medical measures may benefit from a long esophageal myotomy.

10.3 Achalasia

This uncommon primary motility disorder is characterized by aperistalsis in the body of the esophagus and absent or incomplete LES relaxation in response to swallowing. Resting LES pressures may also be elevated. Failure of LES relaxation leads to progressive proximal dilation of the esophagus with consequent elevated resting intraesophageal pressures. On x-ray the esophagus is dilated, and retained food and fluid may be present. The distal esophagus narrows in a beak-like fashion (Figure 9). This "beak" represents the hypertonic, nonrelaxing LES. In some patients there are associated vigor-

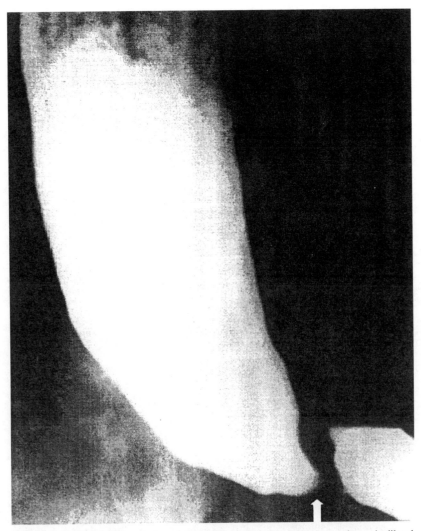

FIGURE 9.   Typical barium x-ray in a patient with achalasia. Note that the esophagus is dilated and there is stasis of barium and food debris in the esophagus. At the gastroesophageal junction (arrow) there is a beak-like narrowing, which is caused by the nonrelaxing LES. The mucosal contour at this narrow area appears normal, which helps distinguish this from a stricture caused by malignancy or reflux disease.

ous nonperistaltic contractions in the esophageal body, a condition called *vigorous achalasia*. Achalasia is caused by degeneration of inhibitory nitric oxide neurons within the esophageal and LES myenteric plexus. Nerve damage may also be found in the vagal nerve trunks and the dorsal motor nuclei. The parasite Trypanosoma cruzi, which is endemic in Brazil, can cause achalasia by destroying myenteric neurons (Chagas' disease). Neoplastic disease can also interfere with esophageal and LES nerve function and cause "secondary" achalasia. In most cases, however, the cause of the degeneration is unknown.

The cardinal symptom of achalasia is dysphagia, although chest pain and even heartburn may be present. The heartburn is not due to gastroesophageal reflux. It may be caused by lactic acid formed by fermentation of stagnant esophageal contents. Another common symptom of achalasia is regurgitation of esophageal contents.

In mild cases treatment can begin with the use of calcium channel blockers or long-acting nitrates, which have been shown to decrease LES pressure. This is rarely successful in the long term, however. The treatment then usually performed is pneumatic balloon dilation of the LES. This consists of passing a balloon across the sphincter and inflating it rapidly so that the sphincter is forcefully dilated. Pneumatic dilation is successful in alleviating the dysphagia and improving esophageal transport in 60–90% of patients, although repeated dilations may be required to achieve the highest success rate. Patients who do not respond to pneumatic dilation should be treated with Heller myotomy. This consists of a longitudinal incision through the muscle of the LES, which in many centers is now done via a laparoscopic or thoracoscopic approach. Following either pneumatic dilation or Heller myotomy, the patient can develop severe GERD, because the pressure barrier preventing reflux has been destroyed. This tends to be worse after Heller myotomy and has led some surgeons to perform a modified antireflux procedure at the time of myotomy. Because of this problem all patients having successful myotomy or pneumatic dilation should be instructed regarding lifelong antireflux therapy. Usually dietary and posture-type treatment are all that is needed, but in some patients drug therapy is required.

Recent studies have found that injection of botulinum toxin into the muscle of the LES can alleviate dysphagia in approximately two-thirds of patients with achalasia. This therapy is limited because the response is not sustained (average duration is approximately one year), but it may be a useful treatment option in elderly patients who would not tolerate the complications of more invasive therapy. Achalasia patients have an increased risk of developing esophageal cancer and need to be carefully evaluated if new esophageal symptoms develop.

10.4 Scleroderma Esophagus
Patients with scleroderma frequently have esophageal involvement. This may occur even in the absence of obvious skin and joint involvement, although in

such cases, Raynaud's phenomenon is almost always present. The initial event is damage to small blood vessels, which in turn leads to intramural neuronal dysfunction. With time, actual muscle damage and fibrosis occur. This results in a very hypotensive LES, as well as weak nonpropulsive esophageal contractions. Scleroderma may also involve the stomach and cause delayed gastric emptying. As a result, patients develop gross GERD. They present with heartburn and regurgitation, as well as dysphagia. The dysphagia can be due to poor esophageal propulsion and/or reflux-induced stricture. These patients need very aggressive treatment for GERD, often requiring twice-daily PPI therapy. Because they have very poor peristaltic function, increasing the barrier at the LES with antireflux surgery may markedly worsen the dysphagia.

11. THE ESOPHAGUS AS A CAUSE OF ANGINA-LIKE CHEST PAIN

At least one-third of the patients referred to a cardiologist or admitted to a coronary care unit because of angina-like chest pain will have cardiac causes excluded. Because in most of these patients an alternative etiology is not apparent, they are often labeled as having "noncardiac chest pain." Lack of a specific diagnosis may lead to ongoing anxiety, changes in lifestyle and frequent medical consultations if the patient continues to worry that serious heart disease may be present. In such patients esophageal disease or dysfunction should be considered. The pathophysiology of angina-like chest pain of esophageal origin is poorly understood. In some patients acid reflux is the cause: these patients experience angina-like chest pain under circumstances in which most people would experience heartburn. In others, the pain is caused by abnormal "spastic" contractions of the esophagus that either occur spontaneously or are secondary to acid reflux. Many of these patients appear to have an abnormal esophageal pain threshold; pain episodes may be triggered by multiple different stimuli that in normal subjects would not be perceived as painful.

The diagnostic approach to patients with noncardiac chest pain is controversial. In the past, full esophageal testing was usually recommended, including upper GI endoscopy, esophageal manometry with provocative testing (Figure 10) and/or 24-hour ambulatory esophageal pH monitoring (Figure 3). More recently the value of such testing has been called into question. Endoscopy is performed primarily to look for evidence of reflux esophagitis, but the diagnostic yield in this setting is low, and a negative result does not rule out acid reflux as a cause of pain. Esophageal manometry with "provocative testing" (e.g., esophageal acid perfusion, balloon distention or administration of muscarinic agonist) may be used in an attempt to reproduce the patient's chest pain and possibly relate it to induced esophageal muscle

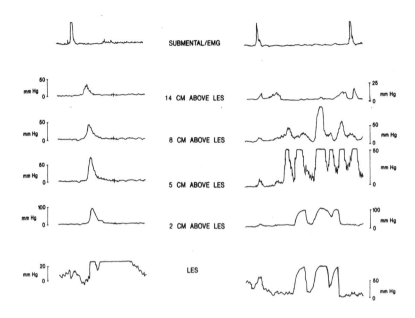

FIGURE 10.   Example of esophageal manometry with provocative testing in a patient with angina-like chest pain and normal coronary angiography. The baseline tracing (left) is within normal limits. During acid perfusion (right) a pattern of diffuse esophageal spasm is induced, which coincided with the patient experiencing her typical angina-like pain. The patient also developed marked esophageal spasm with coincident pain following the injection of bethanechol (not shown). The top tracing is the submental electromyogram (EMG), which records the onset of deglutition. This is followed in sequence by intraluminal side hole pressure recordings from 14, 8, 5 and 2 cm above the lower esophageal sphincter (LES). The lowermost tracing is the pressure recorded by the Dent sleeve, which straddles the LES.

SOURCE: Paterson WG, Marciano-D'Amore DA, Beck IT, et al. Esophageal manometry with provocative testing in patients with non-cardiac angina-like chest pain. Can J Gastroenterol 1991; 5(2):51–57. Reproduced with permission of the *Canadian Journal of Gastroenterology*.

spasm. However, this test appears to lack specificity, as the patient with a positive provocative test may experience seemingly identical spontaneous pain episodes that are unrelated to esophageal dysfunction. Ambulatory 24-hour pH monitoring can be extremely useful in correlating pain episodes with reflux events, but patients must have frequent (i.e., daily) pain attacks if one is likely to be captured during the monitoring period.

Because GERD is probably the most common, specifically treatable cause of noncardiac chest pain, it has been recommended that these patients first receive intensive treatment for GERD (i.e., twice-daily proton pump inhibitor therapy). If symptom resolution occurs, then a diagnosis of reflux-induced pain can be presumed and the patient managed accordingly. More in-depth esophageal testing can then be reserved for those patients who fail this empiric therapy and have persisting troublesome pain, especially if associated with considerable anxiety surrounding the diagnosis.

Management of angina-like chest pain of esophageal origin should be directed at the specific pathophysiological process. If the pain is triggered by gastroesophageal reflux, then antireflux treatment may be quite helpful. If the pain is due to esophageal spasm, smooth-muscle relaxants such as nitrates and calcium channel blockers may help, although few controlled clinical trials have demonstrated any significant benefit. Tricyclic antidepressants in relatively low dosage have been shown to be beneficial and should be tried in patients with frequent pain episodes that are not caused by reflux or severe esophageal spasm. These are most likely to be useful in patients with abnormal visceral nociception, or the so-called irritable esophagus. Simple reassurance and education are probably the most important part of treatment. Symptoms often improve once the patient is given a positive diagnosis and no longer fears that underlying heart disease is the cause.

12. ESOPHAGEAL NEOPLASMS

A large number of different tumors can involve the esophagus (Table 5). The vast majority are extremely rare and often do not produce clinical disease. Unfortunately, the most common esophageal neoplasm is squamous cell carcinoma, which has a five-year survival rate (< 10%) that is among the lowest for any neoplastic disease.

12.1 Benign Tumors

Leiomyoma is the most common benign esophageal tumor. Esophageal leiomyomas may produce dysphagia and retrosternal chest pain, but in most cases are asymptomatic. Unlike gastric leiomyomas, they rarely hemorrhage. On barium x-ray a characteristic smooth, round luminal defect is seen projecting from one wall. Its endoscopic appearance is a clearly demarcated projection into the lumen; the overlying mucosa is normal. Endoscopic biopsy is not helpful, as the lesion is submucosal and cannot be reached with biopsy forceps. If leiomyomas are symptomatic, surgical enucleation is indicated.

Squamous cell papillomas consist of frond-like projections of the lamina propria that are covered by squamous epithelium and develop at several sites simultaneously. They rarely grow large enough to produce dysphagia. They occur in association with acanthosis nigricans and tylosis. Except when asso-

TABLE 5.   Classification of esophageal tumors

Benign tumors
Epithelial origin
  Squamous cell papilloma
Non-epithelial origin
  Leiomyoma
  Granular cell tumor
  Hemangioma
  Lymphangioma

Malignant tumors
Epithelial origin
  Squamous cell carcinoma
  Adenocarcinoma
  Adenoid cystic carcinoma
  Mucoepidermoid carcinoma
  Adenosquamous carcinoma
  Undifferentiated carcinoma; small-cell carcinoma
Non-epithelial origin
  Leiomyosarcoma
  Carcinosarcoma
  Malignant melanoma
Secondary tumors
  Malignant melanoma
  Breast carcinoma

Tumor-like lesions
  Fibrovascular polyp
  Heterotopia
  Congenital cyst
  Glycogen acanthosis

---

ciated with tylosis, these lesions are not considered to be precursors of squamous cell carcinoma.

Fibrovascular polyps consist of a core of loose fibrous connective tissue, fat and blood vessels covered by a thick layer of squamous epithelium. Such a polyp may become quite large, with a very long stalk that permits the lesions to flop back and forth in the esophageal lumen. Patients with this lesion have presented with regurgitation of the free end of the polyp into the mouth; in other instances, the regurgitated polyp has caused sudden death by obstructing the larynx.

Granular cell tumors are submucosal lesions with intact mucosal covering that are usually picked up incidentally at endoscopy. They may originate from neural elements. They rarely cause symptoms, although there have been occasional reports of dysphagia due to large granular cell tumors. There have also been rare reports of malignant granular cell tumors in the esophagus. Symptomatic tumors need to be removed surgically.

12.2 Malignant Tumors

Carcinoma of the esophagus is a relatively uncommon malignancy in Canada, with only 3 to 4 new cases per 100,000 population per year in males and just over 1 new case per 100,000 population per year in females. Nevertheless, because of its poor prognosis, esophageal cancer ranks among the 10 leading causes of cancer death in Canadian men 45 years of age and older.

Although several different types of primary and secondary malignancies can involve the esophagus (Table 5), squamous cell carcinoma and adenocarcinoma are by far the most common esophageal malignancies.

12.2.1 *ADENOCARCINOMA*

Adenocarcinoma used to make up approximately 10% of all esophageal cancers. However, its incidence has been increasing in recent decades such that now it comprises up to 30–40% of esophageal cancers in North America. Rarely, primary esophageal adenocarcinomas arise from embryonic remnants of columnar epithelium or from superficial or deep glandular epithelium. In most instances, adenocarcinoma arises from metaplastic Barrett's epithelium in the distal esophagus. Adenocarcinoma of the cardia of the stomach may also involve the distal esophagus and give the appearance that the cancer arises from the esophagus.

The true incidence of Barrett's-related cancer is uncertain, but most studies suggest that patients with Barrett's esophagus will develop adenocarcinoma at a rate of about 0.5% per year. This is a significant problem given the large number of reflux patients with Barrett's metaplasia. Because dysplasia develops prior to frank carcinoma in Barrett's epithelium, most experts suggest that these patients should undergo surveillance endoscopy with multiple biopsies every two years to identify those who are likely to progress to cancer (Section 7).

The clinical presentation and diagnostic evaluation of patients with adenocarcinoma of the esophagus are similar to those of squamous cell carcinoma (Section 12.2.2). These lesions are relatively insensitive to radiotherapy and their response to various chemotherapeutic agents is also not very satisfactory. Surgical resection may be performed with curative intent. However, surgical resection for palliation, or palliation with laser, photodynamic therapy, peroral dilation and/or stent placement are more often required, since curative

TABLE 6.   Esophageal squamous cell carcinoma: possible etiological factors

Alcohol
Tobacco
Nutritional exposures
   Nitrosamines; "bush teas" containing tannin and/or diterpene phorbol esters
Nutritional deficiencies (riboflavin, niacin, iron)
Chronic esophagitis
Achalasia
Previous lye-induced injury
Tylosis
Plummer-Vinson (Paterson-Kelly) syndrome

surgery is feasible in only 20% of patients. The prognosis is similar to that for gastric adenocarcinoma – i.e., an overall five-year survival rate of < 10%.

12.2.2 SQUAMOUS CELL CARCINOMA

The occurrence of squamous cell carcinoma of the esophagus shows striking geographic variability, with high frequencies in certain regions of Iran, Africa, China and the former USSR. This has led to several theories concerning certain environmental agents that may be important etiologically (Table 6). In North America, squamous cell carcinoma is associated with alcohol ingestion, tobacco use and lower socioeconomic status. It is also significantly more common in blacks and in males.

Characteristically these cancers, similarly to adenocarcinoma, extend microscopically in the submucosa for substantial distances above and below the area of the gross involvement. They also have a propensity to extend through the esophageal wall and to regional lymphatics quite early. Furthermore, they usually produce symptoms only when they have become locally quite advanced. For these reasons approximately 95% of these cancers are diagnosed at a time when surgical cure is impossible.

In most studies, the mid-esophagus is the most common site of origin (Figure 11); however, others have reported distal cancers to be most common. The lungs, liver and bones are the most common sites of distant metastases.

Most patients present with progressive, predictable dysphagia and weight loss. Other symptoms include odynophagia, chest pain (which may radiate to the mid-scapular region), hoarseness (due to recurrent laryngeal nerve involvement) and blood loss. Pulmonary complications due to either direct aspiration or esophagorespiratory fistulas are also quite common during the course of the disease. Physical examination is usually negative aside from signs of weight loss. Hepatomegaly or enlarged cervical or

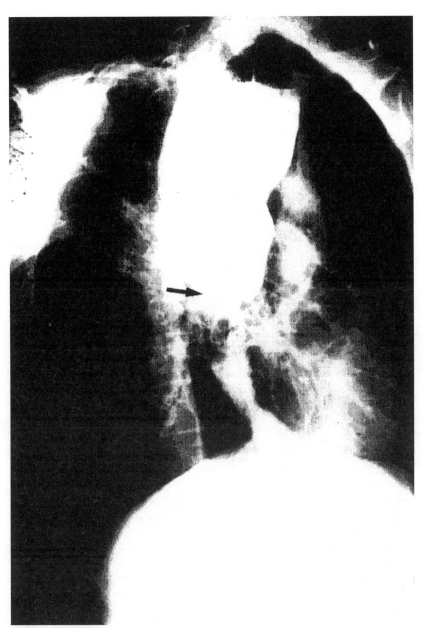

FIGURE 11.   Barium swallow radiograph in a patient with squamous cell carcinoma of the mid-esophagus. Note narrowing of the esophageal lumen with irregular mucosal contour. (Radiograph courtesy of Dr. M. Jabbari.)

supraclavicular lymph nodes may be detected in cases of disseminated metastases.

Barium swallow is usually diagnostic, although small cancers can be missed in up to 30% of cases. Endoscopy with multiple directed biopsies combined with brush cytology is required to confirm the diagnosis. This should be followed by careful attempts to stage the disease prior to deciding on therapeutic intervention. In addition to a careful physical examination, chest x-ray and blood tests for transaminases, alkaline phosphatase and bilirubin, an ultrasound of the abdomen should be performed to look for liver metastasis. If this is negative, one should proceed to a CT scan of the thorax in order to define the extent of local spread. Unfortunately the CT scan lacks sensitivity in this regard. Endoscopic ultrasound appears promising in accurately assessing depth of tumor involvement and presence or absence of enlarged mediastinal lymph nodes. If the above investigations are negative, some experts recommend bronchoscopy, mediastinoscopy and scalene node biopsy prior to attempting surgical resection when the cancers are localized to the mid or upper esophagus.

Treatment results of squamous cell carcinoma of the esophagus are discouraging. These tumors are quite radiosensitive; however, most centers give radiotherapy to patients who have advanced unresectable tumors or other health problems that make them poor surgical candidates. This understandably leads to very poor overall survival following radiotherapy. In the few reports where radiotherapy is used as the primary mode of therapy in patients who might otherwise be considered surgical candidates, the five-year survival rate is as high as 17%, which compares quite favorably to surgical results. Both forms of treatment have significant morbidity, but the surgical mortality following esophageal resection is 5–10%. Controlled trials are needed, but in only a small proportion of the total population of esophageal cancer patients is cure a realistic goal. In the majority the disease is too far advanced. New regimens that combine radiotherapy and chemotherapy, with or without surgery, are currently being evaluated and show promise in improving cure rates and disease-free survival. However, the toxicity and morbidity from combined treatment can be substantial.

The goal of treatment has to be palliation in most patients. Both radiotherapy and palliative surgery can be used in this setting; however, other modalities are often necessary. The dysphagia can be relieved with peroral dilation, but in many patients this becomes exceedingly difficult as the disease progresses. If this is the case, a prosthetic device can sometimes be placed across the tumor to maintain luminal patency. These stents can work quite well, although tube blockage, tube migration, erosion through the esophageal wall and sudden massive aspiration are important complications. These prosthetic devices are the best treatment for an esophagorespiratory fistula. Endo-scopic Nd-YAG laser therapy has been used to thermally destroy and vapor-ize tumors that obstruct the esophageal lumen. This appears to be a very use-ful form of palliation, but it is expensive and has not as yet been documented to be superior to dilation and stent placement. Photodynamic therapy has recently been approved for palliation of neoplastic dysphagia. This involves using a photosensitizing compound that accumulates in cancer cells, which leads to their destruction when they are exposed to light of a certain wave-length. The caring physician must also provide emotional support, nutritional support and adequate pain therapy for these unfortunate patients.

13. MISCELLANEOUS DISORDERS OF THE ESOPHAGUS

13.1 Webs and Rings

Webs are thin, membrane-like structures that project into the esophageal lumen. They are covered on both sides with squamous epithelium and are most commonly found in the cervical esophagus. Webs are usually detected incidentally during barium x-rays and rarely occlude enough of the esoph-ageal lumen to cause dysphagia. The etiology of these webs is unclear. Most are probably congenital in origin. In some instances postcricoid esophageal webs are associated with iron deficiency and dysphagia – the so-called *Plum-mer-Vinson* or *Paterson-Kelly* syndrome. This syndrome is associated with increased risk of hypopharyngeal cancer and should be managed with bougienage, iron replacement and careful follow-up. Esophageal webs may also form after esophageal injury, such as that induced by pills or lye inges-tion, and have also been reported in association with graft-versus-host dis-ease.

The lower esophageal or *Schatzki's ring* is also a membrane-like structure, but unlike webs is lined by squamous epithelium on its superior aspect and columnar epithelium inferiorly. Such a ring is quite common, being detected in up to 10% of all upper GI barium x-rays. Few produce sufficient luminal obstruction to cause dysphagia (yet a lower esophageal ring is a common cause of dysphagia). When the lumen is narrowed to a diameter of 13 mm or less, the patient will experience intermittent solid-food dysphagia or even epi-sodic food-bolus obstruction. Treatment of a symptomatic Schatzki's ring involves shattering the ring with a large-diameter bougie or a balloon dilator.

13.2 Diverticula

Pharyngoesophageal diverticula are outpouchings of one or more layers of the pharyngeal or esophageal wall and are classified according to their loca-tion.

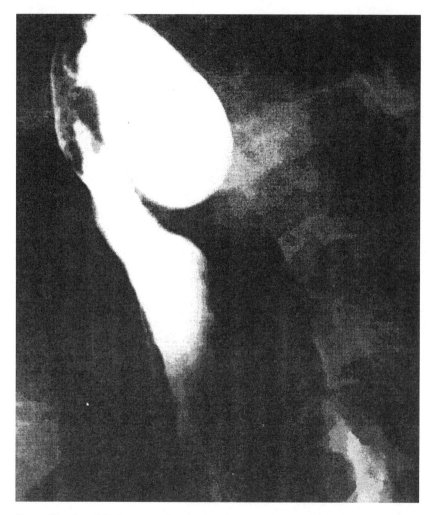

FIGURE 12.   Lateral barium x-ray of a Zenker's diverticulum. These diverticuli form just above the cricopharyngeus muscle and extend posteriorly. Most of these diverticuli shift to the left of the midline as they enlarge.

13.2.1 *ZENKER'S DIVERTICULUM* (Figure 12)

This diverticulum arises posteriorly in the midline between the oblique and transverse (cricopharyngeal) fibers of the inferior pharyngeal constrictor muscles. As this diverticulum enlarges, it usually shifts to the left of the midline. Zenker's diverticulum forms because of decreased compliance of the cricopharyngeal muscle, which results in abnormally high pressures in the hypopharynx during deglutition. If large, the diverticulum may cause dysphagia secondary to external compression of the cervical esophagus. In addition to oropharyngeal-type dysphagia, Zenker's diverticulum may be associated with effortless regurgitation of stagnant, foul-tasting food, as well as aspiration. A very large diverticulum can produce a neck mass, usually on the left side.

Treatment of a symptomatic Zenker's diverticulum is surgical. Most surgeons will either resect the diverticulum or suspend it (diverticulopexy) so that it cannot fill. This is combined with cricopharyngeal myotomy. In many cases, particularly if the diverticulum is small, cricopharyngeal myotomy alone will alleviate symptoms. Once the cricopharyngeal myotomy has been performed, the patient has lost an important defense mechanism to prevent the aspiration of refluxed material. The patient should therefore be instructed to elevate the head of the bed in order to minimize this risk. For the same reason patients with gross GERD should not undergo cricopharyngeal myotomy unless the reflux can be controlled either medically or surgically.

13.2.2 MIDESOPHAGEAL DIVERTICULA

Traditionally, midesophageal diverticula have been called "traction" diverticula because of their supposed etiology. They were believed to arise secondary to old mediastinal inflammation, such as tuberculosis, that caused adherence of mediastinal structures to the outer esophageal wall so that outward traction occurred during peristalsis. It now appears likely that very few midesophageal diverticula arise this way. In most there is an associated motility disorder and it is likely that this is actually a "pulsion" diverticulum formed when a peristaltic wave deteriorates into a simultaneous or spastic contraction in the smooth-muscle esophagus. Midesophageal diverticula rarely require specific therapy. Rather, only the associated motor disorder requires treatment if symptomatic.

13.2.3 LOWER ESOPHAGEAL OR EPIPHRENIC DIVERTICULA

These "pulsion" diverticula form just above the LES and are invariably associated with an esophageal motor disorder – usually diffuse esophageal spasm, with or without abnormal relaxation of the LES. Patients with these diverticula usually present with dysphagia and/or angina-like chest pain. In addition, they may complain of nocturnal regurgitation of large quantities of stagnant fluid.

If symptoms are present, treatment with nitrates or calcium channel blockers may be helpful. If this is not successful, surgery is indicated. Any surgical attack on these diverticula should involve a myotomy of the spastic distal esophagus and/or LES. Resection of the diverticula alone seldom affords long-term benefit.

13.2.4 *INTRAMURAL DIVERTICULOSIS*

This disorder has a characteristic radiologic appearance consisting of numerous tiny, flask-shaped outpouchings from the esophageal lumen. There is usually an associated smooth stricture in the proximal esophagus. Patients typically present with dysphagia that responds to peroral dilation. The outpouchings are actually dilated ducts coming from submucosal glands and thus are not true diverticula. The etiology is obscure. Some cases are associated with esophageal candidiasis, but this organism does not appear to be of etiological importance.

13.3 Esophageal Trauma

Blunt or penetrating trauma to the chest can cause esophageal injury. In addition, esophageal instrumentation such as that used in bougienage, endoscopy or stent insertion may cause perforation or mucosal laceration. Severe retching or vomiting can also cause esophageal perforation (*Boerhaave's syndrome*) or mucosal laceration (*Mallory-Weiss tear*). Boerhaave's syndrome is a life-threatening condition that requires immediate surgery to drain the mediastinum and repair the defect in the esophageal wall. Patients, typically alcoholics, present with sudden epigastric and/or chest pain following a bout of vomiting and usually have fever and signs of hypovolemia or shock. The diagnosis is established by having the patient swallow a small amount of water-soluble contrast material (e.g., Gastrografin®), which is seen to leak into the mediastinum or pleural cavity through the esophageal perforation.

The mucosal laceration of the Mallory-Weiss tear is probably better classified as a disorder of the stomach, because in most cases the laceration starts at the GE junction and extends down into the stomach. These patients present with hematemesis or melena following a bout of retching or vomiting. The bleeding usually stops spontaneously and only supportive therapy is required. If bleeding persists, endoscopically applied hemostasis or surgical intervention may be necessary.

13.4 Food-Bolus Obstruction and Foreign Bodies

A surprising variety of foreign bodies can lodge in the esophagus after being swallowed either inadvertently or deliberately. The three most common sites where foreign bodies become stuck are the piriform sinuses, at the aortic arch and just above the LES. The patient can usually localize the site of the obstruction quite accurately, and this can be confirmed using routine x-rays if the object is radiopaque. (However, as mentioned above, some patients may perceive the obstruction in the throat region when it is really in the distal esophagus.) Otherwise, x-rays using small amounts of water-soluble contrast media may be necessary. Most foreign bodies can be removed by an expert endoscopist. Surgery is rarely required, except when perforation has occurred.

A more common clinical problem is esophageal food-bolus obstruction. This typically occurs when a patient with a motility disorder, stricture or Schatzki's (lower esophageal) ring swallows a large solid-food bolus. The patient notices immediate chest pain, usually well localized to the site of obstruction. Attempts to swallow anything further are unsuccessful and usually lead to prompt regurgitation.

Many physicians will initially treat these patients with smooth-muscle relaxants such as intravenous glucagon, sublingual nitroglycerin or nifedipine; however, there is little evidence that this approach is efficacious. If the food bolus does not pass on spontaneously within a few hours, endoscopy should be performed, at which time the bolus can either be removed per os or pushed through into the stomach. These patients should not be left too long, as the bolus is capable of causing significant maceration to the esophageal mucosa. Giving the patient meat tenderizer, in an attempt to dissolve the bolus, is probably of no value and may be very harmful; papain can digest the esophageal mucosa and has been reported to cause severe hemorrhagic pulmonary edema when aspirated.

SUGGESTED READING LIST

Beck IT, Champion M, Lemire S, et al. (guest eds.). Second Canadian gastroesophageal reflux disease consensus conference. Can J Gastroenterol 1996; 11(Suppl B).

Clouse RE, Diamant NE. Motor physiology and motor disorders of the esophagus. In: Feldman M, Scharschmidt BF, Sleisenger MH (eds.), Sleisenger and Fordtran's gastrointestinal and liver disease: pathophysiology/diagnosis/management, vol. 1. 6th ed. Philadelphia: WB Saunders, 1997:467–497.

DeVault KR, Castell DO. Guidelines for the diagnosis and treatment of gastroesophageal reflux disease. Arch Intern Med 1995; 155:2165–2173.

Goyal RK, Paterson WG. Esophageal motility. In: Wood JD (ed.), Handbook of physiology: motility and circulation, vol. 4. Washington, DC: American Physiological Society, 1989:865–908.

Kahrilas JP, Clouse RE, Hogan WJ. American Gastroentological Association technical review on the clinical use of esophageal manometry. Gastroenterology 1994; 107:1865–1884.

Kahrilas PJ, Quigley EMM: Clinical esophageal pH recording: a technical review for practice guideline development. Gastroenterology 1996; 110:1982–1996.

McCallum RW, Mittal RK (eds.). Gastroesophageal reflux disease. Gastroenterol Clin North Am 1990; 19(3):501–781.

Mercer CD. Management of esophageal cancer. Annals RCPSC 1989; 22(6):407–410.

Paterson WG. Canadian Association of Gastroenterology practice guidelines: management of noncardiac chest pain. Can J Gastroenterol 1998; 12:401–407.

Wong RK (ed.). Mucosal diseases of the esophagus. Gastroenterol Clin North Am 1991; 20(4):635–890.

OBJECTIVES

Anatomy and Physiology
1. Know the anatomy and physiology of the normal esophagus and esophagogastric junction.
2. Describe the process of deglutition and esophageal peristalsis.
3. Understand the different physiological control mechanisms between the upper striated-muscle esophagus and distal smooth-muscle esophagus.
4. Understand the mechanisms underlying LES tone and relaxation.

Congenital and Anatomic Abnormalities
1. Define esophageal atresia and tracheoesophageal fistula, and describe how they present.
2. Define hiatus hernia with regard to anatomic type (sliding versus para-esophageal).

Gastroesophageal Reflux Disease (GERD)
1. Outline the clinical symptoms of GERD.
2. Describe the anatomic and physiological factors predisposing to GERD.
3. Discuss the procedures used in the diagnosis of GERD.
4. Discuss medical management of GERD.
5. List the indications for operative management of GERD and discuss the physiological basis for the antireflux procedures.
6. List the complications of gastroesophageal reflux disease.

Nonreflux-Induced Esophagitis
1. List the major infectious causes of esophagitis (Candida, herpetic) and describe how they present.
2. List other causes of esophagitis.

Disorders of the Oropharyngeal Phase of Deglutition
1. Categorize the major causes of oropharyngeal deglutition.
2. Describe how oropharyngeal dysphagia can be differentiated from esophageal dysphagia based on history.
3. Describe the investigations required in the assessment of oropharyngeal dysphagia.
4. What are the complications of oropharyngeal dysphagia?

Motor Disorders of the Esophagus

1. List the major primary and secondary esophageal motor disorders.
2. Describe the clinical symptoms typically associated with different esophageal motor disorders.

Esophageal Tumors

1. List the symptoms suggestive of an esophageal malignancy.
2. Outline a diagnostic plan for evaluating a patient with suspected esophageal tumor.
3. Describe the natural history of malignant esophageal neoplasms.
4. Describe the treatment options for esophageal malignancy.
5. List the common types of benign esophageal tumors.

Miscellaneous Esophageal Disorders

1. Be able to describe the presenting symptomatology and typical x-ray findings of esophageal webs, and Zenker's and esophageal diverticula.
2. Outline the clinical presentation and management of patients presenting with (a) Boerhaave's syndrome and (b) esophageal foreign body or food-bolus obstruction.

Skills

1. Demonstrate the ability to read a barium swallow in patients with sliding and paraesophageal hiatus hernia, esophageal cancer, Zenker's diverticulum, esophageal diverticulum and achalasia.
2. Describe the motility abnormalities in achalasia, diffuse esophageal spasm, "nutcracker" esophagus and scleroderma esophagus.
3. Develop an approach for the diagnostic evaluation of a patient with dysphagia.

6
The Stomach and Duodenum
B.J. Salena and R.H. Hunt

1. INTRODUCTION

Diseases of the GI tract are common, accounting for one out of seven complaints, and disorders of the stomach and duodenum make up a large part of these.

It has been known for many centuries that the gastric juice is acid in nature, but it was not until 1824 that William Prout established that the acid in the stomach is hydrochloric acid. Since then physicians have been fascinated by the ability of the healthy stomach and duodenum to withstand hydrochloric acid and pepsin. In particular the mechanisms controlling gastric secretion have been extensively studied in the hope of finding a satisfactory way to explain and treat peptic ulcer disease. Further studies turned to the role of mucus, bicarbonate and prostaglandins in maintenance and defense of the gastric mucosa against acid injury. In 1983 Marshall and Warren isolated the bacteria now known as Helicobacter pylori from gastric biopsies in duodenal ulcer patients and a new era in the understanding and treatment of gastroduodenal disease was born. This chapter will review the anatomy, physiology and related common disorders of the stomach and duodenum.

2. ANATOMY

2.1 General Anatomy
The stomach is the most capacious part of the GI tract and lies between the distal esophagus and the duodenum. It is situated entirely within the abdomen below the diaphragm (Figure 1). The body of the stomach lies slightly to the left of the midline, the antrum across the spinal vertebrae at the level of T10–L1

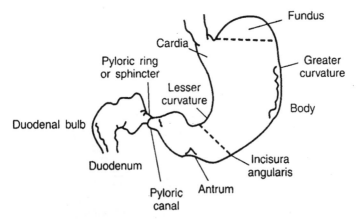

FIGURE 1. Anatomic divisions of the stomach.

and the pylorus to the right of the vertebral column. The duodenum is predominantly retroperitoneal and comprises the cap, descending and distal portions.

The greater curvature is some three or four times the length of the lesser
curvature. A point known as the angulus or incisura may be defined on the
lesser curvature. This point is relatively constant and marks a change from the
prominent rugal folds of the body of the stomach to the smoother, less prominent folds of the antrum.

The stomach and duodenum lie in close proximity to a number of important anatomic structures. Anterosuperiorly are the left diaphragm and left lobe
of the liver, while the body and tail of the pancreas lie posteriorly. Laterally to
the left are the hilum of the left kidney, the left adrenal gland and, above that,
the spleen. These organs form the stomach bed and are separated from it by
the lesser omentum and the lesser sac. The duodenum, apart from the cap, lies
retroperitoneally. The second and distal parts surround the head of the pancreas while the cap, which is attached to the lesser omentum, lies anterior to
the head of the pancreas.

2.2 Blood Supply

The main arterial blood supply (Figure 2) arises from the celiac axis. The
common hepatic artery gives rise to the gastroduodenal artery and the right
gastric artery, which then anastomoses with the left gastric artery. The splenic
artery gives rise to the short gastric arteries that supply the body along the
greater curvature of the stomach. The right and left gastroepiploic arteries also
form an anastomosis along the greater curvature.

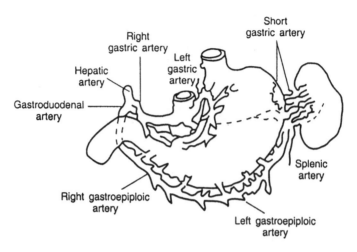

FIGURE 2.   Blood supply to the stomach.

Venous drainage essentially follows the arterial supply but passes to the portal venous system and its tributaries, the splenic vein and the superior mesenteric vein. Veins from the fundus communicate with veins draining the lower third of the esophagus and form a connection between the systemic and portal venous systems. This connection assumes clinical importance if portal venous pressure rises, when venous flow is reversed through the esophageal veins, leading to esophageal or fundal varices.

Lymphatic drainage is to the pancreaticosplenic nodes, the left gastric nodes and the pyloric nodes, and then via the celiac group to the preaortic lymph nodes and the cisterna chyli.

2.3 Nerve Supply

The nerve supply is both sympathetic and parasympathetic. The vagal supply arises via the anterior and posterior trunks, which pass through the diaphragm on either side of the esophagus before giving rise to the hepatic and celiac branches. The hepatic branch supplies further branches to the anterior surface of the body of the stomach and to the pyloric region, while the celiac branch passes to the celiac plexus and the posterior aspect of the body of the stomach. The vagal fibers anastomose with ganglion cells of the stomach within the muscle layers, forming Auerbach's plexus or, in the submucosa, forming Meissner's plexus.

The sympathetic nerve supply arises from the spinal cord between T6 and T10 and passes to the sympathetic ganglia. The parasympathetic supply contracts the stomach, relaxes the pylorus and stimulates acid, pepsin and mucus

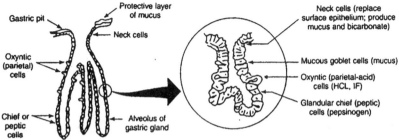

FIGURE 3.   Microscopic appearances of gastric pit and glands.

secretion, whereas sympathetic stimulation constricts the blood supply and reduces gastric motor activity and secretion while the pylorus is contracted.

2.4 Structure of the Stomach and Duodenum

The stomach and duodenum comprise an outer serosal coat, a muscular layer, submucosa and mucus membrane. The mucosal surface is ridged by the rugal folds created by contractions of the muscularis mucosa, especially prominent in the body of the stomach and less obvious in the antrum. The glands of the stomach are of two main types — gastric and pyloric — both of which are closely packed in the columnar epithelium. The gastric glands (known as oxyntic glands) make up 70–80% of the total and are responsible for secreting mucus, pepsinogen, hydrochloric acid and intrinsic factor (Figure 3). The pyloric glands, which secrete mucus and gastrin, make up only about 15%. A line of demarcation can usually be seen between the gastric and pyloric glands in the region of the incisura.

The gastric glands differ in cell type: the chief or peptic cells secrete pepsinogen, while the parietal or oxyntic cells secrete hydrochloric acid and intrinsic factor. The endocrine cells of the antrum secrete gastrin and 5-hydroxytryptamine. In the duodenum the first 4–5 cm of mucosa are smooth, but in the descending duodenum the mucosa is thrown into crescentic folds. The mucosa is lined with columnar, goblet, Paneth's and endocrine cells. The columnar cells line the villi and crypts, which increase in size in the second and third parts of the duodenum. A characteristic feature in the duodenal submucosa is the presence of Brunner's glands, which are similar to pyloric glands.

3. PHYSIOLOGY

The stomach has three major functions: motor, secretory and endocrine (Table 1). The motor functions include temporary storage of food and fluid, mixing of

TABLE 1. Functions of the stomach

Motor
Vagus-mediated and gastrin-induced receptive relaxation
Mixing and emptying

Secretory
Acid, pepsin, intrinsic factor, volume, water, electrolytes

Endocrine
Gastrin, serotonin, somatostatin

---

ingested materials with gastric juice and regulated emptying of gastric contents. The most important substances secreted into the lumen of the stomach include hydrochloric acid, pepsin, mucus, bicarbonate, intrinsic factor and water. The stomach releases two hormones into the blood: gastrin and somatostatin. Serotonin-staining (ECL) cells are also present in the gastric fundus and antrum. Gastrin stimulates acid secretion by the stomach, and somatostatin inhibits the release of gastrin. More recently, it has become clear that inflammation in the stomach due to infection with H. pylori inhibits release of somatostatin, resulting in an increased secretion of gastrin. H. pylori is a spiral bacillus found in the upper gastrointestinal tract, particularly the gastric antrum.

3.1 Gastric Motility

The motor functions of the stomach include serving as a reservoir, mixing its contents, kneading and churning solid food, and regulating the emptying of its contents into the duodenum. The reservoir function involves temporary storage of ingested and secreted substances. Above a certain threshold volume, the stomach is "full" (whether the volume is large or small); i.e., the intragastric pressure increases very little with the addition of more food and fluid because the walls of the stomach relax to accommodate the load. The stomach also mixes ingested substances with gastric juice to dissolve and dilute food, kneads solid materials to a particle size of less than 1 mm diameter, and finally, empties its contents into the duodenum slowly and in small volumes.

Gastric motility is controlled centrally and by local neurohormonal control of muscle. The muscle layers include the outer longitudinal, middle circular and inner oblique fibers. Neuronal control involves the intrinsic myenteric plexus, the extrinsic postganglionic sympathetic fibers of the celiac plexus, and the preganglionic parasympathetic fibers of the vagus nerve. The vagal afferents are both relaxatory and excitatory. These vagal fibers are neither cholinergic nor adrenergic.

Factors that influence gastric motility may be classified as myogenic, neural and chemical. The resting potential difference of the gastric smooth muscle is 5–15 mV and there is a rhythmic depolarization, with this basic electrical rhythm being set by the gastric pacemaker, which gives rise to slow-wave activity. The action potential produces peristalsis and is influenced by gastrin. The force of the contraction is increased with vagal activity, gastrin and motilin, and is decreased with gastric secretion.

Gastric distention by food or liquid stimulates both intrinsic nerves and vagal afferents. There are increased spike burst activity, more forceful peristaltic contractions and increased gastric emptying. Pyloric sphincter relaxation occurs so that the antral lumen is not occluded by peristaltic waves. Gastric contents are propelled both forward and backward toward the body of the stomach and are thoroughly mixed. Gastrin delays gastric emptying by decreasing gastric motility and at the same time increasing duodenal motility and pyloric tone (events that are mediated by fat, protein or acid in the duodenum). This increase in duodenal motility and pyloric tone is effected by stimulation of duodenal osmoreceptors and by the release of secretin, cholecystokinin (CCK) and gastric inhibitory polypeptide (GIP).

Gastric motility is inhibited for the stomach to accommodate food. Vagal relaxatory fibers are stimulated by swallowing, esophageal or gastric distention, and neurogenic stimulation. Sympathetic and adrenergic fibers influence these cholinergic neurons.

The emptying of the stomach is influenced by the substance, volume, osmolality and composition of the ingested meal. Liquids empty more rapidly than solids. The rate of gastric emptying is related to the square root of the volume, so that a constant proportion of the gastric contents empties per unit time. Stimulation of duodenal osmoreceptors with triglycerides, fatty acids or hydrochloric acid slows gastric emptying.

The gastric body serves as a reservoir, whereas the antrum has the function of mixing, churning and emptying. A high-pressure gradient exists at the gastroduodenal junction, with the pyloric sphincter playing an important role in the coordinated activity of emptying the antral contents into the duodenum.

When the volume of the stomach increases with relaxation, the intragastric pressure does not increase, because of receptive relaxation mediated by way of a vagal reflex and the splanchnic nerves. Receptive relaxation occurs primarily in the gastric fundus and body. Vagotomy, fundoplication and extensive involvement of the stomach by adenocarcinoma result in a loss of this capacity, leading to early satiety. Gastric fundal contractions are infrequent, and of large amplitude and long duration (45 seconds). These contractions propel contents to the body and antrum for mixing to occur.

The distal two-thirds of the stomach is under intrinsic myogenic control. Electrical slow-wave activity can be detected on the greater curvature, with aboral contractions passing from the greater to the lesser curvature at a rate of about 3 per minute. Although antral contractions occur only in response to neural stimulation, the muscle will contract only when a slow wave occurs. The gastric pacemaker controls the frequency and direction of propagated contractions. This control can be altered by the insertion of an electrical pacemaker, potentially changing the frequency of contraction and reversing its direction. It is possible that some clinical disorders of gastric emptying may give rise to chronic nausea, vomiting, fullness and distention.

As antral contractions pass distally, velocity increases, with near simultaneous contractions of distal antrum and pylorus. A small amount of gastric chyme may enter the duodenum, but most passes back into the stomach, where further mixing and churning takes place.

The pyloric sphincter is recognized macroscopically by thickening of the distal circular antral muscle, forming a muscular ring. However, it is difficult to accept this as a true physiologic sphincter, since in its resting phase it is open, and the rapid closure with antral peristalsis serves more to retard than to facilitate the aboral passage of gastric chyme. The pylorus acts to limit duodenogastric reflux. Duodenal acidification or infusion of secretin results in an increase in pyloric sphincter pressure. Patients with gastric ulcer or bile gastritis experience increased reflux of duodenal contents (including bile and pancreatic enzymes) into the stomach, apparently secondary to a pyloric defect. If the sphincter is ablated by pyloroplasty for duodenal ulcer disease, bile reflux is inevitable.

3.2 Gastric Secretion

Gastric juice contains many substances. The six most important of these are hydrogen ion, pepsin, mucus, bicarbonate, intrinsic factor and water. Hydrochloric acid and the enzyme pepsin participate in the digestion of proteins. Mucus lubricates ingested solids. Mucus and bicarbonate probably protect the mucosal lining against digestion by acid and pepsin. The intrinsic factor is required for normal absorption of ingested cobalamin (vitamin B_{12}). Each day the stomach secretes about 2 L of water in an adult.

3.2.1 *GASTRIC ACID SECRETION*

It is generally accepted that acid secretion is activated by three separate pathways: the neural, hormonal and paracrinal (local) pathways. The major chemical transmitter substances are acetylcholine, gastrin and histamine.

The vagus and branches from the celiac plexus and ganglia traveling along the celiac artery are the major extrinsic nervous supply to the acid-secreting portion of the stomach. The postganglionic neurons of the vagi that terminate in the oxyntic gland near the oxyntic cells are predominantly cholinergic. These cholinergic fibers are rarely seen in contact with the oxyntic cells, and therefore acetylcholine released by these nerve endings must diffuse a relatively long distance to the cells. There are two types of muscarinic binding sites on oxyntic cells: M_1 and M_2 receptors. The cholinergic binding results in a dose-dependent acid secretory response. Additionally, there may be muscarinic receptors on histamine-containing cells resulting in indirect stimulation of paracrine cells by histamine release.

Histamine has a direct stimulatory action on oxyntic cells via an H_2 receptor. The stimulatory action of histamine on oxyntic cells is competitively antagonized by a group of histamine analogues (such as cimetidine, ranitidine, famotidine, nizatidine and others) that specifically interact with the H_2 receptor. The histamine antagonists binding to the H_1 receptor can decrease gastric histamine, but at much higher doses.

Gastrin, the other major secretagogue, also interacts with oxyntic cells via a gastrin receptor. The weak stimulatory effect of gastrin on acid production can be competitively inhibited by proglumide, a glutamic acid derivative known to antagonize CCK. Since CCK binds with the same affinity and produces a similar weak secretory response, the question has been raised whether the receptor may be a CCK receptor instead of a gastrin receptor, or whether the receptor may be related to the well-known trophic effect of gastrin rather than the acid-secreting effects.

The binding of secretagogues to the oxyntic cell receptors is coupled to at least two possible intracellular messengers, Ca^{++} and cyclic AMP. Cholinergic action controls the influx of extracellular Ca^{++} into the oxyntic cell, with subsequent activation of undefined intracellular events resulting in acid secretion. The weak stimulatory effect of gastrin is also Ca^{++} dependent. Histamine does not require extracellular Ca^{++} for stimulation of acid secretion. Cyclic AMP is the intracellular messenger coupling the effect of histamine to hydrogen ion production and secretion.

After the oxyntic cells have been stimulated, intracellular endoplasmic tubular structures known as tubulovesicles disappear from the cytoplasm, while the microvilli in the secretory canaliculi increase in length to enlarge the secretory surface. The tubulovesicle membranes contain H^+/K^+-ATPase, the enzyme responsible for driving the H^+ pump, exchanging K^+ for H^+. These membranes have a low permeability to K^+ and, at rest, prevent sufficient K^+ from entering the lumen of the tubulovesicles, thus preventing H^+ transport. Stimulatory activity occurs only with a cellular signal from secretagogues.

It is evident that the overall process of acid secretion is controlled by a complex interaction of a number of pathways that will be further elucidated in the future.

3.2.2 PEPSINOGEN SECRETION

Pepsinogens are present in the mucous cells of cardiac glands, in the chief and mucous neck cells of oxyntic glands, in the mucous cells of pyloric glands and in the mucous cells of duodenal Brunner's glands. These proenzymes are secreted and activated by acids to the active form, pepsin. Furthermore, pepsin can activate additional pepsinogen autocatalytically.

The mucosal lining of the stomach contains four types of immunologically distinct pepsinogens with the ability to digest proteins at acid pH. Pepsinogens and hydrochloric acid secretion respond to much the same stimulants. Cephalic-vagal stimulation strongly stimulates pepsinogen secretion. Anticholinergics, histamine H_2-receptor antagonists and vagotomy decrease pepsinogen secretion. Elevated serum type 1 pepsinogen has been associated with duodenal ulcer and gastrinoma, while atrophic gastritis, with or without pernicious anemia, or as a consequence of H. pylori infection, has been associated with low levels of type 1 pepsinogen.

3.2.3 INTRINSIC FACTOR SECRETION

Intrinsic factor (IF) is a glycoprotein secreted by oxyntic cells. It is important in vitamin B_{12} absorption. B_{12} is released from dietary protein by gastric acid and pepsin; it binds to IF and to R protein, which is secreted into saliva. B_{12} binds more efficiently to the R proteins at low pH, so most of the B_{12} is initially complexed with the R proteins. In the upper small bowel, pancreatic enzymes cleave the complexes and the free B_{12} binds to IF, which eventually binds to a specific ileal receptor and is subsequently absorbed and transported to the tissues by another B_{12}-binding protein, transcobalamin II.

Stimulants of acid secretion also stimulate IF secretion. Patients with low or absent acid secretion often have reduced IF secretion. Continued IF secretion is low but the amounts may be adequate to prevent vitamin B_{12} deficiency and pernicious anemia. Rarely, IF secretion can be absent with normal acid secretion. Circulating antibodies to IF and oxyntic cells are found in many patients with atrophic gastritis, achlorhydria or hypochlorhydria, and pernicious anemia.

3.3 Gastric Mucosal Barrier

Healthy gastric mucosa has the ability to resist high intraluminal concentrations of hydrochloric acid and peptic activity. The physiologic basis of this barrier involves several factors.

The tight junctions between the surface epithelial cells seal off the paracellular route for transport between cells. Transport can also occur across the bilipid layer membrane at the apical surface of the mucosal epithelial cells. The fluidity of this membrane can vary and influence permeability to various macromolecules. While there is active and passive transport of H^+, Na^+ and K^+ ions, an electric potential difference exists across the mucosa. With disruption of this barrier, a fall in potential difference occurs.

In the presence of luminal acid, the gastroduodenal pH approaches pH 2, while the immediately adjacent epithelium may be near neutral (pH 7). This pH gradient, which plays some role in protection from acid-peptic digestion, is probably dependent on the combined secretion of mucus and bicarbonate. How the gastric mucosa secretes acid while maintaining a near-neutral pH adjacent to the surface epithelium requires elucidation.

Gastric mucus consists of about 95% water and 5% glycoprotein. It provides lubrication for food particles and its gel-like nature retains water and bicarbonate close to the surface epithelium. Mucus is secreted by exocytosis, apical expulsion and exfoliation, and formed with bicarbonate in the surface epithelial cells, in the epithelial cells of the gastric gland neck and by the Brunner's glands of the duodenum. The mucus layer varies in thickness but averages about 100 μm. The role of mucus in protection against acid-peptic activity is unclear. It does provide a relatively thick unstirred layer adjacent to the mucosa, allowing a rate of diffusion of H^+ ions four times slower than through a similar thickness of unstirred water. This contributes to the maintenance of a hydrogen ion gradient between the gastric lumen and the surface epithelium. That is, when the pH in the gastric lumen is 2, the pH at the gastric membrane will be 6.8 to 7. ASA and nonsteroidal anti-inflammatory agents inhibit mucus synthesis and release, while prostaglandins increase mucus synthesis. Mucus synthesis is decreased after stress and may play a role in stress ulceration. Mucus limits the diffusion of pepsin and other large molecules, thus preventing further injury.

Bicarbonate secretion is an active process dependent on the metabolic integrity of a healthy epithelium. Secretion is stimulated by acetylcholine, prostaglandins, glucagon and cyclic GMP, and inhibited by α-adrenergic agonists and GIP. Luminal acid also appears to stimulate gastric and duodenal bicarbonate secretion. Low concentrations of bile salts in the stomach inhibit gastric bicarbonate secretion.

Prostaglandins probably play an important role in mucosal defense. These saturated, oxygenated fatty acids are derived from arachidonic acid. They may protect the mucosa by maintaining or increasing gastric mucosal blood flow and hence stimulating mucus production and bicarbonate secretion, and increasing protein synthesis (which is necessary for the maintenance and regeneration of cells). It is not known whether prostaglandins play a role in the maintenance of normal membrane function and tight junctions, but they probably maintain sulfhydryl groups, which act as oxidative scavengers. The development of gastritis and gastric ulcer is thought to arise as a result of defective defense mechanisms. There may be increased degradation of mucus by pepsinogen 1, bile or pancreatic secretions; by infection with H. pylori; or through mechanical factors. A quantitatively or qualitatively defective secretion of mucus is also possible. Bicarbonate secretion may be reduced or mucosal blood flow and/or mucosal metabolism compromised, as occurs in stress ulceration.

3.4 Gastric Endocrine Secretion

The stomach produces regulatory peptides, including gastrin and somatostatin. Each agent is a polypeptide; gastrin is known to exist in multiple forms in the body. These peptides are produced by enterochromaffin cells of the gastric mucosa. The cell that produces gastrin is called the "G cell" and is found in large numbers in the antral mucosa.

Gastrin is the most important peptide in the regulation of gastric acid secretion. Under physiologic conditions gastrin is released continually, with increased amounts appearing in the blood at mealtimes. Gastrin is a hormone that increases the rate of oxyntic cell secretion of H^+ and peptic cell secretion of pepsinogen. Gastrin increases contraction of antral smooth muscle and increases mucosal blood flow. Gastrin secretion is increased in the presence of H. pylori infection, and this is associated with an increase in the AUC (area under the concentration curve) for gastrin (see Section 8.2.3.1).

Extragastric actions of gastrin include contraction of the lower esophageal sphincter, stimulation of pancreatic enzyme secretion, gallbladder contraction, increased small intestine motility, and the regulation of glucose-stimulated insulin release. Gastrin is a trophic hormone that stimulates protein synthesis and growth of certain gastrointestinal tissues, such as the mucosal lining of the stomach and gut, and the parenchyma of the pancreas.

Somatostatin inhibits the release of gastrin from the G cells, probably acting as a paracrine substance. H. pylori infection is associated with inhibition of somatostatin release from the gastric D cells. Thus the brake to gastrin release from the G cells is lost and gastrin secretion continues unimpeded.

In addition, the nerves of the gastric mucosa contain vasoactive intestinal peptide (VIP) and gastrin-releasing peptide (GRP or bombesin). VIP is probably responsible for mediating the relaxation of gastric smooth muscle. Bombesin mediates the release of gastrin in response to vagal stimulation.

3.5 Assessment of Gastric Acid Secretion

Basal acid output (BAO) refers to the quantity of hydrochloric acid (HCl) secreted per hour by the stomach in the unstimulated basal state, expressed in milliequivalents of HCl per hour. The normal range is 1–5 mEq of HCl per hour. The acid output is the product of the volume of gastric juices (in liters) multiplied by the concentration of hydrogen ion (in milliequivalents per liter).

Maximal acid output refers to the total acid output during the hour after stimulation with pentagastrin (6 μg/kg IM or SC) or histamine (40 μg/kg SC). This value is determined by adding the results of either four 15-minute or six 10-minute sample collections after stimulation. The normal range is 25–55 mEq HCl per hour.

Peak acid output reflects the two highest consecutive 15-minute periods of stimulated output, multiplied by a factor of 2 to yield a value for a one-hour output.

Gastric secretory studies may be useful in patients with suspected gastric hypersecretion and in the evaluation of the efficacy of medical and surgical therapy in the reduction of gastric acid output. In suspected Zollinger-Ellison syndrome, elevated basal hypersecretion may point to the diagnosis, but usually gastric acid secretory studies are more useful in establishing the therapeutic response to acid-suppressive pharmacotherapy.

4. PATHOPHYSIOLOGY OF PEPTIC ULCER DISEASE

4.1 Gastric Ulcer Disease

Acute ulcers may occur in patients with burns (Curling's ulcer), midbrain disease (Cushing's ulcer) and chronic debilitating disease. ASA-containing analgesics and nonsteroidal anti-inflammatory drugs may also induce acute ulcer bleeding. There is epidemiologic evidence suggesting that the incidence and behavior of chronic peptic ulcers vary according to the site at which they occur. Therefore, gastric and duodenal ulcers will be considered separately, although the basic defects that cause either relate to an imbalance of aggressive and protective factors.

Numerous pathophysiologic defects have been identified in gastric ulcer disease (Table 2A). Not all of these factors are present in each patient. These defects include decreased acid secretion, decreased parietal cell mass and back-diffusion of acid. Many patients with chronic gastric ulcers have associated gastritis. There may be increased concentration of bile acids and pancreatic juice in the stomach as a result of duodenogastric reflux. Delayed gastric emptying has also been identified in some patients with gastric ulcers, and this may accentuate the release of gastrin and the secretion of hydrochloric acid. It has yet to be determined whether delayed gastric emptying is one causative factor or a secondary effect of gastric ulcer disease. However, as a result of

TABLE 2.   Pathophysiologic defects in some patients with:

A. *Peptic ulcer disease/gastric ulcer disease*
Decreased acid secretion, decreased parietal cell mass (PCM), back-diffusion of acid
Chronic superficial and atrophic gastritis
Increased concentration of bile acids and pancreatic juice in stomach (duodenogastric reflux)
Delayed gastric emptying
Inappropriately decreased pyloric sphincter pressure under basal conditions and in response to
    acid (secretin) or fat (cholecystokinin) in the duodenum

B. *Duodenal ulcer disease*
Increased parietal cell mass
Increased sensitivity of parietal cells to gastrin and secretagogues
Increased secretory drive
Decreased acid-induced inhibition of meal-stimulated gastrin release
Increased gastric emptying
Increased duodenal acid/pepsin loads
Chronic active gastritis

---

back-diffusion of acid, the actual concentration of acid in the gastric lumen may be underestimated. Hypergastrinemia and hyperchloremia are less commonly associated with gastric ulcers. The pressure of the pyloric sphincter may be inappropriately decreased under basal conditions and may fail to respond normally to acid or fat in the duodenum, thereby predisposing to duodenogastric reflux.

4.2 Duodenal Ulcer Disease (Figure 4)

A number of pathophysiologic defects have also been identified in some patients with duodenal ulcer disease (Table 2B). These include increased parietal cell mass (leading to increased maximal and peak acid output); increased sensitivity of the parietal cells to gastrin; increased secretory drive; decreased acid-induced inhibition of meal-stimulated gastrin release; and increased gastric emptying (leading to increased duodenal acid and pepsin loads).

In duodenal ulcer patients the gastric mucosa usually shows antral gastritis owing to H. pylori infection, and an increased parietal cell population (and possibly G-cell hyperplasia). By contrast, in gastric ulcer the nonparietal mucosal area is usually increased, especially on the lesser curvature, and there is histologic pangastritis. Biliary reflux back through the pylorus is also a common finding in patients with gastric ulcers, and the combination of bile and acid may be particularly damaging to the mucosa, probably by causing back-diffusion of hydrogen ions and thus disrupting intracellular organelles.

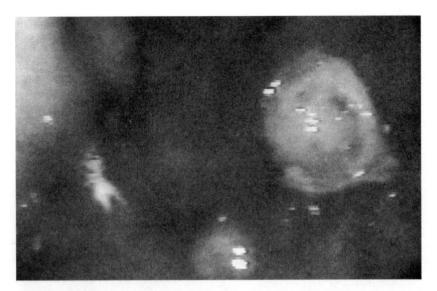

Figure 4.   Duodenal ulcer, posterior wall.

4.3 Hereditary Factors

Hereditary factors are important in the pathogenesis of peptic ulcer disease, as suggested by a higher prevalence of peptic ulcer disease in certain genetic syndromes. A number of familial aggregations have been noted in patients with peptic ulcer disease. These include hyperpepsinogenemia 1, normal pepsinogenemia 1, antral G-cell hyperfunction, rapid gastric emptying, childhood duodenal ulcer and immunologic forms of peptic ulcer disease. Heredity also plays a role in the development of ulceration and is associated with the syndrome of multiple endocrine adenomatosis 1 (adenomas of the pancreas, pituitary and parathyroid). Parents, siblings and children of ulcer patients are more likely to have peptic ulcer disease than control individuals. There is greater concordance for ulcer disease in identical than in fraternal twins. Hyperpepsinogenemia 1 appears to be an autosomal dominant trait. Families have been described in which a number of physiologic abnormalities associated with the development of ulcer disease have been noted, including increased meal-stimulated gastrin release and altered gastric emptying. There is increasing evidence to suggest that familial peptic ulcer disease is related to H. pylori infection amongst family members.

4.4 Interplay of H. pylori Infection, Acid, Pepsin and Other Factors

Peptic ulcer disease is thought to occur as a result of an interplay between H.

TABLE 3.   Environmental factors in pathogenesis of peptic ulcer disease (PUD)

Infection Helicobacter pylori
Drugs NSAIDs
Smoking Prevalence of PUD Healing of duodenal ulcer (DU) and gastric ulcer (GU) Death rates from PUD
Alcohol and caffeine-containing beverages Acid secretion

pylori infection, other environmental factors, inflammation, and changes in acid and pepsin. Peptic ulcers occur more commonly in the duodenum and less commonly in the stomach and esophagus. They usually occur near mucosal junctions. Rarely, peptic ulcers occur in the jejunum; this should raise the possibility of the Zollinger-Ellison syndrome. When gastric mucosa is present in a Meckel's diverticulum in the ileum, peptic ulceration and bleeding can occur. The ulceration occurs in the ileum adjacent to the diverticulum.

4.5 The Patient and the Environment
When considering the pathogenesis of any disease, we need to examine environmental factors, hereditary associations and pathophysiologic abnormalities. Environmental factors (Table 3) that have been examined include H. pylori infection, drugs, smoking, alcohol, caffeine-containing beverages and stress. Of these, H. pylori infection is the most important. Nonsteroidal antiinflammatory agents such as ASA are also thought to cause ulceration, mostly as a result of damage to the protective mucosal barrier. Smoking is associated with a higher prevalence of peptic ulcer disease and may be associated with impaired healing of duodenal and gastric ulcer disease. Also, death rates from peptic ulcer disease are higher in individuals who smoke. Alcohol and caffeine-containing beverages may affect acid secretion, and have been considered in the pathogenesis of peptic ulcer disease. However, it is fair to say that the role of coffee, alcohol, nonsteroidal anti-inflammatory agents and corticosteroids in the pathogenesis of peptic ulcer disease remains unclear.

Both patients and physicians often express the concern that "stress" is important in the initiation or perpetuation of peptic ulcer disease. Some patients with duodenal ulcer disease may have an exaggerated sense of self-sufficiency and demonstrate overambitiousness and aggressiveness. Some psychiatric views suggest that these attitudes represent a defense against an awareness of dependency. It is possible but unproven that patients exposed to excess stress may have more frequent ulceration, may be more sensitive to the symptoms of peptic ulcer disease, and may be more likely to develop perforations. This could be explained by a reduction in immunity to H. pylori infection occurring as a result of stress and immune factors being "overwhelmed." This hypothesis has not been tested as yet.

Recent studies from Israel and the United States have identified a number of other predictors of duodenal ulcer disease in men. These include psychosocial and biological factors. The important psychosocial factors include anxiety – stress, brooding (i.e., difficulty coping and difficulty expressing emotions) and inadequate caring, particularly lack of family support. Biological factors include age, lower blood pressure, use of cigarettes and leanness.

4.6 The Molecular Level

At a molecular level, the pathogenesis of ulcer disease reflects an imbalance between increased aggressive factors and decreased protective factors. In considering the possible aggressive factors, we need to review the normal mechanism of acid secretion. Acid secretion is considered under the cephalic, gastric and intestinal phases. As a result of vagal stimulation arising from the sight, smell, taste or thought of food, acetylcholine is released and acts on the parietal cells to produce acid. In addition, vagal afferents stimulate the antral G cells to release gastrin. Food in the stomach gives rise to antral distention, and this along with peptide breakdown products also stimulates the antral G cells to produce gastrin. In the presence of H. pylori infection these effects are exaggerated. The gastrin and acetylcholine act directly on the parietal cells or the mast cells. The mast cells in turn release histamine, which stimulates gastric acid secretion.

Once acid secretion has been initiated, how is further acid secretion limited? Clearly, there will be loss of vagal stimulation, loss of antral distention and loss of stimulated release of gastrin as food is virtually digested and emptied from the stomach into the duodenum. Also, the acid released from the parietal cells acidifies the antrum and thereby inhibits the further release of gastrin. This inhibitory mechanism is compromised in the presence of H. pylori infection. The presence of food in the intestine further stimulates the release of a number of gastrointestinal hormones (including secretin, somatostatin, GIP and VIP) that inhibit the secretion of acid by parietal cells.

In health, a basal acid output obtained under unstimulated conditions is 5–10 mmol/hr. Following the administration of 6 mg/kg of pentagastrin, the parietal cell mass will be stimulated to produce hydrochloric acid. The maximal acid output will be less than 35 mmol/hr, and the peak acid output will be less than 60 mmol/hr. In health, the ratio of basal to maximum acid output or basal to peak acid output will be less than 0.25. The peak or maximum acid output reflects the parietal cell mass, whereas the ratio of BAO/PAO reflects the parietal cell function under basal conditions.

In disease, acid secretion may change. With gastric atrophy, most often due to H. pylori infection and pangastritis, both the basal and stimulated acid outputs are reduced. Peak acid output is increased in approximately one-half of patients with duodenal ulcer disease, whereas in patients with the Zollinger-Ellison syndrome, the major change is in the increased basal acid output. In patients with gastric ulcers, basal and peak acid output are usually normal or reduced. It must be stressed that this represents the acid measured in the gastric lumen and does not necessarily reflect the acid-secreting ability of the parietal cells in patients with gastric ulcer disease. That is, as a result of associated gastritis and back-diffusion of acid, these patients may secrete normal amounts of acid, which then diffuse back into the parietal cell. Therefore, the amount of acid measured in the gastric lumen would be normal or reduced.

Gastrin, histamine, acetylcholine and unspecified inhibitors influence the gastric secretory drive. Gastrin concentrations may be increased physiologically following food intake, with an increase of less than 100% above basal or fasting values. Secretory drive may be increased in the Zollinger-Ellison syndrome, G-cell hyperplasia or retained antrum. In the short bowel syndrome, temporary gastric hypersecretion may occur. The pathogenesis of this abnormality is unknown, and may relate to the loss of gastrin inhibitory factor in the small bowel. Gastrin levels are commonly increased in H. pylori infection, renal failure and pernicious anemia, and more rarely in diabetes mellitus and rheumatoid arthritis. In the latter two conditions, it is presumed that the gastrin levels are increased as a result of hypochlorhydria.

Once the stimulants of acid secretion (gastrin and acetylcholine) have been released, parietal cells are stimulated to secrete acid. The receptor for acetylcholine and gastrin may be on the mast cells, which are then stimulated to release histamine, which acts directly on the parietal cells to produce acid. Alternatively, there may be three separate receptors on the parietal cell: those for gastrin, acetylcholine and histamine. The histamine acts on adenylate cyclase in the parietal cell membrane to increase the production of cyclic AMP. In the presence of calcium, a protein kinase is stimulated, which then acts on the H^+/K^+-ATPase to secrete hydrochloric acid. This H^+/K^+-ATPase is known as the "proton pump." It represents the final common pathway for hydrogen ion secretion. Acetylcholine may act on the mast cells to release histamine, but may also act on the parietal cells to increase the influx of calcium ions, which then stimulate the protein kinase. The intracellular mechanism of gastric-mediated acid secretion is not known, although gastrin may stimulate the mast cells to release histamine, which further stimulates acid secretion. This discussion of the mechanism of acid secretion provides the basis for understanding the pathogenesis of peptic ulcer disease. The parietal cell mass may be increased, and this may be reflected by an increase in the peak acid output or in serum pepsinogen 1. Secretory drive may be increased, and this is reflected by an increase in the ratio of BAO/PAO. Stimulated secretion is abnormal, as reflected by an increased parietal cell sensitivity to gastrin and possibly to histamine. Finally, the acid load in the duodenum is increased (as a result of increased acid secretion, as well as an increased rate of gastric emptying) in duodenal ulcer disease.

4.7 Diagnosis

Radiology for the diagnosis of peptic ulcer disease should be replaced by upper gastrointestinal endoscopy (esophagogastroduodenoscopy, or EGD) because of its greater sensitivy and specificity. A chronic lesser-curve ulcer is usually seen as a distinct niche or pocket of barium projecting out from the line of the barium-filled stomach. The crater has a clean, smooth outline, and often its upper part contains a fluid level between the barium below and gastric juice or gas above. A posterior-wall gastric ulcer is often best seen *en face* as a barium-filled niche after a small amount of the barium suspension has been drunk, and when the abdomen has been compressed. A spastic notch on the greater curvature opposite the ulcer is a common feature of chronic gastric ulcer. Occasionally, a gross horizontal fibrous contracture in association with long-standing ulceration can cause a permanent hourglass constriction, or the lesser curvature can shorten longitudinally. Antral or prepyloric ulcers present special diagnostic difficulties to the radiologist, because the associated spasm or inflammatory swelling cannot always be distinguished from the appearance of gastric cancer. Greater-curvature ulceration is uncommon, and is seldom malignant. Lesser-curvature ulcers above the angulus can usually confidently be separated from malignant disease by their regularity and relative absence of mucosal distortion within the line of the barium-filled viscus (except by the classical appearances of fibrous contracture). The size of a gastric ulcer is not a guide to the presence of malignancy or to the severity of symptoms; furthermore, large gastric ulcers often respond better to medical treatment than small ones (Figure 5A, 5B).

The radiologic diagnosis of duodenal ulcer is complicated by the problem of distinguishing simple deformity (scarring) in the duodenal bulb (due to previous and now healed ulceration) from deformity with active ulceration. Ulceration in an undeformed cap is relatively uncommon. It may be seen either as a niche in profile on one border of the bulb (Figure 6A, 6B) or *en*

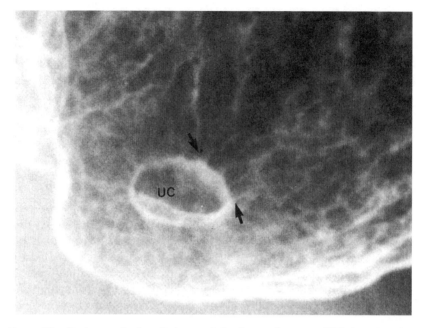

FIGURE 5A.   Benign gastric ulcer. Barium meal showing an ulcer crater (UC) situated on the greater curvature of the stomach, in the gastric antrum. The ulcer is visualized *en face* with a slightly oblique projection. Smooth mucosal folds radiating from the edge of the crater (arrows) in a regular fashion are a pathognomonic sign of a benign gastric ulcer. (Courtesy of Dr. J. Rawlinson.)

face through the bulb when the bulb contains a small quantity of barium suspension and is compressed or examined in air contrast films (e.g., in a posterior view with the patient lying slightly on the left side). Scarring of the bulb can induce a number of deformities, such as trefoil deformity following ulceration at the base of the bulb, and pseudodiverticulum formation. A minority of ulcers occur in the immediate postbulbar region of the duodenum. Close attention to this region is needed if they are to be found.

4.8 Endoscopy

Modern fiberoptic instruments used in endoscopic examination have greatly increased its safety and diagnostic range, and the patient's comfort. The available instruments are either end- or side-viewing. The former are good general-purpose instruments that allow an adequate view of the esophagus, stomach and upper duodenum. Distal duodenal lesions can be viewed using an enteroscope or pediatric colonoscope through the upper gastrointestinal tract.

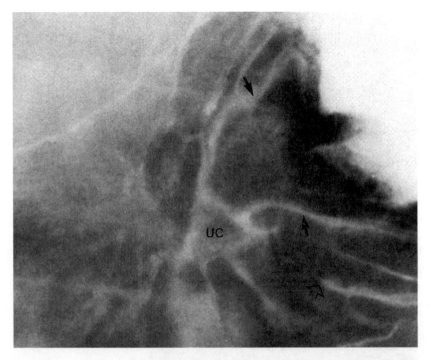

FIGURE 5B. Malignant gastric ulcer. Barium meal demonstrating an ulcer crater (UC) on the lesser curvature of the stomach, also visualized *en face*. In this case the radiating mucosal folds are irregularly thickened (e.g., between closed arrows) and do not extend to the edge of the crater (open arrow) – features indicating a local infiltrative, malignant process. (Courtesy of Dr. J. Rawlinson.)

The presence of H. pylori can be determined noninvasively using serology for IgG, or by a ^{13}C or ^{14}C urea breath test, or with endoscopic biopsy using urease testing and histology demonstrating inflammation and the presence of H. pylori. The absence of chronic inflammation excludes H. pylori infection. Culture is specific but not sensitive for diagnosis, but is useful in determining antibiotic sensitivities and resistance. Several medications, including acid or proton pump inhibitors (e.g., omeprazole, lansoprazole, pantoprazole), bismuth and antibiotics, suppress H. pylori and can contribute to false-negative tests. (See also Section 8.2.3.1.)

4.9 Therapy of Peptic Ulcer Disease

The treatment and eradication of H. pylori infection is the first choice in the therapy of peptic ulcer disease. Eradication of H. pylori leads to the cure of peptic ulcer – i.e., ulcer healing without relapse or recurrence. Currently, the

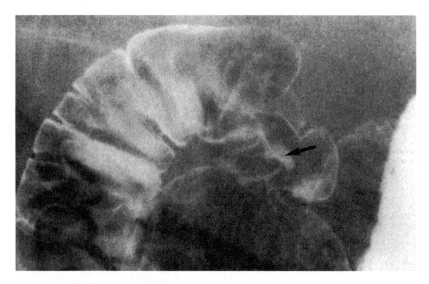

FIGURE 6A.   Duodenal ulcer. Situated at the base of the duodenal cap, the ulcer crater is filled with barium (arrow). The surrounding inflammatory process has considerably distorted the normal bulbar configuration of the proximal duodenum. (Courtesy of Dr. J. Rawlinson.)

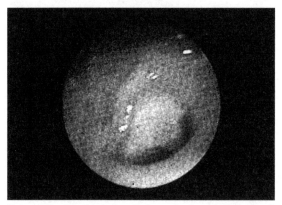

FIGURE 6B.   Duodenal ulcer. Endoscopic view of the duodenal cap ulcer.

best treatment combinations achieve eradication of H. pylori in 85–95% of patients. The most effective regimens combine twice-daily proton pump inhibitors (PPI) with clarithromycin and either metronidazole (PCM) or amoxicillin (PCA) for one week. Either omeprazole 20 mg b.i.d., lansoprazole

TABLE 4. H. pylori treatments of choice

PCA:	PPI	+ clarithromycin 500 mg bid
		+ amoxicillin 1 g bid
PCM:	PPI	+ clarithromycin 500 mg bid
		+ metronidazole 500 mg po bid

All medication given for 7 days
PPI = omeprazole 20 mg bid, lansoprazole 30 mg bid or pantoprazole 40 mg bid

TABLE 5. H. pylori alternative therapy

PBMT:	PPI	+ bismuth subsalicylate 2 tablets qid
		+ metronidazole 250 mg qid
		+ tetracycline 500 mg qid

All medication given for 7 days

RBC (ranitidine bismuth citrate):   RBC 400 mg bid   + clarithromycin 250 mg qid
                                                                    or clarithromycin 500 mg qid

All medication given for 14 days
PPI = omeprazole 20 mg bid, lansoprazole 30 mg bid or pantoprazole 40 mg bid
PBMT = PPI (P); bismuth (B); metronidazole (M); tetracycline (T)

30 mg b.i.d. or pantoprazole 40 mg b.i.d. can be selected as the PPI (Table 4). A one-week course results in cost-effective eradication.

A recommended alternative therapy is one week PPI with bismuth triple therapy (Table 5). Unfortunately this regimen requires 18 pills each day with a difficult q.i.d. dosing. Eradication rates are comparable. Another alternative therapy is a two-week course of ranitidine bismuth citrate (RBC) 400 mg b.i.d. combined with clarithromycin 250 mg or 500 mg b.i.d., achieving eradication rates of 70–82%. The most frequent side effects include taste disturbance, diarrhea, pseudomembranous colitis and vaginal candidiasis. Amoxicillin should not be used in patients with an allergy to penicillins. Metronidazole should not be taken with alcohol, as serious disulfiram-like or hypertensive effects can occur.

What is the practical approach to the management of patients with ulcer disease? A consensus is growing for a "test and treat" approach in the management of peptic ulcer disease. That is, in patients with active peptic ulcer or

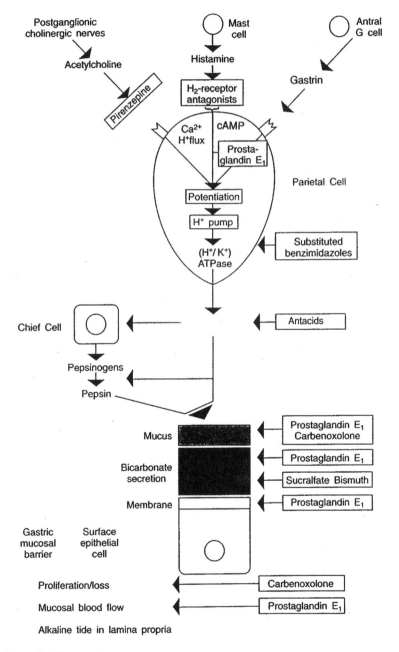

FIGURE 7.   Therapeutic intervention in a pathophysiologic scheme.

proven past peptic ulcer, H. pylori infection is confirmed and eradication treatment is prescribed. Additionally, patients with proven ulcer disease on maintenance therapy or with ulcer complications should be treated.

The need for proof of eradication remains controversial. It is likely not necessary to retest, as the efficacy of antibiotic regimens approaches 85–95% (see Table 12). Reinfection rates in adults are less than 1% annually.

4.10 Test and Treat Approach

The consensus approach to the treatment of peptic ulcer disease is to test for H. pylori and if positive, treat with an H. pylori eradication regimen. The peptic ulcer will heal with eradication of H. pylori with no further therapy required. With antibiotic treatment regimen efficacy in the range of 85%–95%, retesting will be helpful in only 5–15% of cases (see Section 4.9).

Recurrent or refractory ulcers and ulcers complicated by bleeding, obstruction or perforation should be retested before maintenance therapy with antisecretory drugs is discontinued. Bleeding ulcers will not recur with successful eradication of H. pylori. Recurrent or refractory ulcers that remain H. pylori–positive after a breath test should be re-treated with an alternative regimen. H. pylori testing and treatment is recommended for active gastric or duodenal ulcers, proven past ulcers, proven ulcers on maintenance therapy, ulcer complications and MALT (mucosa-associated lymphoid tissue) lymphoma.

4.10.1 *PROTON PUMP INHIBITORS (PPIs)*

PPIs (omeprazole, lansoprazole, pantoprazole, rabeprazole) are substituted benzimidazoles that are acid labile and can be inactivated if dissolved in gastric juice (Figure 7). These prodrugs are enteric-coated, permitting dissolution and subsequent absorption in the small bowel at a pH above 6. PPIs are secreted in the stomach and activated by gastric acid, with the activated molecule inhibiting the H^+K^+-ATPase enzyme of the parietal cell and thus inhibiting acid secretion. There is some minor variability in the pharmacokinetics of the various PPIs, although the clinical effectiveness of these agents remains comparable. These drugs are metabolized hepatically with varying affinity for clearance by the cytochrome P-450 enzyme system (pantoprazole and rabeprazole have least affinity). PPIs have an excellent safety profile. The effects of prolonged acid inhibition, including hypergastrinemia and hyperplasia of enterochromaffin-like (ECL) cells, appear inconsequential, similar to the effects of H_2-receptor antagonists.

TABLE 6.   Side effects of anti-secretory therapy

	H_2 blockers	Proton pump inhibitors
CNS	Confusion, dizziness	Headache
CVS	Bradycardia	—
Endocrine	Gynecomastia	Gynecomastia
	Antiandrogenic	
	Prolactinemia	
Blood	Neutropenia	—
	Immune system	
Liver	Blood flow	Hepatitis
	Increased serum transaminases	
	Cytochrome P-450 (cimetidine)	
Kidney	Increased plasma creatinine	—
	(1–2% of patients)	
Intestine	Diarrhea	Nausea, diarrhea, constipation
Skin	Rash	Rash, alopecia, urticaria
Muscle	Pain	Pain

4.10.2 H_2-RECEPTOR ANTAGONISTS

Cimetidine, ranitidine, famotidine and nizatidine inhibit acid secretion by blocking H_2-receptors on the parietal cell. They are well absorbed after oral dosing, with peak concentrations occurring 1 to 3 hours after dosing. They all cross the blood–brain and placental barrier and are excreted in breast milk. All four drugs are eliminated by a combination of hepatic and renal metabolism excretion. They are safe and well tolerated (see Table 6 for a list of side effects).

4.10.3   SUCRALFATE

Sucralfate is a sulfated polysaccharide, sucrose octasulfate complexed with aluminum hydroxide. It can prevent acute, chemically induced mucosal injury and heal chronic ulcers without buffering or altering gastric acid or pepsin secretion. Sucralfate stimulates angiogenesis and granulation tissue formation, probably by binding epidermal growth factor. Sucralfate binds to injured tissue, providing some protection from the inurious effects of acid and pepsin. It can suppress but not kill H. pylori. Sucralfate is safe, with minimal side effects, but can bind other drugs if taken simultaneously, although clinical consequences are insignificant.

4.11   General Recommendations

What therapeutic recommendations can be made? The proportion of patients whose ulcers heal after six weeks of cimetidine, ranitidine, sucralfate or pros-

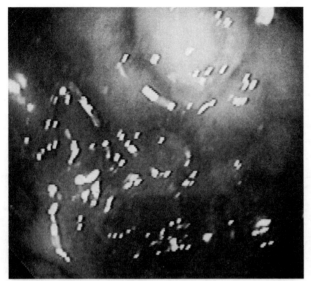

FIGURE 8. Pylorus – pre-dilation.

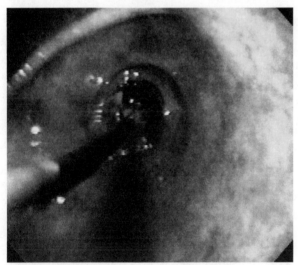

FIGURE 9. Pyloric dilation.

taglandin is comparable. Recommendations must therefore be made on other factors, including convenience, side effects, cost and maintenance of healing. Liquid antacids are inconvenient to take, and patient compliance is poor. Side

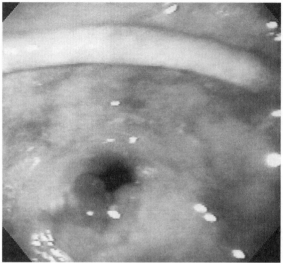

FIGURE 10. Pylorus – post-dilation.

effects from the anticholinergics are frequent, and cimetidine should be avoided in the older patient or in the individual taking multiple drugs. A therapeutic dose of each of these agents – that is, a dose necessary to obtain ulcer healing – is comparable and expensive (about $60 to heal an ulcer).

Peptic ulcer disease has a natural history of recurrence. Once an ulcer has healed, there is a 75% chance that the ulcer will recur in 12 months; 50% will be symptomatic, whereas 25% will be asymptomatic. H. pylori is associated with an antral gastritis seen in 95% of duodenal ulcer patients. Eradication of H. pylori infection associated with duodenal ulcer disease through antibiotic therapy eliminates ulcer recurrence in the majority of cases (see Sections 4.9, 4.10 and 8.2.3).

Complications of peptic ulcer disease such as pyloric stenosis can be treated with endoscopic balloon dilation (Figures 8–10).

4.12 Failure of Medical Therapy

The eradication of H. pylori in the treatment of peptic ulcer has profoundly influenced the natural history of ulcer recurrence. Previously, 50–100% of ulcers recurred after having been healed. After H. pylori eradication peptic ulcer does not recur, except in cases of treatment failure. In these cases, maintenance with antisecretory therapy, such as a PPI, may be necessary.

An additional rare cause of failure of medical therapy and failure of ulcer

TABLE 7. Causes of hypergastrinemia

With acid hypersecretion
Gastrinoma
Isolated retained gastric antrum
Antral G-cell hyperplasia
Massive small bowel resection
Pyloric outlet obstruction
Hyperparathyroidism

With variable acid secretion
Hyperthyroidism
Chronic renal failure
Pheochromocytoma

With acid hyposecretion
Atrophic gastritis
Pernicious anemia
Gastric cancer
Postvagotomy and pyloroplasty

---

healing is the presence of a hypersecretory state, possibly due to hypergastrinemia. It is disputed whether G-cell hyperplasia occurs in patients with duodenal ulcer disease. Clearly, however, a small proportion of patients with ulcer disease would have a hypersecretory state due to the presence of a gastrinoma (which will lead to basal and/or stimulated hypergastrinemia). Other conditions leading to basal hypergastrinemia include retained antrum, pyloric obstruction, pernicious anemia, hypercalcemia, renal failure, massive small bowel resection and portacaval anastomoses (Table 7). Peptic ulcer disease does not occur in patients with pernicious anemia, because they lack parietal cells. However, these other conditions associated with basal hypergastrinemia may also be associated with hyperchlorhydria and associated peptic ulcer disease. It is unclear whether hypergastrinemia also occurs in patients with diabetes mellitus or rheumatoid arthritis.

For the complications of hemorrhage, obstruction, perforation or intractability, surgery may be necessary. There is no consensus regarding the procedure of choice, but generally some form of vagotomy (e.g., truncal, selective or parietal cell) with a drainage procedure (pyloroplasty or antrectomy) is advised. It is not clear that patients who have failed H. pylori eradication will respond well to a surgical procedure to reduce acid secretion.

In general, a vagotomy is performed with a gastric draining procedure (pyloroplasty/gastroenterostomy) and/or a gastric resection to avoid gastric

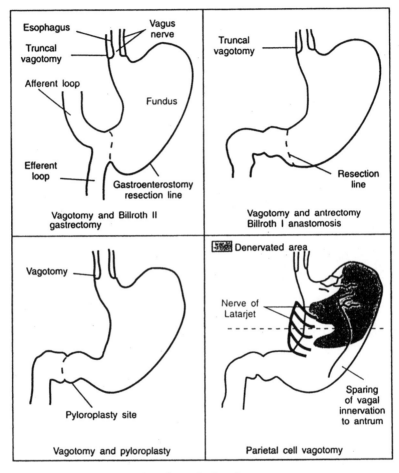

FIGURE 11.   Some surgical procedures for peptic ulcer disease.

stasis (Figure 11). Three forms of vagotomy are in vogue: truncal, selective and parietal cell. A Billroth I or Billroth II anastomosis may also be performed, particularly when the antrum or portions of the body of the stomach are resected. A drainage procedure is needed to avoid the gastric atony resulting from the vagotomy and associated delayed gastric emptying.

4.13 Gastrinoma

The Zollinger-Ellison (ZE) syndrome is characterized by autonomous gastrin production by an adenoma or adenocarcinoma of the pancreas or duodenum.

Patients may present either with severe acute ulcer disease or recurrent ulcer disease; the ulcers will often occur in unusual sites and be associated with diarrhea. The Zollinger-Ellison syndrome is distinguished from peptic ulcer disease by the demonstration of fasting hypergastrinemia. There are many causes of fasting hypergastrinemia (gastritis, vagotomy and pyloroplasty, the short bowel syndrome, rheumatoid arthritis, retained antrum, G-cell hyperplasia), but only two conditions – atrophic gastritis and renal failure – are associated with gastrin levels increased several times above the upper limit of the normal range. However, in a patient with peptic ulcer disease and hypergastrinemia, it is important to exclude the Zollinger-Ellison syndrome. Gastric analysis may be helpful: the finding of a dramatically increased basal output relative to a modestly increased maximal acid output (i.e., BAO/MAO greater than 0.6) is suggestive of this syndrome. Ingestion of a protein-containing meal normally produces a doubling of the gastrin concentration (a.c. versus p.c.), but an exaggerated response is seen in G-cell hyperplasia rather than in gastrinoma syndrome. Infusion of calcium intravenously results in an increase in gastrin concentration in normal individuals and an exaggeration of this response in patients with the Zollinger-Ellison syndrome. However, the most useful diagnostic test is the secretin infusion. In normal individuals or those with G-cell hyperplasia, injection of secretin results in a rapid decline in plasma gastrin concentrations, whereas in patients with the Zollinger-Ellison syndrome, the gastrin concentration will increase in response to secretin.

The Zollinger-Ellison syndrome arises from a gastrinoma, a tumor in the pancreas. This may be a localized or diffuse tumor. The presence of hypergastrinemia leads to hypersecretion; while the maximal acid output may be increased, the major defect is basal hypergastrinemia and a marked increase in the basal acid output. The patient will have aggressive peptic ulcer disease with ulceration in unusual sites, or multiple ulcers that fail to heal on medical therapy. Hypertrophic gastric folds and diarrhea may be prominent features (see Section 6.5). The presence of a gastrinoma should be suspected from the history, and confirmed with provocative tests. A protein meal will increase the serum gastrin concentration in patients with G-cell hyperplasia; a calcium infusion will markedly increase the gastrin concentration in patients with gastrinoma, and have a lesser effect in normal patients and patients with G-cell hyperplasia. The best test to diagnose a gastrinoma is a secretin test in which the basal gastrin concentration increases dramatically, in contrast to the reduction in gastrin concentration that occurs following secretin infusion in patients with G-cell hyperplasia or a normal stomach. A CT scan or an angiogram may be useful in identifying the gastrinoma, although these tumors are often small and difficult to identify. A laparotomy will be necessary to determine whether there is a localized tumor. Since one-half of these tumors are malignant, it is worthwhile to undertake surgery in the hope that resection of the tumor will produce a cure.

If the high dose of H_2-receptor antagonists does not sufficiently relieve the patient's pain, then nighttime anticholinergics can be used. A trial of parietal cell vagotomy is under way, but this is not yet accepted therapy.

5. POSTGASTRECTOMY PROBLEMS

Numerous problems follow peptic ulcer surgery, although these syndromes are less common now because of the effectiveness of modern pharmacotherapy over the past 25 years. These postgastrectomy problems may occur early after surgery or many months later. The early problems relate to the surgery itself. There are many late postgastrectomy syndromes (Table 8); these may be more disabling than the dyspeptic symptoms that led to the surgery in the first place.

5.1 Esophageal Symptoms
The incidence of gastroesophageal reflux after vagotomy or partial gastric resection is unknown, although it is a common symptom even in unoperated patients. The effect of vagotomy on lower esophageal sphincter pressure is uncertain, but operations involving mobilization and manipulation of the proximal stomach can damage the sphincter. Operations that involve the antrum and pylorus may allow duodenal juice to reflux into the stomach. From there it may enter and damage the esophagus, an additional factor that may contribute to therapeutic problems. Assessment of patients with symptoms of gastroesophageal reflux should include a barium swallow and endoscopy. If the patient's acid output is low, then the esophagitis may be due to the reflux of bile and pancreatic juice from the duodenum into the stomach and esophagus. If the bile-induced esophagitis does not respond to bile acid binding agents (cholestyramine, sucralfate, aluminum hydroxide antacid), then surgical revision with a Roux-en-Y anastomosis may be necessary.

One of the more troublesome postgastrectomy syndromes is that of dysphagia. This usually occurs in the early postoperative period. Although spontaneous improvement is the rule, occasionally esophagitis and stricture may occur. This dysphagia may result from trauma to the esophagus at the time of surgery, the development of a periesophageal hematoma, or a vagotomy.

5.2 Delayed Gastric Emptying
Delayed gastric emptying may result from recurrent ulceration, stomal edema, fibrosis or decreased gastric tone and motility, and may lead to bezoar

TABLE 8.   Complications of gastric surgery

Esophagus
Gastroesophageal reflux
Dysphagia

Stomach
Delayed gastric emptying
Bezoars
Outlet obstruction
Stomatitis
Recurrent ulcers
Stump carcinoma
Afferent loop syndrome

Small intestine
Diarrhea
   Dumping syndrome
   Bacterial contamination syndrome
   Unmasked celiac disease, unmasked pancreatic
      insufficiency or unmasked lactase deficiency
Weight loss and malabsorption
   Iron
   Folate
   Vitamin B_{12}
   Calcium
   Fats
Anemia

Gallbladder
Cholelithiasis

---

formation. The patient may suffer early satiety or postprandial fullness. Gastric bezoars are secretions of food or foreign material in the stomach. Vegetable bezoars are called phytobezoars; those composed of hair are called trichobezoars. These develop following antrectomy and vagotomy, and probably relate to inadequate chewing, hypochlorhydria, and a high-fiber diet. Bezoars may be suspected on plain film of the abdomen or upper GI series and may be confirmed at endoscopy. It is occasionally possible at endoscopy to fragment the bezoar, but therapy with papain (an enzyme that digests protein, and thus helps dissolve either type of bezoar) is usually necessary.

If stomal fibrosis is present, surgery is usually indicated. Intravenous therapy may be required if the obstruction is severe, but if the outlet is patent,

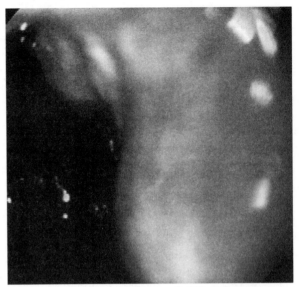

FIGURE 12.   Bleeding ulcer at the site of a Billroth II anastomosis.

metoclopramide or domperidone may improve gastric emptying. Alternatively it may be necessary to revise the surgical anastomosis.

5.3 Recurrent Ulcers

Ulcers that recur following gastric surgery bear many names (e.g., stomal ulceration, recurrent ulcers, postgastrectomy ulcers). These recurrent ulcers may be due to incomplete vagotomy, incomplete resection of G cells or acid-producing cells, retained antrum, delayed gastric emptying, duodenogastric reflux, ulcerogenic drugs or gastrinoma (Figure 12). Naturally, these benign conditions must be excluded from a stump ulcer. Recurrent ulceration with edema and partial obstruction may benefit from a trial of an H_2-receptor antagonist.

5.4 Carcinoma

Carcinoma of the gastric stump may develop 20 or more years following gastric surgery for benign peptic ulcer disease. Stump carcinoma appears to be more common following a Billroth II anastomosis. The carcinoma develops at the anastomosis, or in the gastric body or fundus. The pathogenesis is thought to be related to the development of chronic atrophic gastritis. Initially, there may be metaplasia of the Paneth's and goblet cells, and then subsequent dysplasia. These morphologic changes seem to relate to chronic bile and alkaline reflux.

5.5 Afferent Loop Syndrome

In patients with a gastrojejunostomy or a Billroth II anastomosis, obstruction of the afferent loop may occur. Symptoms may be acute or chronic and due to the presence of an internal hernia, kinking, the formation of adhesions or stenosis of the stoma. The acute afferent loop syndrome occurs in the early postoperative period. There may be partial or complete obstruction of the afferent loop, giving rise to pain, nausea, vomiting of nonbilious material, the palpation of an abdominal mass, and occasionally elevation in the serum amylase and liver function tests. The chronic afferent loop syndrome is due to partial obstruction of the afferent loop. The patient will complain of postprandial bilious vomiting without food. This vomiting will be intermittent, severe and painful.

5.6 Diarrhea

Diarrhea commonly occurs immediately after truncal vagotomy; various mechanisms have been suggested, including the dumping syndrome, the bacterial overgrowth syndrome, use of excessive amounts of magnesium-containing antacids, the Zollinger-Ellison syndrome, unmasked celiac disease, unmasked lactose intolerance and unmasked pancreatic insufficiency. Other causes of diarrhea seen in patients without previous gastric surgery or vagotomy also need to be considered.

Most cases of postvagotomy diarrhea improve with time. Antidiarrheal agents such as loperamide and diphenoxylate may improve symptoms; in those patients who do not respond, cholestyramine or antibiotics are sometimes helpful. More persistent diarrhea should be fully investigated to rule out infection, malabsorption or gastrin-secreting tumors. In extreme cases, surgical intervention may be necessary.

"Early dumping" occurs 10 to 20 minutes after meals and has three components: gastrointestinal, vasomotor and cardiovascular. The patient may develop pain, nausea, vomiting, fullness and diarrhea. Vasomotor symptoms include weakness, dizziness, faintness, pallor and sweating; cardiovascular symptoms include palpitations and tachycardia. The early dumping syndrome is caused by rapid emptying of gastric contents with osmotic fluid shifts, abdominal distention and release of vasoactive substances. The intestinal distention produces the pain, nausea and vomiting, whereas the vasomotor and cardiovascular symptoms are due to the release of serotonin and bradykinin.

The "late dumping" syndrome occurs 1 to 3 hours after meals, particularly meals containing large amounts of carbohydrate. The late dumping syndrome is characterized by evidence of sympathetic discharge due to hypoglycemia. These symptoms include weakness, sweating, hunger and confusion. The pathophysiologic basis for this dumping syndrome is straightforward: rapid gastric emptying, rapid absorption of glucose, release of large amounts of insulin, rapid decline in blood sugar levels due to the rapid cessation of glucose absorption, and excessively high insulin levels.

The dumping syndrome may be treated with dietary therapy: six small meals per day containing high-protein, low-carbohydrate foods, and the ingestion of liquids between rather than with meals. This is effective for most patients, but in some individuals anticholinergics will be necessary before meals, or the serotonin antagonist cyproheptadine may be prescribed. Tolbutamide or pectin may be useful in some individuals. When all else fails, a Billroth II anastomosis will need to be converted into a Billroth I. If the patient already has a Billroth I, then in rare cases an antiperistaltic loop of small bowel will need to be inserted.

5.7 Weight Loss and Malabsorption

Weight loss occurs after surgery in 30–60% of patients; it is less common with vagotomy alone than with vagotomy and antrectomy. The most common cause is decreased caloric intake because of early satiety, but in patients with severe malnutrition or persistent diarrhea, an investigation of malabsorption should be undertaken.

5.8 Anemia

Anemia is common following gastric surgery. Iron deficiency may be due to a preoperative iron deficiency, surgical blood loss inadequately replaced during or following surgery, postoperative GI or GU losses, or malabsorption of iron resulting from reduction in gastric acid (necessary for the absorption of food iron) or bypassing of the duodenum (the optimal site for the absorption of all forms of iron). In some patients, an associated malabsorption syndrome unmasked by the gastric surgery will result in folate deficiency from inadequate intake or malabsorption of folate. B_{12} deficiency may occur if a sufficient number of intrinsic-factor–producing cells have been resected. B_{12} deficiency may also occur if there is associated bacterial overgrowth syndrome, and rarely if there is pancreatic insufficiency. In patients with pernicious anemia, the urinary excretion of vitamin B_{12} (Schilling test) will increase to normal when the intrinsic factor is given together with a low dose of vitamin.

5.9 Cholelithiasis

Cholelithiasis occurs more frequently following a truncal than other types of vagotomy. The mechanism is thought to be decreased bile flow and gallblad-

TABLE 9. ABC classification of gastritis

Autoimmune	Congenital pernicious anemia
Bacterial	Helicobacter pylori
Chemical	Bile reflux
Drug-induced	NSAIDs, alcohol
Eosinophilic	Eosinophilic gastroenteritis
Follicular	Helicobacter pylori
Granulomatous	Tuberculosis, Crohn's disease
Hypertrophic	Ménétrier's disease

der contraction, associated with increased gallbladder size and the development of lithogenic bile.

6. GASTRITIS

6.1 Acute Gastritis

Acute infection with H. pylori causes a neutrophilic gastritis with transient hypochlorhydria manifesting clinically with a one- to four-day illness with mild to moderate epigastric pain, anorexia, nausea and/or vomiting. Acute gastritis can also be caused by irritation of the gastric mucosa by alcohol, corrosive poisons and the various bacterial and oral causes of food poisoning.

6.2 Chronic Gastritis

Three main types of gastritis are recognized by histological examination: superficial gastritis, atrophic gastritis and gastric atrophy. Chronic gastritis, most commonly due to infection with H. pylori, is characterized by mononuclear and polymorphonuclear cell infiltration of mucosa, glandular atrophy and intestinal metaplasia. In superficial gastritis inflammation is marked and glandular atrophy is minimal, whereas in gastric atrophy inflammatory cells are few and glandular atrophy is extensive. These represent different degrees of gastritis, though not necessarily all cases that progress to atrophy must be preceded by the two lesser lesions.

With progressive gastritis that involves the body and antrum, there is degeneration of the mucosa, and gastric secretion progressively fails. Hydrochloric acid secretion fails first, followed by pepsinogen secretion and finally by the secretion of intrinsic factor. As intrinsic factor secretion fails, the body becomes depleted of vitamin B_{12} and pernicious anemia develops. Antibodies to parietal cells and intrinsic factor appear in the serum. The presence of these

TABLE 10.   Causes of hypochlorhydria

Chronic gastritis (Table 9)
Gastric ulcer or cancer or polyposis
Resection

antibodies together with a partial response to steroids suggests that autoimmunity may play an etiologic role.

Chronic gastritis is most commonly due to H. pylori infection and aggravated by a combination of genetic and acquired factors (Table 9). Among the latter may be included repeated minor trauma due to alcohol and analgesics, reflux of duodenal contents and gastric irradiation. Deficiencies of vitamin B_{12}, folic acid and iron interfere with the regenerative and functional capacity of the gastric mucosa.

Predisposition to gastric cancer results from H. pylori infection. H. pylori has been designated a class I carcinogen because of its effect on gastric epithelial cellular degeneration and on development of gastric carcinoma. While most of the causes of hypochlorhydria are associated with gastritis, it remains disputed whether gastritis is necessarily associated with an increased risk of gastric cancer. Gastric cancer is 5 to 10 times as common as expected in those with chronic atrophic gastritis; the same increased incidence is also found in first-degree relatives of patients with gastric cancer and pernicious anemia.

It is uncertain whether chronic gastritis causes symptoms. Chronic gastritis can be diagnosed only by gastric biopsy of body or fundic mucosa, and H. pylori should be sought. Marked gastric hyposecretion or anacidity is present if the lesion is diffuse.

6.2.1 COMPLETE GASTRIC ATROPHY AND PERNICIOUS ANEMIA

There are many causes of hypochlorhydria (Table 10). The ability to produce acid, pepsin and intrinsic factor is lost altogether in patients with complete gastric atrophy as a result of loss of epithelial cells. However, vitamin B_{12} deficiency – which may lead to pernicious anemia or (much more rarely) to subacute combined degeneration of the spinal cord – takes several years to supervene because of the large liver stores of the vitamin. In the complete atrophy of pernicious anemia, gastric glandular and all parietal cells are lost, and the mucosa is infiltrated by large numbers of plasma cells and lymphocytes. Pentagastrin stimulation will demonstrate that the patient is achlorhydric. Studies will demonstrate antibodies to intrinsic factor and to parietal cells in serum, gastric secretions and mucosa in most patients. Though the presence of such antibodies is a useful marker, it is not diagnostic: intrinsic factor antibodies can be demonstrated occasionally (and parietal cell antibodies frequently) in patients with simple atrophic gastritis or chronic superficial gastritis without vitamin B_{12} malabsorption.

Hydroxocobalamin has replaced cyanocobalamin for the treatment of pernicious anemia, because it is better retained in the body. A dose of 100 µg by injection every month is more than sufficient to maintain body stores after loading treatment with 200 µg on three alternate days.

6.2.2 CONGENITAL PERNICIOUS ANEMIA

Congenital pernicious anemia is a rare condition, inherited as a Mendelian recessive, and is due to an inherited inability to secrete intrinsic factor in adequate amounts. It presents as megaloblastic anemia in infancy and is associated with normal acid secretory potential. The specific failure of intrinsic factor synthesis in this condition must be distinguished from congenital ileal receptor deficiency for the vitamin B_{12}-intrinsic factor complex (the Imerslund-Graesbeck syndrome) and from vitamin B_{12} deficiency due to gastric failure in the hypoparathyroidism-candidiasis syndrome.

The cause of pernicious anemia is unknown. The presence of autoantibodies, mucosal infiltration by plasma cells and reversibility of the gastric lesion by corticosteroids suggest an autoimmune process. There is also a small but definite genetic predisposition; like gastric cancer, the disease is slightly more common in individuals of group A than in those of the remaining ABO groups. Exogenous factors that predispose to gastric cancer also seem likely to predispose to pernicious anemia. It is unclear why most patients present with pernicious anemia while a few develop the neurological condition of subacute degeneration of the spinal cord without anemia.

6.3 Chronic Superficial Gastritis

In this form of gastritis, inflammatory cells, mainly polymorphonuclear, infiltrate the superficial mucosa but gastric glands are well preserved. It is due to H. pylori infection and has been found with increased frequency in those who smoke excessively or who consume large amounts of alcohol or hot beverages. No specific symptom pattern has been correlated with it, and it does not necessarily predispose to gastric atrophy. Chronic superficial gastritis is commonly found in patients with chronic gastric ulcer.

6.4 Chronic Atrophic Gastritis

Chronic atrophic gastritis is usually due to H. pylori infection. In addition to cellular infiltration, predominantly lymphocytic and plasma cell in pattern, there is a loss of gastric glands, and acid and pepsin secretory capacity is

TABLE 11.   Differential diagnosis for intrinsic causes of thickened gastric folds

Lymphoma
Mucosa-associated lymphoid tissue (MALT) syndrome
Gastric adenocarcinoma
Linitis plastica
Ménétrier's disease
Acute H. pylori gastritis
Lymphocytic gastritis
Eosinophilic gastritis
Gastric varices
Gastritis cystica profunda
Gastric antral vascular ectasia
Kaposi's sarcoma
Zollinger-Ellison syndrome
Gastric Crohn's disease

reduced in parallel. It does not cause symptoms, but in a minority of patients there is progression to the complete atrophy of pernicious anemia. Patients with atrophic gastritis may progress to eventual gastric cancer as often as those with pernicious anemia.

6.5 Giant Mucosal Rugal Hypertrophy

Giant mucosal rugal hypertrophy is a histologic change occurring in association with the Zollinger-Ellison syndrome and rarely as an isolated entity. Ménétrier's disease (giant hypertrophic gastritis), a rare condition associated with mucosal hypertrophy, involves reduced acid secretion. Hypertrophic-hypersecretory gastropathy, another associated condition, involves increased acid secretion. These conditions may be associated with H. pylori infection. In giant mucosal rugal hypertrophy, as a result of protein loss into the gastric lumen, the serum albumin concentration will be reduced. The condition usually occurs in males between the ages of 30 and 50, and the patient will present with pain, nausea, vomiting, weight loss, bleeding, or edema as a result of hypoalbuminemia. The condition is suspected from the presence of large rugal folds identified on upper GI series or at endoscopy. A biopsy will demonstrate hyperplasia of the parietal, chief and mucus cells. There may be cystic structures in the mucosa and submucosa as well. The condition must be distinguished from giant hypertrophic gastritis, the Zollinger-Ellison syndrome, gastric carcinoma, lymphoma and amyloidosis (Table 11). H. pylori infection should be sought and treated if present. The protein loss may be reduced with anticholinergics. If gastric hypersecretion occurs, as in the case of hypertrophic-hypersecretory gastropathy, H_2 blockers will prove useful. If pain, bleeding and protein loss persist, then a vagotomy and pyloroplasty or subtotal gastrectomy is necessary.

6.6 Granulomatous Gastritis

Chronic inflammatory changes in the gastric mucosa may occur in Crohn's disease, tuberculosis, syphilis and sarcoidosis, and granulomas may be present. These diseases are all uncommon.

6.7 Eosinophilic Gastritis

The cause of eosinophilic gastritis is unknown. There is extensive infiltration of the gastric and often the small intestinal mucosa by eosinophils, in association with peripheral eosinophilia. The disease produces nonspecific dyspeptic symptoms, and antral distortion is radiographically visible. Spontaneous cure is common, but some patients require steroid therapy and in a few the disease is progressive.

6.8 Bile Gastritis

The common occurrence of gastritis following gastric surgery is thought to be due to the effect of bile and alkaline duodenal secretion damaging the gastric mucosal barrier and giving rise to an inflammatory reaction. Some patients will respond to medical treatment with cholestyramine, aluminum hydroxide or sucralfate. Cholestyramine and aluminum hydroxide act by binding bile acids and pepsin, and providing a protective surface to the gastric mucosa. When the condition persists and is associated with pain or bleeding, a surgical procedure (Roux-en-Y) will be necessary.

6.9 Miscellaneous

There are two forms of gastritis that fall outside the classifications listed above. One is intestinal metaplasia, where a large number of cells with the histochemical properties of intestinal mucosal cells are found in the stomach. This is commonly associated with chronic gastritis. The second is Ménétrier's disease or giant hypertrophic gastritis, where the giant mucosal folds may be confused with neoplastic disease (Table 11); excess protein loss from the folds may cause a syndrome of protein depletion (protein-losing enteropathy). Erosive gastritis and hyperplastic atrophic gastritis are less well defined entities.

7. PREMALIGNANT CONDITIONS OF THE STOMACH AND GASTRIC CANCER

7.1 Premalignant Conditions

Possible premalignant gastric conditions include pernicious anemia, chronic

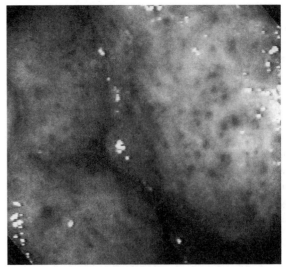

Figure 13.   Fundal (type A) gastritis.

atrophic gastritis, adenomatous polyps and previous gastric surgery. People with a family history that is positive for gastric cancer also have an increased risk of developing this disease. Benign gastric ulcer is not a premalignant condition, but can appear so because of the long natural history of some ulcerating cancers. Regular endoscopy is not necessary for most patients with conditions predisposing to gastric ulcer. A high index of suspicion for cancer, however, must be maintained. If endoscopy and biopsy have been performed and distinct dysplastic changes are found in the epithelium, regular follow-up endoscopy and biopsy are advised.

7.1.1 PERNICIOUS ANEMIA
Patients with pernicious anemia have long been considered at risk for gastric cancer, but the risk is likely to be low and does not justify intensive endoscopic screening. Pernicious anemia is invariably associated with fundal gland atrophy, usually with intestinal metaplasia and sometimes with polyps. When cancer develops, it tends to occur in the body or fundus of the stomach.

7.1.2 CHRONIC ATROPHIC GASTRITIS
There are two main types of atrophic gastritis: fundal gland (type A), and pyloric (antral) gland (type B). These occur in older people. Antral gastritis increasingly involves the fundal gland area with advanced age. Both types A

and B are associated with intestinal metaplasia and a predisposition to gastric cancer. Type A gastritis (Figure 13) is less common and its distribution in the stomach resembles that of pernicious anemia. Type B gastritis is predominant in those areas of the body where gastric cancer is common and appears to be a risk factor mainly for the intestinal type of gastric cancer. H. pylori, which is the cause of type B gastritis, is a risk factor for gastric cancer (see Section 6.2).

7.1.3 GASTRIC POLYPS
There are two main types of gastric polyps: hyperplastic and adenomatous. Hyperplastic polyps are small, often multiple, and do not become malignant. Adenomatous polyps are uncommon and are usually larger than 2 cm in diameter. They are premalignant, and a substantial minority show areas of cancer at the time of detection. Endoscopic or surgical excision is recommended.

7.1.4 PREVIOUS GASTRIC SURGERY
Patients who have had a partial gastrectomy for peptic ulcer disease may have an increased probability of developing gastric cancer some 15 to 20 years after the operation. Endoscopic surveillance of these patients does not appear to be justified in North America, since the risk is low.

7.2 Other Conditions
Individuals with a parent or sibling with gastric cancer are three times as likely to develop gastric cancer as the general population. People born in a country where gastric cancer is common (e.g., Japan or Eastern Europe) are also at increased risk, even if they have lived in North America for many years. Although regular screening is not warranted in either case, minor symptoms should be promptly and thoroughly investigated.

Barrett's epithelium (columnar cell lining of the lower esophagus) is a proven precursor of esophageal adenocarcinoma, and there is increasing suspicion that lesser degrees of Barrett's epithelium may predispose to the much more common adenocarcinoma of the gastric cardia.

7.3 Gastric Cancer
The association of gastritis and gastric adenocarcinoma has long been known. The discovery of H. pylori as the cause of acute and chronic gastritis and subsequent atrophic gastritis has implicated H. pylori as a co-carcinogen in gastric cancer. This is strengthened by the epidemiologic association of H. pylori infection and gastric cancers of the gastric body and antrum. The progress of acute infection with H. pylori to gastric adenocarcinoma in the ferret model further strengthens its role as co-carcinogen.

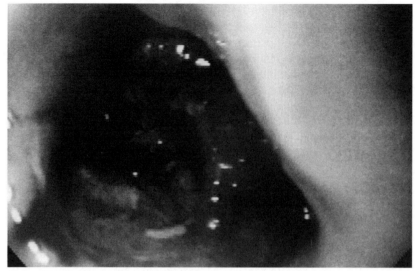

FIGURE 14.   Carcinoma of the gastric cardia.

MALT (mucosa-associated lymphoid tissue) lymphoma is also associated with H. pylori infection, and when MALT is diagnosed, H. pylori should be sought on biopsies. Eradication of H. pylori with antibiotic regimens has led to remission in about 60% of cases.

Adenocarcinoma is the most common gastric cancer, but lymphoma and leiomyosarcoma also occur. The frequency of gastric cancer has decreased considerably over the past 50 years in North America, but it still ranks as the second most common GI malignancy (after colon cancer). Most patients are over 60 years of age. Men are affected about twice as often as women. The cancer usually involves the antrum, body or cardia with about equal frequency. (Figure 14 shows carcinoma of the cardia.) The three main macroscopic types are polypoid, ulcerative and infiltrative. The two main microscopic types are intestinal and diffuse. The intestinal type is often associated with atrophic gastritis and intestinal metaplasia; the diffuse type is often manifest as a linitis plastica.

Most patients have advanced incurable disease by the time they have significant complaints, but some patients with early gastric cancer may have mild epigastric discomfort or ulcer-like symptoms. Physical examination is usually normal but may reveal a mass or a succussion splash in a minority of patients. There may be evidence of metastases, such as a supraclavicular node, hepatomegaly, ascites, a "shelf" on a rectal examination, an ovarian mass or an umbilical node. Iron deficiency anemia is found in about 50% of patients and occult blood is present in the stool in about 75% of cases. Occasionally, the neurological signs of subacute combined degeneration of the spinal cord from associated pernicious anemia will be found. Measurement of gastric acid secretion or carcinoembryonic antigen (CEA) is not helpful. Barium radiograph is usually the first diagnostic procedure. Experienced radiologists can show some abnormality in up to 90% of patients, particularly if double contrast techniques are used. While there are distinguishing clinical and radiological features, every patient with a presumed benign gastric ulcer should have biopsies obtained to exclude a malignant ulcer. Endoscopy and biopsy, with or without brush cytology, are required to establish the diagnosis.

The diffuse type of gastric cancer often manifests itself as a linitis plastica. It is harder to diagnose than the intestinal type, particularly in the earlier stages. Thus, although diagnostic techniques have improved, some gastric cancers are still missed on the initial investigation. Although routine endoscopic screening is not feasible in North America, minor symptoms should be thoroughly investigated in people with predisposing conditions. It is also important to ensure that only benign gastric ulcers are treated medically; if a gastric ulcer fails to heal after three months of intensive medical therapy, surgery is generally recommended.

Early surgery offers the only hope for cure, but is not performed if there is evidence of metastatic disease, unless the patient suffers from gastric outlet obstruction. Cancers of the distal and mid-stomach are treated by subtotal gastrectomy. In order to remove the regional lymph nodes, the lesser and greater omenta are resected and, if necessary, the spleen is removed. Cancers of the proximal stomach are usually treated by esophagogastrectomy. With the increased proportion of diffusely infiltrating cancer, total gastrectomy with biliary diversion is being performed more often. Palliative resection, bypass, surgery or laser photoablation is justified in those patients with gastric outlet obstruction.

Palliative esophagogastrectomy or total gastrectomy is not recommended. The prognosis after surgical treatment is related to the depth of the tumor's penetration. Overall, about 10–15% of patients survive five years. Occasionally, patients have a long course without treatment or with only palliative surgery.

Therapy includes chemotherapy with 5-fluorouracil (5-FU), doxorubicin and mitomycin (FAM). This approach achieves a response rate of up to 40% but gives a disappointing median survival of less than one year. Occasionally, good responses are obtained, and a trial is recommended for patients in good condition and with advanced disease. Adjuvant chemotherapy or radiotherapy remains of unproven value, but palliative radiotherapy is useful to control bleeding, to alleviate pain from bone metastases and to relieve dysphagia. Esophageal dilation and endoscopically placed plastic tubes can also help dysphagia caused by persistent spread of a cardia tumor.

General supportive care is important, including dietary advice, replacement of iron and vitamin B_{12}, judicious use of analgesics, antiemetics, and antacid support. Emotional support is particularly important and increasingly includes guidance in interpreting the common, overoptimistic "breakthroughs" reported in the press.

8. OTHER GASTRIC DISEASES

8.1 Acute

Partial (antral) or total gastric volvulus is a rare cause of acute upper abdominal pain and vomiting. These obstructions can arise by themselves, or as torsion within a hiatus hernia. Volvulus within a hernia is not uncommon in the elderly, when there may be no symptoms. The belief that twisting obstruction poses an important risk to the blood supply is probably unjustified. Gastric aspiration is followed by surgical relief of the volvulus in those who present with obstruction.

Sudden gross gastric distention and acute dilation of the stomach can arise after any form of upper abdominal surgery, including cholecystectomy, and especially after vagotomy, after childbirth and in diabetic coma. The causes are uncertain. Vomiting of relatively clear gastric contents is succeeded by the production of dirty brown or feculent material and the development of abdominal distention. Prompt decompression with a large-bore stomach tube and intravenous fluid replacement are required. After a variable interval the condition should then resolve spontaneously.

8.1.1 GASTRIC RUPTURE

Acute, nontraumatic, spontaneous rupture of the stomach is a rare, catastrophic and poorly understood event. The majority of ruptures occur on the lesser curvature. They have also been reported to occur during upper gastrointestinal radiography using barium, sodium bicarbonate ingestion, nasal oxygen therapy, cardiopulmonary resuscitation and labor, and during the postpartum period.

8.2 Chronic

Hypertrophic pyloric stenosis is an idiopathic condition that may occur in infants or adults. The muscle of the pyloric canal is unduly hypertrophied. Infantile hypertrophic pyloric stenosis is more common in boys than in girls (the sex ratio is approximately 10:1), is a frequent anomaly (its incidence is about 3 per 1,000 live births) and is thought to be due to a combination of genetic predisposition and some abnormality of fetal or early postnatal development. Symptoms usually develop in the first few weeks after birth and characteristically consist of copious projectile vomiting of the gastric contents after feeding. On examination there is usually visible gastric peristalsis; a lump can be felt abdominally in the region of the pylorus. Barium-meal examination is not usually necessary but will confirm the presence of a narrow segment, 1–2 cm long, at the pylorus. The condition must be distinguished clinically from esophageal atresia (which involves onset at birth of difficulties with swallowing) and duodenal obstruction/atresia (which involves bile-stained vomitus). A minor proportion of all cases settle in the first two to three months with conservative management with anticholinergic drugs, but most patients will require early surgery with Ramstedt's procedure (pyloromyotomy).

Occasionally, adult patients present with obstructive symptoms resulting from pyloric stenosis associated with muscular hypertrophy. This is rarely if ever caused by recurrence of infantile pyloric stenosis; it is usually associated with juxtapyloric peptic ulceration, but sometimes the problem seems to be due to primary hypertrophic stenosis arising in adult life. The differential also includes pyloric mucosal diaphragm and annular pancreas. Pyloric obstruction requires pyloroplasty together with a procedure such as vagotomy if there is an associated ulcer.

8.2.1 GASTRIC DIVERTICULA
Gastric diverticula occur most commonly near the cardia on the lesser curve, but occasionally are found in the prepyloric region. They seldom cause symptoms. Their principal importance lies in the likelihood of confusion with gastric ulceration.

8.2.2 PSEUDOLYMPHOMA
Localized lymphoid hyperplasia of the stomach is also known as pseudolymphoma. The lesions are raised, flat or nodular folds, and are often associated with gastric ulceration. The etiology of this condition remains unclear, but H. pylori infection has been implicated. It is difficult to exclude lymphoma using radiology or endoscopic biopsy; thus, a resected specimen is required for diagnosis.

8.2.3 GASTRIC INFECTIONS AND INFESTATIONS
Gastric acid provides a bactericidal barrier against infection. Acid-suppressive pharmacotherapy, hypochlorhydria or gastric surgery may increase the risk of bacterial infection. Recent attention has been turned to H. pylori, which is highly associated with chronic gastritis in addition to peptic ulcer disease.

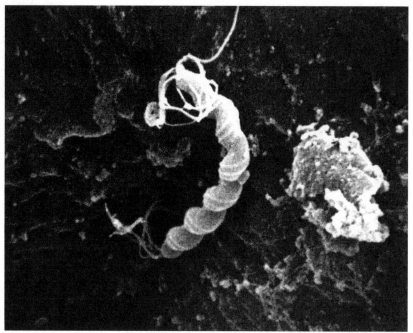

FIGURE 15.   Helicobacter pylori. (Courtesy of McMaster University Medical Centre Electron Microscopy Lab.)

H. pylori infection is recognized to be a major causative factor associated with a spectrum of gastroduodenal disease. It is found in about 95% of patients with gastritis and 100% with chronic active gastritis. It is found in 70–95% of patients with duodenal ulcer and 60–80% of patients with gastric ulcer. It is also highly associated with gastric carcinoma and gastric lymphoma (see Sections 6.2 and 7.3). The association of H. pylori infection with nonulcer dyspepsia is more controversial and as yet not convincingly substantiated.

Viral infections such as cytomegalovirus (CMV) and herpes simplex virus are very often found in immunocompromised hosts. They are associated with gastric erosions, although CMV has been found in intact mucosa. Cultures or endoscopic biopsies and smears demonstrating intranuclear inclusions are helpful in establishing a diagnosis. Candida albicans is commonly found in the gastric ulcers or erosions of immunocompromised hosts. Candidal infection should be a consideration in an ulcer that fails to heal. In the immunocompromised host, parasites such as Strongyloides stercoralis may become overwhelmingly disseminated. Histoplasmosis and mucormycosis involving the stomach are rare causes of gastric ulceration and bleeding.

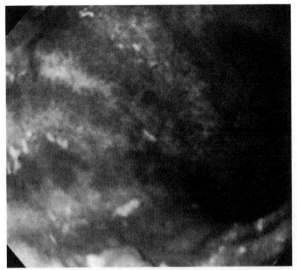

FIGURE 16.   Chronic H. pylori gastritis.

8.2.3.1 *H. pylori gastritis*

H. pylori is a small (3 × 0.5 μm) gram-negative, microaerophilic urease-producing rod-shaped bacillus, which has been closely linked to both acute and chronic active type B gastritis, especially of the antrum (Figure 15). H. pylori is the most important pathogenic factor in peptic ulcer disease.

H. pylori is present in almost all cases of chronic active gastritis, which most commonly involves antral inflammation but may spread to the whole stomach over time (Figure 16). H. pylori does not colonize areas of intestinal metaplasia, but has been seen in the distal esophagus of some patients with Barrett's esophagus.

The source of H. pylori is unknown, although person-to-person spread is probably demonstrated by intrafamilial clustering and a high prevalence of seropositivity in institutionalized persons, those of low economic status, and populations in less developed countries. The prevalence of H. pylori infection increases with age; in Western countries it is uncommon before the third decade but thereafter increases with seropositivity at the rate of approximately 1% per year of age.

Most people with H. pylori–associated gastritis are asymptomatic and have normal-appearing gastric mucosa at endoscopy. The histologic spectrum of H. pylori–associated gastritis ranges from minimal to severe inflammation, but the organisms noted in the mucous layer are associated with severe depletion of mucus and an intense inflammation, which most often is chronic, although neutrophils can be noted in some instances. Eradication of H. pylori with antibiotics has resulted in a marked lessening in the severity of the gastritis.

8.2.3.1.1 *Diagnosis*   The organism can be identified on histology with conventional hematoxylin- and eosin-stained sections at high-power magnification, but is more easily seen with the Warthin-Starry or the modified Giemsa stains. The enzyme-linked immunosorbent assay (ELISA) is the most widely employed serologic method; its sensitivity and specificity are greater than 90%. Rapid urease tests can be performed on tissue biopsies in the endoscopy unit since H. pylori produces large amounts of urease, which can convert urea into ammonia and carbon dioxide. Rapid urease tests involve urease and pH indicator gel, into which the biopsy is placed. The presence of H. pylori results in an alkaline pH of the medium and a color change when the pH rises. Approximately 75% of the positive tests occur between 20 minutes and 1 hour, and 90% are positive between 6 and 24 hours. Carbon-urea breath tests using carbon ^{13}C and ^{14}C employ carbon-labeled urea that is fed to the patient and is subsequently hydrolyzed by the H. pylori urease, resulting in the formation of ammonia and carbon dioxide. This labeled carbon dioxide in the breath is then measured.

8.2.3.1.2 *H. pylori association with peptic ulcer disease*   Numerous studies have established the close association of antral H. pylori and peptic ulcer disease. Over 90% of patients with duodenal ulcer have H. pylori identified in gastric antral biopsies. The association for gastric ulcer and H. pylori is up to 80%. Although ulcers can be healed with a variety of agents that do not eradicate H. pylori, in these cases relapse is common. However, when the H. pylori organism is eradicated the impact on the subsequent course of duodenal ulcer is dramatic. The recurrence rate in patients in whom H. pylori is eradicated ranges from 0–4% per year. This is in marked contrast to those who remain H. pylori–positive, whose recurrence rates vary from 40–80% per year.

   H. pylori infection is associated with duodenal ulcer by way of an antral-predominant gastritis that is accompanied by a decrease in somatostatin and an increase in gastrin. This may augment gastric acid secretion, which may already be high as a result of genetic factors. Increased gastric acid secretion leads to gastric metaplasia in the duodenum, which can be colonized by H. pylori leading to duodenal bulb inflammation, duodenitis and duodenal ulcer. The ulcer diathesis may reflect more damaging strains of the organisms, greater density of the infecting organisms or an exaggerated host inflammatory response (Figure 17).

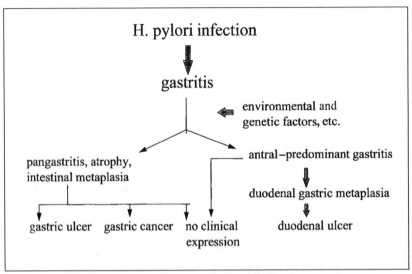

FIGURE 17. Possible mechanisms of H. pylori–associated disease.

TABLE 12. Eradication rates for H. pylori

Bismuth triple therapy (2 weeks)	PPI + 1 antibiotic (2 weeks)	PPI + 2 antibiotics (1 week)
90–98% (metronidazole-sensitive)	70–85% (clarithromycin)	88–94% (metronidazole/clarithromycin)
31–63% (metronidazole-resistant)	55–70% (amoxicillin)	75–96% (amoxicillin/clarithromycin)
		79–90% (amoxicillin/metronidazole)

The therapy for the eradication of H. pylori has evolved over the past decade (see Sections 4.9 and 4.10; Tables 4, 5 and 12). The early regimen of bismuth triple therapy included a bismuth compound (Pepto-Bismol®) plus metronidazole and tetracycline or bismuth plus metronidazole and amoxicillin. The therapy is effective in patients with metronidazole-sensitive H. pylori infection but not very effective in those with metronidazole-resistant strains. This regimen has limited compliance because of dosing frequency and adverse effects.

Therapy later evolved to combinations of a proton pump inhibitor (PPI) and one antibiotic, usually clarithromycin. Eradication rates with a PPI plus clarithromycin are usually between 70 and 85%. The addition of a second antibiotic to the regimen, usually metronidazole, has led to much higher eradication rates, such as 88–94% for a PPI plus metronidazole and clarithromycin. With amoxicillin and clarithromycin the eradication rates are between 75 and 96%; the rates decrease about 10% with amoxicillin and metronidazole compared to the previous two combinations.

8.2.3.1.3 *Nonulcer dyspepsia and H. pylori* The role of H. pylori infection in nonulcer dyspepsia remains an important question. There may be a subset of patients with nonulcer dyspepsia whose symptoms are due to H. pylori infection. However, many patients harboring H. pylori are symptom-free. Acute infection with H. pylori is associated with belching, pyrosis and malaise, and may be associated with decreased gastric acid secretion. At present, there is no evidence to suggest that the presence of H. pylori is associated with any particular symptom cluster related to functional dyspepsia.

SUGGESTED READING LIST

Marshall BJ, Warren JR. Unidentified curved bacilli in the stomach of patients with gastritis and peptic ulceration. Lancet 1984; 1(8390):1311–1315.

Walsh JH, Peterson WI. The treatment of Helicobacter pylori infection in the management of peptic ulcer disease. N Engl J Med 1995; 333:984–991.

Antonioli DA. Chronic gastritis: classification. In: Bayless TM (ed.), Current therapy in gastroenterology and liver disease. 4th ed. St. Louis: CV Mosby, 1994.

Correa P, Fox J, Fontham E, et al. Helicobacter pylori and gastric carcinoma: serum antibody prevalence in populations with contrasting cancer risks. Cancer 1990; 66: 2569–2574.

Hughes R. Diagnosis and treatment of gastric polyps. Gastrointest Endosc Clin North Am 1993; 2:457–467.

Yamada T, Alpers DH, Owyang C, et al. (eds.). Textbook of gastroenterology. Philadelphia: JB Lippincott, 1995.

OBJECTIVES

Anatomy and Physiology
1. Describe the arterial and nerve supply to the stomach.
2. List the three major functions of the stomach.
3. Describe the factors that determine gastric motility and emptying.

Peptic Ulcer Disease
1. What is Helicobacter pylori?
2. How is infection transmitted?
3. What part(s) of the gastrointestinal tract does H. pylori colonize?

4. What is the best method to detect H. pylori in clinical practice?
5. Describe the mechanism(s) by which H. pylori causes damage.
6. Describe the association of H. pylori with histologic gastritis, gastric ulcer and duodenal ulcer.
7. List the causes of ulcer other than H. pylori.
8. What treatment regimens have been used to eradicate H. pylori?
9. List the indications for H. pylori eradication.

Gastritis
1. List 10 causes of thickened gastric folds.
2. What are the cardinal symptoms of gastritis?
3. List the causes of acute gastritis.
4. List the complications of gastric surgery.

Gastric Cancer
1. List the premalignant conditions associated with gastric cancer.
2. Describe the relationship of H. pylori to gastric cancer.
3. Which radiologic features distinguish a benign from a malignant gastric ulcer?

7
The Small Intestine
A.B.R. Thomson, P. Paré and R.N. Fedorak

1. GROSS ANATOMY OF THE SMALL INTESTINE

1.1 Duodenum
The term *duodenum* (a Latin derivation from the Greek *dodekadaktulon*, "12 fingers") is applied to the most proximal segment of the small intestine because of its length – 12 fingers' breadth. The duodenum is subdivided into four portions: the first portion, which corresponds to the radiologic designation of duodenal bulb or cap; the second (descending) portion; the third (transverse) portion; and the fourth (ascending) portion.

Situated immediately above the first portion of the duodenum are the quadrate lobe of the liver and the gallbladder. The gallbladder normally can impinge on the lesser curve of the duodenal cap to produce the smooth concavity seen in radiographs. Behind the first portion of the duodenum is the head of the pancreas. Because of this relationship, the pancreas is the commonest site of penetration by a duodenal ulcer.

The second portion of the duodenum is concave; it hugs the head of the pancreas. A carcinoma or inflammatory mass in the head of the pancreas can occasionally affect the mucosal pattern along the medial aspect of the second portion of the duodenum. Congenital duodenal diverticula are commonly seen extending from the medial aspect of the second portion.

The third portion of the duodenum lies horizontally at the level of the third lumbar vertebra. The superior mesenteric artery, vein and nerve run anterior to its middle segment. In a thin individual or a person with recent massive weight loss, the superior mesenteric vessel sheath may impinge on the third portion of the duodenum, which is associated with chronic, intermittent obstruction of the duodenum.

The fourth portion of the duodenum as it ascends to the level of the second lumbar vertebra is in intimate contact with the aorta. This intimacy of duodenum and aorta can lead to fatal complications of aortic grafting when the graft erodes the duodenal wall, resulting in hemorrhage. Bleeding may be either catastrophic (due to a tiny connection between the aortic lumen and the duodenal lumen) or chronic with iron deficiency and fever (due to erosion of the duodenal mucosa by the exterior of the graft).

The mucosal pattern of the first portion (the duodenal cap or bulb) can be distinguished radiologically and endoscopically from the remaining duodenum. In the cap, shallow folds run longitudinally and are obliterated as the cap is distended. At the junction between the first and second portions of the duodenum begin permanent transverse conniventes, characteristic of the small intestine.

1.2 Jejunum and Ileum

The length of the small intestine is approximately 6 m; the length can vary from 4 to 7 m according to the technique used to make the measurement. The proximal 40% of the small intestine is referred to as the *jejunum* (from the Latin, meaning "empty"), and the distal 60% is designated as the *ileum* (from the Greek *eilein*, "to roll or twist"). The wall of the jejunum is thicker and its lumen wider than are those of the ileum. There is also a gradual diminution in the caliber of the lumen from duodenum to ileum. Because of its narrower lumen, the ileum is more prone to obstruction. There is a characteristic difference in the mesentery between jejunum and ileum. The fat is thicker in the ileal mesentery and extends fully to the intestinal attachment. In Crohn's disease, the thickened mesenteric fat encroaches further beneath the serosa of the small intestine. On x-ray, the mucosa in the proximal and ileal segments of the small intestine also differs. In the jejunum, the valvulae conniventes (also known as plicae circulares) are thick, tall and numerous, giving a feathery mucosal pattern on x-ray. This contrasts with the sausage-shaped ileal loops, where the valvulae conniventes are progressively fewer and less prominent but are more clearly seen as transverse folds on x-ray.

2. SMALL INTESTINAL MOTILITY

The main function of the small intestine is digestion and absorption of nutrients. In this process, the role of small bowel motility is to mix food products with the digestive enzymes, to promote contact of chyme with the absorptive cells over a sufficient length of bowel and finally to propel remnants into the colon. Well-organized motility patterns occur in the small intestine to accomplish these goals in the fed as well as the fasting state. During fasting, a migrating motor complex (MMC) exists. This complex is characterized by a front of intense spiking activity (phase III activity) that migrates down the entire small intestine; as the front reaches the terminal ileum, another front develops in the gastroduodenal area and progresses down the intestine. The purpose of this phase III myoelectric and contractile activity is to sweep remnants of the previous meal into the colon and prevent stagnation and bacterial overgrowth. The MMC often starts in the lower esophagus. Sweeping through the stomach, it removes debris and residual material not emptied with the last meal. Absence of phase III activity is associated with bacterial overgrowth and diarrhea. Thus, the small bowel is active even during fasting.

During meals, this cycle is interrupted and the motility pattern in the small bowel becomes an irregular spiking activity called the fed pattern. This fed pattern of motility does not seem to move intestinal contents forward to any great extent but does mix these contents with digestive juices, spreading them again and again over the absorptive surface of the brush border. Diarrhea can thus occur when this normal fed pattern is replaced by aggressive propulsive contractions.

3. PRINCIPLES OF ABSORPTION

Understanding the pathophysiology of diarrhea and malabsorption is based on understanding the normal steps in the digestion and absorption of food. The normal gastrointestinal tract is a finely integrated system geared to carry out the assimilation of ingested foodstuffs. Assimilation (the process by which ingested foods reach body fluids and cells) consists of two stages: (1) digestion (the breakdown of large molecules in the lumen of the intestine into their component small molecules) and (2) absorption (the transport across the intestinal mucosa to systemic body fluids).

Many disease processes directly or indirectly alter gastrointestinal physiology in such a manner that normal absorptive mechanisms are compromised, resulting in maldigestion or malabsorption of one or more dietary constituents. Too simplistic an approach to these diseases may be confusing because of the large number of illnesses involved and because of the plethora of diagnostic tests. This chapter will (1) present a classification of malabsorption and (2) outline the usefulness and potential pitfalls of common tests of intestinal function.

4. ABSORPTION OF VITAMINS AND MINERALS

4.1 Folic Acid (Pteroylglutamic Acid, PteGlu$_1$)

4.1.1 *FOOD SOURCES*
Dietary folates (folacins) are synthesized by bacteria and plants. They occur

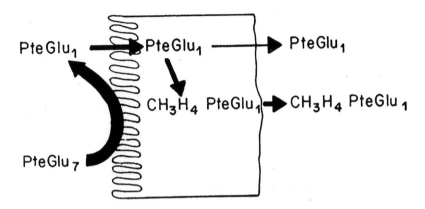

FIGURE 1. Proposed scheme of the digestion and absorption of dietary pteroylglutamates. Hydrolysis of polypteroylglutamates (shown here as $PteGlu_7$) probably occurs outside the intestinal epithelial cell. The overall rate of absorption into the mesenteric circulation is governed by the rate of transport of the monoglutamyl product ($PteGlu_1$). At physiologic doses, a substantial amount of $PteGlu_1$ is reduced and then methylated to $CH_3H_4PteGlu_1$ in the intestinal cell before release to the circulation.
SOURCE: Rosenberg IH. Folate absorption and malabsorption. N Engl J Med 1975; 293:1303.

mostly as polyglutamates, which are not absorbed intact. All folacins, or polypteroylglutamates ($PteGlu_n$), are hydrolyzed to folic acid, or pteroylglutamic acid ($PteGlu_1$), during absorption. Pteroylglutamic acid ($PteGlu_1$) is absorbed at a faster rate than larger polymers ($PteGlu_n$). Only 25–50% of dietary folacin is nutritionally available; boiling destroys much of folate activity. Therefore, uncooked foods with a large portion of the monoglutamate form ($PteGlu_1$) – e.g., bananas, lima beans, liver and yeast – contain the highest availability of folacin. Average Canadian diets contain about 240 μg of folate a day. The daily requirement for folate is approximately 100 μg, although the recommended dietary allowance is 400 μg. Tissue stores of folate are only about 3 mg; therefore, malabsorption can deplete the body of folate within one month.

4.1.2 HYDROLYSIS AND ABSORPTION OF POLYGLUTAMATE FOLATES

Polyglutamate forms of folate ($PteGlu_n$) hydrolyze sequentially down to the monoglutamate form ($PteGlu_1$). This hydrolysis takes place at the brush border by the enzyme folate conjugase (Figure 1). Folic acid ($PteGlu_1$) is absorbed from the intestinal lumen by a sodium-dependent carrier, which has been cloned. Once in the intestinal epithelial cell, folic acid is methylated and reduced to the tetrahydro form ($CH_3H_4PteGlu_1$).

Interference with folic acid absorption at the brush-border carrier site occurs with drugs such as phenytoin and sulfasalazine. In addition, folic acid deficiency itself can impair folic acid absorption by producing "megaloblastic" changes in columnar epithelial cells of the gut – an abnormal epithelium.

4.2 Cobalamin (Vitamin B_{12})

4.2.1 FOOD SOURCES

Cobalamin refers to cobalt-containing compounds with a corrin ring: these have biological activity for humans. Vitamin B_{12} is the generic term for all of these compounds with bioactivity in any species. Cobalamin is therefore the preferred term to distinguish those compounds that are active in humans from the many analogues produced by bacteria. Cobalamin enters animal tissues when the animal ingests bacteria-containing foods or from production in the animal's rumen. Microorganisms in the human colon synthesize cobalamin, but it is not absorbed. Thus, strict vegetarians who do not eat cobalamin-containing foods will develop cobalamin deficiency. The average Western diet contains 10–20 μg per day. The daily requirement for cobalamin is 1 μg. The human liver is the repository of approximately 5 mg of cobalamin. These large hepatic stores account for the delay of several years in the clinical appearance of deficiency after cobalamin malabsorption begins.

4.2.2 ROLE OF THE STOMACH, PANCREAS AND ILEUM

Once cobalamin is liberated from food, it is bound at acid pH to R proteins (so called because of their rapid movement during electrophoresis). R proteins are glycoproteins present in many body secretions, including serum, bile, saliva and gastric and pancreatic juices. Most of the gastric R protein is from swallowed saliva. The R proteins cannot mediate the absorption of cobalamin alone, and their physiologic function is incompletely understood. Rare cases of complete R-protein deficiency have occurred without obvious clinical effect on the patient.

The cobalamin/R protein complex leaves the stomach along with free intrinsic factor (IF) (Figure 2). In the duodenum, pancreatic proteases in the presence of bicarbonate (i.e., neutral pH) hydrolyze the R protein, thereby liberating free cobalamin. The cobalamin now combines with gastric intrinsic factor. A conformational change takes place, allowing the cobalamin/intrinsic-factor complex to be resistant to proteolytic digestion. This resistance allows

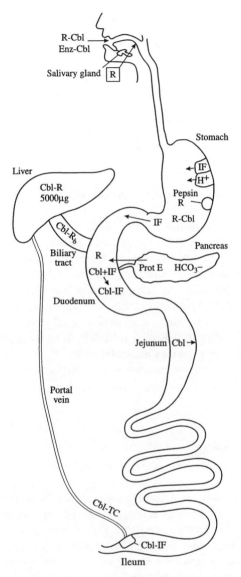

FIGURE 2.   Absorption of cobalamin (Cbl) requires proteolysis and intrinsic factor (IF). The intrinsic factor secreted is far in excess of that needed for binding the available cobalamin. R protein derived from saliva is also present in great abundance. Note that Cbl binds initially to R protein in the stomach at acid pH. Only after R protein is degraded by protease does Cbl bind to IF. After Cbl is absorbed in the ileum, it is bound to transcobalamin II.

SOURCE: Kalser MH. Absorption of cobalamin (vitamin B_{12}), folate, and other water-soluble vitamins. In: Berk JE (ed.), Bockus gastroenterology, vol. 3. 4th ed. Philadelphia: WB Saunders, 1985:1556.

TABLE 1.   Abnormalities of cobalamin absorption that produce deficiency

Physiologic step	Disorder
Decreased IF secretion	Pernicious anemia, gastrectomy, achlorhydria
Impaired transfer to IF (acidic pH)	Pancreatic insufficiency
Competition for uptake	Bacterial overgrowth
Impaired attachment to ileal receptor	Ileal disease or resection
Impaired passage through the ileal cell wall	Familial cobalamin malabsorption
Impaired uptake into blood	Transcobalamin II deficiency

the complex to safely traverse the small intestine and reach the ileum, its site of active absorption.

Since transfer of cobalamin from R protein to intrinsic factor depends upon pH, pancreatic insufficiency (with deficient bicarbonate production) or the Zollinger-Ellison syndrome (with excess hydrogen ion production) interferes with this process and may result in cobalamin deficiency.

In the ileum, the cobalamin/intrinsic-factor complex binds to a specific receptor located on the brush border. Free cobalamin does not bind to the ileal receptor. In the enterocyte the cobalamin is released from the instrinsic factor. After passage across the enterocytes, cobalamin is transported in blood bound to circulating proteins known as transcobalamins.

Understanding the normal absorptive processes allows an appreciation of a suggested classification of cobalamin malabsorption and deficiency (Table 1).

4.3 Iron

4.3.1 FOOD SOURCES

Iron is available for absorption from vegetables (nonheme iron) and from meats (heme iron). Heme iron is better absorbed (10–20%) and is unaffected by intraluminal factors or its dietary composition. Nonheme iron is poorly absorbed, with an efficiency of 1–6%, and absorption is largely controlled by luminal events. The average dietary intake of iron is 10–20 mg/day. Men absorb 1–2 mg/day, while menstruating women and iron-deficient patients absorb 3–4 mg/day. In acute blood loss, increased absorption of iron does not occur until three days later. Nonheme iron (in the ferric, Fe^{+++} state), when ingested into a stomach unable to produce acid, forms insoluble iron complexes, which are not available for absorption (Figure 3). In the presence of gastric acid and reducing agents such as ascorbic acid, however, ferrous iron (Fe^{++}) forms. The ferrous iron complexes bind to a mucopolysaccharide of about 200,000 MW_r and are transported as an insoluble complex into the duo-

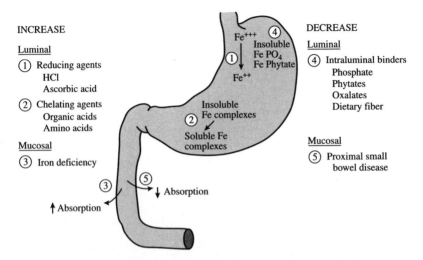

INCREASE

Luminal

① Reducing agents
  HCl
  Ascorbic acid

② Chelating agents
  Organic acids
  Amino acids

Mucosal

③ Iron deficiency

Fe^{+++} ④
Insoluble
① Fe PO_4
Fe Phytate

Fe^{++}

Insoluble
② Fe complexes

Soluble Fe
complexes

③ ⑤
↓ Absorption

↑ Absorption

DECREASE

Luminal

④ Intraluminal binders
  Phosphate
  Phytates
  Oxalates
  Dietary fiber

Mucosal

⑤ Proximal small
  bowel disease

FIGURE 3.   Factors that affect iron absorption. Nonheme iron absorption is affected both by intraluminal factors (1, 2 and 4) and by the total iron body content (3) as well as by small bowel disease (5). Heme iron absorption is altered only by those factors that affect the mucosa itself (3 and 5).
SOURCE: Alpers DH. Absorption of water-soluble vitamins, folate, minerals, and vitamin D. In: Sleisenger MH, Fordtran JS (eds.), Gastrointestinal disease: pathophysiology, diagnosis, management. 3d ed. Philadelphia: WB Saunders, 1983:835.

denum and proximal jejunum. Here, with the assistance of ascorbic acid, glucose and cysteine, the iron is absorbed. Dietary factors such as phosphate, phytate and phosphoproteins can render the iron insoluble and so inhibit nonheme iron absorption.

Heme iron (ferrous, Fe^{++}) is ingested as myoglobin and hemoglobin. In the presence of gastric acid, the globin molecule is split off, and ferrous iron is liberated and transported with its phosphorin ring from the stomach into the duodenum and jejunum for absorption.

Both heme and nonheme iron are absorbed most rapidly in the duodenum. Some of the iron taken up is deposited as ferritin within the enterocyte, and the remainder is transferred to the plasma-bound transferrin. When the enterocyte defoliates, iron deposited as ferritin is lost into the intestinal lumen. This mechanism for loss is probably overwhelmed by the large amounts of iron ingested. The amount of iron entering the body depends largely upon two factors: (1) total body iron content and (2) the rate of erythropoiesis. The mechanism of intestinal iron absorption is shown in Figure 4.

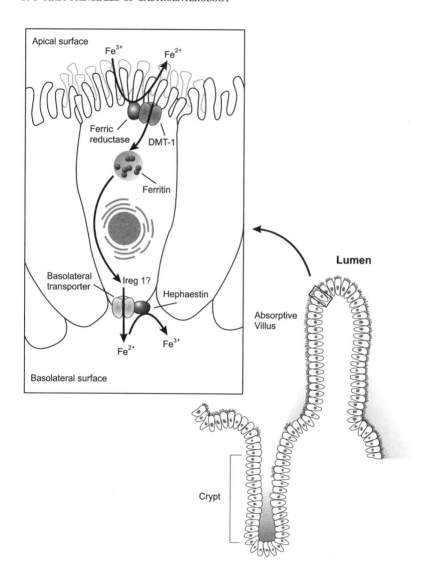

FIGURE 4.   Intestinal absorption of iron. Iron is being transported across the brush-border membrane (BBM) by DMT (duodenal metal-transporter), and across the basolateral membrane possibly by Ireg 1, in conjunction with hephaestin, a ceruloplasmin-like molecule. Ferrureductase already in the BBM reduces Fe^{3+} to Fe^{2+} for transport by DMT. Absorption of iron is regulated by the amount of iron in the diet, by body iron stores and by the activity of the bone marrow erythropoiesis.

5. ABSORPTION OF WATER AND ELECTROLYTES

5.1 Passive Permeability to Ions and Water

The epithelium of the small intestine exhibits a high passive permeability to salt and water that is a consequence of the leakiness of the junctions between epithelial cells. Some water absorption may occur as the result of carrier-mediated transport of solutes. Osmotic equilibration between plasma and lumen is fairly rapid; therefore, large differences in ion concentration do not develop. These intercellular junctions are more permeable to cations than anions, so that lumen-to-blood concentration differences for Na^+ and K^+ are generally smaller than those for Cl^- and HCO_3. The colonic epithelium displays lower passive permeability to salt and water. This ionic permeability diminishes from cecum to rectum. It also decreases from duodenum to ileum. One consequence of this lower passive ionic permeability (higher electrical resistance) is that electric potential differences across the colonic epithelium are an order of magnitude greater than those in the small intestine (remember Ohm's law, $E = IR$, where E is electrical potential, I is electrical current, and R is electrical resistance). Active Na^+ absorption, which is the main transport activity of the distal colon, generates a serosa-positive charge or potential difference (PD). Under the influence of aldosterone (i.e., salt depletion), this PD can be 60 mV or even higher. A 60 mV PD will thus sustain a 10-fold concentration difference for a monovalent ion such as K^+. Most of the high K^+ concentration in the rectum is accounted for, therefore, by the PD. Despite the high fecal K^+ level, little K^+ is lost in the stool, since stool volume (about 200–300 mL per day) is normally so low. In contrast, during high-volume (several liters per day) diarrhea of small bowel origin, the stool K^+ concentration is considerably lower (10–30 mmol) but stool K^+ loss is nonetheless great because of the large volumes involved. In such states, the stool K^+ concentration is low (and the Na^+ concentration relatively high) because diarrheal fluid passes through the colon too rapidly to equilibrate across the colonic epithelium.

5.2 Active Electrolyte Absorption along the Intestine

The small intestine has the largest capacity for secreting water and electrolytes of any organ system in the body. In both the small bowel and the colon, secretion appears to arise predominantly, if not exclusively, in crypts; the more superficial villous tip epithelium is absorptive. Disease processes that result in damage to the villus or to superficial portions of the intestinal epithelium (e.g., viral enteritis) inevitably shift the overall balance between absorption and secretion toward secretion. This is especially important in patients with celiac disease, where there is villous atrophy as well as hypertrophy of the crypts of Lieberkühn.

   In the small intestine, active electrolyte and fluid absorption can be conceived of as either *nutrient-dependent* or *nutrient-independent*.

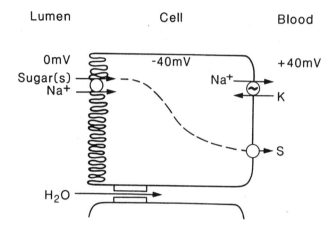

FIGURE 5. Na^+-coupled sugar absorption in the small intestine. This model presents the mechanism for sodium-coupled absorption of sugar. In addition to sugar, many amino acids, certain B vitamins and bile salts are absorbed through this mechanism. Sodium is taken up across the apical membrane in association with glucose (SGLT1) and exits by means of the basolateral sodium/potassium-ATPase. Glucose exits through a facilitated diffusion pathway in the basolateral membrane (GLUT2). Details of the model are described in the text.

5.2.1 NUTRIENT-DEPENDENT TRANSPORT

The absorptive processes for the nutrients glucose and neutral amino acids are Na^+-dependent – i.e., one Na^+ molecule is translocated across the brush border with each glucose or amino acid molecule (Figure 5). The sodium pump (Na^+/K^+-ATPase), which is located exclusively in the basolateral membrane of the enterocyte, extrudes Na^+ that has entered the enterocyte from the lumen, thereby maintaining a low intracellular Na^+, a high intracellular K^+ and a negative intracellular electric potential. This Na^+/K^+ pump provides the potential energy for uphill sugar and amino acid absorption. Glucose is cotransported with sodium. Patients in intestinal secretory states such as cholera can absorb glucose normally. Na^+ (and thus water) are also absorbed, accompanying the transport of glucose. As a consequence, the fluid losses incurred by these patients can be replaced by oral glucose-electrolyte solutions[1] and do not require intravenous fluids unless the patient is comatose or too nauseated to

[1] The WHO oral rehydration solution contains in mmol/L: glucose, 111; Na^+, 90; K^+, 20; Cl^-, 80; HCO_3^-, 30.

Lumen   Cell   Blood

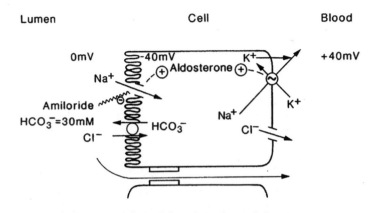

FIGURE 6. Electrogenic Na⁺ absorption in the distal colon. Sodium enters the cell at the apical membrane through sodium channels and leaves the cell at the basolateral membrane through the sodium/potassium-ATPase. Details of the model are described in the text.

drink the necessary large volumes of fluid to correct the dehydration. Application of this knowledge has had a major impact on world health, and especially on that of children, since the parts of the world where cholera-like diarrheas are prevalent generally have very limited hospital facilities and insufficient supplies of sterile electrolyte solutions.

5.2.2 NUTRIENT-INDEPENDENT TRANSPORT

Nutrient-independent active absorption of electrolytes and water by intestinal epithelial cells occurs through several specific mechanisms, located at different levels of the mammalian intestinal tract. All of these mechanisms have in common the Na^+/K^+-ATPase pump, located on the basolateral membrane, and also a requirement for luminal Na^+.

In the distal colon (Figure 6), the luminal membrane contains Na^+ channels, which can be blocked by low concentrations of the pyrazine diuretic amiloride. The Na^+ entering through these channels in the luminal membrane is then extruded across the basolateral membrane by the Na^+/K^+-ATPase pump. Aldosterone increases the number of these channels and also, more slowly, increases the number of Na^+/K^+-ATPase pumps. Aldosterone therefore enhances active Na^+ absorption in the distal colon. To a more limited extent, aldosterone also causes the appearance of Na^+ channels more proximally in the colon and even in the distal ileum. Cl^- is absorbed along with Na^+ and traverses the epithelium by both cellular and paracellular routes. Its transcellular

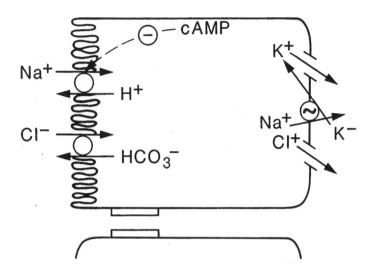

FIGURE 7.   Electroneutral sodium chloride absorption in the small intestine and colon. Apical sodium chloride entry through sodium/hydrogen and chloride/bicarbonate permits sodium and chloride to enter the cell in an electroneutral fashion. Sodium exits the cell through the basolateral sodium/potassium-ATPase. The route of chloride efflux remains relatively speculative, but likely occurs through some basolateral channel. Details of the model are described in the text.

route involves a Cl^-/HCO_3^- exchanger in the luminal membrane and Cl^- channels in the basolateral membrane. Intracellular mediators such as cyclic AMP (cAMP) do not appear to affect these Na^+ channels. Thus, patients with secretory diarrheas, especially those who are salt-depleted and therefore have elevated blood levels of aldosterone, are able to reabsorb some of the secreted fluid in their distal colon. Spironolactone, which inhibits the action of aldosterone, can increase the severity of diarrhea in such patients.

In the more proximal colon and in the ileum, the luminal membrane contains Na^+/H^+ exchangers that permit net Na^+ entry (Figure 7). A family of Na^+/H^+ exchangers has been identified and cloned. The colon and the ileum (but not the jejunum) also have Cl^-/HCO_3^- exchangers in their luminal borders. Cell pH adjusts the relative rates of these two exchangers. Thus, H^+ extrusion by Na^+/H^+ exchange can cause cell alkalinization, which then stimulates Cl^- entry and HCO_3^- extrusion by this Cl^-/HCO_3^- exchange. The latter exchanger increases cell H^+, thereby sustaining Na^+/H^+ exchange. Increases in cell concentrations of cAMP and free Ca^{2+} inhibit the Na^+/H^+ exchange.

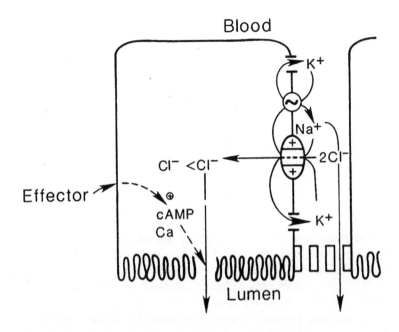

FIGURE 8. Electrogenic chloride secretion in both small and large intestine. A cyclic AMP–activated channel in the apical membrane permits hormone-stimulated chloride secretion. The chloride channel is coded by a gene (cystic fibrosis transmembrane conductance regulator [CFTR]) that is responsible for cystic fibrosis. Chloride enters the cell through a sodium/potassium transport along the basolateral surface. Details of this model are discussed in the text.

Cyclic AMP and its agonists thereby cause cell acidification – which, in turn, inhibits Cl^-/HCO_3^- exchange. Therefore, electrolyte absorption in small and large intestinal segments (except the distal colon) can be down-regulated by hormones, neurotransmitters and certain luminal substances (bacterial enterotoxins, bile salts, hydroxylated fatty acids) that increase cell concentrations of cAMP or free Ca^{2+}. For this reason, body fluid secreted in response to these stimuli cannot be effectively reabsorbed in the absence of amino acids and sugars, except in the distal colon. In the jejunum, where Cl^-/HCO_3^- exchange does not appear to be present, Na^+/H^+ exchange can be well sustained by anaerobic glycolysis, which generates H^+ as well as some ATP.

There is also some evidence for a direct cotransport of Na^+ and Cl^-, although this is difficult to separate experimentally from dual exchangers. This entry mechanism may exist in the ileum and proximal colon.

TABLE 2. Hormones and neurotransmitters that stimulate intestinal secretion

	Intracellular mediator	
cAMP	Ca^{2+}	Unknown
Vasoactive intestinal peptide	Bradykinin	Bombesin
Prostaglandins	Acetylcholine	Lipoxygenase products
Bradykinin	Substance P	Thyrocalcitonin
	Neurotensin	Histamine
	Serotonin	Vasopressin

Only agents found effective in vitro have been listed. Several other hormones have been found to stimulate secretion in vivo, but it is unclear whether they act directly on the intestinal mucosa. The latter include glucagon and pentagastrin.

5.3 Active Electrolyte Secretion along the Intestine

In the secretory cell, the entry of Cl$^-$ from the contraluminal bathing medium (blood or serosal side of the enterocyte) is coupled to that of Na$^+$ and probably also K$^+$ by a triple cotransporter with a stoichiometry of 1 Na$^+$, 1 K$^+$ and 2 Cl$^-$. Na$^+$ entering in this fashion is then recycled to the contraluminal solution by the Na$^+$/K$^+$ exchange pump (Figure 8). K$^+$, entering via the pump and also the triple cotransporter, diffuses back to the contraluminal side through K$^+$ channels. Owing to the Na$^+$ gradient, Cl$^-$ accumulates above electrochemical equilibrium and can either (1) recycle back to the contraluminal solution through the Na$^+$/K$^+$/2 Cl$^-$ cotransporter or through basolateral membrane Cl$^-$ channels, or (2) be secreted into the lumen through luminal membrane Cl$^-$ channels. When Cl$^-$ is secreted into the lumen it generates a serosa-positive electric potential difference, which provides the driving force for Na$^+$ secretion through the paracellular pathway between cells. In the resting secretory cell, the luminal Cl$^-$ channels are closed. When secretion is stimulated by a hormone or neurotransmitter, these channels open. Secretion is initiated, therefore, by opening the Cl$^-$ "gate" in the luminal membrane of the secretory cell.

The known intracellular mediators of secretion are cAMP, cGMP and Ca^{2+} (Table 2). These can arise from the blood; nerve endings; endocrine cells in the epithelium (APUD cells); mesenchymal elements such as lymphocytes, plasma cells and mast cells; or the enterocytes themselves. Except for the cAMP agonists, lipoxygenase products and calcitonin, the actions of the other agonists are short-lived; desensitization rapidly develops. They operate to fine-tune electrolyte transport rather than invoke persistent secretion.

Predictably, since there are hormones and neurotransmitters that stimulate active electrolyte secretion in the gut, there are also agonists that inhibit secretion and/or stimulate absorption. These include adrenocorticosteroids, norepinephrine, somatostatin, enkephalins and dopamine. Glucocorticoids enhance electrolyte absorption throughout the intestinal tract, but the mechanisms involved are less well understood than for aldosterone. They may act in part by inhibiting phospholipase A_2 and therefore the arachidonic acid cascade. The adrenergic receptors on enterocytes are almost exclusively α_2 in type. The sympathetic nervous system in the intestinal mucosa releases norepinephrine (an α_2 antagonist) and so inhibits electrolyte secretion and stimulates absorption. Sympathectomy, whether chemical or surgical, leads to diarrhea, at least transiently. Chronic diabetics with autonomic neuropathy sometimes develop persistent diarrhea that is associated with degeneration of adrenergic nerve fibers to the gut. Somatostatin and endogenous enkephalins are also antisecretory.

6. ABSORPTION OF FAT

The overall process of fat digestion and absorption consists of four distinct phases, related to the respective functions of the pancreas, liver, intestinal mucosa and lymphatics (Figure 9). Physiologically, these involve (1) lipolysis of dietary triglyceride (TG) to fatty acid (FA) and β-monoglyceride (MG); (2) micellar solubilization with bile acid; (3) uptake into the mucosal cell, with re-esterification of the MG with FA to form TG, and chylomicron formation in the presence of cholesterol, cholesterol esters, phospholipids and protein; and (4) delivery of chylomicrons in lymphatics to the body for utilization of fat.

The average North American diet contains 60–100 g of fat each day, mostly in the form of neutral fat or triglycerides. In the proximal intestine, TG comes under hydrolytic attack by lipases, producing glycerol, FA and MG. These products of lipolysis first form an emulsion and later a micellar solution.

Following the entry of food and particularly fat into the duodenum, cholecystokinin (CCK) is released from mucosal cells, causing gallbladder contraction. Bile acids, along with other biliary constituents, are released into the proximal small intestine. Bile acids chemically resemble detergent molecules, in that a portion of the molecule is polar and water-soluble, while another portion of the molecule is nonpolar and fat-soluble. When the bile acids are present in sufficient amounts, known as the critical micellar concentration (CMC), they form negatively charged spheres, called simple micelles. Incorporation of FA and MG forms a larger, polymolecular aggregate, a mixed micelle. All this is necessary to solubilize fat and disperse it in small packets more effectively, setting the stage for further digestion by pancreatic lipase. This enzyme acts only at oil–water interfaces and requires a large surface area. Pancreatic lipase is secreted into the duodenual lumen where it acts on ingested food.

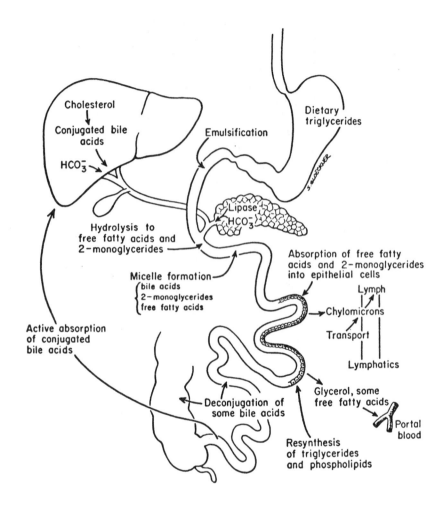

FIGURE 9.   Diagram of the major steps in the digestion and absorption of dietary fat. These include (1) the lipolysis of dietary triglyceride (TG) by pancreatic enzymes; (2) micellar solubilization of the resulting long-chain fatty acids (FA) and β-monoglycerides (βMG; shown in figure as 2-monoglycerides) by bile acids secreted into the intestinal lumen by the liver; (3) absorption of the fatty acids and β-monoglycerides into the mucosal cell with subsequent re-esterification and formation of chylomicrons; and, finally, (4) movement of the chylomicrons from the mucosal cell into the intestinal lymphatic system. During the process of chylomicron formation, small amounts of cholesterol (C), cholesterol ester (CE), and phospholipid (PL) as well as triglyceride are incorporated into this specific lipoprotein fraction.

SOURCE: Wilson FA, Dietschy JM. Differential diagnostic approach to clinical problems of malabsorption. Gastroenterology 1971; 61:912.

Adequate concentrations of bile acid must be present within the jejunal lumen for effective micellar solubilization and lipolysis by pancreatic lipase, a preliminary to esterification and uptake. Such adequate concentrations of bile acids are maintained by the constant reutilization of a relatively small pool of bile acid. In the liver, about 0.6 g of new bile acid is produced daily from cholesterol. This is added to the total bile acid pool of 3.0 g, which cycles 6 to 10 times daily from passive absorption in the jejunum and active absorption in the ileum. Approximately 96% of the bile acid is absorbed through these mechanisms with each cycle; the remainder is lost in the stool. The bile acid transporter has been cloned. A deficiency of this transporter may lead to bile salt malabsorption and diarrhea. Bile acids return to the liver via the portal vein and are excreted once more. This recirculation of bile acid between the intestine and the liver is called the enterohepatic circulation.

The principal role of the bile salt micelle is to facilitate lipid absorption by maintaining the lipid in a water-soluble form, overcoming the resistance of the unstirred water layer and maintaining a high concentration of a local source of fatty acid and cholesterol, which leave the micelle and enter the mucosal cell. Lipid uptake across the brush-border membrane is passive, but a number of lipid-binding proteins have been isolated; their role in lipid absorption remains to be determined.

Two important events occur within the mucosal cell: re-esterification and chylomicron formation. The fatty acids are first reattached to the monoglycerides through re-esterification, and the resultant triglyceride is then combined with small amounts of cholesterol and coated with phospholipids and apolipoproteins to form a specific class of lipoproteins known as chylomicrons. The intestine produces four apolipoproteins, apo A-I, A-IV, B and C. The chylomicrons are then released from the basal portion of the columnar epithelial cell and find their way into the central lacteal of the intestinal villus. From there, chylomicrons travel in lymph up the thoracic duct and eventually reach the general circulation. Chylomicrons are then transported in the blood to the sites of disposal and utilization in the periphery (e.g., liver, muscle and adipose tissue). A small amount of lipid may be absorbed into the portal circulation, bypassing the lacteals.

From these physiological considerations, malabsorption of fat due to impaired lipolysis or micellar solubilization would be expected to occur in the following circumstances: (1) rapid gastric emptying and improper mixing – e.g., following vagotomy or postgastrectomy; (2) altered duodenal pH – e.g., the Zollinger-Ellison syndrome, where excessive duodenal acidification inhibits the action of lipase; (3) pancreatic insufficiency; (4) cholestasis – e.g., biliary obstruction, liver disease; and (5) an interrupted enterohepatic circulation – e.g., ileal disease or loss, and bile salt deconjugation due to the bacterial overgrowth syndrome.

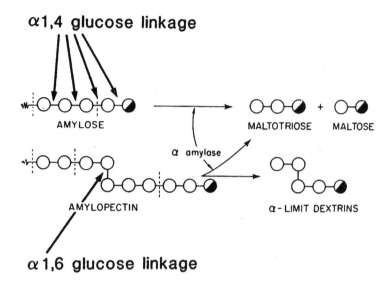

FIGURE 10.   The action of pancreatic α-amylase on linear (amylose) and branched (amylopectin) starch. Circles indicate glucose residues and the reducing glucose unit.
SOURCE: Gray GM. Mechanisms of digestion and absorption of food. In Sleisenger MH, Fordtran JS (eds.), Gastrointestinal disease: pathphysiology, diagnosis, management. 3d ed. Philadelphia: WB Saunders, 1983:851.

Fat malabsorption due to impaired mucosal uptake, assembly or delivery would be expected to occur following (1) generalized impaired enterocyte function – e.g., celiac disease, Whipple's disease; (2) failure of the packaging process – e.g., abetalipoproteinemia, which represents a genetic defect of lipoprotein B synthesis with consequent impairment of chylomicron formation; (3) disorders of lymphatics – e.g., intestinal lymphangiectasia, retroperitoneal fibrosis or lymphoma; and (4) loss of mucosal surface area – e.g., the short bowel syndrome.

7. ABSORPTION OF CARBOHYDRATES

Starch, sucrose and lactose constitute the main carbohydrates in the human diet. All are inexpensive sources of food. Together they constitute the major source of calories when considered worldwide. People in the Western world consume about 400 g of carbohydrates daily: 60% as starch, 30% as sucrose and 10% as lactose (milk contains 48 g of lactose per liter).

Starch present in wheat, rice and corn is a polysaccharide whose molecular weight ranges from 100,000 to greater than 1,000,000. The straight chain of glucose molecules in starch is bridged by an oxygen molecule between the first carbon (C_1) of one glucose unit and the fourth carbon (C_4) of its neighbor ($\alpha 1,4$ glucose link). This type of starch is called amylose and makes up as much as 20% of the starch in the diet. The glucose-to-glucose bridge is of the alpha type – in contrast to the beta type, which connects glucose units in cellulose, an indigestible saccharide. The remaining 80% of the starch that humans ingest has a branch point every 25 molecules along the straight $\alpha 1,4$ glucose chain. This starch is called amylopectin. These branches occur via an oxygen bridge between C_6 of the glucose on the straight chain and C_1 in the branched chain ($\alpha 1,6$ branch points), which then continues as another $\alpha 1,4$ glucose-linked straight chain (Figure 10).

Salivary and pancreatic α-amylases act on interior $\alpha 1,4$ glucose–glucose links of starch but cannot attack $\alpha 1,4$ linkages close to a 1,6 branch point. The products of amylase digestion are therefore maltose and maltotriose. Since α-amylase cannot hydrolyze the 1,6 branching links and has relatively little specificity for 1,4 links adjacent to these branch points, large oligosaccharides containing five to nine glucose units and consisting of one or more 1,6 branching links are also produced by α-amylase action. These are called α-limit dextrins, and represent about 30% of amylopectin breakdown.

The responsibility for digesting the oligosaccharides, including α-limit dextrins, and the amylose and amylopectin rests with the hydrolytic enzymes on intestinal epithelial cells (Figures 11 and 12). These hydrolytic enzymes are called disaccharidases, but most are in fact oligosaccharidases: they hydrolyze sugars containing three or more hexose units. They are present in highest concentration at the villous tips in the jejunum and persist throughout most of the ileum, but not in the colon. Lactase breaks down lactose into glucose and galactose. Glucoamylase (maltase) differs from pancreatic α-amylase since it sequentially removes a single glucose from the nonreducing end of a linear $\alpha 1,4$ glucose chain, breaking down maltose into glucose. Sucrase is a hybrid molecule consisting of two enzymes – one hydrolyzing sucrose and the other, the $\alpha 1,6$ branch points of the α-limit dextrins. This enzyme is commonly called sucrase-isomaltase, because the isomaltase moiety hydrolyzes isomaltose, the $\alpha 1,6$ glucosyl disaccharide. However, the only products containing $\alpha 1,6$ linkages after amylase action on starch are the α-limit dextrins. Thus no free isomaltose is presented to the intestinal surface and the term "isomaltase" is a misnomer. The sucrase moiety thus breaks down sucrose into glucose and fructose.

Humans normally are born with a full complement of brush-border-membrane disaccharidases. Intake of large amounts of sucrose results in an increase in sucrase activity, probably as the substrate stabilizes the enzyme

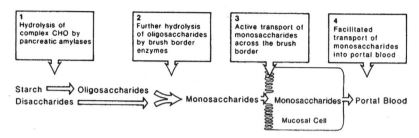

Starch ⟹ Oligosaccharides
Disaccharides ⟹ ⟹ Monosaccharides → Monosaccharides → Portal Blood

Mucosal Cell

FIGURE 11.   Major steps in the digestion and absorption of dietary carbohydrate.

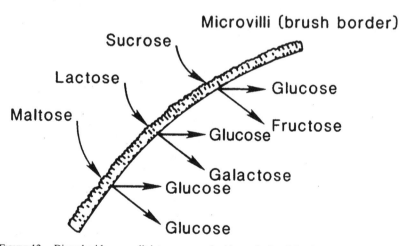

FIGURE 12.   Disaccharides are split into monosaccharides at the brush border.

and reduces its rate of breakdown. In contrast, there is no evidence that dietary manipulation can regulate the activities of human lactase or maltase.

Once the disaccharides are broken down, how are the monosaccharides absorbed? Sodium facilitates glucose uptake by binding to the brush-border membrane carrier (SGLT1) along with glucose. Since intracellular Na^+ concentration is low, the Na^+ ion moves down its concentration gradient into the cell, to be pumped out subsequently at the basolateral membrane by Na^+/K^+-ATPase, an active process that utilizes energy derived from the hydrolysis of ATP. The electrochemical gradient thus developed by Na^+ provides the driving force for glucose entry. Glucose accompanies Na^+ on the brush-border carrier and is released inside the cell, where its concentrations may exceed those in the intestinal lumen. Glucose then exits from the basolateral membrane of the cell into the portal system by a non–Na^+-dependent carrier (GLUT2).

Fructose, released from the hydrolysis of sucrose, is transported by facilitated diffusion, a carrier-mediated process in the brush-border membrane (GLUT5) that is independent both of Na^+ and of the glucose transport mechanism. The glucose and fructose are transported out of the enterocyte by GLUT2, a sodium-independent carrier in the basolateral membrane.

From these physiological considerations, carbohydrate malabsorption can occur in the following circumstances: (1) severe pancreatic insufficiency; (2) selective deficiencies of brush-border disaccharidases – e.g., lactase deficiency; (3) generalized impairment of brush-border and enterocyte function – e.g., celiac disease, tropical sprue, gastroenteritis; and (4) loss of mucosal surface area – e.g., the short bowel syndrome.

Although infants often have a deficiency of amylase, starch is not usually fed for the first few months of life. In the adult, there is a great excess of pancreatic amylase secreted into the intestinal lumen, so that even in patients with severe fat malabsorption due to pancreatic exocrine insufficiency, residual salivary and pancreatic amylase output appears to be sufficient to completely hydrolyze starch to the final oligosaccharides by the time a meal reaches the mid-jejunum. Hence, severe maldigestion of starch rarely occurs in humans.

Secondary deficiency of disaccharidases results from anatomic injury of the small intestine, as in celiac disease, tropical sprue and gastroenteritis. When disaccharidase levels are sufficiently low, the particular oligosaccharide or disaccharide remains unhydrolyzed within the intestinal lumen and augments intraluminal fluid accumulation by virtue of its osmotic effect. Bacterial fermentation of disaccharides that reach the colon produces fatty acids (butyric, formic, acetic and propionic acids), alcohols and gases (H_2 and CO_2) (Figure 13). The benefits of this bacterial fermentation to the host are twofold. First, the bulk of the caloric value present in carbohydrates remains in the fermentative products. Reabsorption of fatty acids and alcohols in the colon "salvages" calories from malabsorbed carbohydrates. Second, this colonic "salvage" reduces the number of osmoles in the lumen and hence lessens the water lost in feces. During the fermentation of carbohydrates to organic acids, colonic bacteria liberate H_2 and CO_2 gas. In general, the passage of large quantities of rectal gas suggests that excessive carbohydrates are reaching the colon.

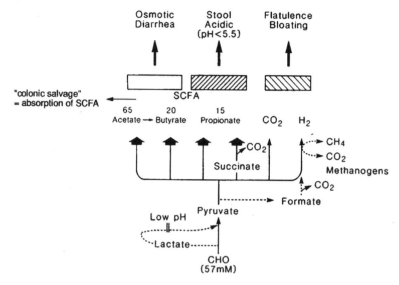

FIGURE 13.   Intermediate and end products of anaerobic bacterial fermentation of carbohydrates.
Minor pathways are depicted by dashed lines.
SOURCE: Soergel KH. The role of the colon in case of inhibition of carbohydrate absorption. In:
Creutzfeldt W, Fölsch UR (eds.), Delaying absorption as a therapeutic principle in metabolic diseases. Stuttgart and New York: Thieme Verlag, 1983:854.

Other primary (congenital) deficiencies of disaccharidases are unusual.
Such entities can be differentiated from a secondary defect, since general
tests of absorption and mucosal histology are normal; however, assay of an
intestinal biopsy reveals the absence of hydrolytic activity for a single disaccharide. Primary lactase deficiency is very common in certain ethnic groups,
such as persons from South East Asia, and may limit the intake of milk in
some adults.

8. ABSORPTION OF PROTEIN

8.1 Intraluminal Digestion
Digestion of protein begins in the stomach under the influence of pepsin. This
lasts for only one to two hours, while the pH is acidic following meal-stimulated acid secretion. Most dietary protein, however, is hydrolyzed by pancreatic proteases secreted into the proximal duodenum in inactive form. Activation of each protease is initially catalyzed by the duodenal mucosal surface

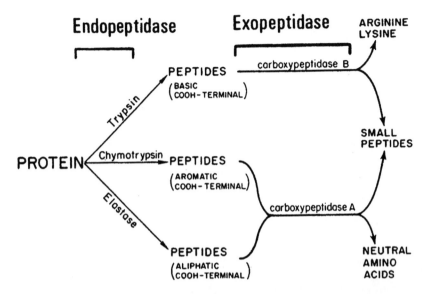

FIGURE 14. Sequence of events leading to hydrolysis of dietary protein by intraluminal proteases.
SOURCE: Gray GM. Mechanisms of digestion and absorption of food. In Sleisenger MH, Fordtran JS (eds.), Gastrointestinal disease: pathphysiology, diagnosis, management. 3d ed. Philadelphia: WB Saunders, 1983:854.

enzyme enterokinase and by activated trypsin (Figure 14). Activation is virtually instantaneous in the first and second portions of the duodenal lumen. Intraluminal digestion of dietary protein occurs in the duodenum by sequential action of pancreatic endopeptidases and exopeptidases. The endopeptidases trypsin, chymotrypsin, elastase, DNAase and RNAase act on the peptide at the interior of the protein molecule. These peptides are then acted upon by the exopeptidases carboxypeptidase A and B, which remove a single amino acid from the carboxyl terminal end of the peptide, yielding basic and neutral amino acids (AAs) as well as small peptides.

8.2 Cellular Digestion
Peptidases in the brush border then hydrolyze the residual di-, tri- and tetrapeptides that contain neutral AAs. Peptides consisting primarily of glycine, proline, hydroxyproline or dicarboxylic AA appear to be hydrolyzed inside the cell. AA and dipeptides are then transported into the mucosal cell interior. The transport system for neutral AA absorbs aromatic (phenylalanine, tyrosine, tryptophan) and aliphatic (valine, leucine, isoleucine, methionine) AAs.

The basic AAs (arginine, lysine) are absorbed by a separate mechanism. There is a third mechanism for glycine, proline and hydroxyproline, and a fourth for dicarboxylic AAs (aspartic and glutamic AA).

From these physiological considerations, protein malabsorption would be expected in diseases causing (1) pancreatic insufficiency; (2) generalized impaired enterocyte function – e.g., celiac disease; and (3) loss of mucosal surface – e.g., the short bowel syndrome.

A transporter for dipeptides has been cloned. The absorption of amino acids from dipeptides may be faster than from amino acids, and the peptide transporter may be more resistant to disease-associated damage than are the amino acid transporters.

9. MALDIGESTION AND MALABSORPTION: THE MALASSIMILATION SYNDROMES

Normal digestion and absorption of foods is essential for life and well-being. Given the length of the gastrointestinal tract, the number of organs involved in digestion, and the large number of nutrients that must be taken into our bodies, it is not surprising to find a large number of disease states that impair the processes of food digestion and absorption. Clinical malassimilation occurs in only one of two ways: (1) through intraluminal disorders (maldigestion of food) and (2) through intramural disorders (malabsorption of food).

9.1 Clinical Manifestations

The list of diseases that can cause malassimilation is long (Table 3), necessitating logical history-taking and investigation.

Clinical suspicion, as always, comes from the patient's history and physical examination. A patient with malassimilation may have symptoms and signs of specific nutrient deficiencies or those of the underlying disease process itself (e.g., Crohn's disease). Furthermore, considering that malassimilation usually involves multiple nutrients, the symptoms and signs of a malassimilation state can vary from a straightforward presentation to myriad symptom complexes (Tables 4 and 5).

The patient who gives a history of progressive weight loss, polyphagia, excessive flatus, diarrhea, bulky and foul-smelling stools, food particles or fat in the stool, abdominal distention, muscle wasting, bone pain, bleeding, weakness, tetany, paresthesia, glossitis, cheilosis or dermatitis is giving you the "classical" history of severe intestinal malassimilation. Rarely will you hear such a history from a patient in North America. It is far more common to see patients who will have vague symptoms for which there is some abnormality in their blood chemistry that alerts you to the presence of disease.

TABLE 3. Classification of malassimilation syndromes

Defective intraluminal digestion	*Defective intramural absorption*
Mixing disorders	Inadequate absorptive surface
Postgastrectomy	Intestinal resection or bypass
	Mesenteric vascular disease with mas-
Pancreatic insufficiency	sive intestinal resection
Primary	Regional enteritis with multiple bowel
Cystic fibrosis	resections
Secondary	Jejunoileal bypass
Chronic pancreatitis	Mucosal absorptive defects
Pancreatic carcinoma	Biochemical or genetic abnormalities
Pancreatic resection	Celiac disease
	Disaccharidase deficiency
Reduced intestinal bile salt concentration	Hypogammaglobulinemia
Liver disease	Abetalipoproteinemia
Hepatocellular disease	Hartnup disease
Cholestasis (intrahepatic or extrahepatic)	Cystinuria
Abnormal bacterial proliferation in the	Monosaccharide malabsorption
small bowel	Inflammatory or infiltrative disorders
Afferent loop stasis	Regional enteritis
Strictures	Amyloidosis
Fistulas	Scleroderma
Blind loops	Lymphoma
Multiple diverticula of the small bowel	Radiation enteritis
Hypomotility states (diabetes, scleroder-	Eosinophilic enteritis
ma, intestinal pseudo-obstruction)	Tropical sprue
Interrupted enterohepatic circulation of	Infectious enteritis (e.g., salmonellosis)
bile salts	Collagenous sprue
Ileal resection	Nonspecific ulcerative jejunitis
Ileal inflammatory disease (regional	Mastocytosis
ileitis)	Dermatologic disorders (e.g., dermatitis
Drugs (by sequestration or precipitation of	herpetiformis)
bile salts)	Lymphatic obstruction
Neomycin	Intestinal lymphangiectasia
Calcium carbonate	Whipple's disease
Cholestyramine	Lymphoma

Early symptoms of the disease may easily be overlooked, and a severely malnourished state may come to exist. Often a patient will have noticed "early" symptoms, which will become apparent only when questioned directly. Hence, the physician must inquire about minor changes in bowel habits occurring before the onset of weight loss, hyperphagia, pain, anorexia or gross changes in bowel habits. Subtle changes in stool volume or bulk (manifested by a slight increase in the number of bowel movements per day), consistency

TABLE 4.   Clinical signs and symptoms of malassimilation

	Clinical sign or symptom	Deficient nutrient
General	Weight loss	Calorie
	Loss of appetite, amenorrhea, decreased libido	Protein energy
Skin	Psoriasiform rash, eczematous scaling	Zinc
	Pallor	Folate, iron, vitamin B_{12}
	Follicular hyperkeratosis	Vitamin A
	Perifollicular petechiae	Vitamin C
	Flaking dermatitis	Protein energy, niacin, riboflavin, zinc
	Bruising	Vitamin K
	Pigmentation changes	Niacin, protein energy
	Scrotal dermatosis	Riboflavin
	Thickening and dryness of skin	Linoleic acid
Head	Temporal muscle wasting	Protein energy
Hair	Sparse and thin, dyspigmentation Easy to pull out	Protein
Eyes	History of night blindness	Vitamin A
	Photophobia, blurring, conjunctival inflammation	Riboflavin, vitamin A
	Corneal vascularization	Riboflavin
	Xerosis, Bitot's spots, keratomalacia	Vitamin A
Mouth	Glossitis	Riboflavin, niacin, folic acid
	Bleeding gums	Vitamin C, riboflavin
	Cheilosis	Riboflavin
	Angular stomatitis	Riboflavin, iron
	Hypogeusia	Zinc
	Tongue fissuring	Niacin
	Tongue atrophy	Riboflavin, niacin, iron
	Scarlet and raw tongue	Niacin
	Nasolabial seborrhea	Pyridoxine
Neck	Goiter	Iodine
	Parotid enlargement	Protein
Thorax	Thoracic "rosary"	Vitamin D

(cont'd)

TABLE 4.   Clinical signs and symptoms of malassimilation (cont'd)

	Clinical sign or symptom	Deficient nutrient
Abdomen	Diarrhea	Niacin, folate, vitamin B_{12}
	Distention	Protein energy
	Hepatomegaly	Protein energy
Extremities	Edema	Protein, thiamine
	Softening of bone	Vitamin D, calcium, phosphorus
	Bone tenderness	Vitamin D
	Bone ache, joint pain	Vitamin C
	Muscle wasting and weakness	Protein, calories
	Muscle tenderness, muscle pain	Thiamine
	Hyporeflexia	Thiamine
Nails	Flattening, brittleness, luster loss, spooning	Iron
	Transverse lines	Protein
Neurologic	Tetany	Calcium, magnesium
	Paresthesias	Thiamine, vitamin B_{12}
	Loss of reflexes, wrist drop, foot drop	Thiamine
	Loss of vibratory and position sense, ataxia	Vitamin B_{12}
	Dementia, disorientation	Niacin
Blood	Anemia	Iron, vitamin B_{12}, folate
	Hemolysis	Phosphorus

or odor are early manifestations of malassimilation. A slight increase in the frequency of stools occurring at a time when the patient is mildly anorexic occurs a long time before disease becomes clinically apparent. An early increase in bulk of the stool and floating of the stool is caused by increased water and gas content and leads to an inability to flush the stool easily. It is not uncommon for the patient to think the toilet is malfunctioning because several flushings are needed to remove the stool. A greasy character and truly rancid odor are indicative of increased stool fat, but are often absent until late. These complaints are often readily passed over by the busy physician. At such time, physical findings are usually absent, but hyperactive bowel sounds may be noted, especially in small intestinal disease. If symptoms are intermittent or if they progress slowly over many years, patients may exhibit vague, seemingly unrelated symptoms such as chronic fatigue and depression, long before the physician considers the possibility of serious organic disease.

TABLE 5.   Specific vitamin and mineral deficiencies

Vitamin/mineral		Clinical manifestation
Vitamin A	Eyes	Night blindness
		Xerosis (dry bulbar conjunctiva)
		Bitot's spots (conjunctiva plaques)
		Keratomalacia (corneal ulceration)
	Skin	Hyperkeratosis
Vitamin B$_{12}$	Hematologic, neurologic systems	Anemia
		Nonreversible loss of vibratory and position sense
		Paresthesia
	Gastrointestinal	Diarrhea
Vitamin C	Skin	Perifollicular papules (brittle hair)
		Perifollicular hemorrhages
		Gum bleeding
		Skin purpura, ecchymosis
Vitamin D	Bone	Bone pain and softening
		Joint pain
		Rickets
		Proximal myopathy
Vitamin K		Bruising
		Bleeding
Vitamin B$_6$ (Pyridoxine)	Skin	Seborrheic dermatitis
		Cheilosis
		Glossitis
Niacin		Dermatitis
		Diarrhea
		Dementia
Thiamine	CVS	Congestive heart failure
	CNS	Wernicke's encephalopathy
		Wernicke-Korsakoff syndrome
Zinc	Skin	Acrodermatitis enteropathica
		Alopecia
	Taste	Hypogeusia
Folate	Hematologic, neurologic systems	Anemia
		Reversible loss of position and vibratory sense

CVS = cardiovascular system; CNS = central nervous system

9.2 Manifestations of Carbohydrate Malassimilation

Carbohydrate malassimilation will result in both specific and generalized symptoms. Specific to the maldigestion and malabsorption of carbohydrates are diarrhea and excess flatus. Unfortunately, everyone has flatus, and a definition or measure of excessive "wind" is lacking. Malabsorbed carbohydrates that enter the colon are fermented by colonic bacteria to gases (CO_2, H_2 and CH_4) and organic acids (Figure 13). These organic acids produce diarrhea by acting directly on colonic epithelium to stimulate fluid secretion and by their osmotic effect, which further draws water into the lumen. The presence of organic acids in the stool reduces the pH below 6 and suggests carbohydrate malassimilation. The gas produces flatulence, with associated borborygmi and abdominal distention. The presence of intraluminal H_2 gas, eventually absorbed into the circulation and exhaled, forms the basis of the hydrogen breath test to detect carbohydrate malabsorption. Physical examination often reveals a distended tympanitic abdomen with hyperactive bowel sounds. Stools float on the water because of their increased gas content (not because of their fat content).

Generally, lack of carbohydrate as an energy source will result in decreased plasma insulin levels, increased plasma glucagon and cortisol levels and decreased peripheral T_4-to-T_3 conversion. Given sufficient time, the body will enter a state of oxidative metabolism: fat and muscle will be catabolized. Physical examination may reveal signs of weight loss from both fat stores and lean body mass. The patient will be weak and will easily develop fatigue. Fat loss will generally be noted as sunken cheeks and flat buttocks, with wrinkled or loose skin indicative of loss of subcutaneous fat stores. The loss of muscle mass is easily noted as thenar mass reduction and sunken soft tissues between the extensor tendons on the dorsum of the hands. There may be direct evidence of a reduced metabolic rate secondary to decreased T_3 conversion. The patient will often be mentally slowed.

9.3 Manifestations of Fat Malassimilation

Failure to digest or absorb fats results in a variety of clinical symptoms and laboratory abnormalities. These manifestations are the result of both fat malassimilation per se and a deficiency of the fat-soluble vitamins. In general, loss of fat in the stool deprives the body of calories and contributes to weight loss and malnutrition. More specific is the action of unabsorbed long-chain fatty acids, which act on the colonic mucosa to cause diarrhea by an irritant effect on the colon. In addition, fatty acids bind calcium, which would normally be available to bind oxalate. In fat malabsorption, oxalate is not bound to calcium and remains free (undissociated) within the colonic lumen, where it is readily absorbed. This results in oxaluria and calcium oxalate kidney stones. This occurs in Crohn's disease more readily than in other cases of fat malabsorption (steatorrhea).

Failure to absorb the fat-soluble vitamins A, D, E and K also results in a variety of symptoms. Vitamin K deficiency presents as subcutaneous, urinary, nasal, vaginal and gastrointestinal bleeding. Deficiencies in factors II, VII, IX and X produce defective coagulation. Vitamin A deficiency results in follicular hyperkeratosis. Vitamin E deficiency leads to a progressive demyelination of the central nervous system. Malabsorption of vitamin D causes rickets and osteopenia, as discussed later.

9.4 Manifestations of Protein Malassimilation

Severe loss of body protein may occur before the development of laboratory abnormalities. Impaired protein synthesis from liver diseases and excessive protein loss in renal diseases can further aggravate protein deficiencies. Clinically, protein deficiency results in edema and diminished muscle mass. Since the immune system is dependent upon adequate proteins, protein deficiency can manifest as recurrent infections. Protein deficiency in children results in growth retardation, mental apathy and irritability, weakness and muscle atrophy, edema, hair loss, deformity of skeletal bone, anorexia, vomiting and diarrhea. Protein-calorie malnutrition is known as marasmus, whereas protein malnutrition by itself is known as kwashiorkor.

9.5 Manifestations of Iron Deficiency

Hypochromic microcytic anemia characterizes iron deficiency. Since malassimilation may result in folate or B_{12} deficiency (producing megaloblastic red cells), the microcytosis of iron deficiency may be obscured with automated cell counters; a dimorphic picture is present. Rarely accompanying the development of anemia may be symptoms of pica and dysphagia. Pica originally referred to the eating of clay or soil; however, the commonest "pica" in North America is the eating of ice. Dysphagia may be due to the Plummer-Vinson (Paterson-Kelly) syndrome (with atrophic papillae of the tongue and postcricoid esophageal webs), and/or cheilosis (reddened lips with angular fissures, also known as cheilitis or angular stomatitis). Weakness, fatigue, dyspnea and edema also can occur. Physical examination often reveals pallor, an atrophic tongue and koilonychia (brittle, flat or spoon-shaped fingernails).

The clinical picture of vitamin B_{12} and folic acid deficiency includes the nonspecific manifestations of megaloblastic anemia and its sequelae – i.e., anemia, glossitis, megaloblastosis, and elevated serum lactate dehydrogenase (LDH). In addition, deficiency of B_{12} may induce neurologic abnormalities consisting of symmetrical paresthesias in the feet and fingers, with associated

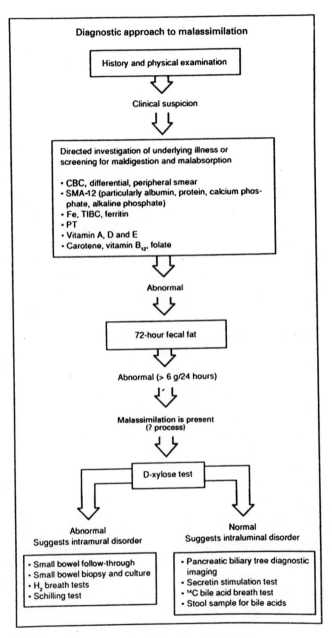

FIGURE 15.   Diagnostic approach to the patient with malassimilation.
SOURCE: Fedorak RN. Maldigestion and malabsorption. Medicine North America 1988; 3:3400.

disturbances of vibration sense and proprioception, progressing to ataxia with subacute combined degeneration of the spinal cord. This subacute combined spinal cord degeneration includes cortisospinal as well as dorsal column damage. Neurologic manifestations are not part of folic acid deficiency alone.

9.6 Manifestations of Calcium, Vitamin D and Magnesium Malabsorption

Impaired absorption of calcium, magnesium and vitamin D may lead to bone pain, fractures, paresthesias and tetany. In latent tetany, the neuromuscular instability can be brought out by provocative tests. Chvostek's sign and Trousseau's sign are provocative tests of clinical manifestations of hypocalcemia that are caused by neuromuscular instability. Osteomalacia resulting from vitamin D deficiency principally affects the spine, rib cage and long bones with or without fractures (Milkman's fractures), and may cause extreme pain, particularly in the spine, pelvis and leg bones. A child with calcium or vitamin D malabsorption will present with classical rickets. Hypomagnesemia may cause seizures and symptoms identical to those of hypocalcemia. In addition, hypomagnesemia may reduce the responsiveness of the parathyroids to calcium and impair parathyroid regulation of calcium homeostasis.

9.7 Initial Diagnostic Approach to Malassimilation

To avoid embarking on the shotgun approach to investigation, there are several questions one must ask. First, does malassimilation exist? And second, if so, is it due to a disorder of intraluminal digestion or a disorder of intramural absorption? Physicians should attempt to restrict the use of laboratory tests to those that establish the presence and cause of malassimilation (Figure 15).

To determine if malassimilation exists, one begins with the simplest, least invasive and least expensive tests. A complete blood count (CBC) and differential might reveal a macrocytic or microcytic anemia. A peripheral smear may demonstrate megaloblastosis, microcytosis and/or lymphopenia. Serum calcium, phosphorus and alkaline phosphatase may suggest the presence of osteomalacia. Serum albumin can assess protein stores. Serum cholesterol, carotene and prothrombin time (vitamin K) indirectly assess fat assimilation. Body iron stores may be assessed from the measurement of serum iron, total iron binding capacity (TIBC) and ferritin. The presence of depleted body iron stores suggests malabsorption of iron or depletion as the result of bleeding. More sensitive testing for osteoporosis using a bone scan (DEXA scan) may be necessary. Serum B_{12} is an index of body stores of B_{12}, which may be depleted because of reduced intake, deficient intrinsic factor, abnormal luminal pH, bacterial overgrowth or impaired ileal absorption. Red cell folate measures folate stores.

If their results are abnormal, the above tests suggest the presence of malassimilation and may indicate the deficient nutrient(s). Steatorrhea is the most important feature in the diagnosis of generalized malassimilation. Accurate measurement of fecal fat is important. Qualitative Sudan stain for fat globules on suspension of stool will give an indication of possible steatorrhea. However, this test cannot substitute for a quantitative fecal fat determination for a definitive diagnosis.

Quantitative fecal fat determination is the most reliable measure of steatorrhea. In the normal individual, the amount of fat appearing in the stool is relatively constant despite small changes in the quantity of dietary fat. Even when the daily fat intake is zero, the fecal fat output equals about 2.9 g/day. Presumably this is the amount of fat that is derived from endogenous sources, such as sloughed mucosal cells, excreted bile lipids (cholesterol and bile acids) and bacterial lipids. As the dietary intake of fat is increased, the fecal fat will increase to about 5 g/day on a 100 g fat diet. Fecal fat (FF) bears some relation to dietary fat: normally, the fecal fat loss is usually less than 5% of dietary intake. A defect at one of the steps in the overall process of fat assimilation dramatically increases this fat loss. A number of conditions should be met in order to obtain a reliable quantitative stool fat output. The patient should be on a steady dietary intake of a known 60–100 g fat, there must be a regular pattern of stooling, and all stool must be collected for 72 hours.

There are numerous possible artifacts for this test. Poor food intake, interrupted food intake, constipation or incomplete stool collection all give rise to a spuriously low value for the 24-hour fecal fat output. An artifactually high value will be seen when castor oil or nut oils have been consumed, but not petroleum mineral oils. The Van de Kamer method is the most commonly used procedure to chemically determine fecal fat output. This method, however, may lead to incomplete extraction and quantitation of medium-chain triglycerides (MCT) and thus may underestimate (by 10%) the quantity of fecal fats in patients whose diet has been supplemented with MCT. Steatorrhea does not indicate into which category of malassimilation the patient falls. An elevated fecal fat may be due to intraluminal maldigestion or intramural malabsorption. Therefore, further investigations are required to fully characterize the problem (Figure 16).

9.8 Investigating Suspected Intraluminal Maldigestion
Intraluminal maldigestion will occur with (1) inadequate mixing; (2) pancreatic insufficiency; and (3) reduced bile salt concentration. If the small bowel x-rays are normal, then it is likely but not absolutely certain that malassimilation is due to an intraluminal disorder. Pancreatic function is assessed by the secretin stimulation test used to measure secretory capacity of the exocrine

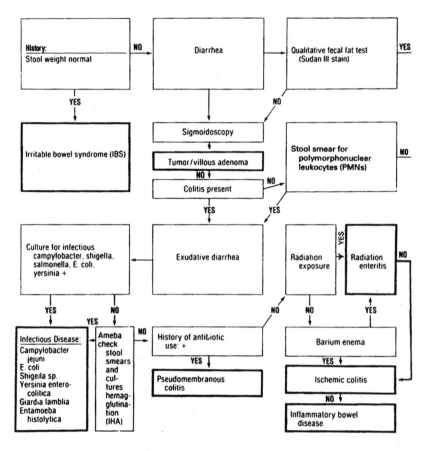

FIGURE 16. Diagnostic approach to chronic diarrhea.
SOURCE: Knapp AB, Farkas PS. Diagnostic diagrams: gastroenterology. Baltimore: Williams and Wilkins, 1985:54–55.

pancreas. A tube placed in the duodenum adjacent to the ampullae of Vater collects pancreatic juice to measure volume, bicarbonate and enzyme (amylase) output. Maximal secretion should reach 2 mL/min at 90 minutes after injection of 2 units of secretin/kg of body weight, and bicarbonate concentration is normally 90 mEq/L. Both enzyme and bicarbonate secretion are diminished in chronic pancreatitis. Partial duct obstruction resulting from pancreatic cancer often reduces the volume of secretion without reducing bicarbonate concentration. The test is cumbersome and not very sensitive.

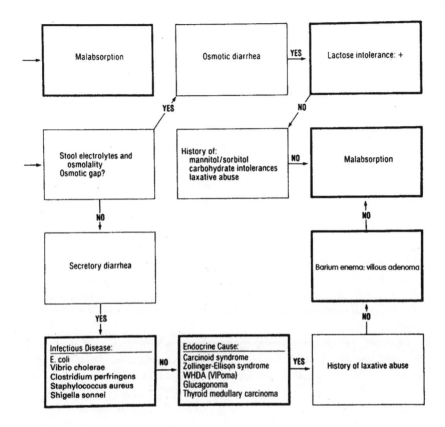

Assessment of biliary disease includes liver biochemistry, abdominal ultrasound and, where indicated, transhepatic or endoscopic cholangiography to ensure patency of the ductal system. In the bacterial overgrowth syndrome, bile acids are deconjugated and rapidly absorbed in the small intestine, and are not available or active for micellar solubilization. With bacterial overgrowth, the Schilling test for vitamin B_{12} is abnormal, even with the addition of intrinsic factor. Bile salt concentration may be diminished as a result of failure of reabsorption in a diseased ileum, adding to the malabsorption from gut loss. A ^{14}C-labeled bile acid breath test detects bile acid deconjugation in the bacterial overgrowth syndrome; an isotope scan with a radiolabeled bile acid analogue measures bile acid absorption. The presence of bacterial overgrowth in the small bowel (small bowel bacterial contamination) may be demonstrated by the hydrogen breath test: a nonabsorbed carbohydrate (lactulose) is ingested, and a breath sample is assessed for H_2; if the H_2 level is increased, then bacterial overgrowth is present. The H_2 breath test may also be used with lactose to demonstrate lactose malabsorption due to lactase deficiency.

The bile acid breath test is used if one suspects bile acid malabsorption due to ileal dysfunction (decreased absorption) or bacterial overgrowth (deconjugation and thus diminished absorption). The basis of the test is that the amino acid (glycine) part of the bile salt is labeled with ^{14}C-glycine. Bacteria deconjugate the glycine and metabolize this amide to $^{14}CO_2$, which is then exhaled. With ileal dysfunction, an excess of bile salts reaches the colon, where colonic bacteria split off the glycine, producing $^{14}CO_2$. With bacterial overgrowth, the excess coliform bacteria in the jejunum metabolize these bile salts to $^{14}CO_2$. The bile acid breath test is beginning to be replaced by the hydrogen breath test, which assesses the presence of an abnormal increase in the concentration of breath H_2 after the subject has ingested a nonabsorbable sugar such as lactulose. This is an inexpensive and sensitive test for bacterial overgrowth. The type of sugar used in the breath test may be changed to test for malabsorption of various carbohydrates. The H_2 breath test is not used to test for bile salt malabsorption.

Disordered mixing of ingested food with endogenous enzymes results from the rapid transit in postgastrectomy syndromes. Small bowel x-rays with transit times sometimes help to demonstrate rapid transit or abnormal anatomy such as may occur with gastric surgery or with congenital or acquired conditions, such as multiple jejunal diverticula or small bowel strictures.

9.9 Investigating Suspected Intramural Malabsorption
Malabsorption from an intramural defect occurs as a result of (1) inadequate absorptive surface – e.g., the short gut syndrome; (2) mucosal absorptive defects – e.g., celiac disease; or (3) lymphatic obstruction. Since the pentose sugar D-xylose does not require intraluminal digestion, D-xylose absorption tests serve to separate patients with intramural malabsorption from those with intraluminal maldigestion. An abnormal result points toward intramural malabsorption, while a normal result points toward intraluminal maldigestion. Remember that patients with renal impairment (who cannot excrete the sugar), delayed gastric emptying, bacterial overgrowth (who metabolize the sugar in the lumen) and advanced age may have spuriously low measurements of D-xylose absorption. Because of its low sensitivity and specificity, the D-xylose test is seldom performed. Aspirin (ASA) or nonsteroidal anti-inflammatory drugs (NSAIDs) inhibit the renal excretion of xylose and may lead to a false-negative test. The presence of ascites may also lead to a false-negative

test by increasing the volume of distribution of the sugar and thereby decreasing its renal clearance. Measurement of the serum level of xylose may be a better test of xylose absorption because it avoids these issues of renal function. Indeed, clinicians may elect to omit a xylose test and advance to specific intramural or intraluminal investigations (Figure 15).

Following an abnormal D-xylose test, the next evaluation should be barium contrast x-rays of the small intestine. They may demonstrate structurally abnormal bowel patterns, dilation of bowel lumen, segmentation of barium or a dilution of barium because of increased intraluminal fluid. Although segmentation and flocculation of barium have been used as indications of malassimilation in the past, the use of nondispersible barium sulfate in recent years rarely allows us to observe such signs. Additionally, x-ray films may demonstrate multiple diverticula as sites of bacterial overgrowth or thickening of folds resulting from infiltration or edema.

Following the x-ray, endoscopic or suction biopsy of the small intestine will identify evidence of specific mucosal disease. If there is a high clinical suspicion of celiac disease, a blood test for antigliadin antibody may be performed, and if this is positive, then a test for anti-endomysial antibody may be performed. If this is positive, the suspected diagnosis of celiac disease may be confirmed with a small bowel biopsy. Once the etiology of the intramural disease is known, further tests can be carried out to determine the extent of functional derangement. Tests can help define unabsorbed carbohydrate as a result of disaccharidase deficiency, generalized mucosal damage, inadequate surface area or bacterial overgrowth. Unabsorbed carbohydrate produces stool with an acid pH, easily tested on pH paper strip. This is a useful test in children but less so in adults. The hydrogen breath test will detect an increase in exhaled hydrogen, which might result when an ingested carbohydrate is not absorbed. This test is used to diagnose suspected disaccharidase deficiencies or bacterial overgrowth. The basis of the test is that bacteria ferment sugars to fatty acids and H_2, which is exhaled. Normally, sugars are absorbed as monosaccharides in the small intestine and no H_2 is exhaled. In lactase deficiency, exhaled H_2 is elevated after ingestion of the test sugar lactose, since the unabsorbed sugar reaches colonic bacteria and is catabolized. In bacterial overgrowth, bacteria in the jejunum ferment the sugar before it can be absorbed and H_2 is exhaled. The hydrogen breath test is reliable, noninvasive and helpful in establishing the diagnosis of carbohydrate malabsorption and/or the bacterial overgrowth syndrome.

Vitamin B_{12} absorption is tested by the Schilling test. Radiolabeled vitamin B_{12} with intrinsic factor (labeled with ^{58}Co) and without intrinsic factor (labeled with ^{57}Co) are simultaneously administered orally. The excretion of both compounds is then measured in the urine over a 24-hour period. Excre-

TABLE 6.   Therapy for malassimilation syndromes

Site of defect	Therapy
Pancreas	Enzyme supplements; insulin; dietary counseling; surgery for pancreatic duct obstruction or cancer
Hepatobiliary	Endoscopic therapy or surgery for obstruction of biliary tree
Mucosa	Diet, such as gluten withdrawal or milk-free diet; nutrient supplements; 5-ASA compounds or steroids for Crohn's disease; antibiotics for bacterial overgrowth or Whipple's disease
Lymphatics	Low-fat diet; medium-chain triglycerides (MCTs)

tion of both radiolabeled compounds is normal. Failure to excrete ^{57}Co-labeled vitamin B_{12} indicates absent gastric intrinsic factor – e.g., pernicious anemia or gastrectomy, while failure to excrete ^{58}Co- and ^{57}Co-labeled vitamin B_{12} indicates ileal disease or loss, or absent ileal B_{12} receptors.

9.10 Treatment

The specific treatments for malabsorption or maldigestion are given in Table 6. The nutritional therapies necessary for any associated deficiencies are given in Table 7.

10. ACUTE DIARRHEA

With a complaint of "diarrhea," the physician must establish if this represents a change in the patient's bowel habit and if the complaint arises from a perception of increased frequency of stool, increased volume or both. To the patient, the term *diarrhea* usually means a change in the frequency or fluid-nature of the stools.

If the diarrhea is acute (i.e., lasting less than two weeks), the malabsorption of fluid and electrolytes probably has an infectious or toxic cause (Table 8). When diarrhea lasts for a longer period of time, other explanations need to be considered. In the absence of prior gastric surgery, the four most common causes of chronic diarrhea are (1) the irritable bowel syndrome; (2) inflammatory bowel disease; (3) malabsorption; and (4) carcinoma of the colon. The physician also must consider altered bowel function due to drug or alcohol abuse (see Section 11). Associated tenesmus, urgency or a sense of incomplete evacuation suggests involvement of the rectum or sigmoid colon. The passage of blood, pus and mucus suggests bowel inflammation, ischemic bowel disease or cancer. Malassimilation syndromes (discussed in the previous section) are suspect if there is passage of food and oil droplets,

TABLE 7.   Representative doses for agents used in replacement therapy in patients with malassimilation syndromes

Minerals

Calcium   PO: requires at least 1,000 mg elemental calcium daily as:
              (a) Calcium gluconate (93 mg Ca^{2+}/500 mg tablet)
              (b) Calcium carbonate (200 mg Ca^{2+}/500 mg tablet)
              IV: Calcium gluconate, 10 mL (9.3 mg Ca^{2+}/mL) of 10% soln over 5 min

Magnesium   PO: Magnesium gluconate (29 mg Mg^{2+}/500 mg tablet), 2–6 g/day
              IV: Magnesium sulfate (50% soln, 1 mL contains 2.03 mmol Mg^{2+})

Iron   PO: Ferrous fumarate (65 mg elemental Fe/200 mg tablet), 200 mg tid
              Ferrous gluconate (35 mg elemental Fe/300 mg tablet), 600 mg tid
              Ferrous sulfate (60 mg elemental Fe/300 mg tablet), 300 mg tid
              IM: Iron dextran 1 mL once daily (calculated from existing Hb)*
              IV: Iron dextran approx. 30 mL (calculated from existing Hb)* in 500 cc
                    5% D/W over 4 hrs, beginning with slow observed infusion
              *NOTE: IM/IV Fe for deficit replacement only

Zinc   PO: Zinc sulfate (89 mg elemental zinc/220 mg capsule), 220 mg tid

Vitamins

Vitamin A   Water-miscible vitamin A (25,000 IU/capsule), 25,000 IU daily

Vitamin B_{12} 100 µg/IM monthly

Vitamin D_2 (Ergocalciferol) (50,000 IU/capsule), 50,000 IU 3 times per week

Vitamin E   Water-miscible vitamin E (100 IU/capsule), 400 IU daily

Vitamin K_1 (Phytonadione) has caused fatal reactions, thus should be avoided

Vitamin K_3 (Menadione) water-soluble
              PO: 5–10 mg/day
              IV: 5–10 mg/day

Folic acid   PO: 1 mg/day

Other
water-soluble   Multiple vitamin 1/day

(cont'd)

TABLE 7.   Representative doses for agents used in replacement therapy in patients with malassimilation syndromes (cont'd)

Pancreatic supplements

Preparation	Type	Enzyme activity (IU/unit)			
		Lipase	*Trypsin*	*Proteolytic*	*Amylase*
Ku-Zyme HP®	Capsule	2,330	3,082	6,090	594,048
Festal®	Enteric-coated	2,073	488	1,800	219,200
Cotazym®	Capsule	2,014	2,797	5,840	499,200
Viokase®	Tablet	1,636	1,828	440	277,333
Pancrease®	Micro-				
	encapsulated	>4,000	>25,000		

Usually taken as 4–8 capsules with each meal and half that number with snacks. Some patients will need higher doses or will need acid-lowering therapy with an H_2-receptor antagonist or a proton pump inhibitor to alkalize the fluid in the duodenum and achieve greater activity of the pancreatic enzymes

Bile salt binding agents
Cholestyramine 4 g (1 scoop), 3–6 times daily, according to response
Psyllium and aluminum hydroxide gel may also be effective
Colestipol 1 g 3–6 times daily, according to response

(cont'd)

or if the patient develops symptoms suggestive of nutrient deficiency, particularly weight loss.

In Western societies, stool weight is approximately 200 g/day. Since stools are 70–90% water, regardless of their consistency, excess fecal water must accompany diarrheal diseases with elevated stool weight. This concept leads directly to consideration of the mechanisms responsible for the malabsorption or stimulated secretion of water.

Two caveats need to be remembered. First, fecal bulk varies with the diet, being influenced most notably by the content of indigestible carbohydrates (dietary fiber). Stools are smaller in developed countries than they are among societies whose members regularly ingest large amounts of dietary fiber. Second, disease of the distal colon or rectum can lead to the frequent, often painful passage of small stools (due to limited capacity as a reservoir), yet there may be little fecal water and no increase in stool weight. In fact, "constipation" may be common in patients with proctitis.

Acute diarrhea is thus defined as stool weight > 200 g/day for less than 14 days' duration. It always will represent a change in bowel habit for the individual and will often be associated with an increased frequency of bowel movements.

TABLE 7. Representative doses for agents used in replacement therapy in patients with malassimilation syndromes (cont'd)

Caloric supplements
Medium-chain triglyceride oil: (8 cal/mL), 60 mL/day po, 480 cal/day
Portagen®: medium-chain triglyceride + other oils: (1 cal/mL), 1 L/day
Enteral supplements:

Product	Kcal*/ 1,000 mL	Grams of protein/ 1,000 mL	Na mg/L	K mg/L	Osmolality mOsm/kg Water
Ensure®	1,060	37	740	1,270	450
Isocal®	1,040	34	530	1,320	300
Osmolite®	1,060	37	540	1,060	300
Precision					
Isotonic Diet®	960	29	800	960	300
Precision LR Diet®	1,110	26	700	810	525
Travasorb STD®					
(unflavored)	1,000	45	920	1,170	450
Standard Vivonex®					
(unflavored)	1,000	21	470	1,170	550
High-Nitrogen Vivonex®					
(unflavored)	1,000	44	530	1,170	810
Meritene Powder®					
in milk	1,065	69	1,000	3,000	690
Compleat B®	1,000	40	1,200	1,300	390
Formula 2®	1,000	38	600	1,760	435–510

*When prepared in standard dilution
Parenteral supplements: Intralipid® 1 L/day IV (10 mL/kg/day)
Travasol® 2 L/day IV (mix as per patient's protein requirements)

10.1 Bacterial Diarrhea

In immunocompetent individuals, enteric infections are usually self-limiting and resolve in less than two weeks. Acute bacterial diarrheas can be classified into *toxigenic types*, in which an enterotoxin is the major pathogenic mechanism, and *invasive types*, in which the organism penetrates the enterocyte as a primary event, although an enterotoxin may be produced as well. Enterotoxins are either *cytotonic* (producing intestinal fluid secretion by activation of intracellular enzymes, without damage to the epithelial surface) or *cytotoxic* (causing injury to the enterocyte as well as inducing fluid secretion). Three major clinical syndromes caused by bacterial infections are (1) food poisoning, (2) infectious gastroenteritis and (3) traveler's diarrhea.

TABLE 8.   Common causes of acute diarrhea

Drugs	*Bacteria (toxin-mediated, cytotoxic)*
Laxatives	Clostridium difficile
Antacids	Staphylococcus aureus
Antibiotics	Shigella dysenteriae
Cholinergic drugs	Campylobacter jejuni
Lactose	Yersinia enterocolitica
Guanethidine	
Quinidine	*Bacteria (invasive)*
Digitalis	Salmonella
Colchicine	Enteroinvasive Escherichia coli
Potassium supplements	
Lactulose	*Bacteria (unknown mechanism)*
	Enteropathogenic Escherichia coli
	Enteroadherent Escherichia coli
	Viruses
Bacteria (toxin-mediated, cytotonic)	Parvovirus (Norwalk agent)
Enterotoxigenic Escherichia coli	Reovirus (rotavirus)
(both heat-labile and heat-	
stable toxins)	*Protozoa*
Vibrio cholerae	Cryptosporidia
Vibrio parahaemolyticus	Giardia lamblia
Clostridium perfringens	Entamoeba histolytica
Bacillus cereus	
	Parasites
	Strongyloides
	Trichuris

10.1.1 *FOOD POISONING*

The food poisoning syndrome characteristically features the development of a brief but explosive diarrheal illness in subjects following exposure to a common food source contaminated with bacteria or bacterial toxins. Staphylococcus aureus, Salmonella, Clostridium perfringens and Bacillus cereus are responsible for 90% of these outbreaks.

Staphylococcus aureus produces a heat-stable, odorless and tasteless enterotoxin that is generated in poorly refrigerated desserts and seafoods. Ingestion of the preformed enterotoxin causes nausea, vomiting and profuse diarrhea within 4 to 8 hours. Spontaneous resolution occurs within 24 hours. No specific therapy is available or necessary.

Clostridium perfringens produces a preformed toxin from spores that germinate in contaminated meats cooked to less than 50°C. Symptoms are diarrhea and crampy abdominal pain without vomiting, beginning 8 to 24 hours after the meal. The illness lasts less than 24 hours. No specific therapy is indicated.

Bacillus cereus produces either a diarrheal syndrome or a vomiting syndrome, depending upon the enterotoxin. The vomiting syndrome is always associated with ingestion of rice and is caused by a preformed toxin that is elaborated when rice is left to cool unrefrigerated. Flash-frying later does not generate enough heat to destroy the toxin. The diarrheal syndrome occurs after ingestion of the organism itself. Both illnesses are short-lived and require no specific therapy.

The diagnosis of food poisoning is usually made by history. Except in special circumstances (e.g., botulism), isolation of the toxin is not cost-effective.

10.1.2 GASTROENTERITIS

The organisms responsible for bacterial gastroenteritis exert their predominant effects by invading and destroying the intestinal epithelium or by producing various enterotoxins.

10.1.2.1 Toxin-mediated, cytotoxic bacterial gastroenteritis

Vibrio cholerae is the prototypic cause of toxigenic diarrhea. The Vibrio cholerae organisms elaborate a toxin that attaches to the inner cell membrane and activates adenylate cyclase (formerly "adenyl cyclase"). The presence of adenylate cyclase then elevates cyclic AMP (cAMP) levels. Cyclic AMP then stimulates the enterocyte to secrete fluid and electrolytes while at the same time impairing their absorption. Stool output can exceed 1 L/hour. Treatment is based on restoring fluid and electrolyte balance and maintaining intravascular volume. Even though fluid and electrolyte transport is impaired, glucose transport is intact. Since glucose absorption carries Na^+ (and thus water with it), an oral rehydration solution containing glucose, sodium and water will enhance water absorption during the profound dehydration stage of cholera.

Several types of Escherichia coli (E. coli) are intestinal pathogens. Each exerts its effects through different mechanisms (Table 9). Invasive forms of E. coli may cause colitis that resembles colitis from other bacterial infections and also may resemble ischemia clinically, endoscopically and histologically.

Enterotoxigenic E. coli (ETEC) colonizes the upper small intestine after passing through the acid barrier of the stomach. The organisms colonize the surface without penetrating the mucus layer. Like cholera, ETEC causes no mucosal damage and no bacteremia. Two types of enterotoxins are produced by ETEC: the heat-labile toxin (also called "labile toxin" or LT) and the heat-stable toxin (also called "stable toxin" or ST). ETEC can elaborate LT only, ST only, or both toxins. ST produces diarrhea by stimulating intestinal secretion through guanylate cyclase and subsequently cyclic GMP. LT produces

TABLE 9. Types of Escherichia coli intestinal pathogens

Name	Toxin	Mechanism
Enteropathogenic (EPEC)	Shiga-like toxin	Adherence
Enterotoxigenic (ETEC)	Labile toxin (LT)	Activates adenylate cyclase
	Stable toxin (ST)	Activates guanylate cyclase
Enteroinvasive (EIEC)	Shiga-like toxin	Penetrates epithelium
Enteroadherent (EAEC)	—	Adherence
Enterohemorrhagic (EHEC)	Shiga-like toxin (verotoxin)	Unknown

diarrhea by a similar mechanism, except that it acts through adenylate cyclase and cyclic AMP. After a 24- to 48-hour incubation period, the disease begins with upper abdominal distress followed by watery diarrhea. The infection can be mild (with only a few loose movements) or severe (mimicking cholera). Treatment is symptomatic. Antibiotic therapy is ineffective and favors the emergence of resistant ETEC strains.

Vibrio parahaemolyticus causes acute diarrheal disease after consumption of seafood: raw fish or shellfish. The common factor in most outbreaks appears to be storage of the food for several hours without proper refrigeration. Explosive, watery diarrhea is the cardinal manifestation, along with abdominal cramps, nausea and vomiting. Fever and chills occur in 25% of cases. The duration of illness is short, with a median of three days. Treatment is symptomatic; there is no role for antimicrobial therapy.

After ingestion, Shigella dysenteriae organisms attack the colon, sparing the stomach and small bowel. Shigella organisms adhere to the mucosal surface, penetrate the mucosal surface, and then multiply within epithelial cells, moving laterally through the cytoplasm to adjacent cells by filopodium-like protrusions. Shigella organisms rarely penetrate below the intestinal mucosa and almost never invade the bloodstream. Both attached and intracellular organisms elaborate toxic products.

Even a small inoculum of 200 organisms (as contrasted with Salmonella, which requires greater than 10^7 organisms) will lead to crampy abdominal pain, rectal burning and fever associated with multiple small-volume bloody mucoid bowel movements. Intestinal complications include perforation and severe protein loss. Extraintestinal complications include respiratory symptoms, meningismus, seizures, the hemolytic uremic syndrome, arthritis and rashes. Ampicillin 500 mg q.i.d. or co-trimoxazole 2 tablets b.i.d. for 5 days is the treatment of choice. Amoxicillin, interestingly, is not effective therapy for shigellosis.

Salmonella food poisoning has been attributed to an enterotoxin similar to that of Staphylococcus aureus, but none has been clearly identified. Within 12 to 36 hours after ingestion of contaminated foods (usually poultry products), there is a sudden onset of headaches, chills and abdominal pain, with nausea, vomiting and diarrhea. These symptoms may persist for one to four days before subsiding. Antibiotic therapy of nontyphoidal Salmonella gastroenteritis fails to alter the rate of clinical recovery. In fact, antibiotic therapy will increase the duration of intestinal carriage of the Salmonella and is thus contraindicated.

Campylobacter jejuni–induced diarrhea is more common than diarrhea from either Salmonella or Shigella. Infection is from consumption of improperly cooked or contaminated foodstuffs. Campylobacter attaches to the mucosa and releases an enterotoxin that destroys the surrounding epithelia. Clinically, there is often a prodrome of constitutional symptoms along with headache and generalized malaise. A prolonged diarrheal illness follows – often with a biphasic character, with initial bloody diarrhea, slight improvement, then increasing severity. The illness usually lasts less than one week, although symptoms can persist for a longer period, and relapses occur in as many as 25% of patients. Erythromycin 500 mg q.i.d. for 7 days is optimal therapy.

Yersinia enterocolitica is often transmitted to humans from pets or food sources. The organism invades epithelial cells and produces an enterotoxin. Clinically, the spectrum of illness ranges from simple gastroenteritis to invasive ileitis and colitis that needs to be distinguished from Crohn's disease or ulcerative colitis (Chapter 10). This organism causes diarrheal illness most frequently in children less than 5 years of age. Children over 5 years of age develop mesenteric adenitis and associated ileitis, which mimic acute appendicitis. Yersinia is less likely to cause disease in adults; if it does, the illness is an acute diarrheal episode that may be followed two to three weeks later by joint symptoms and a rash (erythema nodosum). Treatment is symptomatic. There is no evidence that antibiotics alter the course of the gastrointestinal infection.

Clostridium difficile causes antibiotic-associated colitis (Section 10.4).

10.1.2.2 *Invasive bacterial gastroenteritis*

Certain strains of E. coli are invasive, producing an illness indistinguishable from shigellosis. Isolates of E. coli 0157:H7 have been identified in the stools of patients with a diarrheal illness clinically designated as "hemorrhagic colitis." Infection has been traced to contaminated hamburger meat obtained from a variety of sources, including large national restaurant chains. E. coli 0157:H7 infection may be complicated by thrombotic thrombocytopenic purpura, or by the hemolytic uremic syndrome, which sometimes leads to death.

Ingestion of this organism results in severe crampy abdominal pain and fever, followed within 24 hours by bloody diarrhea that lasts five to seven days. Since the organism is shed in the stool for only a short period of time, early stool collections are critical for the diagnosis. Treatment is symptomatic, as antibiotics do not appear to alter the disease course. In severe cases with possible toxic megacolon, systemic antibiotics may be in order.

Approximately 1,700 serotypes and variants of Salmonella are potential pathogens for humans. A dose of approximately 10^7–10^9 organisms is required to produce a clinical illness. Salmonella organisms invade the mucosa of the small intestine and (particularly) the colon. This form of gastroenteritis produces nausea and vomiting followed by abdominal cramps and diarrhea that lasts three to four days and then gradually subsides. In 10% of the cases bacteremia of the Salmonella organism occurs, and in approximately 5% there are disseminated infections to bones, joints and meninges. Certain conditions increase the risk of salmonellosis: hemolytic anemia, malignancy, immunosuppression, achlorhydria and ulcerative colitis. With uncomplicated Salmonella gastroenteritis, treatment is symptomatic. In fact, antibiotic therapy increases the duration of intestinal carriage of these organisms. Patients with complicated Salmonella gastroenteritis (e.g., those with predisposing conditions or sepsis, or who are very young or very old) should be treated with ampicillin or co-trimoxazole.

10.1.2.3 *Bacterial gastroenteritis of unknown mechanism*
Enterohemorrhagic E. coli–induced diarrhea tends to occur in neonates and young children. Only occasionally does it affect older children and adults. The pathogenic mechanism of this diarrhea is unclear; adherence of the organism to the intestinal epithelial cell seems to cause intestinal damage. There is no indication for specific treatment except for neonates in a nursery epidemic. In this case, oral nonabsorbable aminoglycosides should be used.

10.1.3 *TRAVELER'S DIARRHEA*
Traveler's diarrhea is a syndrome characterized by an increase in frequency of unformed bowel movements, typically four to five loose stools per day. Associated symptoms include abdominal cramps, nausea, bloating, urgency, fever and malaise. Traveler's diarrhea usually begins abruptly, during travel or soon after returning home, and is generally self-limiting, lasting three to four days.

TABLE 10.   Traveler's diarrhea: recommendations for treatment

---

General
Avoid ice cubes, raw vegetables and fruits, raw fish and shellfish, unrefrigerated food.
Drink canned pop and beer, boiled water.
Drink oral replacement solutions for acute attacks.
Avoid over-the-counter preparations sold locally for acute attacks.

Specific
To provide symptomatic relief of acute attack:
  Diphenoxylate 1 tab, 2.5 mg, after each bowel movement to max 8 tab/day
  Loperamide 1 cap, 2.0 mg, after each bowel movement to max 8 cap/day
  Pepto-Bismol® 30 mL q 30 min × 8 doses

To decrease severity of acute attack:
  Co-trimoxazole 1 tab bid po × 3 days
  Doxycycline 100 mg bid po × 3 days

Prophylaxis:
Not recommended except for persons who are immunosuppressed or suffer chronic illness. If
indicated, then:
  Co-trimoxazole 1 tab bid po × 3 days
  Doxycycline 100 mg bid po × 3 days
  Ciprofloxacin 500 mg bid po × 7 days

Ten percent of cases persist longer than one week, approximately 2% longer
than one month and very few beyond three months. Enterotoxigenic E. coli
(ETEC) is the most common causative agent of traveler's diarrhea. These
organisms adhere to the small intestine, where they multiply and produce an
enterotoxin that causes fluid secretion and hence diarrhea. Salmonella gastroenteritis, Shigella dysentery, and viral enteric pathogens (rotavirus and
Norwalk-like virus) are less common causes of traveler's diarrhea.

   Since traveler's diarrhea is usually mild and self-limiting, with complete
recovery even in the absence of therapy, therapy should be considered option-
al (Table 10). The value of prophylaxis for travelers is unclear. Bismuth preparations are helpful, but their use is limited by the large volumes necessary and
by their taste. Antibiotic prophylaxis can reduce the likelihood of developing
diarrhea, but carries its own risks.

10.2 Viral Gastroenteritis
At least two groups of viruses are capable of producing an acute diarrheal illness.

10.2.1 NORWALK VIRUS
The Norwalk virus causes a self-limiting syndrome that affects children and

adults, mainly in winter. An incubation period of 24 to 48 hours is followed by a variable combination of fever, anorexia, nausea, vomiting, myalgia, abdominal pain and diarrhea. Spontaneous recovery occurs two to three days later. Immune electron microscopy of fecal filtrates demonstrates a characteristic 27 nm viral particle (the Norwalk agent). No specific treatment is available. The vomiting represents delayed gastric emptying; there are no morphologic features of gastritis.

10.2.2 ROTAVIRUSES

Rotaviruses are the most common causes of acute nonbacterial gastroenteritis in infancy and childhood. Rotaviruses invade mucosal epithelial cells. The resulting illness is more severe than that caused by the Norwalk virus. Rotavirus infection commonly requires hospital admission and intravenous fluids. Infection occurs mainly in children from 6 to 24 months old, and almost always in winter. Virus excretion is maximum three to four days after the onset of symptoms and disappears after a further three to four days. The stability of the virus and the large number of viral particles excreted make environmental contamination inevitable, with a high risk of secondary infection in susceptible contacts. For example, 20% of the rotavirus infections diagnosed in pediatric hospitals are acquired in the hospital. Most older children and adults have antibodies to rotaviruses, so any subsequent infection is generally mild.

10.3 Parasitic Enteritis

The parasites that infect the intestine may be divided into three broad groups. These include protozoa, roundworms and flatworms. The flatworms may be further divided into cestodes (tapeworms) and trematodes (flukes). This chapter will focus upon only a few protozoa seen in immunocompetent Canadian residents (infections seen in immunocompromised persons are discussed in Chapter 9).

10.3.1 GIARDIA LAMBLIA

Giardia lamblia is endemic in many areas of the world, including Canada. Some patients with giardiasis ("beaver fever") present with an abrupt, self-limiting illness that develops one to three weeks after infection and lasts three to four days. Others may develop chronic and episodic diarrhea associated with bloating and, at times, steatorrhea and a malabsorption syndrome clinically like celiac disease. Diagnosis is made by recovery of the organism; it is found in the stool of approximately 50% of patients and in 90% of histologically examined smear preparations obtained from small bowel biopsy specimens (Figure 17A, B). The treatment of choice in both asymptomatic and symptomatic patients is metronidazole 250 mg t.i.d. for 7 days. Repeat thera-

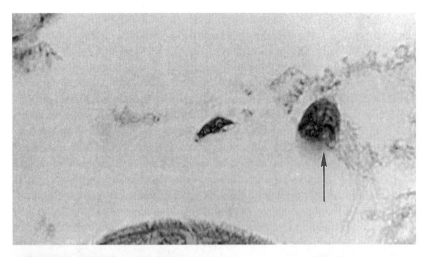

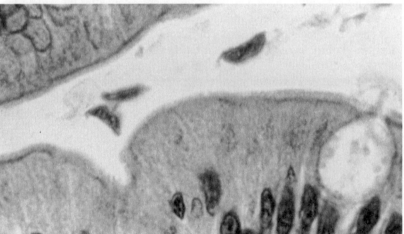

Figure 17. Two high-power views of giardiasis show the typical appearance in cross-section. The crescentic shape and double nuclei are characteristic. One cut shows the organism in longitudinal section (arrow); the organism has the pear shape more familiar from smear preparations. Only one of the two nuclei is visible.

py will occasionally be needed to totally eradicate the organism. Quinacrine 100 mg t.i.d. for 7 days also is effective.

10.3.2 AMEBIASIS
This is an acute and chronic disease caused by the organism Entamoeba his-

tolytica. Although there are numerous species of ameba that inhabit the human intestinal tract, E. histolytica seems to be the only variety that is pathogenic for humans. Its manifestations vary from the asymptomatic carrier state to a severe fulminating illness with mucosal inflammation and ulceration. Asymptomatic patients harbor only cysts in their stools and have no evidence of tissue invasion. Since the cysts are resistant to the outside environment, the disease can be transmitted by individuals unaware of their infective potential. This is in contrast to patients with acute or chronic invasive disease, who harbor a trophozoite that cannot survive outside the host.

The acute illness is characterized by diarrhea with the passage of blood and mucus, and by variable degrees of abdominal pain. In its most severe form it may mimic fulminating ulcerative colitis and may progress to a toxic dilation (toxic megacolon) and perforation of the colon. During the acute illness, trophozoites may be recovered in the stool, from biopsies of shallow ulcers in the rectum, or from smears of rectal mucus.

Chronic infectious features may develop many years after the patient has left an endemic area. Patients present with nonspecific bowel complaints and may show radiologic changes in the distal small bowel and colon that mimic ulcerative colitis, cancer or tuberculosis. Diagnosis necessitates recovering trophozoites from the stool. As an adjunct, the indirect hemagglutination test can help detect patients with invasive disease.

Intestinal complications of amebiasis include massive intestinal hemorrhage, which is rare; ameboma formation in any part of the colon, which may lead to obstruction or intussusception; permanent stricture formation during the healing stage; and postdysenteric colitis, which usually resolves over several weeks or months without specific therapy.

Systemic dissemination of the ameba may involve other organs, such as the brain, lung, pericardium and liver. Liver abscess is the most common extraintestinal infection by the ameba.

Therapeutic agents used for the treatment of amebiasis act at selected sites: intraluminally, intramurally or systemically. Treatment must therefore be individualized to the location of the disease. Asymptomatic carriers are treated with iodoquinol 650 mg t.i.d. for 20 days; this agent acts against amebas located intraluminally. Acute or chronic intestinal disease is treated with metronidazole 750 mg t.i.d. for 10 days. However, because metronidazole is less effective against organisms within the bowel lumen, iodoquinol (650 mg t.i.d. for 20 days) must be added.

10.3.3 CRYPTOSPORIDIA

Cryptosporidia are a genus of protozoa classified within the subclass Coccidia. In immunocompetent persons cryptosporidia infection presents as a

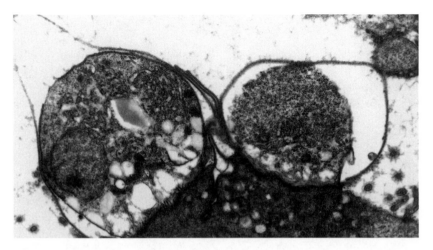

Figure 18. This electron micrograph of cryptosporidiosis in the small bowel shows the characteristic intracellular but extracytoplasmic location of the organisms.

transient, self-limiting diarrheal state lasting from one to seven days. Adults are less commonly affected than young children. In most, the illness is mild and medical help is not sought. With immunological incompetence (e.g., AIDS, neoplasia, hypogammaglobulinemia or concurrent viral infection), a persistent chronic watery diarrhea may occur. Diagnosis is made by demonstrating Cryptosporidia oocysts in the stool or, better still, by mucosal biopsy and examination of the microvillus border for embedded Cryptosporidia oocysts (Figure 18).

A successful treatment for Cryptosporidia has not yet been found. Spiramycin and hyperimmune bovine colostrum remain experimental, as does thalidomide.

10.4 Drug-Related Diarrhea

Since almost every drug can cause diarrhea, the first question to ask a patient is "What medications, both prescribed and over-the-counter, are you currently taking?" Discontinuing the drug is often the only therapeutic move required. Although many drugs can cause diarrhea, little is understood about the ways in which they do so. The common causes of drug-induced diarrhea with pathogenic mechanisms follow.

10.4.1 *ANTIBIOTIC-ASSOCIATED DIARRHEA AND PSEUDO-MEMBRANOUS COLITIS*

Antibiotics are the most common cause of drug-induced diarrhea. In many cases, the condition is self-limiting. The development of pseudomembranous

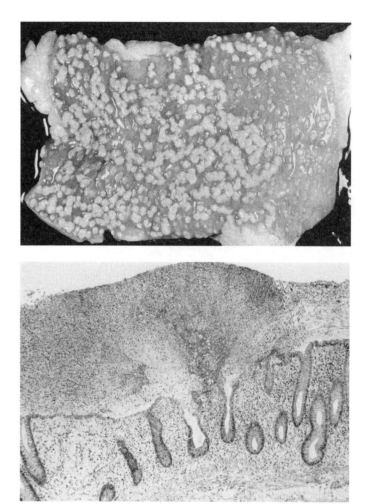

Figure 19.   The confluent white patches of pseudomembraneous colitis are typical. In Figure 19B the pseudomembrane is seen to arise like a volcano from a point of mucosal damage and is composed of an exudative fibrin and neutrophils.

colitis (PMC) in association with antibiotics may be a serious and sometimes life-threatening condition.

PMC can follow virtually any antibiotic use. It may occur months after antibiotic exposure, and may rarely occur without a past history of antibiotic use. The frequency of diarrhea or colitis does not appear to be related to dose or route of administration of the antibiotic. Symptoms can occur while the patient is on the antibiotic or within six weeks following its discontinuation. Only increasing age is clearly identifiable as a risk factor. The diarrhea is usually loose with mucus. Frank bleeding is uncommon. The diarrhea can be devastating, with up to 30 bowel movements in a 24-hour period. The diarrhea may be associated with varying degrees of abdominal pain and low-grade fever. Depending on the severity of the diarrhea and the amount of fluid loss, hypotension, shock and even death have been reported. In many patients the problem is self-limiting and resolves spontaneously with discontinuation of the antibiotic. Further investigation is required in those patients who have severe diarrhea associated with systemic symptoms and those whose diarrhea persists despite discontinuing the implicated antibiotic.

An accurate history is usually sufficient to suggest the diagnosis of PMC, and a sigmoidoscopy may be all that is required for confirmation. The presence of copious amounts of mucus and typical raised white pseudomembrane plaques are characteristic features on sigmoidoscopy. Biopsies help confirm the diagnosis (Figure 19A, B). The distal colon is involved in most cases so that sigmoidoscopy is usually adequate. Sometimes the pseudomembrane lesions may be restricted to the right colon, necessitating colonoscopy to identify the PMC lesions.

Isolation of C. difficile toxin in the stools provides the diagnosis. If it is certain that there is no other likely cause for the diarrhea, treatment can be undertaken while awaiting assay results, although it is usually possible to quickly obtain a sigmoidoscopy to demonstrate the pseudomembranes. If symptoms are resolving with discontinuance of the antibiotic, no further therapy may be indicated. In mild cases, metronidazole 250 mg p.o. t.i.d. for 7–10 days is effective. In severe hospitalized cases the drug of choice is vancomycin 125 mg p.o. q.i.d. for 14 days. Vancomycin is poorly absorbed and central nervous system and renal toxic effects are uncommon. The high cost of this medication limits its use, even though the eradication rate is high. If oral therapy cannot be used, as with severe ileus or recent surgery, parenteral metronidazole is preferred. Some 20% of treated patients will have a recurrence of symptoms, PMC or C. difficile, usually within 4 to 21 days of stopping treatment. In this case, another course of metronidazole or vancomycin should be given. Cholestyramine (Questran®) binds the toxin and can provide symptomatic relief even though it will not eliminate the microorganism.

10.4.2 MAGNESIUM-CONTAINING ANTACIDS

Usually, the osmotic diarrhea produced by Mg^{++} is mild; it may even be welcomed by previously constipated patients. A change to a magnesium-free, aluminum-containing antacid is all that is required to control the situation in some. The use of antacids is a common cause of diarrhea in dyspeptic patients. Magnesium can be used to induce diarrhea by the rare patient with the Münchausen syndrome seeking medical attention for self-induced problems.

10.4.3 ANTIARRHYTHMIC DRUGS
The antiarrhythmic drugs most commonly associated with diarrhea include quinidine, procainamide and disopyramide. The mechanism involved is unknown. Changing the antiarrhythmic drug may halt the diarrhea.

10.4.4 OTHER MEDICATIONS
Colchicine, often administered for acute gout, produces diarrhea as a common side effect. It resolves with discontinuance of the medication. The mechanism of the diarrhea is unknown, but may relate to an intestinal cytotoxic effect of colchicine. Antimetabolites (e.g., methotrexate) often cause diarrhea as a result of damage to the small or large bowel mucosa. This type of diarrhea can be devastating and difficult to control. Except for rehydration and stopping the drug, little can be done.

11. CHRONIC DIARRHEA

11.1 Pathogenesis
The four basic mechanisms that cause chronic diarrhea are osmotic, secretory and exudative factors, and abnormal intestinal transit (Table 11).

If the diarrhea ceases when fasting, or if there is a significant osmotic gap in the stool water, then an osmotic cause for the diarrhea is suspect. Examples include diarrhea after ingesting milk (a result of lactase deficiency) or drugs such as laxatives and antacids, or the excessive use of artificial sweeteners such as sorbitol and mannitol, which contain polycyclic alcohols.

If the patient's diarrhea persists when fasting (such as may occur at nighttime when the diarrhea awakens the person from sleep), a secretory diarrhea is likely. Secretory diarrhea usually arises from infection or inflammation associated with toxigenic and invasive bacteria. Secretory diarrhea may also result from the spillage of excess bile acids into the colon (choleretic enteropathy) or from the cathartic effect of hydroxy fatty acids arising from the colonic bacterial action on malabsorbed fat. Very rarely, secretory diarrhea can arise from a tumor producing an intestinal secretagogue (e.g., pancreatic islet cell tumor producing vasoactive intestinal peptide or gastrin).

Exudative diarrhea results from mucosal damage to the small or large bowel, which interferes with absorption of salt and water, and may be associated with the exudation of serum proteins, blood, and mucus and sloughed cells. This mechanism is seen in infectious, inflammatory and neoplastic disorders.

Disorders of intestinal transit may give rise to diarrhea secondary to abnor-

TABLE 11. Pathophysiologic mechanisms of chronic diarrhea

Major disturbance	Probable mechanisms	Examples/Associated conditions
Osmotic*	Ingestion	Antacids, laxatives
	Maldigestion	Pancreatic insufficiency, disaccharidase deficiency
	Malabsorption	Carbohydrate malabsorption, congenital chloridorrhea
Disorders of intestinal transit	Slow transit ("blind loop syndrome") – excessive contact time	Fistulas, strictures (such as in the patient with Crohn's disease), diabetic neuropathy
	Rapid transit – insufficient contact time	Intestinal resection, hyperthyroidism, irritable bowel
Secretory**	Bacterial enterotoxins	Vibrio cholerae, enterotoxigenic E. coli
	Secretagogues	Bile acids, fatty acids, ethanol, prostaglandins, phenolphthalein, dioctyl sodium sulfosuccinate, VIP, gastrin, calcitonin
Exudative	Increased passage of body fluids into lumen	Ulcerative colitis, Crohn's disease

*See Table 12. **See Table 13.

mal intestinal motility in hyperthyroidism or diabetic neuropathy. Scleroderma leads to bacterial overgrowth and steatorrhea (as can the rapid transit in hyperthyroidism). The mechanism of diarrhea in these conditions relates to a combination of bacterial overgrowth, bile salt wastage and disorders of motility (slow or rapid intestinal transit).

11.1.1 OSMOTIC DIARRHEA

Retention of solute molecules within the bowel lumen generates osmotic forces that retard the normal absorption of water (Table 12). Practical examples include poorly absorbed carbohydrates or a divalent ion. Poorly absorbed divalent ions (e.g., phosphate, sulfate and magnesium) are the laxative constituents of several common antacids and saline purges. Since the "pores" through which ions are absorbed are highly charged, these polyvalent ions tend to be absorbed slowly. Thus, they accumulate within the intestinal lumen, raise the osmolality, and so retard the normal absorption of water or even act to draw water from the circulation into the intestinal lumen.

TABLE 12.   Causes of osmotic diarrhea

Carbohydrates
Specific disaccharidase deficiencies
Glucose–galactose malassimilation
Fructose malassimilation
Mannitol, sorbitol ingestion ("chewing gum diarrhea")
Lactulose therapy

Divalent ions
Magnesium sulfate (Epsom salts)
Sodium sulfate
Sodium phosphate
Sodium citrate
Magnesium-containing antacids

Carbohydrates constitute the other major group of osmotic agents. Some are poorly absorbed by everybody; lactulose, for example, was developed to be a nonhydrolyzable, nonabsorbable disaccharide that would act as a cathartic. The action of lactulose mimics the effects of *primary lactase deficiency*. This condition normally develops after weaning in the majority of African-, Caribbean- or Asian-Canadians and occurs in 30% of persons with southern European ancestry. The unabsorbed lactose acts osmotically to retain water in the small intestine. In fact, any disease that interferes with carbohydrate absorption (e.g., impaired intraluminal digestion due to pancreatic disease, primary disaccharidase deficiencies, and secondary disaccharidase deficiencies due to small bowel disease) will lead to osmotic diarrhea. Since carbohydrates are not inert in the colon, their metabolism leads to further osmotic forces. Once carbohydrate reaches the fecal flora, anaerobic fermentation occurs (Figure 13). Intermediary products are ethanol and formic, succinic and lactic acids. These products are further consumed to varying degrees. CO_2 and H_2 are rapidly absorbed, and CO_2 rises in exhaled air. (Exhaled H_2 is the basis for the hydrogen breath test described earlier.) Excess gas production causes borborygmi and flatus rich in H_2. Short-chain fatty acids (SCFAs) are also produced (acetic acid, propionic acid and butyric acid) and account for the acidic stool pH noted in diarrhea of carbohydrate malabsorption. The caloric loss due to carbohydrate malabsorption is diminished to the extent that short-chain fatty acids can be absorbed from the colon (where they may be used as nutrients by the colonocytes), thus "salvaging" some of the malabsorbed carbohydrates that enter the colon.

The consequences of malabsorption are as follows: With minor impairment of sugar absorption, colonic fermentation is complete and only small amounts of excess solute are present in stool water. Stool volume and stool pH do not change much initially, and up to three-quarters of the glucose energy is returned to the body in the form of short-chain fatty acids (colonic "salvage"). As the extent of carbohydrate malabsorption increases, more short-chain fatty acids are formed than can be reabsorbed. This results in diarrhea due to the presence of osmotically active short-chain fatty acids. The stool pH consequently begins to fall, which further decreases colonic salvage.

Clinically, osmotic diarrhea should stop when the patient stops ingesting the poorly absorbed solute. Stool analysis should not reveal fat, RBC or WBC. There should be a positive osmotic gap – that is, stool osmolality minus stool Na^+ plus stool K^+ times 2 (multiplied by 2 to account for anions) is greater than 50, the size of the osmotic gap being approximately equivalent to the concentration of poorly absorbed solutes in fecal water.

11.1.2 INTESTINAL TRANSIT AND DIARRHEA

The basal electrical rhythm of the small intestine alters the excitability of the muscle cells. The motility patterns of the small intestine consist of three essential patterns: (1) migrating motor complex (MMC), periodic bursts of contractile activity lasting at least 5 minutes that are succeeded by periods of quiescence and appear to migrate down the small intestine at a slow rate of less than 5 cm/min; (2) minute rhythm, regular groups of between 3 and 10 contractions that occur at intervals of 1 to 2 minutes, separated by periods of quiescence, and appear to migrate down the small intestine at a rapid rate of 60–120 cm/min; (3) migrating action potential complex, a single ring contraction or single burst of spike potentials that migrates down the intestine at a rate exceeding 90 cm/min.

These forms of small intestinal motility control the rate at which material travels along the intestine and hence arrives at the anus. Gastrointestinal motor activity also determines the time and thus the degree of contact between gut contents, the digestive enzymes and the absorptive epithelium. Accelerated transit of material through the gut produces diarrhea by limiting digestion and absorption.

Understanding of motility-associated diarrhea remains limited, and only rudimentary measures of intestinal myoelectrical activity exist for humans. The oral–anal transit times of radiolabeled markers, radiopaque tubing, or nonabsorbable carbohydrate markers provide the only clinical assessments. Even small intestinal motility, unlike esophageal motility, remains a research tool.

The ileocecal valve is important to gut function. The ileocecal sphincter extends over a 4 cm length of distal small intestine and produces a high-pressure zone of about 20 mm Hg. Distention of the ileum results in a decrease in the ileocecal sphincter pressure, whereas distention of the colon results in an increased pressure in this area. The ileocecal valve slows down intestinal transit (ileal "break") and prevents backwash from the colon. By this mechanism the ileocecal valve is important in regulating intestinal transit. Removal of the ileocecal valve during surgery will result in marked intestinal hurry as well as the potential for bacterial overgrowth from fecal "backwash." Disorders that impair peristalsis in the small gut allow bacterial overgrowth, resulting in diarrhea. Lastly, premature evacuation of the colon because of an abnormality of its contents or because of intrinsic colonic "irritability" or inflammation results in a reduced contact between luminal contents and colonic mucosa and, therefore, in more frequent, liquid stools.

11.1.3 SECRETORY DIARRHEA

The small intestine normally secretes as well as absorbs fluid and electrolytes; the secretion rate is lower than the absorption rate. Therefore, the net effect of small bowel transport is absorption of fluid. This is an important concept, because it means that a pathophysiologic event may reduce the net absorption rate in either of two ways: by stimulating secretion or inhibiting absorption. Either or both can result in what is clinically recognized as secretory diarrhea. It is not usually possible to ascertain which of the two events is predominant. For clinical purposes, it seems best to consider inhibition of ion absorption and stimulation of ion secretion together.

The prototype of secretory diarrhea is Vibrio cholerae; its clinical description first aroused interest in the secretory process as a mechanism for diarrhea (Table 13).

Bacterial secretagogues fall into two major classes. The first class comprises large (MW 84,000), heat-labile proteins, of which cholera enterotoxin is the prototype. These toxins appear to stimulate secretion by activating mucosal adenylate cyclase and thus increasing cyclic AMP levels in the mucosa. The intracellular "messenger" for secretion is less well defined; cyclic AMP is considered important, though there are additional steps that might also involve intracellular levels of Ca^{++} and the calcium regulatory protein, calmodulin. A second class of secretagogues comprises smaller proteins that are heat-stable. The best studied is the ST (heat-stable toxin) of E. coli, which stimulates secretion by activating mucosal guanylate cyclase, leading to higher levels of cyclic GMP in the mucosa.

Bacterial toxins, however, are only part of the story. Secretion is also stimulated experimentally by hormones, peptides acting locally (paracrine hormones), luminal factors (e.g., dihydroxy bile acids and fatty acids), neurotransmitters, prostaglandins and physical factors (e.g., distention). Bile

TABLE 13.   Causes of secretory diarrhea

Pathophysiologic mechanisms
Enterotoxins
Circulating secretagogues (VIP, calcitonin, prostaglandins, serotonin)
Increased hydrostatic pressure and tissue pressure
Gastric hypersecretion (Zollinger-Ellison syndrome)
Pancreatic hypersecretion
Laxatives (ricinoleic acid, bisacodyl, phenolphthalein, oxyphenisatin, dioctyl sodium sulfo-
    succinate, aloe, senna, danthron)
Bile salts
Fatty acids

Clinical syndromes
Acute secretory diarrhea
Chronic secretory diarrhea
    Surreptitious laxative ingestion
    Pancreatic cholera syndrome (VIP)
    Medullary carcinoma of the thyroid (calcitonin)
    Ganglioneuroma, ganglioneuroblastoma, neurofibroma
    Zollinger-Ellison syndrome (gastrin)
    Malignant carcinoid syndrome (serotonin)
    Idiopathic secretory diarrhea
    Congenital chloridorrhea (some cases)
    Secreting villous adenoma
    Total villous atrophy of small bowel mucosa
    Niacin deficiency
    Intestinal lymphoma
Miscellaneous
    Intestinal obstruction
    Intestinal distention/ileus

---

acids and fatty acids not absorbed in the small intestine evoke secretion of electrolytes and water by the colon. The exact mechanism(s) for this are uncertain. Both groups have multiple effects on the bowel, including stimulation of secretion, increased intestinal permeability and transient alterations in morphology.

One or more humoral stimuli can elicit a massive secretion of water and electrolytes from the small bowel. The colon is usually not involved directly, but it may be unable to adequately reabsorb the fluid load imposed on it. A key question, difficult to answer, is "What is the responsible hormone?" Putative secretagogues include vasoactive intestinal peptides in the pancreatic cholera syndrome, calcitonin in medullary carcinoma of the thyroid, gastrin in the Zollinger-Ellison syndrome, serotonin in the malignant carcinoid syndrome, and glucagon in glucagonomas. Prostaglandins are also potent stimulators of intestinal secretion. Diarrhea secondary to prostaglandin-stimulated intestinal secretion is a common side effect of orally administered prostaglandin analogues.

The intestinal distention that occurs with obstruction or ileus also produces a local secretory state proximal to the obstruction. The mechanism is not entirely clear and may be related to changes in permeability (as tight junctions are stretched and broken) as well as to direct, perhaps neural, stimulation of secretory mechanisms.

Secretory diarrhea is recognized clinically by four features: (1) the stools are large-volume, watery and often >1 L/day; (2) the diarrhea persists during fasting; (3) there is a measured stool osmolar gap of <50 mOsm/L; and (4) patients with secretory diarrhea do not have excessive fat, blood or pus in their stools, but often develop depletion in fluid, Na^+ and K^+.

Therapeutically, the offending agent must be removed. A variety of empirical therapies that influence the secretory process (e.g., somatostatin, prostaglandin inhibitors, phenothiazines, calcium channel blockers, α_2-adrenergic agonists and lithium) may be effective but should be reserved for use in a research center. Oral glucose-saline replacement therapy is useful for maintenance of hydration. For bile acid–induced diarrhea, cholestyramine works well unless there has been a greater than 100 cm resection of the terminal ileum. With more extensive resections (>100 cm) there will be both steatorrhea and bile salt wastage, and treatment must be focused on the steatorrhea.

11.1.4 EXUDATIVE DIARRHEA
Exudation is a far simpler concept. Structural disruption of the intestinal wall by diffuse ulceration, inflammation, infiltrations and tumors will add cellular debris, mucus, serum proteins and blood to the lumen. The effects on stool volume will be most pronounced when the lesions also involve the colon, since there will be little opportunity for normal mechanisms of colonic fluid and electrolyte absorption to compensate for the increased volume of chyme.

11.1.5 SELF-INDUCED DIARRHEA
The possibility that the diarrhea is self-induced must be considered when a patient complains of chronic diarrhea and when the routine investigations are negative. In general, abusing laxatives, diuretics and sometimes thyroid hormones will induce diarrhea. Often the diarrhea is sufficiently severe to cause electrolyte disturbances, acid-based problems and dehydration. The diagnosis can be extremely difficult since the history is often misleading or not obtained. The usual investigations (including sigmoidoscopy and radiographs) will be negative, unless the patient is taking a drug that can cause melanosis

TABLE 14.   Anatomic approach to the causes of chronic diarrhea

---

Gastric
Excessive use of antacids*
Hypergastrinemia/Zollinger-Ellison syndrome
Postoperative unmasked celiac disease, lactase deficiency or pancreatic
  insufficiency
Postoperative dumping syndrome*

Small intestine
Crohn's disease*
Celiac disease*
Lymphoma
Whipple's disease
Bacterial, viral or parasitic infection*
Abnormal intestinal integrity: scleroderma, amyloidosis, diabetes

Large bowel
Colon neoplasia*
Irritable bowel syndrome*
Inflammatory bowel disease*: ulcerative colitis, Crohn's disease

Drugs
Antacids*
Antibiotics*
Alcohol*
Antimetabolites
Laxatives
Digitalis
Colchicine

Metabolic
Hyperthyroidism
Hypoparathyroidism
Addison's disease
Diabetes*
Carcinoid syndrome
VIPoma syndrome

---

*Common causes within the group

coli (brown-black pigmentation of the colonic mucosa), such as the anthracene laxatives senna or aloe. Stool analysis for Mg^{++}, sennas or phenolphthalein may reveal the culprit. Finding packages of laxatives and other drugs in room searches is often the only method that permits the diagnosis; this approach has been criticized because of ethical considerations, but may be the only way to uncover the problem. Ethical issues and respect for the patient's privacy must be carefully considered before embarking on a room or locker search.

11.2 Investigation of the Patient with Chronic Diarrhea

For a patient with chronic diarrhea, a careful history and physical examination can help define the site in the intestinal tract responsible (Table 14). This may avoid the expense and frustration of the unproductive "shotgun" approach. One possible diagnostic approach appears in Figure 16.

12. DISACCHARIDASE DEFICIENCIES

Disaccharide intolerance is a characteristic symptom complex resulting from the ingestion of ordinary dietary quantities of disaccharides, which produces a symptomatic diarrhea. The cause is a deficiency of one or more disaccharidases, but not all people with such a deficiency will experience symptoms.

Dietary carbohydrates are presented to the surface of the jejunal mucosa in the form of isomaltose, maltotriose and three major disaccharides – maltose, sucrose and lactose. Trehalose, a disaccharide contained in young mushrooms and in certain insects, is a minor component of modern Western diets. Deficiencies of disaccharidases may be *primary* (hereditary) or *secondary* (acquired) deficiencies. Characteristically in primary deficiencies, which are rare, only one enzyme is involved; the deficiency is present at birth (with the exception of the common adult-onset form of lactase deficiency), not associated with intestinal disease, and irreversible. Secondary deficiencies usually involve all the disaccharidases, may occur at any age, are associated with a disorder of the small intestinal mucosa, and may be reversed if the intestinal disorder (e.g., celiac disease, stasis syndromes or acute enteritis) heals. Because primary lactase deficiency is uncommon in Canadians with northern European ancestors, the appropriate tests need to be performed to exclude secondary causes such as celiac disease.

The clinical manifestations of enzyme deficiency result from the osmotic diarrhea following ingestion of the disaccharide. The affected individual develops crampy, abdominal distress and distention, relieved by the expulsion of liquid stool and flatus. The severity of the diarrhea varies with the disaccharide load, the degree of deficiency of enzyme activity and any associated/ causal intestinal disease. The clinical diagnosis can be confirmed by direct enzyme assay of jejunal mucosal biopsies or by indirect methods for detecting disaccharide malabsorption (e.g., the breath hydrogen test). Treatment of hereditary deficiencies is usually by elimination diets. For children and adolescents (who have high nutritional requirements) and for adults who enjoy milk, low-lactose milk is available. It can also be prepared by adding yeast lactase (available in commercial form, Lactaid®) to milk and refrigerating it for 24 hours.

Delayed-onset (adult-onset) hereditary lactase deficiency is extremely common and probably "normal" for humans. Beginning as early as age 2 years in some racial groups, and as late as adolescence in others, the activities of lactase in the majority of the world's populations drop sharply. This is the result of the genetically controlled "switching off" of lactase synthesis by intestinal cells. Individuals of northern European ancestry maintain lactase activity throughout adulthood.

13. GLUTEN-INDUCED ENTEROPATHY (CELIAC DISEASE)

In celiac disease (gluten-induced or gluten-sensitive enteropathy) the mucosa of the small intestine is damaged by gluten-containing foods (i.e., those containing wheat, rye, barley and possibly oats). This causes a characteristic though nonspecific lesion and subsequent malabsorption of most nutrients. The precise mechanism of gluten toxicity is unknown, but there is likely both a genetic and an immunological component. Fractionation of cereal proteins reveals that the component that is toxic to the intestinal mucosa is a portion of the gluten molecule called gliadin. Although gliadin can be inactivated in a test tube by enzymatic degradation, digestion to smaller peptides by pepsin and trypsin does not alter its toxicity in humans. In susceptible people, symptoms and pathologic changes occur within 12 hours of gluten intake. The immune system is also involved. The small intestine in patients with untreated celiac disease shows an increase in lamina propria lymphocytes, plasma cells and intraepithelial lymphocytes. Immunocytochemical studies indicate that cells producing IgA, IgG and particularly IgM are increased. Increased levels of serum IgA and decreased levels of serum IgM have also been reported and appear to revert toward normal with treatment.

Genetic studies indicate that about 10% of the patient's first-order relatives have asymptomatic disease. HLA-B8 and HLA-DW3, generally associated through linkage disequilibrium, are present in 80% of patients (compared to 20% of the general population). In addition, a specific antigen is present on the surface of B lymphocytes in approximately 80% of celiac disease patients (compared to 10–15% of controls). It is found in all parents of affected individuals, which suggests that this antigen is inherited by an autosomal recessive method. Celiac disease is also present in about 2% of insulin-dependent diabetics.

TABLE 15. Intestinal and extraintestinal symptoms of celiac disease in adults

Manifestations	Probable causes or deficiencies
Common	
Anemia	Iron, folate, B_{12}, pyridoxine
Glossitis	Iron, folate
Weight loss/weakness	Malassimilation – Negative nitrogen balance
Diarrhea/flatulence	Fat and carbohydrate malassimilation
Abdominal pain	Increased intestinal gas production secondary to carbohydrate malassimilation
Occasional	
Follicular hyperkeratosis and dermatitis	Vitamin A, folate
Pigmentation	Associated adrenal insufficiency
Edema	Hypoproteinemia
Tetany	Vitamin D, calcium, magnesium
Osteomalacia	Vitamin D, calcium
Purpura	Hypoprothrombinemia (vitamin K)
Rare	
Spinal cord degeneration	B_{12}
Peripheral neuritis	B_{12}, vitamin E, thiamine, pyridoxine
Psychosis and other psychological disturbances	B_{12}; other causes likely
Malignancy (usually small bowel lymphoma)	Unknown

13.1 Clinical Features

13.1.1 CHILDHOOD PRESENTATION

In children, onset of symptoms suggestive of celiac disease is gradual with failure to thrive after the introduction of cereals in the diet. The affected infant is irritable, anorexic, pale and wasted. Physical examination discloses generalized hypotonia and abdominal distention. The stools are soft, bulky, clay-colored and offensive. In the slightly older child, abdominal pain may be the presenting complaint. The pain may be sufficiently severe to simulate an intestinal obstruction. Older children may also present with anemia, rickets and failure to grow normally. Quite often, adolescents have a clinical quiescence of the disease. Even if relatively asymptomatic in childhood, affected people often do not attain their normal growth potential, being shorter than their sibs.

13.1.2 *ADULT PRESENTATION*

Celiac disease can present at any age, even after 70 years, but in adults it usually occurs between 20 and 60 years. In adult and adolescent patients, presentations with classical features of diarrhea, weight loss and malnutrition, or bone pain (osteomalacia) have become much less common (Table 15). Mild and subclinical forms are frequent, occurring in more than 50% of patients. The sole presentation may be an otherwise unexplained hematologic abnormality (iron deficiency with or without anemia, folate deficiency, macrocytosis), constitutional symptoms or fatigue with minimal weight loss and no intestinal symptoms, or mild abdominal or digestive complaints. The entity is most common in those of Irish and Scottish background or those who have a family history.

Diarrhea is common but many patients experience normal bowel habits, alternating diarrhea and constipation, and even constipation. The diarrhea is usually mild, with fewer than three bowel movements per day in most. Floating stools, also common in healthy subjects excreting high amounts of stool gas, are often not reported. Indeed, stools suggesting steatorrhea (i.e., unformed, bulky and hard to flush, greasy, sticky, pale and foul-smelling) are quite uncommon. Flatulence, abdominal distention, abdominal cramps and borborygmi are common complaints. Fatigue is the most frequent symptom at presentation. Weight loss is usually moderate (averaging 10 kg) and may be absent in mild cases. Clinically overt metabolic (tetany) and bone (osteomalacia) diseases have become uncommon with our generous Western diets, but these situations are hallmarks of celiac disease. A clue to the diagnosis of celiac disease is the development of lactose intolerance in person whose heritage is northern European.

Patients with dermatitis herpetiformis have gluten enteropathy but often without clinical impact. Overall, mucosal involvement in celiac disease progresses from duodenum to jejunoileum and is most severe proximally; the length of bowel involved determines to a great extent the clinical picture of the disease.

13.2 Laboratory Findings

Laboratory findings, as clinical signs and symptoms, vary widely. The definitive diagnosis of celiac disease requires the demonstration of small bowel mucosal villous atrophy that improves upon gluten withdrawal. In practice, several tests can be used to strengthen the suspicion of celiac disease and/or evaluate the possible biochemical consequences. The tests that are most useful to point to a diagnosis of celiac disease are hematological, serological and stool examination. The definitive diagnostic test is a small bowel biopsy.

13.2.1 HEMATOLOGICAL TESTS
Anemia is present in less than 50% of adult patients and may be secondary to iron, folate or (very rarely) vitamin B_{12} deficiency. Since celiac disease involves the proximal small bowel (i.e., the duodenum, where iron absorption occurs) most severely, iron deficiency is the most common laboratory abnormality. Folate deficiency also commonly occurs. Decreased absorption of B_{12} and malabsorption of vitamin K (with prolonged prothrombin time) are uncommon.

13.2.2 SEROLOGICAL TESTS
The demonstration of antibodies in the serum to gliadin, reticulin or endomysium suggests the presence of celiac disease. Anti-endomysial IgA antibody measurement has proved to be a sensitive test for celiac disease, even in screening studies of asymptomatic children. Tests of antibodies to transglutaminase are being developed as diagnostic markers.

13.2.3 STOOL EXAMINATION
Steatorrhea can be confirmed by a 72-hour fecal fat study. It is usually mild (10–20 g/24 hours) and may be absent in some patients. Its severity correlates with the extent of the intestinal lesion, so that patients whose disease is limited to the proximal small intestine often have normal stool fat excretion.

13.2.4 BLOOD CHEMISTRY TEST
Depletion of minerals (zinc, magnesium) and ions (potassium) occurs only with severe disease. Plasma proteins are often within normal limits but this protein-losing enteropathy (leakage of serum protein into gut lumen) and possible malnutrition may result in decreased serum albumin. A low serum carotene (and sometimes cholesterol) level may be a clue to the presence of the disease.

13.2.5 CARBOHYDRATE TOLERANCE TEST
Approximately two-thirds of patients with celiac disease exhibit an abnormal D-xylose test. D-xylose is an aldopentose that is absorbed in the upper small intestine and is excreted in the urine almost completely within the first five hours after ingestion. Abnormal D-xylose absorption is best evaluated by the serum concentration after ingestion and points specifically to small bowel disease or luminal bacterial overgrowth. Similarly, the absorptive cell lesion also results in secondary lactase deficiency; thus, the H_2-lactose breath test may be abnormal in celiac disease. Because of the low sensitivity and specificity of the D-xylose test for celiac disease, it is not recommended.

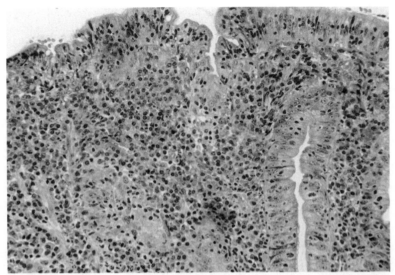

Figure 20. The high-power view of the small intestinal mucosa in gluten-induced enteropathy shows complete flattening of the mucosal surface, crypt expansion, increased numbers of intra-epithelial lymphocytes, and lamina propria plasmacytosis.

13.2.6 *RADIOGRAPHIC STUDIES*
Barium studies of the small bowel may show dilation of the bowel and slight thickening of the mucosal folds. Intraluminal signs of malabsorption with flocculation, segmentation and clumping of the barium (features due to excess amount of fluid present within the lumen) are variable and not common. (The new barium suspensions now used have made this a rare finding.) Radiographic findings in celiac disease are not specific for this syndrome of malabsorption.

13.2.7 *PERMEABILITY TESTS*
The intestine of patients with celiac disease may be "leaky" and allow passage from the lumen into the blood and then into the urine of sugars such as mannitol or lactulose. The finding of increased amounts of these sugars in the urine after an oral dose suggests an abnormal intestinal permeability barrier. Such a finding of increased permeability may suggest the presence of celiac disease or other small intestinal disorders.

13.2.8 *SMALL BOWEL BIOPSY*
Small intestinal biopsies can be obtained endoscopically from the distal

duodenum. Rarely, when diagnostic uncertainty persists, a larger mucosal specimen may be needed and obtained from the duodenojejunal area using the peroral Rubin tube or the Crosby capsule.

A flat mucosal biopsy from a white adult in the Western world is almost certain to indicate celiac disease, although other disorders can be associated with similar changes (e.g., tropical sprue, diffuse lymphoma of small bowel, immunoglobulin deficiency syndromes and the Zollinger-Ellison syndrome with gastric hypersecretion). In infants, soy protein intolerance, cow's milk protein intolerance and viral gastroenteritis produce a similar appearance. Therefore, to establish unequivocally the diagnosis of celiac disease, clinical improvement with a gluten-free diet is needed. Proving this improvement with a second biopsy is usually not necessary in adults. Mucosal small bowel atrophy improves similarly, although reversion of histology toward normal requires many months of gluten withdrawal and often is not complete.

Microscopically the characteristic "flat" lesion of celiac disease will demonstrate absence of villi, an abnormal cuboidal surface epithelium, markedly lengthened crypts and increased numbers of plasma cells and lymphocytes in the lamina propria. The lesion may be very subtle and include increased intraepithelial lymphocytes and a change in the normal position of the nuclei in the enterocyte (Figure 20). In a subtle lesion with shortened villi, proper orientation of the specimen is important in order to correctly estimate the height of the villi. The proximal small bowel is most severely involved, while the lesion decreases in severity toward the distal small intestine. The lesion may be patchy. Celiac disease will not spare the proximal small intestine while involving the distal small intestine, however. Sometimes the gross appearance of the mucosa observed at the time of an upper endoscopy may alert the physician to the possibility of celiac disease (scalloping or loss of folds) and direct her/him to obtain a duodenal biopsy.

13.3 Treatment

The mainstay of therapy for celiac disease is the gluten-free diet, which requires avoiding wheat, rye, barley and oats but allows widely diversified foods. Expert dietetic counseling is a major determinant of successful treatment. Supplements of iron and folic acid are often needed. If milk products cause diarrhea, commercially available lactase enzymes may be used for the first few months. Usually, clinical symptoms improve within weeks, but drastic changes may be seen in sicker patients after a few days.

13.4 Complications and Prognosis

A primary failure to respond to treatment is usually due to incomplete (often involuntary) exclusion of gluten from the diet. Revision of the diet is neces-

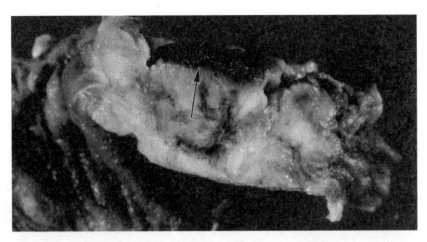

Figure 21A. A gross photograph showing ulcerating (arrow) and infiltrating small intestinal lymphoma.

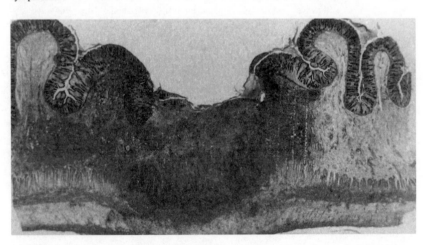

Figure 21B. A very low-power view showing the surface ulceration and infiltration of the lymphomatous tissue through virtually the full thickness of the bowel wall. Note the mucosal flattening adjacent to the neoplasm in this case of enteropathy-associated T-cell lymphoma.

sary. A dietary consultation may help to identify sources of unsuspected gluten such as medications, candies or toothpaste. Motivation for continuing with the gluten-free diet is provided by contacts with the physician and dietitian. Other causes of primary failure include diagnostic error (tropical sprue,

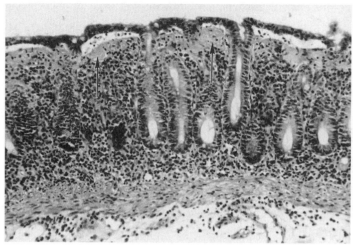

Figure 22. This case of collagenous sprue shows the characteristic thick subepithelial fibrous layer (arrows) as well as the characteristic flattening and surface epithelial damage of sprue.

lymphoma, etc.), dysgammaglobulinemia syndromes, "functional" associated pancreatic insufficiency and so-called refractory sprue. Deterioration after a period of clinical improvement suggests dietary indiscretions, malignancies (there is increased risk of lymphoma) or rare instances of refractory sprue, collagenous sprue and nongranulomatous ulcerative jejunoileitis (Figure 21A, B).

13.4.1 REFRACTORY SPRUE

Refractory sprue is a disease in which malabsorptive symptoms and mucosal small bowel atrophy persist or recur while the patient remains on a strict gluten-free diet. Corticosteroids, total parenteral nutrition and cyclosporine therapy have been used in treatment, but their value is not clear. The prognosis is serious.

13.4.2 NONGRANULOMATOUS ULCERATIVE JEJUNOILEITIS

This very rare complication presents with abdominal pain, intestinal bleeding and diarrhea. Ulcers may lead to small bowel perforations or strictures. The mortality rate for this condition is very high.

13.4.3 COLLAGENOUS SPRUE

This rare disorder is generally associated with severe malabsorption. In addition to the characteristic small intestinal biopsy of untreated celiac disease, a striking trichrome-positive band of collagen is seen beneath the surface epithelium (Figure 22). Changes may be patchy, necessitating multiple biopsies from different sites to confirm the diagnosis. There is no effective therapy other than nutritional supportive care.

13.4.4 MALIGNANCIES

Incidence of malignancies is increased in patients with celiac disease. Most of these are small bowel lymphomas and carcinomas of the esophagus and colon. A strict gluten-free diet decreases this risk – another reason to reinforce a lifetime commitment to gluten avoidance. Overall, the vast majority of patients with celiac disease have a normal life expectancy.

14. SHORT BOWEL SYNDROME

The severity of symptoms following resections of large segments of the small bowel relates to the extent of the resection, to the specific level of the resected small bowel and to the reason for which the resection was undertaken. The level of resection is important because absorption of nutrients is most effective in the proximal small bowel (iron, folate and calcium). Resection of up to 40% of the intestine is usually tolerated provided the duodenum and proximal jejunum and distal half of the ileum and ileocecal valve are spared. In contrast, resection of the distal two-thirds of the ileum and ileocecal valve alone may induce severe diarrhea and significant malabsorption even though only 25% of the total small intestine has been resected. Resection of 50% of the small intestine results in significant malabsorption, and resection of 70% or more of the small intestine will result in severe malnutrition sufficient to cause death unless the patient's malnutrition is aggressively treated.

The most common cause of massive resection of the small bowel is small bowel ischemia due to thrombosis or embolism of the superior mesenteric artery, thrombosis of the superior mesenteric vein, or low flow in the splanchnic vessels. Less commonly, volvulus, strangulated hernias, Crohn's disease, neoplasm and trauma necessitate massive resection.

Two major types of diarrhea can develop after massive ileal resection. One is induced primarily by malabsorbed bile acids, and the other by malabsorbed fat. When the ileal resection is small (less than 100 cm), hepatic synthesis of bile acids is sufficient to compensate for increased fecal losses. The luminal concentrations of bile acids are maintained within the micellar range, and significant steatorrhea does not occur. However, with inadequate absorption in the terminal ileum, bile acids enter the colon, impairing electrolyte and water absorption. Thus the term "bile acid diarrhea" is applied to this circumstance. When the ileal resection is extensive (greater than 100 cm), hepatic compensation for wastage of bile acids is incomplete and the concentration of bile acids in the lumen is too low for adequate micellar solubilization of fat. Steatorrhea results. Here the malabsorbed fat is primarily responsible for the diarrhea. With excessive amounts of fatty acids now in the colon, electrolyte and water absorption are further impaired.

Consistent with these proposed pathogenic mechanisms are the therapeutic observations that a reduction in the dietary intake of long-chain fats will reduce the severity of diarrhea in the second instance (extensive resection and steatorrhea), whereas a sequestrant of bile acids such as cholestyramine, colestipol or aluminum hydroxide is needed for effective therapy of bile acid diarrhea.

Additional metabolic complications arise from the short bowel syndrome. These include hyperoxaluria and subsequent nephrolithiasis. Normally dietary oxalate is excreted in the feces, bound to calcium as an insoluble complex. However, in a patient with steatorrhea, fatty acids in the intestine preferentially bind to calcium, leaving the oxalate soluble and available for absorption in the colon. The short bowel syndrome may also give rise to cholelithiasis. If bile acid malabsorption is extensive, a lithogenic bile will be produced, predisposing to gallstone formation.

15. POSTGASTRECTOMY MALABSORPTION

Postgastrectomy malabsorption frequently follows gastric surgery. The small size of the gastric remnant causes inadequate mixing of food with digestive juices, particularly after a gastroenterostomy. With the loss of the pylorus, there may be rapid gastric emptying ("dumping"), poor mixing of bile and pancreatic secretions, and rapid transit down the small intestine. Incoordinated secretion and poor mixing of bile and pancreatic juice leads to fat maldigestion. Bacterial contamination in a blind loop (with gastroenterostomy) results in maldigestion of fat, carbohydrate, protein, vitamins and minerals. Gastric surgery that allows food to enter into the upper small intestine without dilution and with minimal digestion may "unmask" mild and subclinical celiac disease, lactase deficiency or pancreatic insufficiency.

16. NORMAL SMALL INTESTINAL FLORA

The concentration and population of microorganisms that constitute the normal intestinal flora vary with the location along the intestine. Flora in the stomach, duodenum, jejunum and proximal ileum are sparse, usually less than 10^5/mL. The distal ileum represents a transitional zone between the sparse flora of the proximal small intestine and the luxuriant flora of the lower bowel, where microorganism concentrations reach 10^{11}/mL. The predominant species are strict anaerobes, including bacteroides, anaerobic streptococci, bifidobacteria and Clostridium. The commonest aerobic organisms are E. coli; however, their concentration (10^8/mL) is only 1/1,000 of the usual concentration of anaerobes in the colon.

Normally, bacterial flora are present in the intestinal lumen and in the mucus layer overlying the epithelium, and attached to the mucosal cells themselves. There is a specific tissue or cell type to which each microbial species attaches. For example, Streptococcus mutans, the oral organism that causes tooth decay, attaches only to the enamel surface of teeth; removal of the teeth leads to the disappearance of S. mutans from the oral microflora. This phenomenon of adherence may play an important role in the establishment and maintenance of a normal flora.

What are the mechanisms controlling normal small intestinal flora? First, in the stomach, acid suppresses the growth of most organisms that enter from the oropharynx. Bile added in the duodenum has additional antibacterial properties. Second, small intestinal motility mechanically sweeps bacteria downstream, helping to maintain a low concentration of organisms in the proximal small intestine. Third, the ileocecal valve plays an important role in preventing reflux of large amounts of colonic organisms. Additionally, mucus secreted by goblet cells and immunoglobulins has antibacterial properties.

Whereas the small intestine regulates the number of organisms present, in the colon the microorganisms themselves are responsible for maintaining their own population levels. Volatile fatty acids (e.g., acetic, butyric and propionic acid) are produced by anaerobes as well as by some coliforms. These short-chain fatty acids reduce the intraluminal pH and suppress the growth of certain organisms, thereby serving to control proliferation. In addition, some organisms produce other substances that inhibit bacterial growth, called bacteriocins.

Thus far we have considered what the microorganisms are, where they are located, and how their numbers are controlled. We next examine the concept that the normal flora exert a profound influence on intraluminal constituents, including food, urea, bilirubin, bile salts, drugs and potential toxins. Bacteria ferment dietary carbohydrates, yielding short-chain fatty acids, hydrogen and carbon dioxide. Fatty acids from carbohydrates and those from fat in the diet are hydroxylated by the intestinal flora. The hydroxy fatty acids formed stimulate fluid secretion and are thus cathartics.

Similarly, bacteria alter protein and amino acids. Tryptophan is converted to indole compounds, glycine to ammonia, and methionine to hydrogen sulfide. Urea is converted to ammonia, a reaction that may contribute to hepatic encephalopathy. Bilirubin is metabolized to urobilinogen; bile salts may be deconjugated (removing glycine and taurine) and dehydroxylated (cholic acid

TABLE 16.   Etiology of the bacterial overgrowth syndrome

Breakdown of normal defense mechanisms
Achlorhydria
Stasis: Anatomic (Crohn's disease, multiple small bowel diverticula, lymphoma, strictures)
       Functional (scleroderma, diabetic autonomic neuropathy, pseudo-obstruction)
Loss of ileocecal valve

Contamination
Postinfection
Enteroenteric fistulas, gastrocolic fistulas

---

becomes deoxycholic acid, and chenodeoxycholic acid becomes lithocholic acid). This deconjugation and dehydroxylation renders bile acids more insoluble and less capable of forming micelles. Bacteria also can affect vitamin synthesis and metabolism. Vitamin B_{12} may be bound, thereby becoming unavailable for absorption (hence the abnormal Schilling test in bacterial overgrowth) and vitamin K and folic acid produced.

The normal flora also affect drugs and other ingested materials. Sulfasalazine, a drug used in ulcerative colitis, is unabsorbed in its native form. Intestinal bacteria, however, convert the substance into two moieties, a therapeutically active aminosalicylic acid and an inactive sulfapyridine. The sulfa drug succinylsulfathiazole is itself inactive, but is converted by intestinal bacteria to sulfathiazole, which is an active antimicrobial agent. Another example is cyclamate, unabsorbed and inert in its native form. Intestinal bacteria produce cyclohexylamine, a potential carcinogenic agent. Thus, bacteria can activate pro-drugs and produce carcinogens.

17. BACTERIAL OVERGROWTH SYNDROME

The bacterial overgrowth syndrome (small bowel bacterial contamination syndrome) can result from any disease that interferes with the normal balance (ecosystem) of the small intestinal flora and brings about loss of gastric acidity; alteration in small bowel motility or lesions predisposing to luminal stasis; loss of the ileocecal valve; or overwhelming contamination of the intestinal lumen (Table 16).

The bacterial overgrowth syndrome gives rise to clinical abnormalities arising from the pathophysiological effects on the luminal contents and the mucosa. Bacteria can consume proteins and carbohydrates. In bacterial overgrowth there may be defective transport of sugars, possibly related to the toxic effect of deconjugated bile acids. Steatorrhea results from the deconjugation

TABLE 17. Diagnosis of the bacterial overgrowth syndrome

Jejunal culture

Tests of bile salt deconjugation
^{14}C-glycocholate breath tests
In vitro deconjugation assessment

Tests of malassimilation
Vitamin B$_{12}$ (Schilling test)
D-xylose, glucose, lactulose
H$_2$ breath tests

and dehydroxylation of bile acids; lithocholic acid is precipitated and free bile acids are reabsorbed passively, making them unavailable and incapable of performing micellar solubilization. There may also be mucosal damage. Fats, cholesterol and fat-soluble vitamins are malabsorbed. Vitamin B$_{12}$ is also malabsorbed as a result of the binding and incorporation of this vitamin into the bacteria. Folate deficiency, however, is not a common occurrence in bacterial overgrowth; unlike vitamin B$_{12}$, folate synthesized by microorganisms in the small bowel is available for host absorption. In patients with small bowel bacterial overgrowth, serum folate levels tend to be high rather than low. The enteric bacteria also produce vitamin K, and patients with bacterial overgrowth who are on the anticoagulant warfarin may have difficulty in maintaining the desired level of anticoagulation. In addition to steatorrhea, patients with bacterial overgrowth frequently complain of watery diarrhea. Important mechanisms in producing this diarrhea include (1) disturbances of the intraluminal environment with deconjugated bile acids, and hydroxylated fatty and organic acids; and (2) direct changes in gut motility.

In some patients, symptoms of the primary disease predominate, and evidence of bacterial overgrowth may be found only on investigation. In others, the primary condition is symptomless, and the patient presents with a typical malabsorption syndrome due to bacterial overgrowth. Once diagnosis of bacterial overgrowth is suspected a careful history should be performed to identify possible causes. Physical examination may be normal or may demonstrate signs related to specific nutrient deficiencies.

A small bowel biopsy is of value in excluding primary mucosal disease as the cause of the malabsorption. Histologic abnormalities of the jejunal mucosa are usually not seen in patients with bacterial overgrowth. The sine qua non for the diagnosis of bacterial overgrowth is a properly collected and appropriately cultured aspirate of the proximal small intestine (Table 17). Specimens should be obtained under anaerobic conditions and quantitative colony counts determined. Generally, bacteria concentrations of greater than 10^5 organisms per mL are highly suggestive of bacterial overgrowth. Such methods are difficult and usually undertaken only in a research setting. Alternatively, one can attempt to demonstrate a metabolic effect of the bacterial overgrowth, such as intraluminal bile acid deconjugation by the ^{14}C-glycocholate breath test. Cholylglycine-^{14}C (glycine-conjugated cholic acid with the radiolabeled ^{14}C on the glycine moiety) when ingested circulates normally in the enterohepatic circulation without deconjugation. Bacterial overgrowth within the small intestine splits the ^{14}C-labeled glycine moiety and subsequently oxidizes it to ^{14}C-labeled CO_2, which is absorbed in the intestine and exhaled. Excess $^{14}CO_2$ appears in the breath. The bile acid breath test cannot differentiate bacterial overgrowth from ileal damage or resection where excessive breath $^{14}CO_2$ production is due to bacterial deconjugation within the colon of unabsorbed ^{14}C-labeled glycocholate. This creates clinical difficulties, since bacterial overgrowth may be superimposed on ileal damage in such conditions as Crohn's disease.

Breath hydrogen analysis allows a distinct separation of metabolic activity of intestinal flora of the host, since no hydrogen production is known to occur in mammalian tissue. Excessive and early breath hydrogen production has been noted in patients with bacterial overgrowth following the oral administration of 10 g of lactulose, or a poorly absorbed sugar that is metabolized by the luminal bacteria to H_2.

Another hallmark of bacterial overgrowth is steatorrhea, detected by the 72-hour fecal fat collection.

The Schilling test may also be abnormal. ^{57}Co-B$_{12}$ is given with intrinsic factor following a flushing dose of nonradioactive B$_{12}$ given parenterally to prevent tissue storage of the labeled vitamin. In healthy subjects, ^{57}Co-B$_{12}$ combines with intrinsic factor and is absorbed and >8% excreted in the urine within 24 hours. In patients with bacterial overgrowth, the bacteria combine with or destroy intrinsic factor, the vitamin or both, causing decreased vitamin B$_{12}$ absorption. Following treatment with antibiotics the B$_{12}$ absorption returns to normal.

Treatment of bacterial overgrowth involves removing the cause, if possible. The addition of an antibiotic (tetracycline 250 mg q.i.d., or metronidazole 250 mg q.i.d., for 10 days) will often induce a remission for many months. If the cause cannot be eliminated and symptoms recur, good results can be achieved with intermittent use of antibiotics (e.g., once a day, one day a week, or one week out of every four).

18. PROTEIN-LOSING ENTEROPATHY

Protein-losing enteropathy describes a wide range of gastrointestinal disorders that are associated with an excessive loss of plasma protein into the gut lumen. Normal daily enteric loss of plasma protein corresponds to less than 1–2% of the plasma pool. The route of plasma protein loss across the normal mucosa is not well defined. It is likely that rapid shedding of epithelial cells from the mucosal surface is accompanied by loss of plasma proteins from the lamina propria at the site of cell extrusion.

In virtually any small intestinal disease, excessive transmural loss of plasma proteins may result from several mechanisms: in mucosal disease without ulceration but with increased permeability; in mucosal disease with erosion or ulceration (loss of inflammatory exudate that contains protein occurs); and in lymphatic obstruction with direct leakage of intestinal lymph from obstructed lacteals. Protein-losing enteropathy may also occur as a result of colonic inflammation, ischemia or tumor. Adaptive changes in endogenous synthesis of individual plasma proteins may compensate partially for excessive enteric loss.

Clinically, albumin loss may be manifested by dependent edema. A depression of the levels of thyroid and cortisol binding proteins will lower the total plasma level of these hormones, although normal levels of free hormone will maintain normal hormone function. Excessive enteric loss of plasma proteins other than albumin rarely leads to clinical problems; secondary hypogammaglobulinemia in these patients does not predispose them to infection, and the loss of blood clotting factors is rarely sufficient to impair hemostasis.

Patients with protein-losing enteropathy due to lymphatic obstruction, however, lose not only albumin and other plasma proteins but also intestinal lymph, with loss of long-chain triglycerides, fat-soluble vitamins and small lymphocytes.

Protein-losing enteropathy is considered in patients who exhibit hypoproteinemia and in whom other causes for hypoproteinemia (e.g., proteinuria, protein malnutrition and liver disease) are excluded. Fecal protein loss can then be quantitated using ^{51}Cr-labeled albumin or α_1-antitrypsin clearance into stool.

Management of protein-losing enteropathy involves the appropriate treatment of the disease(s) causing the protein loss. Enteral or parenteral feeding can be used to improve nutrition while the underlying disease is being treated. Enteric protein loss in patients with intestinal lymphangiectasia usually decreases with a low-fat diet. The normal absorption of long-chain triglycerides stimulates intestinal lymph flow; in their absence there is a decrease in the pressure within intestinal lymphatic vessels and hence a diminished loss of lymph into the lumen. Medium-chain triglycerides, which do not require intestinal lymphatic transport, can be substituted for the long-chain triglycerides and further decrease intestinal lymphatic pressure, with subsequent reduction in enteric lymph and protein loss.

19. MECKEL'S DIVERTICULUM

Meckel's diverticulum, an omphalomesenteric duct remnant, is a congenital outpouching usually located in the distal 100 cm of the ileum. Such diverticula are present in 1–3% of the general population. Of these, 30–40% are asymptomatic. Complications of Meckel's diverticulum include hemorrhage, intestinal obstruction, diverticulitis, umbilical discharge, perforation and peritonitis. Bleeding is the most common complication, resulting from ulceration of the ileal mucosa adjacent to ectopic gastric mucosa located within the diverticulum. (However, in the patients with a Meckel's diverticulum but without ectopic gastric mucosa, bleeding does not usually occur.) This bleeding is often painless and is usually encountered in children and young adults. Meckel's diverticulum accounts for nearly 50% of all lower gastrointestinal bleeding in children. Technetium-99m pertechnetate is normally taken by the ectopic gastric mucosa, providing the basis for the Meckel scan. Since only 60% of Meckel's diverticula contain ectopic gastric mucosa, false negative results occur. If the scan is positive, increased sensitivity can be achieved by repeating the scan after a short course of a histamine$_2$-receptor antagonist (H$_2$-RA): the H$_2$-RA releases acid secretion by the ectopic parietal cells in the Meckel's diverticulum and may thereby convert a positive into a negative scan.

20. CARCINOID SYNDROME

Over 90% of carcinoid tumors originate in the gastrointestinal tract. The most frequent sites are the appendix, terminal ileum and rectum. In general, non-metastasized carcinoid tumors are asymptomatic. The carcinoid syndrome is associated only with carcinoid tumors that have metastasized extensively to the liver or are extraintestinal (e.g., lung tumors). Metastasis is infrequent in carcinoids of the appendix, but is common in extra-appendiceal carcinoids.

Although carcinoid tumors differ in their ability to produce and store 5-hydroxytryptamine (5-HT), the excessive production of this substance and its metabolite 5-hydroxyindoleacetic acid (5-HIAA) remains their most characteristic chemical abnormality. Production of this hormone (as well as histamine, catecholamines, kinase and prostaglandins) causes the majority of symptoms. The symptom complex comprises diarrhea, flushing, wheezing, cluster headache, valvular heart disease (particularly pulmonary stenosis) and a pellagra-like skin rash. The carcinoid syndrome can be suspected clinically and confirmed biochemically by the demonstration of increased urinary 5-HIAA or platelet 5-HT.

Once the carcinoid syndrome is apparent, cure is usually impossible, since the tumor has metastasized by this time. Nevertheless, the intestinal origin of the tumor should be removed if it is causing obstruction. Serotonin antagonists (e.g., methysergide and cyproheptadine) can sometimes reduce symptoms. The somatostatin analogue octreotide may prove to be very effective in reducing the patient's symptoms; interferon may also prove to be useful. It is prudent to delay initiation of chemotherapy or radiation in the early metastatic stage of the disease, since the course is often indolent and patients survive many years with diffuse metastatic disease.

21. WHIPPLE'S DISEASE

Whipple's disease characteristically occurs in middle-aged men, who present with weight loss, fever, abdominal pain, arthralgias and intestinal symptoms of diarrhea and malabsorption. Small bowel biopsy characteristically demonstrates PAS-positive macrophages containing the bacillus Tropheryma whippelii plus an enteropathy with villous atrophy (Figure 23A, B). Treatment improves the fever and joint symptoms within a few days; the diarrhea and malabsorption disappear within two to four weeks. Because some patients with Whipple's disease may develop CNS involvement with the recently identified organism, trimethoprim-sulfamethoxazole antibiotics are recommended; treatment is continued for one year. Relapses may occur up to one or two years later and require repeat therapy.

22. IDIOPATHIC INTESTINAL PSEUDO-OBSTRUCTION

Idiopathic intestinal pseudo-obstruction is a disease of the muscular layer or of the enteric nervous system of the intestine. The myogenic form of idiopathic intestinal pseudo-obstruction is an autosomal dominant disease characterized by thinning of the intestinal musculature due to degeneration, fibrosis, malaligned smooth fibers and abnormal contractile filaments. All parts of the intestinal tract may be involved, but usually the small intestine, esophagus and colon are the most severely affected.

The neurogenic form of this disease is characterized by abnormal neuronal and glial cells. The damage may be in the spinal cord or in the splanchnic ganglia. When the splanchnic ganglia are involved, intranuclear inclusion bodies can be identified. The condition is characterized by abnormal systemic neural function, with an inappropriate blood pressure response to phenylephrine,

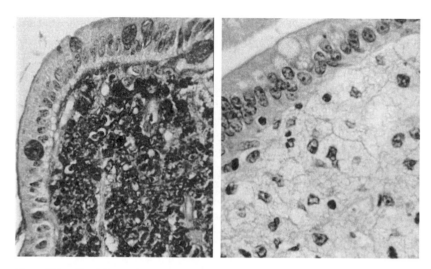

Figure 23A.   The right-hand panel of Figure 23A shows the H & E appearance of Whipple's disease with foamy histiocytes replacing normal lamina propria structures. The enterocytes are normal morphology. The left-hand panel shows the intense PAS positivity of the Whipple cells (as well as goblet cells and the brush border).

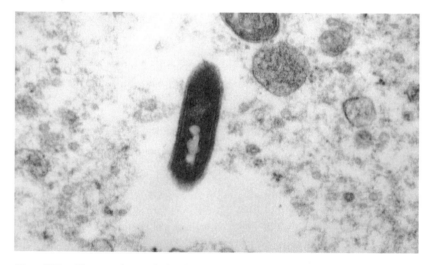

Figure 23B.   Electron micrograph showing the characteristic fine structure of the Whipple bacillus.

Valsalva's maneuver, or achieving the upright posture. There is a lack of sweating on warming of the skin, pupillary denervation hypersensitivity, and lack of intestinal spike activity after small intestinal distention.

Treatment of both the myogenic and neurogenic forms of idiopathic intestinal pseudo-obstruction is generally unsuccessful. Various promotility agents have been tried with only transient success. The somatostatin analogue octreotide may be useful in some patients. Associated bacterial overgrowth may worsen bloating and diarrhea, and should be treated with antibiotics. Surgery only aggravates the disorder and provides long intervals of severe ileus. Home parenteral nutrition may be the only alternative to maintain the patient's nutritional status, reduce the frequency and severity of the associated intestinal complaints, and improve the quality of the patient's life.

23. SMALL INTESTINAL VASCULAR DISORDERS

This topic is considered in detail in Chapter 8, and is only reviewed briefly here.

23.1 Acute Mesenteric Ischemia

The major causes of acute mesenteric ischemia are embolic obstruction thrombosis of the superior mesenteric artery (SMA), mesenteric venous thrombosis and nonocclusive ischemia. The congenital hypercoagulable states due to protein C or S antithrombin III deficiency can also cause thrombosis of the superior mesenteric vein. Embolic obstruction of the superior mesenteric artery is usually associated with cardiac arrhythmias, valvular disease, recent myocardial infarction or mycotic aneurysm. When an embolus lodges at the origin of the superior mesenteric artery, the entire small bowel and proximal colon are affected. Mesenteric venous thrombosis usually involves the superior mesenteric vein or its branches and the portal vein. It can be "primary" or "secondary" to a variety of hypercoagulable states (e.g., polycythemia rubra vera, carcinomatosis, oral contraception); to intra-abdominal sepsis (e.g., cholangitis, diverticular abscess); or to a condition in which blood flow is impaired (e.g., cardiogenic shock).

Nonocclusive bowel ischemia is the most common and lethal form of intestinal vascular insufficiency, accounting for at least 50% of all cases, with a mortality rate approaching 100%. It is commonly associated with reduced cardiac output, intra-abdominal sepsis and advanced malignant neoplasms. Digitalis constricts the splanchnic circulation and may aggravate or even precipitate mesenteric ischemia.

The typical patient is over 50 years of age, with arteriosclerotic or valvular heart disease, poorly controlled long-standing congestive heart failure, hypotension, recent myocardial infarction or cardiac arrhythmias. Abdominal pain is characteristically periumbilical and crampy. In the early stages, physical signs are often minimal. The abdomen is soft, sometimes slightly distended, with mild tenderness on palpation. Abdominal pain of any degree of severity associated with minimal abdominal findings and a high WBC (often over 20,000/mm^2) is an important early clue to the correct diagnosis. Signs of advanced ischemia include nausea, vomiting, peritoneal irritation, leukocytosis and a progressive metabolic acidosis. In a minority, unexplained abdominal distention or gastrointestinal bleeding, or the rapid onset of confusion and acidosis in an elderly patient, may be the first manifestation of small bowel ischemia.

Initial resuscitation is directed at correcting the predisposing or precipitating cause(s). Restoration of cardiac output with IV fluid is paramount. Digitalis, diuretics and vasoconstrictors should be discontinued if possible. Plain radiographs, ultrasound or CT scans as appropriate should exclude other radiologically diagnosable causes of acute abdominal pain. After volume repletion, the key step in the management of acute mesenteric ischemia is abdominal angiography. Remember that angiography in a hypovolemic or hypotensive patient frequently shows mesenteric vasoconstriction; for such patients the technique loses its usefulness as a diagnostic tool. Also, angiography in a volume-depleted patient may precipitate renal failure. If the angiogram is normal, the patient should be carefully observed, and a diagnostic laparotomy performed only if peritoneal signs develop. If the angiogram shows a minor arterial occlusion and clinically there is no peritoneal irritation, papaverine can be infused into the superior mesenteric artery through the catheter used for angiography at a rate of 60 mg/hour. (The role of angioplasty or other angiographic techniques remains unproven.) If peritoneal signs occur at any time, a laparotomy with resection of the ischemic segment is indicated. If the angiogram shows a major obstruction at the origin of the superior mesenteric artery, laparotomy should be carried out immediately. An embolus can usually be easily removed, while thrombotic obstruction requires a bypass graft from the aorta to an area of the artery distal to the site of obstruction. After revascularization, any nonviable bowel should be resected. It is advisable to save all bowel that may be viable and to re-explore the patient 24 hours later. The decision to perform a "second look" operation is made at the initial laparotomy and should not be changed on the basis of a favorable postoperative course. Since acute occlusion of the superior mesenteric artery is associated with prolonged vasospasm, the artery should be perfused with papaverine for 24 hours postoperatively.

If nonocclusive splanchnic vasoconstriction is present, intra-arterial papaverine infusion should be started. If, in spite of the infusion, abdominal pain persists and signs of peritoneal irritation appear, a laparotomy must be performed without delay.

Venous thrombosis is characterized on the angiogram by a prolonged arterial phase and a lack of opacity in the venous system. If a firm diagnosis of venous thrombosis has been made, anticoagulants are appropriate. However, if the patient develops peritoneal signs, immediate laparotomy and resection are indicated.

This systemic approach to the management of ischemia originating in the superior mesenteric artery results in earlier diagnosis and avoidance of surgery. The overall mortality rate has been reduced to about 50%; 90% of the patients who have no peritoneal signs at the time of angiography survive.

23.2 Chronic Mesenteric Ischemia

This uncommon condition occurs in elderly patients with partial occlusion of at least two of the three principal mesenteric vessels (the celiac axis and the superior and inferior mesenteric arteries). Epigastric or periumbilical abdominal pain beginning after a meal and lasting for one to three hours (*"intestinal angina"*) is the most characteristic clinical feature, although it is not often elicited. The pain may lead to a reduction in food intake (sitophobia) and secondarily a significant loss of weight. Bloating, flatulence and diarrhea are common, and steatorrhea is present in 50% of patients. This is the case because chronic mesenteric ischemia can cause mucosal damage. The physical examination is usually not diagnostic. A systolic abdominal bruit is present in 50% of patients but is not pathognomonic. (Epigastric bruits are common in normal persons.) Patients in whom the syndrome is suspected, and who have no other demonstrable abnormality to explain their symptoms, should have abdominal angiography. If angiography shows greater than 90% occlusion of at least two vessels, either angioplasty or an aorto-SMA (superior mesenteric artery) graft is required. The mortality rate for this procedure is less than 10% and the majority of patients will be relieved of their postprandial intestinal angina. It is important to identify and to treat chronic mesenteric ischemia because of the high risk of thrombosis of the SMA.

24. SMALL BOWEL TUMORS

24.1 Benign Small Bowel Tumors

Both benign and malignant small bowel tumors are rare. Adenomas, leiomyomas and lipomas are the three most frequently discovered primary tumors of the small intestine. Hamartomas, fibromas, angiomas and neurogenic tumors are much less common. As a general rule, benign tumors are least common in the duodenum and increase in frequency toward the ileum. Benign tumors often remain asymptomatic and are usually found incidentally.

Symptomatic benign tumors present primarily with obstructive features, giving rise to intermittent colicky abdominal pain or complete bowel obstruction. Bleeding may occur, particularly from leiomyomas that ulcerate centrally. Intussusception occurs with polypoid distal lesions.

24.2 Malignant Neoplasms of the Small Intestine

Adenocarcinomas, lymphomas, leiomyosarcomas and carcinoids are the most common primary small bowel malignant tumors. Metastatic cancer to the small intestine occurs rarely in patients with melanoma, breast cancer and lung cancer. Primary adenocarcinomas occur in the duodenal and proximal jejunum as annular lesions, narrowing the lumen and presenting with the signs and symptoms of obstruction. Adenocarcinomas of the small bowel are more common in patients with Crohn's disease. Leiomyosarcomas are evenly distributed along the small bowel. Symptoms are similar to those of adenocarcinoma – i.e., crampy abdominal pain and bleeding. Lymphoma of the small bowel must be carefully evaluated to determine whether the tumor has originated in the small intestine (primary lymphoma) or whether the small bowel is involved by a diffuse systemic lymphoma. Lymphoma of the small bowel is more common in patients with celiac disease. Primary lymphoma of the small intestine is usually a histiocytic lymphoma. The lymphoma is most often proximal and presents with abdominal pain, weight loss, malabsorption, perforation and anemia. There is an increased incidence of primary lymphoma in patients with long-standing celiac disease or immunodeficiency states and in renal transplant patients receiving chronic immunosuppressive therapy.

A specific form of malignant lymphoma called immunoproliferative small intestinal disease occurs in people of Mediterranean descent. It is characterized by proliferation of mucosal B cells and has a high incidence of α-heavy chain paraproteinemia. It typically involves the duodenum and proximal jejunum, presenting with diarrhea and malabsorption.

SUGGESTED READING LIST

Thomson ABR, Wild G. Adaptation of intestinal nutrient transport in health and disease. Part I. Dig Dis Sci 1997; 453–469, 470–488.
———. Small bowel review. Can J Gastroenterol 1997; 515–531, 607–618.
Thomson ABR, Hasan J, Keelan M, Wild G. Small bowel review. Can J Gastroenterol 1998; 12:487–504.
———. Small bowel review. Can J Gastroenterol 1999; 13:37–54.

OBJECTIVES

1. Discuss the intestinal fluid and electrolyte transport mechanisms.

2. Explain the normal digestion and absorption processes of fat, protein and glucose.
3. Describe the normal pathway of vitamin B_{12}, folate and iron absorption.
4. Locate the absorption sites of Fe, folate and B_{12}.
5. Utilize a proper diagnostic approach to the patient with chronic diarrhea.
6. Discuss normal enterohepatic circulation of bile acids.
7. Discuss normal assimilation of fat-soluble vitamins (A, D, E and K).

Diarrhea

1. Define diarrhea.
2. Classify the causes of diarrhea.
3. Discuss the pathogenic mechanisms of diarrhea.
4. Review diarrhea as altered fluid and electrolyte transport.
5. Differentiate between large and small bowel diarrhea.
6. Discuss diagnostic plans in patients with chronic diarrhea.
7. List conditions that are associated with typical small bowel lesions on biopsy.
8. List the complications of celiac disease.
9. List extraintestinal manifestations of celiac disease.
10. Outline the diagnosis and dietary management of celiac disease.
11. Give the differential diagnosis of "unresponsive" sprue.
12. Discuss the immunologic basis of celiac disease.
13. Recognize the principal manifestation of the carcinoid syndrome.
14. Discuss pharmacologic agents used in the carcinoid syndrome.
15. List biochemical tests used in diagnosing the carcinoid syndrome.
16. Discuss the management of traveler's diarrhea.
17. List the common causes of traveler's diarrhea.
18. Discuss the mechanisms of E. coli–induced diarrhea.
19. List the infectious causes of diarrhea and their management.
20. Discuss the use and mechanisms of antidiarrheal agents.
21. Give the differential diagnosis of abnormal terminal ileum.
22. Describe the radiographic features of small bowel obstruction.
23. Outline the etiology of vitamin B_{12} deficiency with the bacterial overgrowth syndrome.
24. List the underlying conditions associated with bacterial overgrowth.
25. Discuss the mechanisms of steatorrhea associated with the bacterial overgrowth syndrome.
26. Recognize the clinical presentations of the bacterial overgrowth syndrome.
27. Outline the management of the bacterial overgrowth syndrome.
28. Utilize appropriate diagnostic tests for the bacterial overgrowth syndrome.

29. Recognize complications of the short bowel syndrome and their mechanisms.
30. Discuss the adaptive mechanisms of the small bowel following resection.
31. Discuss the management of the short bowel syndrome.
32. Give the indications for the use of medium-chain triglycerides.
33. Outline the diagnosis and treatment of giardiasis.
34. Recognize the clinical presentations and treatment of amebiasis.
35. Describe typical features of Whipple's disease.
36. List the causes of protein-losing enteropathy.
37. List the possible mechanisms of diarrhea in patients with diabetes mellitus.
38. List the possible mechanisms of diarrhea in the Zollinger-Ellison syndrome.
39. List mechanisms of diarrhea following gastric surgery.
40. Discuss diagnostic tests for lactase deficiency/lactose intolerance.
41. List conditions associated with protein-losing enteropathy.
42. Recognize the features of intestinal lymphangiectasia and outline its treatment.

Skills

1. Give the indications for gastroscopy, small bowel biopsy, sigmoidoscopy and colonoscopy.
2. Arrange the proper sequences of GI diagnostic procedures, including radiographic examination (ultrasound, CT scan), and the appropriate order of investigational tests.
3. Utilize proper tests – including malabsorption screen, ^{14}C breath test, H_2 breath test, Schilling test, 72-hour stool collection, x-ray, small bowel biopsy and jejunal aspiration – in the investigation of chronic diarrhea.

8
Ischemic Disease of the Intestine
P.H. Macdonald, D.J. Hurlbut, D. Tomalty
and I.T. Beck

1. INTRODUCTION

Intestinal ischemia occurs when, as a result of inadequate systemic blood flow or local vascular abnormalities, the metabolic demand of the tissue supersedes the delivery of oxygen. In older patients inadequate vascular supply is frequent, and thus ischemic bowel disease occurs most often in the elderly. It may also be seen in young patients suffering from vascular abnormalities – e.g., collagen diseases, vasculitis, diabetes – or in those taking vasoconstrictor drugs. Clinical manifestations are varied, depending on the site of the vascular occlusion and the extent of the bowel necrosis.

2. CLASSIFICATION OF INTESTINAL ISCHEMIA

Many clinicians broadly classify intestinal ischemia into acute or chronic disease. However, because certain acute events may change to a chronic condition, a clear-cut classification of ischemic bowel disease using this two-category system is not always applicable. Since the extent of intestinal ischemia and the pathological consequences depend on the size and the location of the occluded or hypoperfused intestinal blood vessel(s), we find it useful to classify ischemic bowel disease according to the size and type of the vessel(s) that are hypoperfused or occluded (Figure 1). Accordingly, intestinal ischemia may result from occlusion/hypoperfusion of a large mesenteric vessel (mesenteric artery or vein) or from occlusion/hypoperfusion of smaller intramural intestinal vessels. In each of these situations the resultant intestinal ischemia may be acute or chronic. In addition, it is important to point out that vessel occlusion/hypoperfusion may be the result of a mechanical intralumi-

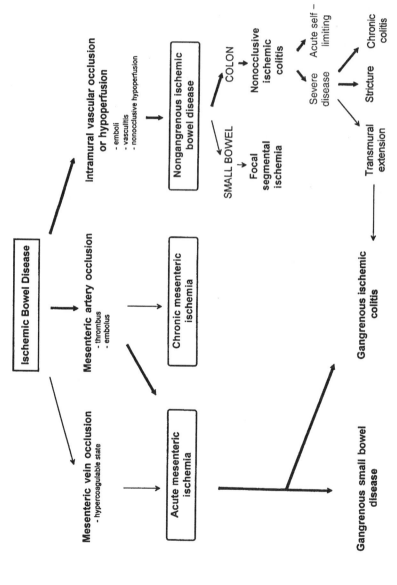

FIGURE 1.   Classification of ischemic bowel disease. The more common pathways are indicated by heavier arrows.

nal obstruction (i.e., embolus or thrombus) or the result of decreased blood flow due to vasospasm, increased blood viscosity, hypotension or other similar conditions. The latter is referred to as *nonocclusive ischemia*. Therefore, the etiology of vessel occlusion/hypoperfusion may be the basis for subclassification of ischemic bowel disease. A clinically important further classification is whether the ischemia-induced necrosis is transmural (*gangrenous ischemia*) leading to peritonitis, or remains intramural (*nongangrenous ischemia*) resulting in localized disease. Figure 1 attempts to combine these different aspects of subdivision in a comprehensive classification.

3. MESENTERIC VASCULATURE

3.1 Anatomy

The blood flow to the splanchnic organs is derived from three main arterial trunks: the celiac, the superior mesenteric and the inferior mesenteric arteries (Figures 2–5). The celiac artery supplies blood to the foregut (stomach and duodenum), the superior mesenteric artery supplies blood to the midgut (duodenum to transverse colon), and the inferior mesenteric artery is responsible for blood to the hindgut (transverse colon to the rectum). Each of these three arterial trunks supplies blood flow to its specific section of the gastrointestinal tract through a vast arcade network. This arcade system is an effective collateral circulation and is generally protective against ischemia, since blood can reach a specific segment of gut via more than one route. As shown in Figure 2, additional vascular protection is obtained from vascular connections between the three arterial systems. Communication between the celiac system and the superior mesenteric system generally occurs via the superior pancreaticoduodenal and inferior pancreaticoduodenal arteries. The superior mesenteric and inferior mesenteric systems are joined by the arch of Riolan and the marginal artery of Drummond, vessels that connect the middle colic artery (a branch of the superior mesenteric artery) and the left colic artery (a branch of the inferior mesenteric artery). In addition, communication also exists between the inferior mesenteric artery and branches of the internal iliac arteries via the rectum. The caliber of these collateral connections varies considerably depending on the existence of vascular disease, but it is important to realize that in chronic states of vascular insufficiency, blood flow to an individual system can be maintained through these collateral connections even when an arterial trunk is completely obstructed. It is not uncommon to find one or even two arterial trunks completely occluded in the asymptomatic patient with chronic vascular disease. In fact, there are reports of occlusion of all three trunks in patients who are still maintaining their splanchnic circulation. However, in up to 30% of people, the collateral connections between the superior

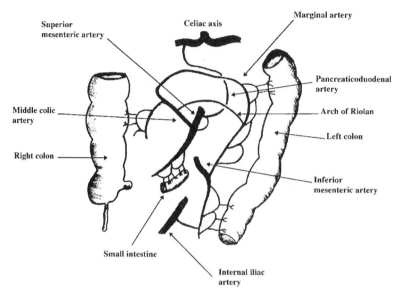

FIGURE 2.   Schematic representation of splanchnic circulation.

and inferior mesenteric arteries, via the arch of Riolan and the marginal artery of Drummond, can be weak or nonexistent, making the area of the splenic flexure particularly vulnerable to acute ischemia. This region of poor collateral circulation is often referred to as a "watershed area."

3.2 Physiology of Splanchnic Blood Flow

The mesenteric circulation receives approximately 30% of the cardiac output. Mesenteric blood flow is less in the fasting state and is increased with feeding. Blood flow through the celiac and superior mesenteric trunks is about equal (approximately 700 mL/min in the adult) and is twice the blood flow through the inferior mesenteric trunk. Blood flow distribution within the gut wall is not uniform, and it varies between the mucosa and the muscularis. The mucosa has the highest metabolic rate and thus it receives about 70% of the mesenteric blood flow. If one compares gut segments of equal weight, the small bowel receives the most blood, followed by the colon and then the stomach.

Much has been written on the control of gastrointestinal blood flow, and many factors are involved in its regulation. A few important highlights of mesenteric vascular resistance will be discussed here. Vascular resistance is proportional to $1/r^4$ (where r = the radius of the vessel). Thus the smaller the

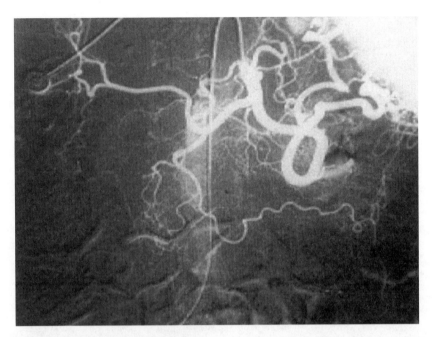

FIGURE 3. Angiogram of the celiac arterial system.

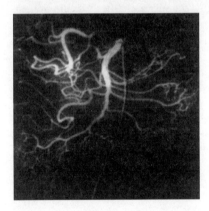

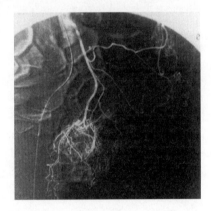

FIGURE 4. Angiogram of the superior mesenteric arterial system.

FIGURE 5. Angiogram of the inferior mesenteric arterial system.

artery, the greater its ability to effect vascular resistance. It is known that the majority of blood flow control occurs at the level of the arterioles, the so-called resistance vessels. Very little control of blood flow occurs at the level of the large arterial trunks. In fact, the diameter of these large arterial trunks can be compromised by 75% before blood flow is reduced. Additional control of blood flow occurs at the level of the precapillary sphincter. In the fasting state only one-fifth of capillary beds are open, leaving a tremendous reserve to meet increased metabolic demands.

Among the most important control mechanisms of splanchnic blood flow are the sympathetic nervous system, humoral factors and local factors. The sympathetic nervous system through α-adrenergic receptors plays an important role in maintaining the basal vascular tone and in mediating vasoconstriction. Beta-adrenergic activity appears to mediate vasodilation, and it appears that the antrum of the stomach may be particularly rich in these β receptors. Humoral factors involved in the regulation of GI blood flow include catecholamines, the renin-angiotensin system and vasopressin. These humoral systems may play a particularly important role in shock states and in some patients may play a role in the pathogenesis of nonocclusive ischemia. Local factors appear to be mainly involved in the matching of tissue blood flow to the metabolic demand. An increased metabolic rate may produce a decreased pO_2, increased pCO_2 and an increased level of adenosine, each of which can mediate a hyperemic response.

The vascular endothelium is a source of potent vasoactive substances, such as nitric oxide (vasodilator) and endothelin (vasoconstrictor). Although these endothelial-derived substances may act systemically, it would appear that their major effect is local in a paracrine hormonal fashion. These vasoactive substances have the potential to dramatically alter mesenteric blood flow. In fact, endothelin is one of the most potent vasoconstrictors identified to date. Regulation of mesenteric blood flow in both health and disease by these potent endothelial-derived vasoactive substances remains to be elucidated.

The integration of these control systems and their alteration by factors such as vascular disease, motor activity, intraluminal pressure and pharmaceuticals remains poorly understood. The key to our understanding and successful treatment of intestinal ischemia lies in a better knowledge of this physiology.

3.3 Pathophysiology of Intestinal Ischemia

Intestinal ischemia occurs when the metabolic demand of the tissue supersedes the oxygen delivery. Obviously, many factors can be involved in this mismatch of oxygen delivery and demand. These include the general hemodynamic state, degree of atherosclerosis, extent of collateral circulation, neurogenic/humoral/local control mechanisms of vascular resistance and abnormal products of cellular metabolism before and after reperfusion of an ischemic segment. Acute occlusion/hypoperfusion of a large mesenteric vessel usually results in transmural (gangrenous) ischemia. On the other hand, acute occlusion of the intramural vessel(s) usually results in intramural (nongangrenous) ischemia. However, there are exceptions in both cases, depending on the severity of occlusion/hypoperfusion. As previously mentioned, the mucosa is the most metabolically active gut wall tissue layer and thus it is the first tissue layer to demonstrate signs of ischemia. The earliest form of intestinal ischemia produces changes at the tip of the intestinal villi. With ongoing ischemia ultrastructural changes begin within 10 minutes and cellular damage is extensive by 30 minutes. Sloughing of the villi tips is followed by edema, submucosal hemorrhage and eventual transmural necrosis.

The intestinal response to ischemia is first characterized by a hypermotility state. It is this intense motor activity that results in the patient experiencing severe pain, even though the ischemic damage may be limited to the mucosa at this stage. As the ischemia progresses, motor activity will cease and gut mucosal permeability will increase, leading to an increase in bacterial translocation. With transmural extension of the ischemia, the patient will develop visceral and parietal inflammation resulting in peritonitis.

An important factor often responsible for, or aggravating, intestinal ischemia is the phenomenon of vasospasm. It has been well demonstrated that both occlusive and nonocclusive forms of arterial ischemia can result in prolonged vasospasm, even after the occlusion has been removed or the perfusion pressure restored. This vasospasm may persist for several hours, resulting in prolonged ischemia. The mechanism responsible for this vasospasm is not clearly defined, but there is preliminary evidence that the potent vasoconstrictor endothelin may be involved. To date, many of the interventional techniques used in the treatment of acute mesenteric ischemia have been directed at counteracting this vasospasm.

A second factor that may be responsible for accentuating ischemic damage is reperfusion injury. This phenomenon has been well demonstrated in the laboratory, where it has been shown to be responsible for a greater degree of cellular damage than that brought about during the actual ischemic period. Parks and Granger have shown in an animal model that the injury after one hour of ischemia and three hours of reperfusion is more severe than that observed after four hours of continuous ischemia. The mechanism responsible for this reperfusion injury appears to be related to the release of harmful reactive oxygen metabolites, which are thought to be released from adhering polymorphonuclear leukocytes. It is not known what role ischemia reperfusion injury plays in humans with occlusive and nonocclusive disease.

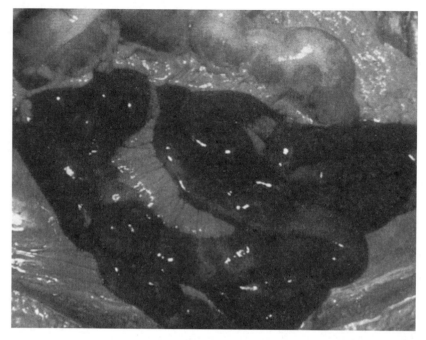

FIGURE 6. Postmortem examination of the abdominal cavity shows extensive small bowel infarction. The intestinal ischemic necrosis was secondary to proximal occlusion of the superior mesenteric artery by thrombus.

4. ACUTE MESENTERIC ARTERIAL OCCLUSION

4.1 Clinical Presentation

Several intra-abdominal disease processes can present in a fashion identical to that of mesenteric ischemia; thus, the key to diagnosis lies in a high index of suspicion. Patients with advanced ischemia present with diffuse peritonitis, shock and severe metabolic derangements. In these patients it is clear that a catastrophic event has occurred. However, ischemia is only one of a few possible diagnoses. In most situations these patients will come to surgery, and in those where the diagnosis was not confirmed preoperatively, the diagnosis will become obvious at the time of surgery. Often these patients can not be salvaged; the mortality is reported to be between 70 and 90% (Figure 6). It must be stressed that the patient with early ischemia is far more challenging to diagnose. Given that the mortality rate is extremely high in advanced ischemia, the best chance of successfully treating a patient with this condition depends on early diagnosis and treatment.

The typical patient is usually over 50 years of age and often has a history of cardiac and peripheral vascular disease. In the early stage of ischemia the patient complains of severe abdominal pain (due to hypermotility and spasmodic contraction of the ischemic gut) in the absence of peritoneal findings. This scenario has been described by clinicians as "pain out of proportion to the physical findings." Other nonspecific symptoms such as nausea, vomiting and altered bowel habit may be present, but they are usually not particularly helpful in the diagnosis.

4.2 Investigation

4.2.1 LABORATORY

Unfortunately, there is no serum marker that can reliably predict early intestinal ischemia. Many studies have attempted to identify such a biochemical marker. Creatinine kinase, alkaline phosphatase, lactate dehydrogenase, diamine oxidase and inorganic phosphate are among those biochemical markers that have been examined. Although all of these will eventually become altered with advanced disease, their alteration with early ischemia is too varied to provide any clinical usefulness.

Although biochemical changes with advanced intestinal ischemia are nonspecific, one can expect to find a leukocytosis. Due to third-space loss of fluid into the abdomen, electrolyte and renal function abnormalities secondary to dehydration are also often seen. Hyperamylasemia may occur secondary to amylase leaking from the infarcted bowel into the abdominal cavity, which may then enter the systemic circulation. In some situations this hyperamylasemia in the setting of abdominal pain may be misinterpreted as an indication of pancreatitis. Finally, in advanced ischemia blood gas analysis will usually show a metabolic acidosis.

4.2.2 RADIOLOGICAL

Initial radiological investigations are aimed at ruling out other causes of abdominal pain and peritonitis. All patients should have an upright and supine plain film of the abdomen. Although these films may support a diagnosis of ischemia, as indicated by bowel wall thickening and "thumb-printing," the main purpose of the films is to rule out visceral perforation or bowel obstruction. In many centers CT scan is being used as a first-line investigation in patients with abdominal pain. Several markers of intestinal ischemia have now been described by radiologists with expertise in CT scans. These include

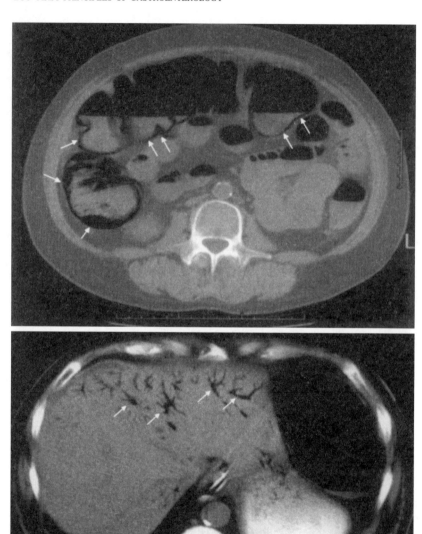

FIGURE 7 (A and B).   CT scan of a patient with mesenteric ischemia secondary to acute occlusion of the ileocolic artery. Arrows point to air in the wall of the ischemic right colon (pneumatosis) (Figure 7A) and secondary accumulation of air in the portal vein system (Figure 7B).

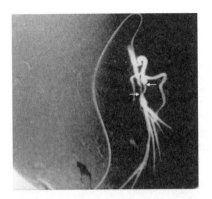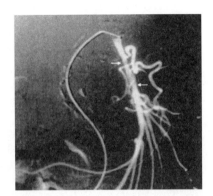

FIGURE 8 (A and B). Mesenteric angiogram demonstrating atherosclerotic narrowing of the superior mesenteric artery (arrows in Figure 8A). Following angioplasty, the diameter of the narrowed area is significantly increased (Figure 8B).

bowel wall thickening, mucosal edema, pneumatosis (Figure 7A) and mesenteric and portal vein gas (Figure 7B). Using large injections of peripheral venous contrast, mesenteric arterial and venous occlusion can now also be identified in some patients. Of course, many of these findings are not specific, and thus we do not at present advocate the CT scan as a diagnostic test for intestinal ischemia. However, the CT scan can play a critical role in ruling out other intra-abdominal disease processes, such as pancreatitis.

Ultrasonography combined with Doppler assessment of blood flow in the splanchnic arterial and venous system is now being used in some centers to screen for mesenteric ischemia. Our personal experience with this technique is limited and the exact role this technique will play is not clearly defined. There is experimental evidence, using a rabbit model of ischemia, that magnetic resonance (MR) scanning may also be of significant use in the diagnosis of mesenteric ischemia. Certainly, both arterial and venous abnormalities as well as the extent of the collateral circulation can be identified in some patients using MR technology; however, further clinical experience is required before this technique can be completely evaluated.

Angiography remains the gold standard in the diagnosis of mesenteric ischemia (Figure 8), and, as will be discussed, it may play a significant role in the treatment of such patients. It is our belief that all patients with suspected mesenteric intestinal ischemia should undergo angiography to confirm the diagnosis and plan treatment. Wherever possible this approach should include even those patients presenting with peritonitis. Often there is a tendency to take patients with peritonitis straight to the operating room without performing angiography. These patients need to be treated in an expedient fashion. However, the short delay to obtain an angiogram may prove to be beneficial. Not only will it identify those patients who may require embolectomy or vascular reconstruction, but it will also provide a means to treat vasospasm in the perioperative period. This type of treatment policy has two implications: First, in order for management to be effective, an invasive radiologist must be available at all times and a system must be in place that will allow the angiography suite to be functioning with a short lead time. Second, the physician must realize that an appreciable number of negative angiograms should be expected with this low angiography threshold.

4.3 Treatment

4.3.1 *RESUSCITATION AND ASSESSMENT*
It must be strongly stressed that if a diagnosis of mesenteric ischemia is being questioned, the subsequent investigation and management must proceed in an efficient and aggressive fashion if morbidity and mortality are to be reduced. Initial management of all patients consists of resuscitation. The degree of resuscitation required varies widely with the degree and extent of ischemia. Patients with early ischemia will require very little resuscitation, whereas those with infarcted intestine may require admission to a critical care unit for invasive monitoring. Insertion of a Swan-Ganz catheter with central pressure monitoring can be very useful in resuscitating the shocked patient with underlying cardiac disease. It must be kept in mind that in patients with extensive and advanced infarction, complete "stability" may never be obtained and thus investigation and treatment should proceed without extensive delay. However, ongoing patient "instability" is no doubt an ominous sign. As a general rule vasopressors to support blood pressure should be avoided, as they may further increase the degree of intestinal ischemia. The role of antibiotics is not clear-cut. Our policy is to administer broad-spectrum antibiotic coverage as soon as possible to those patients presenting with peritonitis. In those without peritonitis, antibiotics are used in the perioperative period, should surgery be required.

The treatment algorithm we recommend is outlined in Figure 9. Essentially, patients are divided into two groups: those with peritonitis and those without. Although all patients with peritonitis will require laparotomy, the exact treatment plan for both groups of patients will be dictated by the angiographic findings. Angiographic findings fall into four major categories:

Thrombotic occlusion. This finding is usually identified with an aortic flush of contrast dye; however, it can sometimes be difficult to differentiate from a proximal arterial embolus. The other pitfall with this finding is that sometimes

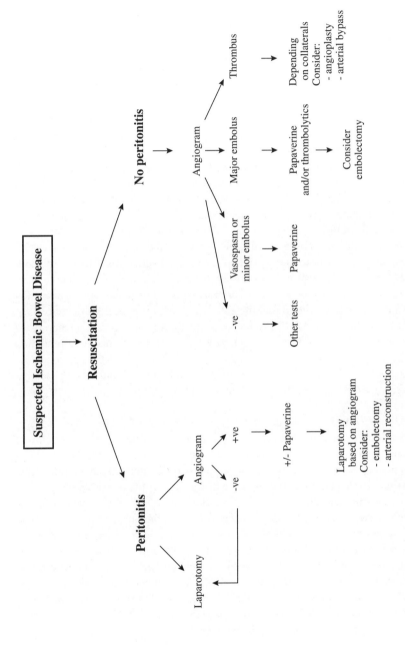

FIGURE 9. Algorithm for the treatment of acute mesenteric ischemia.

it represents a chronic obstruction that is not necessarily related to the patient's present symptoms and findings. In most cases, these patients require arterial reconstruction, although the final treatment plan will be based on the exact vascular anatomy and degree of collateral circulation. Patients with peritonitis will almost always require a bowel resection.

Major embolus. Major emboli are usually located in the proximal portion of the superior mesenteric artery. The majority of these patients should be referred to surgery for consideration of embolectomy regardless of the presence or lack of peritoneal findings. In those patients requiring surgery, intra-arterial papaverine infusion could be used in the perioperative period in an attempt to reduce ongoing vasospasm. Recently, thrombolytic therapy (streptokinase and urokinase) has been used in a selected group of patients with intestinal ischemia secondary to a mesenteric embolus. Data, however, are limited since the literature contains only a handful of case reports describing this technique. Accordingly, the therapeutic efficacy and the potential complications of thrombolytic therapy are unknown at this time.

Minor embolus. These emboli are limited to the branches of the superior mesenteric artery or to that portion of the vessel distal to the origin of the ileocolic artery. Unless peritoneal signs are present, these patients should be managed conservatively or with intra-arterial infusion of papaverine. There may also be a role for intra-arterial thrombolytic therapy in selected patients.

Vasospasm (nonocclusive ischemia). This finding may occur in response to a mechanical arterial obstruction; however, when it represents the sole finding it is diagnostic of nonocclusive ischemia. The recommended management is essentially the same as for patients with minor emboli with the exception that there would be no role for thrombolytics in this group.

4.3.2 *MEDICAL TREATMENT: INTRA-ARTERIAL INFUSION THERAPY*

Intra-arterial infusion therapy has been used in the management of selected patients with intestinal ischemia. Two classes of pharmaceuticals have been employed: smooth-muscle relaxants (papaverine) and thrombolytic agents (streptokinase and urokinase). Although we support the use of these agents, it must be stressed that their efficacy has not been absolutely proven in proper clinical trials. In order to administer intra-arterial therapy, a radiologist skilled in mesenteric angiography must selectively guide a catheter through the femoral artery into the trunk or a branch of the affected mesenteric artery. Once the catheter is properly placed and secured, the chosen pharmaceutical can then be administered. This procedure is not without risk. Complications include injury to the femoral artery, dislodgement of atherosclerotic plaques with embolic accidents in the lower extremities, and the formation of a false femoral artery aneurysm after the catheter is removed.

Papaverine infusion has been recommended as a major component of the medical therapy for mesenteric ischemia. Papaverine is a smooth-muscle relaxant and therefore it is usually used to reduce arterial vasopasm. Vasopasm can occur primarily, as seen in nonocclusive intestinal ischemia, or it may be a secondary event following acute arterial obstruction from an embolus or thrombus. Administered systemically, papaverine will nonspecifically dilate the vascular tree. However, since it is virtually completely metabolized by a single pass through the liver, selective administration into the mesenteric circulation results in very few systemic effects. This allows vasodilation in the mesenteric circulation to occur without a drop in the systemic blood pressure. Papaverine is dissolved in normal saline to a concentration of 1mg/mL, although a higher concentration can be used. Heparin should not be added to the solution, as it will crystallize. The infusion is started at 30 mg/hour and may be increased to 60 mg/hour. In most cases the papaverine infusion is maintained for 24 hours. The catheter is then flushed with normal saline for 30 minutes and the angiogram is then repeated. If vasospasm persists, the cycle should be repeated every 24 hours for a maximum of 5 days. During the papaverine infusion the patient's systemic vital signs must be monitored. A sudden drop in the blood pressure usually suggests that the catheter has slipped out of the mesenteric circulation into the aorta. The papaverine infusion should be stopped until a repeat angiogram is performed to confirm this.

It is generally believed that patients with acute mesenteric ischemia caused by a superior mesenteric artery thromboembolism should undergo surgery with possible embolectomy. However, since many of these patients are elderly and frail, thrombolytic therapy has been used in selected patients as a possible alternative to surgery. To date several case reports have indicated favorable results with either streptokinase or urokinase. Additional experience with these agents is required in order to define their exact role in the management of intestinal ischemia.

4.3.3 SURGICAL TREATMENT

The role of surgery is to evaluate the viability of ischemic bowel, to resect if necessary and if possible to alleviate or bypass a vascular obstruction. If at all possible the vascular surgery should be performed first so that its effect on intestinal viability can be assessed.

One of the most difficult decisions the surgeon has to make is to decide if the bowel injury is reversible or not. Subjective criteria such as the bowel wall color, the presence of peristalsis and the presence of palpable mesenteric pulses are often used. Unfortunately, these criteria can lead to an inaccurate assessment in over 50% of cases. This has led surgeons to adopt a second-look approach. With this approach only the most obviously infarcted gut is resected and any questionable bowel is left in situ. A second look within 24 hours is then used to decide on the necessity for further resection. Several objective measurements have been employed intra-operatively in an attempt to assess bowel viability. These include fluorescence staining, laser Doppler flowmetry, surface oximetry and intramural pH measurements. However, at present, no single technology has been widely adopted.

A second difficult situation for the surgeon is the management of patients with near-total intestinal infarction. Even with resection, the mortality rate in this group of patients is very high, and survivors will be dependent on total parental nutrition indefinitely. In elderly patients with other underlying medical problems, many surgeons would not consider a bowel resection and would treat the patient palliatively. The approach in a younger patient with a catastrophic vascular accident tends to be more aggressive, as advances in bowel transplantation surgery have created some hope for these unfortunate individuals.

5. ACUTE MESENTERIC VENOUS OCCLUSION

Ischemia of mesenteric arterial origin is far more frequent than that of venous disease. It is now recognized that many reported cases of mesenteric vein thrombosis in actuality represented incorrectly diagnosed cases of nonocclusive ischemia. The true incidence of mesenteric vein thrombosis is quite low. Although the etiology of acute mesenteric vein thrombosis may be idiopathic, the thrombosis is usually secondary to another disease process. Conditions that predispose to mesenteric vein thrombosis are (1) severe intra-abdominal sepsis, (2) hypercoagulable state (i.e., polycythemia vera) and (3) portal venous stasis (secondary to portal hypertension associated with hepatic cirrhosis, or to extrinsic compression of the venous system secondary to a tumor mass).

Thrombosis of the superior or inferior mesenteric vein alone is usually not sufficient to produce intestinal ischemia. However, acute thrombosis in a large mesenteric vein has the potential to cause retrograde propagation of the clot up into the venous tributaries within the bowel wall. This resultant venous occlusion within the bowel wall will usually produce ischemia, possibly with infarction. In many cases of venous intestinal ischemia the thrombosis does not begin in a large mesenteric vein. In these situations it appears that the venous thrombosis begins primarily in the small venous intramural tributaries. In either case, if the venous thrombosis becomes extensive, arterial thrombosis may follow, making it very difficult to determine the exact etiology of the intestinal ischemia.

The clinical presentation of patients with venous intestinal ischemia is often similar if not identical to that of patients with acute mesenteric artery occlusion. Accordingly, the diagnosis is often made only at the time of surgery or by the pathologist who examines the resected specimen.

The treatment of this disease is generally surgical, with the infarcted segment of intestine being resected. The surgeon should be aware that the venous thrombosis may extend beyond the limits of the gross infarction. Since any residual thrombosis has the potential to propagate, the resection should include adjacent bowel and mesentery until all grossly involved thrombosed veins are removed. It has been shown that mortality from this disease can be reduced if patients are anticoagulated as soon as possible after surgery.

6. CHRONIC MESENTERIC ISCHEMIA

Because of the extensive collateral arterial network of the gut, chronic mesenteric ischemia is relatively uncommon. It is usually related to extensive mesenteric atherosclerosis. Patients classically present with postprandial abdominal pain, "fear of eating" and weight loss. However, most patients do not present with "classic" symptomatology and are frequently misdiagnosed for other diseases. Until someone with a high index of suspicion proceeds to angiography, these patients may be treated for prolonged periods for suspected peptic ulcer, functional dyspepsia, irritable bowel syndrome, etc. Unfortunately, angiographic evidence of thrombosis of large vessels is not always diagnostic, as two or even three of the major arteries may be thrombosed in apparently asymptomatic patients. Once the diagnosis is clearly established, the treatment is surgical. Many surgical procedures have been described with various results. Endarterectomy and aortovisceral bypass have been employed. More recently balloon angioplasty has appeared to provide good results with a less invasive approach (Figures 8A and 8B).

7. NONGANGRENOUS ISCHEMIC BOWEL DISEASE

7.1 Etiology
In contrast to mesenteric ischemia, where the cause of the disease is occlusion of major vessels, in nongangrenous ischemic bowel disease the hypooxygenation is caused by hypoperfusion of the gut wall microcirculation. Only occasionally is there secondary occlusion of intramural vessels. Many causes may precipitate this disorder. Hypoperfusion is most commonly caused by vascular diseases – e.g., collagen disease, vasculitis, diabetes, atherosclerosis – or by increased viscosity of the blood in sickle cell disease or polycythemia vera. Acute hypotension due to hemorrhage, myocardial infarct, congestive heart failure, sepsis or vasoconstricting drugs may

TABLE 1.   Causes of nonocclusive ischemic bowel disease

A. Acute diminution of intramural blood flow

1. Small vessel disease
Cholesterol embolus (Figure 10A)
Diabetes
Rheumatoid arthritis
Chronic radiation injury (Figure 10B)
Amyloidosis (Figures 10C and 10D)
Systemic vasculitis
Collagen diseases
Allergic granulomatosis
Behçet's syndrome

2. Nonocclusive hypoperfusion
Hypercoagulable states and increased viscosity
   Oral contraceptives
   Polycythemia vera
   Sickle cell disease
   Acute leukemia
   Antithrombin C disease
Shock
   Hemorrhage
   Hypovolemia
   Cardiopulmonary bypass
   Abdominal aortic reconstruction
   Sepsis
   Pancreatitis
   Anaphylaxis
   Cardiogenic shock
   Multiple organ dysfunction syndrome
Congestive heart failure
Portal hypertension
Medications
   Digitalis
   Diuretics
   Catecholamines
   Estrogens
   Nonsteroidal anti-inflammatory agents
   Neuroleptic agents
   Verapamil overdose
   Cocaine abuse
Long-distance running

(cont'd)

TABLE 1.   Causes of nonocclusive ischemic bowel disease (cont'd)

B. Conditions compounding marginal blood flow states

1. Increased metabolic demand secondary to increased motility
Mass lesions
  Carcinoma
  Diverticular disease
Obstruction

2. Compromised blood flow due to increased intraluminal pressure
Obstruction
Fecal impaction
Colonoscopy
Barium enema

C. Idiopathic (spontaneous)

---

precipitate local ischemia in patients who already have impaired local circulation. Because of an adequate collateral circulation, localization is usually segmental. The necrosis of the gut wall is rarely transmural, and as a result, peritonitis is a rare complication. In the small bowel nongangrenous ischemic bowel disease manifests as "focal segmental ischemia" and in the colon as "nongangrenous ischemic colitis." A list of the more common causes of nonocclusive ischemic bowel disease is provided in Table 1, and the histologic appearance of some of these is shown in Figures 10A–10D.

7.2 Focal Segmental Ischemia of the Small Intestine
Ischemia to short segments of the small bowel results in a variable clinical course that depends on the severity of the infarct. For short segment involvement there is usually appropriate collateral circulation, and thus the disease involves only the mucosa and submucosal tissues. Limited necrosis may heal completely. Ongoing repeated injury may cause chronic enteritis, almost indistinguishable from Crohn's disease. In some patients the necrotic ulcer may lead to late stricture formation (Figure 11). Occasionally the process may become transmural, resulting in peritonitis. Diagnosis is difficult, as the symptoms may be those of chronic recurrent abdominal pain, bowel obstruction or frank peritonitis. Unless there is complete spontaneous resolution, the treatment of strictures and persistent ulcers is usually surgical. The diagnosis is often made only on histology of the resected small bowel.

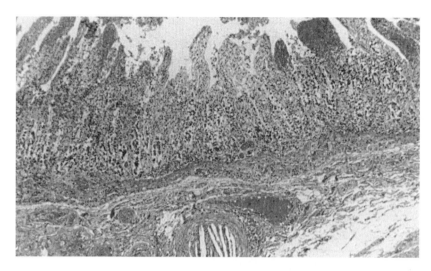

FIGURE 10 (A–D).   Histopathologic examples of small vessel disease producing nonocclusive ischemic bowel disease (see Table 1).

FIGURE 10A.   Cholesterol embolus. A superficial submucosal artery within the small bowel is completely occluded with atheroemboli containing cholesterol clefts. This has caused ischemic necrosis of villus tips of the overlying intestinal mucosa. (H&E stain)

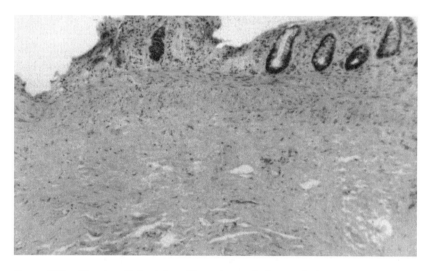

FIGURE 10B.   Chronic radiation injury. Photomicrograph shows colonic mucosal atrophy and marked submucosal fibrosis. The patient had developed a colonic stricture due to the mucosal and submucosal scarring resulting from radiation-induced ischemia. (HPS stain)

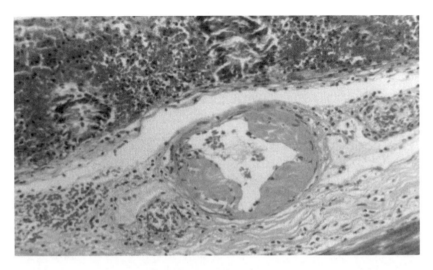

FIGURE 10C. Amyloidosis. Hemorrhagic ischemic necrosis of colonic mucosa associated with mural amyloid deposits within submucosal vessel. (HPS stain)

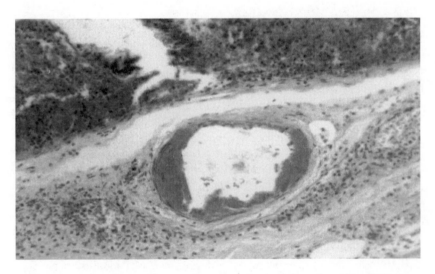

FIGURE 10D. Amyloidosis. Deeper leveled section of colonic tissue from Figure 10C shows positive Congo red staining of amyloid deposits within vessel wall. (Congo red stain)

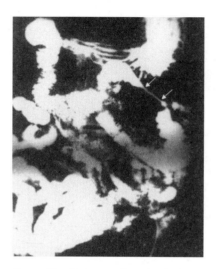

FIGURE 11.   Barium swallow showing a late
ischemic stricture in the proximal small bowel.

7.3 Nongangrenous Ischemic Colitis

7.3.1 *PATHOGENESIS*
There are two major forms of colonic ischemia: gangrenous (transmural) and nongangrenous colitis (disease contained within the colonic wall). These are in fact two different diseases, with different etiologies and clinical courses, and require different approaches to their management. Gangrenous ischemic colitis is caused by obstruction of the major mesenteric vessels and is discussed in Section 4 (see Figure 1). Occasionally, transmural gangrene may develop when nongangrenous ischemic colitis slowly progresses to transmural necrosis. The recognition and management of this complication of the originally nongangrenous disease is crucial, and as discussed below, depends on careful ongoing observation of the patient with nongangrenous ischemic colitis.

In contrast to the rarity of nonocclusive ischemia of the small bowel is the frequency of local vascular hypoperfusion of the colon. The cause of this relative frequency may be related to the following factors: In comparison to the small intestine, the colon receives less blood, has fewer vascular collaterals, has susceptible "watershed areas" and possesses an ongoing forceful motor activity. Elevated intramural pressure during increased motility in patients with constipation, diverticular disease and cancer of the colon may lead to diminished gut wall blood flow. Similarly, distention with air during colonoscopy or barium enema may temporarily reduce blood flow to the colon. The large bowel also has a different neuroendocrine control. Evidence in our laboratory has indicated that the vessels of the canine colon respond more vigorously to hypotension than those of the small intestine and that contrary to the latter, in the colon the major local vasoconstrictory substance is angiotensin.

7.3.2 CLINICAL PRESENTATION

The classic clinical presentation is characterized by a sudden onset of severe crampy abdominal pain, diarrhea mixed with bright red blood, and occasionally melena. Physical examination may reveal a distended abdomen. Bowel sounds are present and there are no signs of peritoneal involvement. The patient is usually elderly and may show signs of one of the associated diseases such as hypotension, congestive heart failure and atherosclerosis. Under specific conditions, nongangrenous ischemic colitis can also occur in the young. This is often due to iatrogenic or patient-induced causes such as contraceptive medication, nonsteroidal anti-inflammatory agents, cocaine abuse, verapamil overdose, etc. (for details see Table 1). In the elderly, the specific event that precipitated the attack occasionally cannot be determined. The early clinical presentation may be so similar to that of infectious colitis, ulcerative colitis, Crohn's colitis and pseudomembranous colitis that the diagnosis can be established only by exclusion of infection, including Clostridium difficile, and by demonstrating the classic radiographic (Figures 12 and 13) and/or colonoscopic (Figure 14) findings of ischemic colitis. Because large vessels are never involved, angiography has no place in the diagnosis of nongangrenous ischemic colitis.

Radiographic and colonoscopic investigations have to be carried out within 24–48 hours of the onset of the disease, as the typical findings tend to disappear and are rapidly replaced by nonspecific signs, and the picture may imitate other conditions such as Crohn's disease (Figure 15). The first radiologic examination should be an abdominal survey film (Figure 12), which may demonstrate the classic intramural hemorrhage-induced thumb-printing in an air-filled segment of the colon. This finding, however, may not always be diagnostic, because occasionally it can be mimicked by mucosal and submucosal edema caused by severe inflammatory processes. Colonic involvement is usually segmental in ischemic colitis. Although any part of the colon may be affected, the "watershed" areas of the splenic flexure and of the rectosigmoid junction are most commonly involved. Thumb-printing can be demonstrated by barium enema (Figure 13), but differentiation between edema and submucosal hemorrhage can be done only by colonoscopy, where hemorrhage can be recognized as large dark red submucosal blebs (Figure 14). Because distention of the colon with air may compress intramural blood

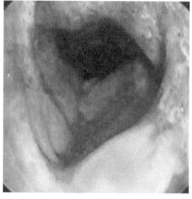

FIGURE 14. Colonoscopic view of a recent-onset ischemic colitis of the splenic flexure. Note the normal mucosa on the left and the dark hemorrhagic mucosal indentation at the right, top and bottom of the image. These blood-filled submucosal blebs in the absence of mucosal damage are diagnostic of the initial stage of ischemic colitis.

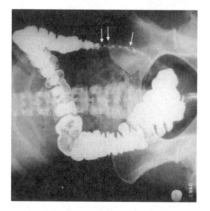

FIGURE 13. Single contrast barium enema. To avoid increased intraluminal pressure the examination was carried out without prepa-ration and no air was insufflated. The multi-ple adjacent areas of indentations provide the appearance of thumb-printing (arrows).

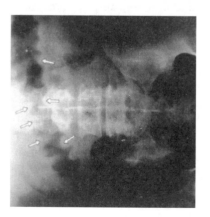

FIGURE 12. Abdominal survey film demonstrating ischemic colitis. This film was taken five hours after the onset of acute hematochezia and severe abdominal pain. Arrows point to areas of submucosal hemor-rhage in the air-filled transverse colon. This appearance is often referred to as "thumb-printing."

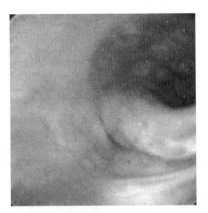

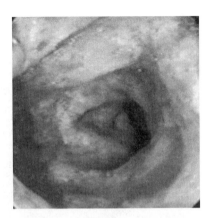

FIGURE 15. Colonoscopic view of ischemic colitis imitating Crohn's disease. Note
the nodularity, erythema and petechiae of
the mucosa.

FIGURE 16. Colonoscopic view of ischemic colitis imitating pseudomembranous
colitis. Note the generalized erythema and
whitish plaques (pseudomembranes).

vessels and thus further decrease blood flow, barium enema is rarely used, unless plain films of the abdomen can not provide a diagnosis and colonoscopy is not available. Colonoscopy must be carried out carefully with minimal air insufflation. After 24–48 hours, the hemorrhage resolves and the mucosa becomes necrotic. If colonoscopy is done at this stage, the endoscopist may be unable to differentiate the necrosis and ulcerations resulting from ischemic colitis from those caused by Crohn's disease (Figure 15) or pseudomembranous enterocolitis (Figure 16). The pathologist reviewing biopsies taken a few days after the onset of the disease may have similar difficulties (Figure 17). Not infrequently, only time will tell whether the patient has inflammatory bowel disease (IBD) or ischemia. It is not impossible that some elderly patients with what is thought to be late-onset IBD or young women on contraceptive medication who are thought to have Crohn's are actually suffering from ischemic colitis.

The disease can progress in four different ways (Figure 1). Mild disease may resolve spontaneously. In patients with involvement of only small segments, the symptoms and physical findings subside within 24–48 hours and complete resolution can occur within two to three weeks. In some, the disease does not resolve and may progress to ongoing or recurrent chronic colitis. As the pathological response of colonic tissue to chronic injury is restricted to a very few modalities, such as infiltration with leukocytes, crypt abscess, hemorrhage, necrosis, ulceration and regeneration of crypts, the pathologist may also have difficulty in differentiating ongoing ischemic colitis from that of

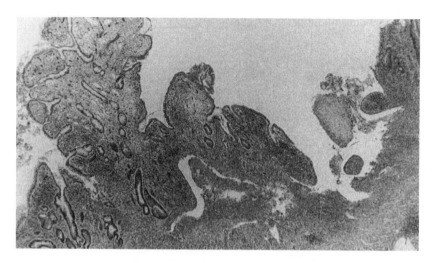

FIGURE 17 (A and B).   Histopathologic mimickers of ischemic bowel disease.

FIGURE 17A.   Photomicrograph of colonic mucosa and superficial submucosa in a patient with chronic ischemic colitis. There is focal ulceration, epithelial regeneration with polypoid mucosal areas, inflammation and distortion of crypt architecture similar to that seen in the chronic colitis of Crohn's disease. (HPS stain)

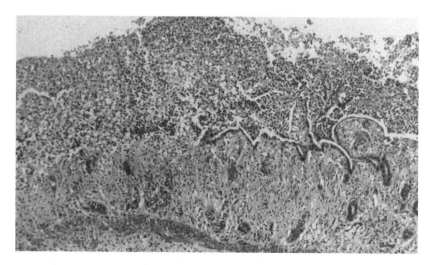

FIGURE 17B.   Photomicrograph showing prominent inflammatory exudate forming a pseudomembrane that covers the colonic mucosa, which is superficially eroded. This intense inflammatory reaction was due to acute mucosal ischemic injury and mimics the histopathology of infectious pseudomembranous colitis. (HPS stain)

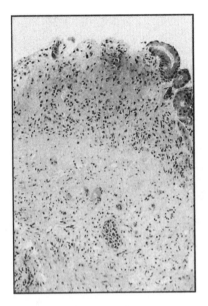
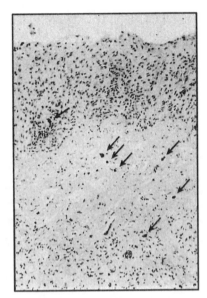

FIGURE 18.   Photomicrograph of mucosal biopsy in patient with ischemic colitis taken five days after onset of disease.
A. Routine HPS stain showing ischemic necrosis of the mucosa and submucosa.
B. Prussian blue stain. Arrows indicate dark blue iron-laden macrophages in the mucosa and submucosa.

Crohn's disease (Figure 17A). Hemosiderin, a sign of previous bleeding, is often considered a typical manifestation of ischemic colitis (Figure 18). Unfortunately, this finding is not restricted to ischemic colonic disease, as it can be found in any type of colitis, including IBD, if hemorrhage has occurred sometime in the past.

Once ischemic colitis has become chronic, it may resolve, relapse or progress to deeper intramural inflammation and necrosis. In severe disease the patient may exhibit toxic symptoms with chills, fever, severe bloody diarrhea and abdominal distention with diminished bowel sounds. The patient may develop leukocytosis, anemia, elevated platelet count and electrolyte disturbances. In some instances the disease progresses to toxic megacolon, and if the intramural necrosis becomes transmural, acute peritonitis will ensue. This progression may take only a few hours or several days to develop, and as the patient must be surgically treated well before peritonitis develops, this process

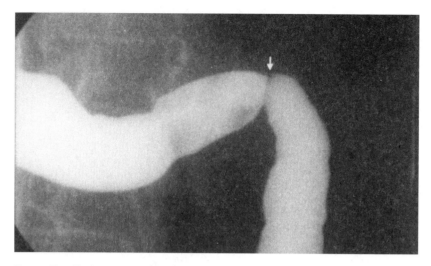

FIGURE 19.   Single contrast barium enema demonstrating a late colonic ischemic stricture.

must be detected early by careful, sometimes hourly, follow-up of the patient. If the necrosis does not progress transmurally, the process will heal first with granulation tissue that is replaced by fibrous tissue, scarring and finally a stricture (Figure 19).

7.3.3 TREATMENT
Infectious enteropathies, IBD and other precipitating causes such as diverticulitis, cancer, etc. have to be detected and appropriately treated. Therapy for ischemic colitis can be considered under the following three categories: (1) nonspecific supportive therapy, (2) specific medical treatment and (3) surgical therapy.

Nonspecific supportive therapy. Fluid and electrolyte balance must be carefully maintained. Oral intake should be restricted according to the severity of disease. Well-nourished patients can be maintained for a few days without specific nutritional support, except for what they receive in intravenous solutions. Severely undernourished patients may require enteral nutrition, or if this is poorly tolerated, total parenteral nutrition (TPN). Bleeding is rarely severe enough to require blood transfusion, but if anemia is present it may have to be corrected even in elderly patients with poor cardiovascular reserve. This requires careful balancing, so that an already precariously maintained circulation is not overloaded. Patients tend to request medication to relieve diarrhea and abdominal pain. However, the use of analgesics, antispasmodic or antidiarrheal agents is contraindicated, because they may lead to an inert bowel, which may result in a toxic megacolon.

As the patient improves, a low-residue diet may be slowly started. If this is not well tolerated, enteric feeding may be required. However, in some patients the diarrhea and abdominal pain may become worse on enteric nutrition. This may be overcome with the use of an iso-osmotic product, dilution of the solution and constant slow administration over 24 hours.

Patients have to be carefully followed to detect deterioration, as they may progress to toxic megacolon or perforation. In patients who show signs of deterioration, the use of antibiotics may be justified. If there is further progression and the patient develops increasing peritoneal signs, surgery becomes imperative, even in an elderly patient who appears to be a poor surgical risk.

Specific medical treatment. There is no need for specific therapy for mild self-limiting disease. For chronic ongoing disease there is no proven specific therapy, and no experimental data exist to assess the usefulness of any of the drugs utilized in IBD. Because of the relatively low incidence of ischemic colitis, up to now it has not been possible to design a valid prospective double-blind study to assess the efficacy of these drugs. However, patients with long-standing progressive disease have been treated with variable results using 5-aminosalicylic acid (5-ASA) by oral and/or (depending on the location of the disease) rectal administration. For patients who do not respond to 5-ASA, a trial with oral or local steroids may be attempted. There is no experience with metronidazole or immunosuppressive agents. In contrast to acute mesenteric arterial occlusion, there is no evidence in nongangrenous ischemic colitis that vasodilators (papaverine, ACE inhibitors, nitrites) and/or fibrinolytic agents (streptokinase, urokinase) are useful. By the time the patient is seen the intramural ischemic injury has already occurred and vasodilators cannot reverse the pathological changes. Treatment of heart disease, change of digitalis to other medication, discontinuation of estrogens, management of diabetes, recognition and treatment of vasculitis, polycythemia, etc., may not necessarily alter the outcome of already established chronic disease, but may prevent future recurrences.

Surgical therapy. Indications for immediate surgery are toxic megacolon and transmural necrosis leading to peritoneal signs. Usually within six months after onset of the disease a considerable number of patients with severe ischemic colitis will develop strictures. They present with symptoms of partial obstruction. One should attempt colonoscopic dilation, but if this fails stricturoplasty or surgical resection may be necessary.

SUGGESTED READING LIST

Gandhi SK, Hanson MM, Vernava AM, Kaninski DL, Longo WE. Ischemic colitis. Dis Colon Rectum 1996; 39:88–100.

Haglund U. Gut ischaemia. Gut 1994; 35(Suppl 1):S73–76.

Howard TJ, Plaskon LA, Wiebke EA, Wilcox MG, Madura JA. Nonocclusive mesenteric ischemia remains a diagnostic dilemma. Am J Surg 1996; 171:405–408.

Levine JS, Jacobson ED. Intestinal ischemic disorders. Dig Dis 1995; 13:3–24.

Panes J and Granger DN. Leukocyte-endothelial cell interactions: molecular mechanisms and implications in gastrointestinal disease. Gastroenterology 1998; 114:1066–1090.

Pastores SM, Katz DP, Kvetan V. Splanchnic ischemia and gut mucosal injury in sepsis and the multiple organ dysfunction syndrome. Am J Gastroenterol 1996; 91: 1697–1710.

Welch M, Baguneid MS, McMahon RF, et al. Histologic study of colonic ischaemia after aortic surgery. Br J Surg 1988; 85:1095–1098.

Yamada K, Saeki M, Yamaguchi T, et al. Acute mesenteric ischemia: CT and plain radiographic analysis of 26 cases. Clin Imaging 1998; 22:34–41.

OBJECTIVES

1. Understand the anatomy and physiology of splanchnic circulation.
2. Understand the pathophysiology of ischemic bowel disease.
3. Realize the importance of differentiating superficial (mucosal and submucosal) from deep (transmural) necrosis.
4. Be aware of the risk factors that may lead to intestinal ischemia.
5. Develop a high index of suspicion for the possibility of acute mesenteric ischemia in an emergent patient with extremely severe abdominal pain.
6. Learn to act immediately when this condition is suspected, as delay may lead to rapid necrosis of the bowel.
7. Understand the value of the different imaging techniques used in acute mesenteric ischemia.
8. Learn the methods of management of acute mesenteric ischemia.
9. Become aware of the possibility of chronic mesenteric ischemia in a certain group of patients who present with unexplained postprandial abdominal pain.
10. Learn to consider nongangrenous ischemia in localized small bowel disease.
11. Suspect nongangrenous ischemic colitis in patients with severe crampy abdominal pain and hematochezia.
12. Learn the risk factors that can lead to nongangrenous ischemic colitis.
13. Understand the differences between imaging techniques used in nongangrenous ischemic colitis and those used in acute mesenteric ischemia.

14. Learn the problems involved in differentiating nongangrenous ischemic colitis from inflammatory bowel disease or infectious colitis.
15. Understand the natural history and evolution of nongangrenous ischemic colitis.
16. Learn to be aware of possible progression of acute ongoing nongangrenous disease to toxic megacolon and occasionally to transmural necrosis.
17. Understand the problems involved in managing nongangrenous ischemic colitis during its acute and chronic phases.

9
Gastrointestinal Manifestations of Human Immunodeficiency Virus Infection
G.R. May

1. INTRODUCTION

Infection with the human immunodeficiency virus (HIV) and the development of the acquired immunodeficiency syndrome (AIDS) represents a significant problem worldwide. As of the end of 1998 it was estimated that over 20 million persons worldwide were infected with the HIV. In Canada, it is estimated that over 30,000 persons are infected with the HIV, giving an approximate prevalence of 191/100,000. The clinical manifestations of HIV infections and AIDS are varied and can involve all organ systems. The gastrointestinal (GI) tract is a common site for opportunistic infections and neoplasms in patients with HIV infection. Over 75% of patients will have significant symptoms related to the gastrointestinal tract at some point during the course of their infection. In many patients GI involvement represents the major manifestation of their HIV infection.

2. BASIC PRINCIPLES OF HIV INFECTION

HIV is a human retrovirus that is acquired predominantly through contact of infected body fluids with the bloodstream, a situation similar to the transmission of hepatitis B virus. It mainly infects the CD4 population of lymphocytes, which perform a helper cell function; immunodeficiency develops as the number of CD4 lymphocytes decreases. Cell-mediated immunity is mainly affected, but there is also impairment in the ability to mount new B-cell–mediated responses. As a result, the patient becomes susceptible to infections and neoplasms. Normal individuals usually have approximately 600–800 × 10⁶/mL CD4 lymphocytes. Patients with HIV infection slowly lose their CD4 cells.

Opportunistic infections and neoplasms rarely occur until the number of CD4 lymphocytes drops below 300×10^6/mL. Certain infections are not seen until CD4 counts are below 100×10^6/mL. HIV is also known to infect other cell populations such as macrophages, nerve cells and possibly enterocytes, where it may be clinically latent and act as a reservoir of virus.

Persons recognized to be at high risk for acquiring HIV infection include homosexual or bisexual men, intravenous drug users, hemophiliacs and others who received blood or blood products prior to universal testing of blood in approximately 1985. Heterosexuals who have unprotected intercourse with infected partners are also at risk and at present represent the group with the fastest-rising incidence of HIV infection in North America. In Africa, where HIV infection is endemic, heterosexual transmission through unprotected intercourse is the commonest mode of HIV transmission. When seeing patients with suspected HIV infection, it is important to get an accurate history of risk factors including sexual orientation and practices, history of intravenous drug use, past exposure to blood and blood products and travel to endemic areas.

Many physicians find it difficult to discuss sexual orientation and sexual practices with patients. It is often best to ask the patient directly whether he or she is heterosexual, homosexual or bisexual. For male patients the question can also be addressed by asking the patient if he has ever had sexual relations with other men. Many persons may classify themselves as heterosexual but may have had same-sex sexual experiences. Sexual activity and practices should be ascertained by inquiring about the number of sexual partners in the past and whether the patient has had anal intercourse. Unprotected receptive anal intercourse represents the highest-risk sexual practice for HIV transmission. A history of other sexually transmitted diseases is also important as it suggests high-risk activity, and the presence of open lesions during unprotected intercourse may increase the risk of HIV transmission. It is important to address these issues in a clinical and nonjudgmental way, as negatively phrased questions or judgmental attitudes toward sexual orientation and practices can interfere with the doctor–patient relationship. Patients who perceive a judgmental or negative attitude are less likely to discuss these issues truthfully with the physician.

The acquired immunodeficiency syndrome (AIDS) results from infection with the HIV and the resultant immunodeficiency. The diagnosis of AIDS is usually made on the basis of demonstrating positive serology for HIV with the presence of an opportunistic infection, neoplasm or a CD4 lymphocyte count less than 200×10^6/mL. At present it appears that most patients with HIV infection will eventually progress to AIDS; however, the rate of progression is variable. It has been well documented that therapy with antiretroviral drugs slows the progression of HIV infection to AIDS and prolongs the life of patients with established AIDS. Several classes of antiretroviral drugs are now available to treat the HIV, including nucleoside reverse transcriptase inhibitors (e.g., AZT, 3TC), protease inhibitors (e.g., saquinavir, ritonavir and indinavir) and non-nucleoside reverse transcriptase inhibitors (e.g., efavirenz, nevirapine). It is clear that combination therapy with two or more drugs is more efficacious than single-drug therapy and reduces the incidence of drug resistance. Combination therapy with these new agents has in many cases had dramatic clinical effects, with patients showing improvement in CD4 counts. Current recommendations for initiation of antiretroviral therapy are that therapy should be started once the CD4 lymphocyte count falls below 500×10^6/mL. With advancing immunosuppression, the common occurrence of certain opportunistic infections such as Pneumocystis carinii pneumonia, Mycobacterium avium-intracellulare and toxoplasmosis has also prompted recommendations for prophylactic therapy.

3. GASTROINTESTINAL INVOLVEMENT IN HIV INFECTION

3.1 General Considerations
The GI tract represents a common site of involvement of opportunistic infection and neoplasms in HIV infection. GI symptoms such as dysphagia, abdominal pain, diarrhea and weight loss are common and affect over 75% of patients with HIV infection at some time during the course of their disease. It is important to remember that HIV-infected patients may also have common gastrointestinal problems unrelated to the HIV infection. The approach to HIV-infected patients with gastrointestinal symptoms should be guided by the CD4 count. In patients with counts greater than 300×10^6/mL an opportunistic infection or neoplasm is very unlikely, and the approach to investigation of these patients should be similar to that in immunocompetent individuals. Once the CD4 count falls below 300×10^6/mL the risk for opportunistic problems increases, and they must be considered in the differential diagnosis.

Other issues that must be considered in the evaluation of HIV-positive patients with gastrointestinal symptoms are drug side effects and problems specific to risk factor groups. Many of the antiretroviral drugs and antimicrobials used in HIV infection have prominent GI side effects, which are often overlooked in the differential diagnosis of GI problems in these patients. Homosexual males are also at risk for a variety of gastrointestinal problems as a result of their sexual practices. This includes an increased risk of gastrointestinal parasitic infections and proctitis resulting from gonorrhea, syphilis or Chlamydia. Patients having receptive anal intercourse are at risk for rectal trauma manifesting as lacerations, fissures, perianal infections and rarely, bowel perforations. Intravenous drug users are also at risk for infection with hepatitis B and hepatitis C viruses.

3.2 Bacterial Infections

Typical enteric bacterial pathogens such as nontyphoidal strains of Salmonella, Shigella species and Campylobacter jejuni occur with only a slightly increased frequency in HIV-infected patients. When they do occur in immunocompromised patients the presentation is often atypical with a high incidence of bacteremia in addition to the typical symptoms of enteritis or colitis. Immunocompromised HIV patients also appear to be unable to effectively eradicate these organisms so that recurrent infection is common, often necessitating the use of chronic antibiotic suppression. Diagnosis is made with stool cultures. Because of the high incidence of bacteremia, blood cultures should also be done in patients presenting with acute diarrhea and fever.

The principles of treatment for acute bacterial enteritis or colitis in HIV-infected patients are generally the same as for other patients, with supportive care and intravenous fluids as required. Immunocompetent patients will usually clear the infection, and indications for antibiotic therapy are the same as for other patients. Immunocompromised patients and those with bacteremia should be treated with appropriate antibiotics (Table 1). Chronic suppressive therapy is often required as a result of the high incidence of recurrent infection.

3.3 Mycobacterial Infections

3.3.1 MYCOBACTERIUM AVIUM-INTRACELLULARE

Mycobacterium avium-intracellulare (MAI) is an atypical mycobacterium of environmental origin that is a common opportunistic infection in immunocompromised HIV-infected patients (CD4 lymphocyte counts $< 100 \times 10^6$/mL) and is an AIDS-defining illness. It usually presents as a chronic systemic illness including fever, night sweats, weight loss and lymphadenopathy in addition to diarrhea. The diarrhea is often mild to moderate in severity and may have features to suggest malabsorption. Hepatosplenomegaly is a common finding on examination, as the liver and spleen are also commonly involved in MAI infection. The organism commonly infects the small bowel mucosa where it causes thickening and blunting of the villi as a result of an increased number of macrophages in the lamina propria. The appearance on hematoxylin and eosin stains is strikingly similar to Whipple's disease. With mycobacterial stains the macrophages can be seen to be filled with acid-fast organisms. In addition to the liver and spleen, the intra-abdominal lymph nodes and bone marrow are also commonly involved with MAI. Diagnosis can usually be made with blood and stool cultures. Blood cultures will usual-

TABLE 1.   Treatment regimens for HIV-related gastrointestinal infections

Organism	Drug of first choice	Alternative treatments
Bacteria		
Salmonella	Ceftriaxone 1–2 g IV q12–24h	Ciprofloxacin 500 mg q12h Trimethoprim-sulfamethoxazole 160 mg/800 mg po bid
Shigella	Ciprofloxacin 500 mg po bid	Trimethoprim-sulfamethoxazole 160 mg/800 mg po bid Ceftriaxone 1–2 g IV q12–24h
Campylobacter	Ciprofloxacin 500 mg po bid or Erythromycin 500 mg po qid	Tetracycline 500 mg po qid
Mycobacteria		
Mycobacterium tuberculosis	Isoniazid 300 mg po qd + Rifampin 600 mg po qd + Pyrazinamide 15–25 mg/kg po qd + Ethambutol 15–25 mg/kg po qd or Streptomycin 15 mg/kg IM qd	Depends upon sensitivity patterns
Mycobacterium avium-intracellulare	Clarithromycin 500–1,000mg po bid + one or more of: Ethambutol 15–25 mg/kg po qd Clofazimine 100–200 mg po qd Ciprofloxacin 750 mg po bid Amikacin 7.5–15 mg/kg IM qd	Rifabutin 450–600 mg po qd + one or more of the other agents
Fungi		
Candida albicans (oral)	Clotrimazole troches 100 mg po 1–3 times/day Fluconazole 100 mg po qd	Ketoconazole 200 mg po qd Itraconazole 200 mg po qd
(esophageal)	Fluconazole 100–200 mg po qd	Ketoconazole or itraconazole 200 mg po qd Amphotericin B 0.3 mg/kg IV qd × 7 days
Histoplasmosis	*Initial therapy:* Amphotericin B 0.5–0.6 mg/kg IV qd for 4–8 weeks *Chronic suppression:* Itraconazole 200 mg po bid	Itraconazole 200 mg po bid Amphotericin B 0.5–0.8 mg/kg IV weekly

(cont'd)

TABLE 1.   Treatment regimens for HIV-related gastrointestinal infections (cont'd)

Organism	Drug of first choice	Alternative treatments
Parasites		
Giardia lamblia	Metronidazole 250 mg po tid	Quinacrine hydrochloride 100 mg po tid
Entamoeba histolytica	Metronidazole 750 mg po tid × 10 d followed by Iodoquinol 650 mg po tid × 20 d	
Cryptosporidium	Supportive fluid therapy Loperamide 2–24 mg po qd	Paromomycin 500–750 mg po qid Octreotide 50–500 µg sq tid
Microsporidium	Supportive fluid therapy Loperamide 2–24mg po qd	Albendazole 400 mg po bid Octreotide 50–500 µg sq tid
Isospora belli	Trimethoprim-sulfamethoxazole 160 mg/800 mg po qid × 10 d then bid × 21 d	Pyrimethamine 50–75 mg qd × 21 d
Viruses		
Herpes simplex virus	*For active lesions:* Acyclovir 200 mg po 5 times/day Famciclovir 500 mg po tid Valacyclovir 1,000 mg po tid *For maintenance therapy:* Acyclovir 400 mg po bid	Foscarnet 40 mg/kg IV q8h × 21 d Foscarnet 40 mg/kg IV qd
Cytomegalovirus	*For active disease:* Ganciclovir 5 mg/kg IV q12h × 14–21 d *For maintenance therapy:* Ganciclovir 5 mg/kg IV qd or 6 mg/kg IV qd 5 times/week	Foscarnet 60 mg/kg IV q8h × 14–21 d Foscarnet 90–120 mg/kg IV qd

ly be positive within 3–4 weeks, as this is a rapidly growing mycobacterium. Barium radiographs of the small bowel will often show dilation of the small bowel and irregular thickening of the small bowel folds. Ultrasound or CT scan of the abdomen will document hepatosplenomegaly, and there will often be enlarged intra-abdominal lymph nodes. Small bowel biopsy showing typical histology can also be used to establish a diagnosis.

Therapy for MAI is difficult and requires combinations of 4–6 antituberculous drugs, and the results are generally poor (Table 1). The organism usually cannot be eradicated; the goal of therapy is chronic suppression. Drug side effects are common, and many patients are unable to tolerate full therapy. Despite treatment, many patients have progressive symptoms and wasting. Because of the difficulty in treating established MAI infection, prophylactic therapy is recommended, and recent studies have shown some benefit to using either rifabutin 300 mg p.o. daily or azithromycin 1,250 mg p.o. weekly, once the patient's CD4 cell count falls below 100×10^6/mL.

3.3.2 MYCOBACTERIUM TUBERCULOSIS
Pulmonary Mycobacterium tuberculosis (TB) is being seen with increased frequency in HIV-infected patients and is especially common in IV drug users. The incidence of multiple-drug-resistant tuberculosis is increasing at an alarming rate. In HIV infection the GI tract may be involved with extrapulmonary TB either as direct extension from pulmonary lesions, where the esophagus is usually involved, or from systemic spread, where any part of the GI tract including liver and pancreas may be involved. Isolated involvement of the GI tract is unusual. Diagnosis should be made with biopsy and culture of the most readily accessible lesions. It is important to culture and do sensitivities on isolates of TB because of the rising incidence of multiple drug resistance. Initial therapy should include three or four antituberculous drugs. Choice of drugs should be determined on the basis of local sensitivity patterns.

3.4 Fungal Infections

3.4.1 CANDIDA ALBICANS
Candida albicans is one of the most common opportunistic infections in HIV-infected patients. Oropharyngeal candidiasis occurs frequently and is often one of the earliest clinical signs of immune impairment. When limited to the oropharynx it is often asymptomatic or associated with mild discomfort. Esophageal involvement is usually associated with dysphagia; however, many patients may have only vague epigastric discomfort during meals. Odynophagia can occur with esophageal candidiasis, but severe pain with swallowing is unusual and suggests other infections such as cytomegalovirus (CMV), herpes simplex virus (HSV) or nonspecific HIV-associated esophageal ulceration. Patients with esophageal involvement usually have evidence for oropharyngeal Candida, commonly seen as whitish plaques on the buccal mucosa and posterior oropharynx. Esophageal involvement may occasionally occur in the absence of oral Candida, but this is unusual.

Candidal esophagitis can be demonstrated with a barium swallow that shows abnormalities ranging from small filling defects on the mucosal surface representing mucosal plaques to thickening of the mucosal folds with a shaggy outline to the wall. Severe or deep ulcerations may be seen but are unusual. Diagnosis is best made with endoscopy, which shows typical white adherent pseudomembranous plaques. In severe cases the entire esophageal mucosa may be covered with a confluent white membrane. The diagnosis is confirmed by brush cytology or mucosal biopsy showing invasion of the candidal pseudohyphae into the squamous epithelium. Cultures are not routinely done, as these organisms are commonly present in normal individuals and tissue invasion should be demonstrated to confirm the diagnosis.

Oropharyngeal candidiasis can be treated with either local therapy using clotrimazole troches 100 mg p.o. 1–3 times/day or with systemic antifungals such as ketoconazole 200 mg p.o. daily, fluconazole 100 mg p.o. daily or itraconazole 200 mg p.o. daily. Esophageal involvement should be treated with one of the oral antifungal agents, as topical agents are generally not effective. Higher doses may be required for initial treatment in symptomatic patients (Table 1). Initial therapy should continue for approximately 14 days. Recurrence is common, and many patients require ongoing therapy with an oral antifungal agent. Resistance to oral antifungal agents is starting to emerge. Intravenous amphotericin B can be used in low doses for those who fail therapy with oral antifungal agents. Esophageal candidiasis is so common in HIV infection that many experts recommend empiric therapy in patients with esophageal symptoms, especially if oral Candida is present. Further investigation with endoscopy can be reserved for those who do not respond to empiric antifungal therapy or for those with atypical symptoms. Disseminated infection with Candida may occur in HIV infection but is unusual, as the infection usually remains mucocutaneous. Disseminated infection has a poor prognosis and is often fatal.

3.4.2 OTHER FUNGAL INFECTIONS

Other fungal infections seen in HIV infection include cryptococcosis, histoplasmosis and coccidioidosis. Disseminated infection of any of these fungi establishes a diagnosis of AIDS when present with a positive HIV antibody test. The incidence of these infections varies, and they are usually seen in patients who have lived in or have visited endemic areas. Clinically, patients usually present with prominent systemic symptoms such as fevers, night sweats and weight loss. Neurologic involvement is usually seen with cryptococcosis. With histoplasmosis, the liver is often involved as part of a disseminated infection producing abnormalities of liver chemistry. Diagnosis of these infections generally depends on the demonstration of fungi through examination or culture of clinical specimens. Serologic tests are not dependable in the immunocompromised patient. Therapy usually requires intravenous amphotericin B in high doses. The response to therapy is generally poor, with a high rate of relapse and a poor overall prognosis.

3.5 Intestinal Parasitic Infections

3.5.1 *GIARDIASIS*

Giardia lamblia is a common intestinal parasitic infection that is commonly seen in homosexual or bisexual males. Its increased frequency in HIV patients is likely due to the high frequency in homosexual men rather than as a direct result of the HIV infection, as it does not appear to have a significantly higher incidence in other risk groups. Transmission occurs via the fecal–oral route. It usually infects the small bowel mucosa where it may be asymptomatic but usually causes diarrhea with abdominal cramping, bloating and nausea. In severe cases it may produce malabsorption and steatorrhea. Dissemination is rare and does not appear to be a significant problem in HIV infection.

The diagnosis depends upon demonstrating Giardia in the stool with an examination for ova and parasites. It may also be diagnosed on a duodenal aspirate or duodenal biopsy taken at the time of endoscopy. Treatment with metronidazole 250 mg p.o. t.i.d. for 5 days is usually effective in eradicating the organism even in HIV-infected patients; alternatively, quinacrine 100 mg p.o. t.i.d. for 5 days can be used.

3.5.2 *ENTAMOEBA HISTOLYTICA*

Entamoeba histolytica is an intestinal ameba that is also seen with increased frequency in HIV-infected patients as a result of its increased frequency in homosexual and bisexual males. It usually causes colitis with bloody diarrhea and abdominal cramps. Asymptomatic carriage is seen more commonly in HIV-infected patients than in patients with amebiasis who are not infected with the HIV. Dissemination is rare and is not seen more frequently in HIV-infected patients than in other Entamoeba histolytica patients. Diagnosis is made by demonstrating ameba on a stool examination for ova and parasites. Sigmoidoscopy may show evidence for colitis, and typically Entamoeba histolytica infection causes punched-out "flask-shaped" ulcers. Diagnosis can be confirmed by demonstrating organisms on biopsy or from a fresh stool aspirate.

Therapy for symptomatic Entamoeba histolytica infection is with metronidazole 750 mg p.o. t.i.d. for 10 days followed by iodoquinol 650 mg p.o. t.i.d. for 20 days. Asymptomatic carriers may just be treated with iodoquinol. Patients should have follow-up stool studies to confirm the eradication of the infection.

3.5.3 CRYPTOSPORIDIUM

Cryptosporidium is a protozoal parasite that is now recognized as a cause of self-limited diarrhea in immunocompetent persons. Several epidemic outbreaks have been identified. In immunocompromised patients it causes chronic watery nonbloody diarrhea that can be severe, leading to significant dehydration with electrolyte disturbances and death. Patients may have associated abdominal cramps and bloating, but these are not usually severe. Cryptosporidiosis is an AIDS-defining illness in HIV-infected patients.

The diagnosis of Cryptosporidium infection is based upon the demonstration of cryptosporidial oocysts in stool or on mucosal biopsy from the small intestine or colon. Involvement of the bowel may be patchy and involve the ileum, so intestinal biopsy from the duodenum or distal colon is not reliable and examination of the stool is the best diagnostic test. Recently, special stains have been developed, which have increased the yield of diagnosis from stool tests. Therapy in immunocompromised patients usually is supportive with the use of intravenous fluids as necessary to correct volume depletion and antidiarrheal agents such as loperamide 2–24 mg per day to keep diarrhea under control. In severe cases where diarrhea cannot be controlled with antidiarrheal agents, the somatostatin analogue octreotide has been used successfully in doses ranging from 50 μg to 500 μg s.q. t.i.d. to control the diarrhea. To date, there is no proven therapy to specifically treat and eradicate Cryptosporidium. Trials using spiramycin and paromomycin have been reported, but the results have been disappointing.

3.5.4 MICROSPORIDIUM

Microsporidia are a group of intracellular protozoans that measure 1–2 μm in size and have been described in HIV-infected patients. The commonest organisms of this group identified are Enterocytozoon bieneusi and Septata intestinalis. They are believed to be pathogenic in most patients, but asymptomatic carriage in HIV patients has been documented. When symptomatic, infection with Microsporidium resembles that of Cryptosporidium, usually with watery nonbloody diarrhea of variable severity, mild abdominal cramps and bloating.

When these organisms were initially described, the diagnosis required electron microscopy of a small bowel biopsy to see the small intracellular parasites. More recently, special stains have been developed to detect Microsporidia in stool samples. Experienced pathologists can usually see the organisms with high-power microscopy of thin plastic sections of mucosal biopsies. Therapy of symptomatic microsporidial infection is similar to that of Cryptosporidium, with the use of supportive therapy and antidiarrheal agents. Octreotide has also been used successfully for severe watery diarrhea.

Metronidazole and albendazole have been used to try to eradicate Microsporidium, but neither has been shown to be reliably effective.

3.5.5 ISOSPORA BELLI

Isospora belli is another intestinal protozoal parasite that has been identified as causing infection in the setting of HIV, and infection with Isospora belli is also an AIDS-defining illness. Uncommon in North America, it has been seen in up to 15% of Haitian patients with AIDS. Clinically it causes a nonspecific nonbloody watery diarrhea similar to that of Cryptosporidium. Diagnosis is usually easily made by examination of stool for ova and parasites. Unlike infection with Cryptosporidium and Microsporidium, isoporiasis can usually be treated successfully with trimethoprim-sulfamethoxazole 160 mg tmp/800 mg smx p.o. q.i.d. for 10 days, then b.i.d. for 3 weeks. Recurrence is common (approximately 50%), and some patients may need chronic therapy.

3.5.6 STRONGYLOIDES STERCORALIS

Strongyloides stercoralis is a nematode endemic in tropical areas. It usually infects a host by penetrating the skin as filariform larvae. The larvae then travel via the bloodstream to the lungs where they leave the alveolar capillaries, are coughed up and swallowed. Once they reach the small intestine they release eggs that develop into infective filariform larvae that burrow into the small bowel mucosa. Pruritus, papillary rashes and edema may occur at the site of skin entry. Intestinal involvement may result in fever, nausea, vomiting, diarrhea, abdominal pain and weight loss. Diagnosis can best be made by examination of duodenal aspirate but can also be done by examination of concentrated stool specimens. Treatment is usually successful with thiabendazole 50 mg/kg/day in 2 doses for 2 days. Disseminated strongyloidiasis may occur in immunocompromised individuals and is recognized as an AIDS-defining illness. Therapy in immunocompromised individuals may need to be continued for at least 7 days, and some may require chronic therapy.

3.5.7 PNEUMOCYSTIS CARINII

Pneumocystis carinii is recognized as a common cause of pulmonary infection. Extrapulmonary infections of Pneumocystis have been recognized especially in patients who have received aerosolized pentamidine rather than systemic therapy for Pneumocystis carinii pneumonia (PCP) prophylaxis. Infection of the liver, spleen, intestine, bone marrow and peritoneal cavity (producing ascites) have all been reported. Diagnosis is made by demonstrating typical organisms on a methenamine-silver stain of clinical specimens. Therapy is similar to that of pneumocystis pneumonia.

3.6 Viral Infections

3.6.1 CYTOMEGALOVIRUS

Cytomegalovirus is a common infection, with greater than 50% of Canadian adults showing serologic evidence of previous exposure to CMV. Homosexual men and intravenous drug users have a seroprevalence of CMV as high as 90%. In immunocompetent patients the infection is latent and rarely causes clinical illness. Reactivation of latent infection occurs as HIV-infected patients become immunocompromised and is usually seen when the CD4 lymphocyte count is below 50×10^6/mL. CMV infection is increasing as an important clinical problem in HIV patients.

The two most common sites for CMV infection in HIV-infected patients are the retina and gastrointestinal tract. The infection can involve any part of the GI tract, where it produces ulcerating lesions. The esophagus and colon are the most common sites of GI involvement. Esophageal involvement usually presents with odynophagia and dysphagia. Endoscopy shows large shallow ulcerations that may be circumferential. Involvement of the colon produces an acute colitis presenting with diarrhea that may be bloody, often with severe abdominal pain. Sigmoidoscopy or colonoscopy shows a colitis with friable edematous mucosa and scattered ulcerations, a picture similar to Crohn's disease. Small intestinal, gastric and hepatic involvement are less common. Since CMV is commonly found in HIV patients, culture of virus from mucosal biopsies is not sufficient to make a diagnosis of CMV infection. The diagnosis is based upon demonstrating the presence of intranuclear inclusion bodies in biopsy specimens. The presence of an accompanying vasculitis with viral inclusions in endothelial cells further supports CMV as the cause of the lesion. Systemic infection can be confirmed by viral cultures of white blood cells from the buffy coat of a centrifuged specimen of blood.

Therapy of symptomatic CMV requires ganciclovir 5 mg/kg IV q12h initially for 14–21 days. Foscarnet 60 mg/kg IV q8h for 14–21 days can be used as an alternative. These treatments usually result in clinical improvement and healing of mucosal lesions. Recurrence is high, however, and many experts recommend chronic suppressive therapy with ganciclovir 6 mg/kg IV daily 5 times per week or foscarnet 90–120 mg IV daily after acute therapy. Chronic therapy appears to be required lifelong. Recently an oral formulation of ganciclovir has been developed and shown to be effective for chronic suppression of CMV retinitis. Its efficacy for suppression of gastrointestinal CMV infections has not yet been established.

3.6.2 HERPES SIMPLEX VIRUS

Herpes simplex virus (HSV) most commonly infects the esophagus to produce multiple esophageal ulcerations. Clinically herpetic esophagitis presents with prominent odynophagia and dysphagia that are indistinguishable from symptoms of CMV esophagitis. Differentiation from other causes of esophagitis in these patients requires endoscopy. The ulcers produced by herpes simplex virus are usually multiple and small. Biopsies will show multinucleated giant cells and Cowdry type A intranuclear inclusion bodies. Viral culture of biopsy material should be positive for HSV.

HSV esophagitis can usually be treated effectively with oral acyclovir 200 mg p.o. 5 times per day, famciclovir 500 mg p.o. t.i.d. or valacyclovir 1,000 mg p.o. t.i.d. In patients unable to take oral medications due to odynophagia, acyclovir can be given intravenously in a dose of 5 mg/kg q8h. Initial therapy should continue for 10–14 days. Recurrence is common, and many patients require chronic therapy with one of the oral agents. Foscarnet has been used as alternative therapy in those who have failed therapy with the other antiviral agents.

3.6.3 HUMAN IMMUNODEFICIENCY VIRUS

It is not clear whether the HIV itself causes gastrointestinal pathology. Two situations where direct pathologic effect of the HIV in the GI tract is suspected are nonspecific esophageal ulcerations and HIV enteropathy. Esophageal ulcerations are most commonly due to CMV and herpes virus, as discussed above. Ulcerations thought possibly to be directly due to the HIV occur as one of the seroconversion syndromes and as the idiopathic nonspecific esophageal ulcers seen in later stages of HIV infection. Acute infection with the HIV is usually associated with a nonspecific viral illness. As part of this seroconversion syndrome some patients develop severe odynophagia and are found on endoscopy to have multiple superficial esophageal ulcers. Electron microscopy of these ulcers has shown viral particles consistent with retroviruses. The ulcerations and odynophagia typically spontaneously resolve.

Later in the course of HIV infection, esophageal ulcerations may occur which are negative for the usual pathogens. These ulcers are usually deep with undermined edges and may be multiple. Although usually found in the esophagus, they can also occur in the posterior pharynx. Symptomatically they present with severe odynophagia that often limits oral intake. Interestingly they usually respond dramatically to treatment with corticosteroids taken orally or injected intralesionally. The etiology of these lesions is not clear; the dramatic response to steroids and other immune modifiers such as thalidomide implies an immunologic basis to the ulcerations.

HIV enteropathy is a term that has been applied to describe chronic diarrhea, often accompanied by weight loss, where no identifiable pathogen can be found. It is unclear if this enteropathy is due to an unidentified pathogen or to a direct effect of the HIV on the gut. The HIV potentially could affect the gut directly by infecting enterocytes, or indirectly by inducing the local release of cytokines and other inflammatory mediators, which then may affect enterocyte function. Improvement in some patients has occurred with anti-retroviral therapy. Otherwise, treatment is symptomatic only.

3.7 Neoplasms

3.7.1 *KAPOSI'S SARCOMA*

Kaposi's sarcoma (KS) is the most common neoplasm seen in HIV-infected patients. It has been more common in homosexual or bisexual males than in other risk groups for HIV infection, and its incidence appears to be decreasing within this risk group over the last 10 years. An infective cofactor has been postulated to explain the epidemiology of HIV-related KS, although such a factor has not been definitely identified. KS predominantly involves the skin and oropharynx; gastrointestinal involvement is seen in up to 40% of patients with skin involvement. Rare cases of visceral KS in the absence of skin lesions have been reported.

In most cases, GI involvement with KS is asymptomatic. Mucosal lesions can occur throughout the GI tract and are usually incidentally found at endoscopy, where they appear as raised red to violaceous macules. Large lesions may be nodular and may ulcerate. Symptoms are usually the result of hemorrhage from ulceration or obstruction from bulky lesions. Diarrhea and protein-losing enteropathy have also been reported. The exact presentation will depend upon the location of the lesions in the GI tract. Visceral KS should be suspected in any HIV patient with skin KS who has GI symptoms.

The diagnosis is made by histologic examination of mucosal biopsies. A recently described infection, bacillary angiomatosis, has similar histology to KS; differentiation is made by demonstrating organisms on silver stains. Gastrointestinal involvement with bacillary angiomatosis has also recently been described. HIV-related KS can be treated by local or systemic therapy. Oral lesions are best treated with local radiation or laser excision. Symptomatic visceral involvement requires systemic therapy, usually with combination chemotherapy. Good responses to subcutaneous or intralesional interferon have also recently been reported.

3.7.2 *LYMPHOMA*

B-cell lymphomas represent the second most common neoplasm occurring in HIV-infected patients. These are usually high-grade lymphomas of the large cell type; however, patients with Burkitt's lymphoma and Hodgkin's disease have also been reported. The gastrointestinal tract represents the second commonest site of involvement after the central nervous system. The lymphomas occurring in HIV infection are commonly extranodal.

Any part of the gastrointestinal tract can be involved, with the presentation and symptoms depending on the particular site. Systemic symptoms of fevers, night sweats and weight loss are commonly associated. The diagnosis is made by histologic examination of material obtained from endoscopy, or ultrasound- or CT-guided biopsy. Treatment requires combination chemotherapy similar to that for other high-grade lymphomas. Tolerance of therapy is generally poor, often as a result of the poor functional status of these patients when they develop lymphoma and the presence of other opportunistic infections. Full remissions can occur in patients who can tolerate combination chemotherapy, but the prognosis is generally poor.

3.7.3 ANAL CARCINOMA

Squamous cell carcinoma of the anal canal is seen with higher frequency in homosexual and bisexual men who practice anoreceptive intercourse. The increased risk is independent of HIV infection and, like cervical carcinoma in women, appears to be related to previous infection with human papilloma virus. Colorectal carcinoma is not seen with higher frequency in this risk group. Anal carcinoma may present with a mass and associated fissure or fistula. Local pain is usually present and there may be bleeding. The differential diagnosis includes infections such as syphilis, lymphogranuloma venereum and condyloma acuminatum, and benign perianal conditions of fissure in ano and anal trauma from intercourse or instrumentation. Definitive diagnosis is made through biopsy of suspicious lesions, especially those that fail to heal after treatment of any secondary infections. Treatment modalities include surgical excision, but many may be treated with combined radiation and chemotherapy, which has effected cures with good preservation of anorectal function.

4. HEPATOBILIARY AND PANCREATIC INVOLVEMENT IN HIV INFECTION

The liver is commonly involved during the course of HIV infection, with hepatomegaly and/or abnormal liver chemistry being seen in approximately 60% of AIDS patients. Involvement of the biliary tree and gallbladder is much less common. Hepatic disease may occur as a result of opportunistic infections (HSV, CMV, MAI, fungi) or neoplasms (KS, lymphoma). In such cases the liver is usually involved as part of more diffuse systemic involvement and is rarely the sole site of infection. Other infections such as hepatitis B and hepatitis C are common as a result of associated risk factors such as intravenous drug use and sexual transmission. Malnutrition, alcohol and hepato-toxicity of medications are other common factors that should be considered in the evaluation of hepatic abnormalities in these patients.

Co-infection of HIV with either hepatitis B or hepatitis C virus is often seen as a result of common risk factors. The effect of HIV-related immunosup-pression on chronic hepatitis B often results in clinical improvement of the chronic hepatitis. Since it is the immune reaction to hepatitis B that causes the hepatic inflammation, biochemical parameters of hepatitis often improve, as does the activity on liver biospy as the HIV-associated immunosuppression progresses. Despite the clinical improvement, hepatitis B viral replication increases. Hepatitis C, on the other hand, is directly hepatotoxic, and advanc-ing immunosuppression is not uncommonly associated with worsening of the hepatitis and progressive liver disease.

Complications resulting from liver disease caused by hepatitis B or C pre-viously were not commonly seen, since patients would often not survive long enough for end-stage liver disease to develop. As a result of this, treatment of hepatitis B or C with interferon was generally not recommended and was associated with a poor response. With the advent of new combination anti-retroviral therapies, patients with HIV infection are surviving longer and those that have co-infection with hepatitis B or C are starting to develop complica-tions of chronic liver disease. Patients with hepatitis B and evidence of active liver disease should receive lamivudine (3TC), as it has potent activity against the hepatitis B virus in addition to its antiretroviral activity. There is current-ly no recommended therapy for hepatitis C in patients with HIV infection, but combination therapy with interferon and ribavirin is presently being studied.

Biliary involvement in HIV infection is commonly termed *AIDS cholan-giopathy* and results from inflammation of the biliary tree and gallbladder. There can be a spectrum of involvement ranging from acute acalculous chole-cystitis to papillary stenosis with bile duct obstruction or more diffuse involve-ment of the biliary tree producing a picture similar to sclerosing cholangitis. Cholangiopathy is most commonly due to CMV infection of the biliary tree but has also been reported to result from biliary infection with Cryptosporidium or Microsporidium. Acute acalculous cholecystitis presents with RUQ pain, fever and tenderness on examination. Cholecystectomy is usually required. Cholan-giopathy may present with less acute RUQ pain, fever and nausea, with cholestatic liver enzyme abnormalities. Diagnosis of cholangiopathy is made by ERCP. Patients with dilated common bile ducts who presumably have pap-illary stenosis secondary to an acute papillitis have responded symptomatical-ly to endoscopic sphincterotomy. Patients in whom CMV is proven or sus-pected as the cause may improve with specific treatment for CMV. Rarely Kaposi's sarcoma or lymphoma can involve the gallbladder or biliary tree.

Symptomatic pancreatic involvement in HIV infection is not common, but clinically will usually present as acute pancreatitis. Asymptomatic elevations of serum amylase or lipase are common and are seen in up to 45% of patients. These are often related to medications but may also be due to asymptomatic involvement of the pancreas with opportunistic infection or neoplasm. Acute pancreatitis presents in a similar manner in patients with and without HIV infection. In addition to the commonly recognized causes of pancreatitis, other possibilities need to be considered in HIV patients. Drugs commonly used in HIV patients, including sulfonamides, pentamidine and the reverse transcriptase inhibitor dideoxyinosine (ddI), are common causes of pancreatitis. Pancreatic involvement with opportunistic infection and neoplasm, although usually asymptomatic, may cause pancreatitis. The principles of treatment of acute pancreatitis are the same for HIV-infected patients as for those without HIV infection. Drugs potentially involved should be stopped. Where no obvious etiology is apparent, CT scan of the pancreas is useful to rule out focal lesions that might indicate infections or neoplasms involving the pancreas.

5. NUTRITIONAL CONSIDERATIONS AND THE WASTING SYNDROME

Weight loss is a common problem in HIV infection, especially in the more advanced stages of AIDS. Weight loss of greater than 40% of lean body mass is an independent predictor of mortality. Weight loss of greater than 10% of body weight with no obvious underlying opportunistic infection or neoplasm has been termed *the HIV wasting syndrome* and is an AIDS-defining illness. The cause of weight loss in HIV-infected patients is multifactorial and includes diminished intake, malabsorption and increased metabolic rate. The major cause for weight loss in most patients has been shown to be inadequate caloric intake. Anorexia is a common result of systemic infection and drug side effects. Patients with oropharyngeal and esophageal pathology have discomfort related to eating and will decrease intake. The presence of gastrointestinal involvement is often associated with variable degrees of malabsorption so that the limited calories that are taken in are not assimilated efficiently. Increased basal metabolic rate as well as inefficient use of energy has been demonstrated in some cases. All of these contribute to weight loss.

Apart from treating the underlying infection there is no specific and effective therapy for wasting. With the new combinations of antiretroviral agents, patients have shown dramatic improvements, including weight gain and some reversal of wasting. Therefore, the control of HIV infection appears to be the most important factor in controlling wasting. Caloric intake should be optimized; the assistance of a dietitian is invaluable in helping patients in this regard. Intervention with enteral or parenteral nutritional support has not been generally effective, but may be used in selective cases.

6. CONCLUSIONS

Care of HIV-infected patients with gastrointestinal involvement represents a clinical challenge. Differential diagnosis and investigations should be guided by the degree of immunosuppression indicated by the CD4 lymphocyte count. As curative therapies for most of the GI problems are not available, therapy is usually directed at symptom relief with the goal to improve the quality of life. Functional status and psychosocial issues need to be considered for the successful management of these patients.

10
Inflammatory Bowel Disease
R.N. Fedorak and A.B.R. Thomson

1. CROHN'S DISEASE

Crohn's disease, or regional enteritis, is a chronic inflammatory disorder that can affect the small intestine and/or the large intestine. Inflammation, which may or may not be accompanied by noncaseating granulomas, extends through all layers of the gut wall to involve adjacent mesentery and lymph nodes. The inflammatory process is frequently discontinuous, with normal bowel separating portions of diseased bowel. This disease is characterized by an indolent variable course, by its diverse clinical manifestations, by its perianal and systemic complications, and by its tendency to recur after surgical resection.

1.1 Pathology
Both ulcerative colitis and Crohn's disease have a characteristic and pathological appearance. However, in any given case the pathological picture may not be specific enough to separate one from the other, or from other diseases such as infectious colitis or ischemic colitis. Therefore, in making the diagnosis the pathological assessment must be correlated with both the clinical and endoscopic assessments.

The key pathological feature of Crohn's disease is an inflammatory process that extends through all layers of the bowel wall. Microscopic examination reveals (1) hyperplasia of perilymphatic histiocytes, (2) diffuse granulomatous infiltration, (3) discrete noncaseating granulomas in the submucosa and lamina propria, (4) edema and lymphatic dilation of all layers of the gut, and (5) monocytic infiltration within lymph nodules and Peyer's patches on the serosal surface of the bowel.

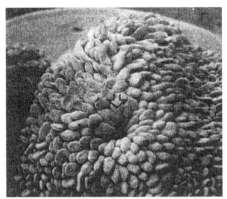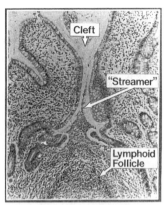

FIGURE 1.   At the endoscopic mucosal level, the earliest visible lesions of Crohn's disease are often minute aphthous ulcers. Aphthous ulcers are tiny mucosal defects that are appreciated on scanning electron microscopy (left panel). The corresponding light microscopic picture (right panel) demonstrates this mucosal defect with a cleft extending down into the lamina propria. SOURCE: Adapted from the AGA clinical teaching project, copyright 1991.

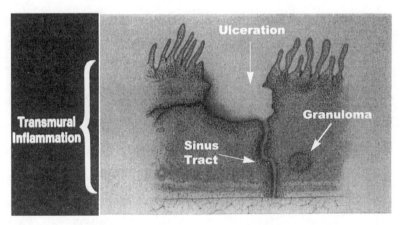

FIGURE 2.   Aphthous ulcers coalesce into larger ulcers that can extend through all layers of the bowel wall and become transmural.
SOURCE: Adapted from the AGA clinical teaching project, copyright 1991.

The mesentery in the vicinity of the diseased bowel is markedly thickened, fatty and edematous. Finger-like projections of thick mesenteric fat characteristically "creep" over the serosal surface of the bowel toward the antimesenteric border.

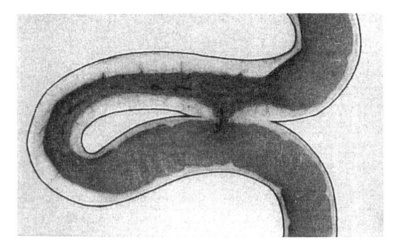

FIGURE 3.   As the inflammatory process of Crohn's burrows through the entire thickness of the bowel wall, sinus tracts are formed and frequently penetrate the serosal surface and extend into adjacent tissues. Since the serosal surface becomes "sticky," the fistulizing segments of bowel tend to adhere to surrounding tissues and the fistulous process can tunnel through into contiguous structures.
SOURCE: Adapted from the AGA clinical teaching project, copyright 1991.

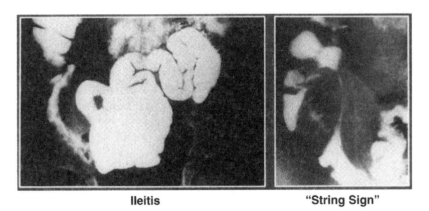

Ileitis   **"String Sign"**

FIGURE 4.   Crohn's disease. Barium contrast x-rays showing (a) ulcerations and narrowing characteristic of terminal ileal involvement and (b) the "string sign" as a consequence of stricturing following ulceration.

The earliest mucosal lesion of Crohn's disease is the aphthous ulcer. An aphthous ulcer is a small, superficial mucosal ulceration that endoscopically has the appearance of a white spot, usually less than 1–2 mm in diameter, surrounded by normal mucosa (Figure 1). In the small intestine aphthous ulcers typically occur over Peyer's patches, and in the colon they occur over lymphoid aggregates. However, aphthous ulcers can occur anywhere along the epithelium, even when there is no lymphoid tissue. As the disease progresses these tiny aphthous ulcers enlarge to coalesce and form longitudinal and transverse linear ulcers (Figure 2). These linear ulcers have a characteristic "cobblestone" appearance, resulting from the combination of deep mucosal ulceration and nodular submucosal thickening. Ulcers are frequently elongated and tend to lie along the long axis of the bowel, giving the mucosa the appearance of having been clawed.

Since the serosa and mesentery are inflamed, a characteristic feature of Crohn's disease is the tendency for involved bowel loops to be firmly matted together by fibrotic bands. This adhesive process is often associated with the fistula formation characteristic of Crohn's disease (Figure 3). Fistulas begin as ulcerations and gradually burrow through the serosa into adjacent organs. Such fistulas communicate between the loops of small bowel themselves, as well as between loops of small bowel and colon, skin, perineum, bladder or vagina, or they may end blindly in indolent abscess cavities located within the peritoneal cavity, mesentery or retroperitoneal structures.

When the lesions of Crohn's disease are discontinuous, the intestine that lies adjacent to or between diseased segments ("skip lesions") shows no gross or histological abnormalities. Skip lesions are characteristic of Crohn's disease.

1.2 Anatomic Distribution

Crohn's disease can affect the gastrointestinal tract anywhere from mouth to anus. Typically, patients with Crohn's disease can be divided into those with small bowel disease alone (30%), those with both small and large bowel involvement (50%), and those with disease involving only the colon (20%) (Table 1). When Crohn's disease involves the small bowel, 80% of the time the terminal ileum is involved (Figure 4). In only 20% of cases are other areas of small bowel also affected. When the colon is involved in Crohn's disease (Crohn's colitis), many will have pancolitis with the typical rectal sparing of Crohn's disease, but approximately 30% will have segmental disease. Much less commonly, Crohn's disease involves more proximal parts of the gastrointestinal tract such as the mouth, tongue, esophagus, stomach and duodenum.

1.3 Epidemiology

Crohn's disease was first described in 1932, although in retrospect, isolated cases were described throughout the 19th century. Since its first description we have seen a remarkable rise in disease incidence, an increase that reflects

TABLE 1. Anatomic distribution of Crohn's disease

Major site of involvement	Percentage
Small bowel only	30
Small bowel and colon	50
Colon only	20

TABLE 2. Epidemiology of inflammatory bowel disease

Factor	Ulcerative colitis	Crohn's disease
Incidence (per 100,000)	2–10	1–6
Prevalence (per 100,00)	35–100	10–100
Racial incidence	High in whites	High in whites
Ethnic incidence	High in Jews	High in Jews
Sex	Slight female preponderance	Slight female preponderance

much more than enhanced awareness and diagnosis of the disease. Figure 5 demonstrates the changes and incidence over 60 years in selective registries. Although some of the increase in incidence could be due to a shortening in the time interval between symptom onset and disease diagnosis or a better appreciation of the disease, it is the general feeling of experts in the field that the increase is real. Given the rapidity of change in disease incidence, it is likely that some environmental factor is responsible, since purely genetic factors do not change as quickly.

Crohn's disease occurs throughout the world, with a prevalence of 10 to 100 cases per 10^5 people (Table 2). The disorder occurs most frequently among people of European origin, is 3 to 8 times more common among Jews than among non-Jews, and is more common among whites than nonwhites. Interestingly, Crohn's disease seems to occur in developed countries and is infrequently found in underdeveloped or developing countries. For instance, in contrast to North America and Europe, South America and South East Asia have very few cases of inflammatory bowel disease. This observation provides one of the most compelling arguments for a yet to be determined environmental influence as a cofactor in the etiology of the disease.

Although the disorder can begin at any age, its onset most often occurs between 15 and 30 years of age. There is a familial aggregation of patients with Crohn's disease, representing the polygenetic influence, such that 20–30% of patients with Crohn's disease have a family history of inflammatory bowel disease.

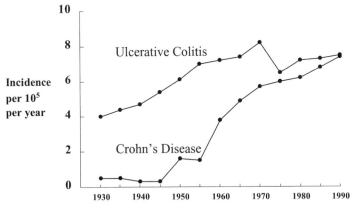

FIGURE 5. The incidence of Crohn's disease has been almost doubling in North America and Europe every decade since the 1940s, while the incidence of ulcerative colitis has remained relatively constant over the past 20 years.

1.4 **Etiology**

The etiological agent responsible for inflammatory bowel disease has not yet been determined. The abnormalities of T cells and/or macrophages and their interaction still remains the most feasible hypothesis [1–4]. In synthesizing existing literature, one could propose the following sequence of pathological events leading to the development of inflammatory bowel disease. The gastrointestinal immune system becomes exposed to a mucosal antigen (this may represent the environmental link), perhaps even an antigen normally present within the lumen – i.e., a bacterial constituent of normal flora. The movement of the luminal antigen across the epithelial barrier and tight junctions into the lamina propria may occur in the presence of an intestinal permeability defect. It is proposed that this permeability defect (either genetically or environmentally determined) causes the normally tight epithelial barrier to become "leaky" and thus permit the movement of the initiating antigen from the lumen into the lamina propria, where it is exposed to antigen-presenting cells. However, on this occasion the antigen does not evoke the typical antigen-specific suppressor T-cell activity, mucosal unresponsiveness. Rather, because of an antigen-specific mucosal immunoregulatory defect, it evokes helper T-cell activity and sets in play an ongoing proinflammatory immune response. Subsequently, in an attempt to down-regulate the antigen-specific response, antigen-nonspecific anti-inflammatory suppressor T cells appear. Initially, these antigen-nonspecific suppressor T cells may prevent disease progression; however, they are gradually depleted, leaving the unregulated proinflammatory antigen-specific helper T-cell activity to predominate (Figure 6). This unreg-

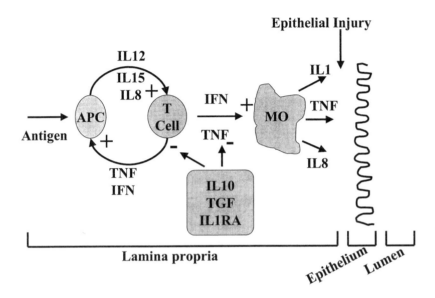

FIGURE 6. An immunological sequence that has been postulated to account for the inflammatory response observed in inflammatory bowel disease starts with an exogenous sensitization to luminal antigens, possibly facilitated by genetic influences. The first cell population involved would be the intestinal macrophage, which would phagocytose and process an antigen and present it to the T lymphocyte. In combination with this signal and cytokines (interleukin-12, interleukin-15, interleukin-8), a population of sensitized and activated T cells capable of interleukin-2, interferon-γ (IFN-γ) and tumor necrosis factor alpha (TNFα) secretion are produced. This in turn stimulates clonal expansion of specific cytolytic T cells, and a helper T-cell/B-cell collaboration, resulting in increased antibody secretion (IgG subcauses). At the same time interferon-γ and TNFα induce further macrophage activation. These macrophages then secrete IL-1, TNFα and IL-8, in addition to other proinflammatory mediators that ultimately lead to epithelial injury.

ulated antigen-specific immune response leads to the unchallenged production of proinflammatory cytokines, which stimulate migration of inflammatory and cytolytic cells to the region. Through this process the microscopic and gross morphological changes of inflammatory bowel disease are manifest.

The initiating antigen in the above process has yet to be identified. Nevertheless, there is a growing body of evidence to suggest that an initiating factor is going to be bacterial (or a bacterial product) in origin and is not likely to be specifically related to an individual food antigen. It is likely that the environmental influence in the etiology of the disease will enter the equation

TABLE 3. Frequency of clinical features in Crohn's disease

	Disease location		
Clinical feature	Ileitis (%)	Ileocolitis (%)	Colitis (%)
Diarrhea	100	100	100
Pain (abdominal)	60	60	50
Rectal bleeding	20	10	50
Weight loss	10	20	50
Perianal disease	10	40	40
Extraintestinal manifestations	5	10	20

at this point, perhaps by altering the bacteria themselves or the bacterial exposure.

1.5 Clinical Features

The typical patient with Crohn's disease is a young adult whose illness begins with right lower quadrant pain, diarrhea and a low-grade fever (Table 3). Examination reveals tenderness, guarding and a palpable mass in the right lower quadrant. If the illness has come on acutely and diarrhea is not prominent, these findings, along with an elevated white blood cell count, often lead to a clinical diagnosis of appendicitis with consequent laparotomy and discovery of the Crohn's disease.

More often, however, the clinical picture is insidious. The patient has recurrent episodes of mild diarrhea, abdominal pain, and fever lasting from days to weeks, and then has a spontaneous improvement in symptoms. If disease is confined to a small segment of intestine, this can go on for many years before a correct diagnosis is made.

The abdominal pain of Crohn's disease is localized to the right lower quadrant. When the colon is involved, crampy pain may occur in one or both lower abdominal quadrants. Fever, in the absence of complications, rarely exceeds 38°C. Diarrhea tends to be moderate in severity, with five to six bowel movements per day when the disease is confined to the ileum. When the disease involves the colon, urgency, incontinence and rectal bleeding may also occur.

If the disease is not diagnosed, gradual deterioration will occur over a period of years; there will be shorter and shorter asymptomatic intervals, along with weight loss and increasing fatigue. A slow and persistent blood loss combined with poor food intake leads to anemia.

Malnutrition and malabsorption, with subsequent weight loss, are common at all stages of Crohn's disease. A variety of factors are responsible. Neverthe-

TABLE 4.   Mechanisms responsible for malabsorption and malnutrition in Crohn's disease

---

Inadequate dietary intake (most important)
Anorexia
Specific dietary restrictions to avoid diarrhea/pain symptoms

Inflammatory involvement of small bowel
Decreased absorption of nutrients
Acquired disaccharidase deficiency
Protein-losing enteropathy
Iron deficiency due to chronic blood loss

Small bowel bacterial overgrowth due to strictures and fistulas
Malabsorption of vitamin B_{12}
Altered bile salt metabolism and fat malabsorption

Intestinal surgery
Loss of absorptive surface area due to resection
Ileal resection causing vitamin B_{12} malabsorption, bile salt deficiency, and steatorrhea

Diarrhea
Fluid and electrolyte losses

Combination of above factors

---

less, a voluntary decrease in food intake for fear of exacerbating abdominal symptoms is the primary cause of weight loss (Table 4).

Approximately 10–15% of individuals present without any of the above abdominal symptoms and are seen for the first time with perirectal disease, fever or one of the extraintestinal manifestations (Table 5).

Physical findings in Crohn's disease also vary with the distribution and severity of the disease. When the disease is active the patient may be pale and appear chronically ill. Palpation of the abdomen reveals tenderness over the area of disease activity. Thickened bowel loops, thickened mesentery or an abscess may cause a sense of fullness or a mass in the area of the Crohn's disease. The presence of perianal Crohn's disease is suggested by fistulous openings, induration, redness or tenderness near the anus.

Whatever the presenting clinical features, only 20% of patients will remain completely asymptomatic during the next 10 years. The remainder will have recurrent attacks of abdominal pain, diarrhea, and low-grade fever as the disease relapses and then enters remission.

If the Crohn's disease is surgically resected it will invariably recur (85% within 15 years), in contrast to ulcerative colitis which, when the colon is

TABLE 5. Manifestations of inflammatory bowel disease

	Crohn's disease	Ulcerative colitis
Local		
Perianal disease		
Anal fissures, rectovaginal fistulas, rectovesical fistulas	+++	+
Pararectal abscess	+++	+
Rectal prolapse	++	+
Hemorrhage		
Mild – may lead to anemia	+++	+
Massive – may be life-threatening	+	+++
Toxic megacolon	+	+++
Perforation		
Free, with or without toxic megacolon	+	+++
Walled-off	+++	–
Stricture		
Fibrous – permanent	+++	–
Muscularis mucosa hypertrophy – reversible	+	+++
Cancer	+	+++
Extraintestinal		
Skin manifestations		
Erythema nodosum	+++	+
Aphthous ulcers of the mouth	+++	–
Pyoderma gangrenosum	+	+++
Eye lesions		
Conjunctivitis	+++	+
Iritis, uveitis, episcleritis	+++	+
Arthritis		
Peripheral joints – migratory, nondeforming, seronegative	+++	+
Ankylosing spondylitis, sacroiliitis	+	+++
Hepatic disease		
Biliary		
Pericholangitis	+	+
Primary sclerosing cholangitis	+	+++
Bile duct carcinoma	+	+
Gallstones	+++	–
Hepatocellular		
Chronic active hepatitis	+	+
Cirrhosis	–	+
Miscellaneous		
Fatty change (malnutrition)	+	+
Amyloidosis	+	–

(cont'd)

TABLE 5. Manifestations of inflammatory bowel disease (cont'd)

	Crohn's disease	Ulcerative colitis
Hematologic manifestations		
Megaloblastic anemia	+++	+
Iron deficiency anemia	+++	++
Autoimmune hemolytic anemia	++	+
Thrombocytosis	++	++
Clotting abnormalities (hypercoagulable state)	+	+++
Renal disease		
Nephrolithiasis	+++	–

removed, will never recur. Interestingly, for reasons that are unknown, the recurrence is almost always at the site of the surgical resection and anastomosis. Additionally, the interval between operations appears to be shorter after the second or third operation than after the initial resection. It is this high rate of recurrence that preferentially directs the management of Crohn's disease along the lines of medical rather than surgical therapy.

1.6 Complications

1.6.1 SMALL BOWEL OBSTRUCTION
Small bowel obstruction is the most common reason for surgery when Crohn's disease involves the small intestine. Acute small bowel obstruction in Crohn's disease is usually due to mucosal thickening and edema from acute inflammation, in addition to muscular hyperplasia as a result of previous inflammation. This process results in progressive narrowing of the lumen to the point where obstruction occurs. The obstruction is often partial and is transient once the edema and inflammation are treated and allowed to resolve. The acute initiating event for the obstruction is often a result of impaction of a bolus of a particularly fibrous material (e.g., popcorn) in the setting of a stable, longstanding narrowing. Obstruction presents with the acute onset of crampy abdominal pain, diarrhea, nausea and vomiting that is worse after meals and resolves with fasting. In some cases the obstruction is not due to luminal narrowing from inflammation and edema but occurs suddenly when the small bowel becomes kinked off as a result of twisting over a surgically or inflammation-induced fibrous adhesion.

1.6.2 FISTULAS AND FISSURES

Perianal and perirectal fistulas and fissures are particularly common in Crohn's disease and may be so severe as to overshadow other intestinal manifestations. Enteroenteric fistulas can develop between loops of bowel and may contribute to nutritional problems if they cause ingested nutrients to bypass areas of small bowel absorptive surface. Additionally, the presence of enteroenteric fistulas may lead to recirculation of intestinal contents and stasis, thus causing bacterial overgrowth within the lumen. More often than not, enteroenteric fistulas are asymptomatic, as they affect only small segments of the intestine and do not cause any clinical problems. Fistulas between loops of bowel and the urinary bladder (enterovesical fistulas) ultimately lead to chronic urinary tract infections. Signs and symptoms of enterovesical fistulas include gas in the urine and recurrent urinary infections. Definitive surgical management of the enterovesical fistulas is usually recommended because of the risks of irreversible kidney damage. Fistulas can also occur between bowel and cutaneous surfaces (enterocutaneous fistulas), bowel and the vagina, or bowel and other internal organs.

1.6.3 PERFORATION

Free perforation is unusual in Crohn's disease, except in areas of longstanding active Crohn's disease with obstruction, where increased luminal pressure resulting from the obstruction readily leads to perforation. When free perforation does occur, it leads to frank peritonitis.

1.6.4 GASTROINTESTINAL BLOOD LOSS

Insidious blood loss occurs with small bowel disease and often leads to an iron deficiency anemia. Frank bleeding of bright red rectal blood occurs with colonic disease and with perianal fistulas.

1.6.5 MALIGNANT NEOPLASMS

Adenocarcinomas occur both in the involved bowel and in the noninvolved bowel of patients with Crohn's disease three times more frequently than in the general population. Nevertheless, the frequency of malignancy is much lower than that observed in patients with ulcerative colitis.

1.6.6 EXTRAINTESTINAL MANIFESTATIONS

Extraintestinal manifestations of Crohn's disease (Table 5) frequently develop alongside colonic involvement and perianal disease. Patients with one extraintestinal manifestation are at increased risk for developing a second.

Arthritis is the most common systemic manifestation and presents as migratory arthritis involving large joints, or as sacroiliitis or ankylosing spondylitis. Arthritis is common with Crohn's colitis and is uncommon with Crohn's disease confined to the small intestine. Deformity of joints rarely occurs and most arthritic flare-ups last only several weeks. The joint pain, swelling and stiffness parallel the course and activity of the bowel disease. Therefore, successful treatment of the intestinal Crohn's disease results in the improvement of the arthritis. Spondylitis or sacroiliitis may occur for many years prior to the manifestation of intestinal disease. In contrast to the peripheral arthritis, the activity of the spondylitis and the sacroiliitis does not follow that of the bowel disease and treatment of the bowel disease does not affect the progression of the spondylitis.

The eye complications of Crohn's disease are uveitis (iritis) and episcleritis. Uveitis is an inflammation of the anterior chamber of the eye presenting with blurred vision, headache, eye pain and photophobia. Episcleritis is less serious and presents with burning of the eyes and scleral injection.

The two cutaneous complications of Crohn's disease are pyoderma gangrenosum and erythema nodosum. Pyoderma gangrenosum is more often seen with colitis and ileal colitis and appears as a deep, discrete ulcer with a necrotic base, usually over the lower limbs. Erythema nodosum is the more common skin manifestation seen in Crohn's disease and consists of red, raised, tender nodules found over the anterior surface of the lower limbs.

Clinically important liver disease is not generally seen with Crohn's disease. Mild abnormalities in liver function studies may be observed in a few patients, and liver biopsy will often show a mild pericholangitis in these cases. Cholelithiasis occurs with a frequency of approximately 30% in patients with ileal disease and/or ileal resection. This high incidence is probably related to a bile salt deficiency that causes the production of a lithogenic bile conducive to cholesterol gallstone formation.

Nephrolithiasis occurs in 30% of patients with Crohn's disease. Oxalate stones and hyperoxaluria are common and are related to fat malabsorption. During fat malabsorption the unabsorbed fatty acids bind calcium in the lumen. When calcium is bound to these malabsorptive fatty acids it is not able to bind to oxalate and thus leaves oxalate free to combine with sodium to form sodium oxalate, which is soluble and absorbed in the colon. The development of calcium oxalate stones in Crohn's disease requires an intact colon to absorb the sodium oxalate. Thus patients with ileostomies do not develop calcium oxalate nephrolithiasis.

1.7 Diagnosis

Diagnosis of Crohn's disease, as of ulcerative colitis, is made through the accumulation of history and physical findings, as well as laboratory, radiologic, endoscopic and histologic findings.

TABLE 6.   Differential diagnosis of Crohn's disease (includes
colonic and/or small bowel involvement)

Infectious
   Yersinia species
   Campylobacter species
   Salmonella species
   Amebiasis
   Tuberculosis
   Balantidium coli
   Cytomegalovirus
   Histoplasmosis
   Anisakiasis
Eosinophilic gastroenteritis
Vasculitis
Solitary rectal ulcer syndrome
Colonic cancer
Appendicitis
Appendiceal abscess
Appendiceal mucocele
Meckel's diverticulitis
Pelvic inflammatory disease
Ectopic pregnancy
Ovarian cysts or tumors
Cecal diverticulitis
Carcinoma of the cecum involving the ileum
Carcinoid tumor
Ileal plasmacytoma
Ischemic bowel disease
Intestinal lymphoma
Nongranulomatous ulcerative jejunoileitis
Pseudomembranous enterocolitis
Ulcerative colitis
Radiation enteritis
Small bowel tumors
Systemic vasculitis
Fabry's disease
Zollinger-Ellison syndrome
Benign lymphoid hyperplasia

Initially, other causes of bowel inflammation must be excluded (Table 6).
In the acute phase of Crohn's disease, infectious gastroenteritis or appendicitis must be excluded. If the Crohn's disease presents as a chronic recurrent illness, then culture of the stools and rectal mucosa for giardiasis, amebiasis and
intestinal tuberculosis must be done to exclude these diseases, which may
mimic Crohn's disease symptoms. If the inflammatory state is limited to the

colon or rectum, ulcerative colitis, ischemic colitis, diverticulitis and occasionally cancer of the colon may simulate Crohn's disease.

1.7.1 LABORATORY INVESTIGATIONS

A complete blood count (CBC) will reveal leukocytosis, an elevated erythrocyte sedimentation rate and thrombocytosis, all of which suggest that an active inflammatory process is present. Indices may be microcytic hypochromic if an iron deficiency anemia exists, macrocytic megaloblastic if a vitamin B_{12} (absorbed in the terminal ileum) or folic acid deficiency exists. If both these states are present then the automated counter will present a normochromic, normocytic–type anemia that must then be investigated through peripheral smear and measurement of serum iron, total iron binding capacity (TIBC), ferritin, vitamin B_{12} and folic acid levels.

Urinalysis may demonstrate a urinary tract infection if a fistula is present and proteinuria if amyloidosis has developed. The serum albumin is a useful indication of the patient's overall condition. It is low in those patients not eating, those with extensive malabsorption, and those whose disease is causing significant enteric loss of proteins. Serum carotene, calcium, phosphorous, Schilling test and stool fat assessment are useful in determining whether or not frank malabsorption is present. Lactose hydrogen breath test and ^{14}C-labeled glycocholate breath test are useful in assessing the degree of lactose intolerance and bacterial overgrowth, respectively. Note that the ^{14}C-labeled glycocholate breath test will also be abnormal in the presence of ileal disease or ileal resection.

1.7.2 ENDOSCOPY

Endoscopy, flexible sigmoidoscopy, and/or colonoscopy are useful for identifying and performing biopsies on discrete mucosal ulcerations. The earliest endoscopic manifestation of Crohn's disease is the aphthous ulcer, a small, discrete, white-based ulcer a few millimeters in diameter surrounded by a red halo of edematous tissue. Aphthous ulcers can coalesce to form large stellate or linear ulcers. Often islands of normal mucosa protrude into the colonic lumen as a result of submucosal inflammation and edema. When prominent islands of mucosa are separated by linear ulcerations, the intestine assumes a cobblestone appearance. This pattern is characteristically different from that seen in ulcerative colitis, where diffuse ulceration extends without patches of normal mucosa.

The decision to perform colonoscopy should take into account the specific diagnosis and/or therapeutic issues that the procedure may be asked to resolve. These include (1) establishing a diagnosis; (2) determining the activity of the disease; (3) establishing the extent of involvement; (4) determining the type of disease; and (5) resolving a suspicion of cancer.

Endoscopy has also become important in the management of Crohn's-induced fibrotic strictures. Strictures that become symptomatic with recurrent obstructions can often be successfully dilated, avoiding surgery, with a balloon dilator passed through the colonoscope.

1.7.3 *RADIOLOGIC FINDINGS*

The plain x-ray of the abdomen will reveal dilated bowel and air fluid loops when an obstruction is present. Intra-abdominal masses resulting from matted inflamed loops of bowel or from abscesses can also be seen on the plain film.

An air contrast barium enema will demonstrate involvement of the colon and show narrowing, ulcerations, strictures or fistula formation. As with colonoscopy, a barium enema should be deferred in patients acutely ill with Crohn's colitis, since the examination is not critical for immediate management decisions and the risk of toxic megacolon and perforation is appreciable.

A barium enema may reveal disease of the terminal ileum as a result of reflux of barium past the ileocecal valve. However, determination of the extent of small bowel involvement requires administration of contrast medium orally or via enteroclysis. The small bowel abnormalities seen on x-ray are similar to those observed in the colon and include the characteristic cobblestone appearance, stenosis, and diseased segments separated by small bowel that appears normal (Figure 4).

It is important to note that changes in the appearance of both the large and small bowel on x-ray film or endoscopy correlate poorly with the clinical course of the disease. There is thus no reason to perform "routine" evaluative x-rays or endoscopy.

1.7.4 *HISTOLOGIC EXAMINATION*

Mucosal biopsies obtained from the rectum, colon, terminal ileum or duodenum at the time of colonoscopy or upper endoscopy provide histologic documentation. Granulomatous inflammation of bowel mucosa strongly supports a diagnosis of Crohn's disease (Figure 2; see Section 1.1).

1.8 **Therapy**

The management of Crohn's disease varies greatly depending upon the clinical status of the individual patient. No single therapeutic regime is considered routine for patients with Crohn's disease, and treatment must be individualized.

When the patient presents with acute Crohn's disease, the history and physical examination are critical in determining the severity of the disease, in addition to gathering evidence of intestinal obstruction, bowel perforation or abscess. The use of steroids or immunosuppressive agents in the presence of gross infection can be disastrous. In mild to moderate cases, diarrhea and abdominal cramps can be managed effectively on an outpatient basis with codeine, diphenoxylate (Lomotil®) or loperamide (Imodium®) while the disease is being treated. In severe cases, the severity of abdominal cramps and diarrhea requires that the patient be admitted to hospital, remain on clear fluids and be maintained with intravenous fluids. When symptoms and findings suggest small bowel obstruction, nasogastric suction is usually required until edema and spasm of the bowel subside. If evidence of abscess formation, fever and leukocytosis suggests a systemic infection, broad-spectrum antibiotic coverage should be initiated after appropriate cultures of blood, urine, fistulas or other possible sources of infection have been collected.

1.8.1 SUPPORTIVE THERAPY

Symptomatic therapy may be necessary to control diarrhea in cases of chronic stable disease. As indicated above, diphenoxylate, loperamide and codeine are useful agents for controlling diarrhea, but they should be used carefully so as not to simply mask disease that requires specific therapy and not to provoke a toxic megacolon.

Additionally, for patients with Crohn's disease, the diarrhea may be due to unabsorbed deconjugated bile acids that enter the colon and cause a cholerrheic diarrhea. Cholestyramine, an ion-exchange resin, effectively binds the unabsorbed bile salts and controls the diarrhea. Bacterial overgrowth proximal to areas of stenosis causes deconjugation of bile salts, again resulting in diarrhea; it responds well to courses of broad-spectrum antibiotics (e.g., tetracycline). Diarrhea may also be caused by lactase deficiency that may occur secondary to the active inflammation. In these cases a trial of lactose-free diet is warranted. Finally, diarrhea may also occur as a consequence of fat malabsorption (i.e., steatorrhea). Unabsorbed fat reaching the bacteria in the colon is hydroxylated to short-chain fatty acids, which in high concentrations lead to a secretory type of diarrhea. In these cases following a low-fat diet or supplementing long-chain fatty acids with medium-chain fatty acids (which can be absorbed in the small intestine directly into the portal vein) may be useful in managing the diarrhea.

The patient with Crohn's disease also requires continuous emotional support for this chronic, complicated illness; this support is necessary not only during acute attacks, but also during periods of remission. Although many consultants may be required to manage the varying aspects of complicated cases, one physician should be directly and continuously responsible for the overall care of the patient. Psychiatric or psychological consultation may occasionally be necessary for specific problems; however, successful management requires that continuous emotional support come from the physician who is directing the overall care of the patient.

1.8.2 NUTRITIONAL THERAPY

Nutritional deficiencies are frequent with Crohn's disease and often result from inadequate food intake by patients who have "learned" that ingestion of food aggravates diarrhea and abdominal pain. In addition, several pathophysiologic mechanisms contribute to nutritional problems in patients with Crohn's disease (Table 4). Nutritional problems may be further aggravated by surgical resection of diseased intestine, which decreases absorptive surface area; this decrease may be sufficient to interfere with an adequate absorption of multiple nutrients. Of particular importance, because of the distal small bowel involvement, is the malabsorption of bile salts and vitamin B_{12}, both of which have receptors located solely in the distal ileum.

Whatever the combination of mechanisms responsible for the impaired absorption and nutritional deficiencies in Crohn's disease, the physician must be attuned to assessing nutritional parameters, including ideal body weight, anthropometrics, serum proteins, and serum vitamin and mineral levels. The consequences of nutritional disturbances are particularly serious in children with Crohn's disease. Delayed growth and sexual maturation can and do occur, and if they are not corrected prior to closure of the epiphysis, permanent shortness of stature will result. Adjunctive nutritional therapy is, as well, required by patients who are malnourished at the time of their Crohn's exacerbation or who are unable to ingest adequate calories because of their disease.

Increasingly, patients with extensive and complicated Crohn's disease are being treated partially or completely with enteral or parenteral nutritional programs as a means of "resting" the gut, allowing fistulas to heal, inducing a positive nitrogen balance, and even causing weight gain. Short-term remission is often achieved through the use of "bowel rest"; however, unless concomitant medical therapy is instituted, relapse rates are high within a few months of discontinuing therapy. Greenberg et al. have demonstrated that disease remission could be induced provided the patient received an adequate number of calories. Furthermore, it did not matter whether these calories were provided through oral intake, oral intake supplemented with enteral elemental feeding, or total parenteral nutrition. This study highlights the fact that the total number of calories and adequate nutrition are more important in aiding disease remission than is delivering these calories intravenously and permitting "bowel rest."

TABLE 7.   Drug therapy in inflammatory bowel disease

Corticosteroids
Rectal
    Suppositories
    Foam
    Enemas
Systemic

Sulfasalazine
Oral
Enemas

Mesalamine (5-ASA)
Oral
Rectal
Enemas
Suppositories

Metronidazole

Immunosuppressive agents
Azathioprine
6-mercaptopurine
Cyclosporine
Methotrexate

1.8.3 *MEDICAL THERAPY IN ACTIVE CROHN'S DISEASE*

Although a small percentage of patients with Crohn's disease enjoy prolonged symptom-free intervals when treatment is not required, the vast majority experience long periods of symptomatic active disease or frequent relapses that necessitate treatment of the disease with anti-inflammatory and immunosuppressive agents (Table 7). Evaluation of the efficacy of such agents is extremely difficult, given the fluctuating activity and unpredictable long-term course of Crohn's disease. Recently, randomized double-blind control studies have attempted to answer some of the questions relating to drug therapy.

1.8.3.1 *Corticosteroids*

1.8.3.1.1 *Rectal corticosteroid preparations*   Rectal instillation of steroid-containing preparations is useful when Crohn's disease involves the rectum (the rectum is frequently spared, however) and the sigmoid region. The topical application of steroids allows for rapid healing of the area and restoration of the rectum and sigmoid to their stool reservoir capacity and, therefore, often leads to fewer episodes of diarrhea. The rectal formulation used will depend upon the distance from the anal verge the corticosteroid is intended to cover, with suppositories, foam and enemas reaching distal extensions of approximately 10, 20 and 60 cm, respectively.

1.8.3.1.2 Systemic corticosteroid preparations   Corticosteroids are beneficial in the management of acute exacerbations of small and large intestinal Crohn's disease, in which they induce remission of symptoms and decrease disease activity indices [5]. Although steroids continue to be used by many practitioners on a chronic basis in the management of Crohn's disease, there is little evidence to support administration to prevent disease relapse. Steroid therapy for acute disease is best begun at prednisone 40 mg/day (outpatient oral treatment in mild cases or inpatient intravenous therapy in severe cases). As improvement occurs, parenteral therapy may be replaced by oral administration of a dosage that is gradually reduced by 5 mg/week to the minimum level needed to suppress signs of the inflammatory process (20 mg) and then by 2.5 mg/week; the ultimate goal is to end steroid therapy. Unfortunately, this objective cannot always be achieved, and up to 40% of patients become symptomatic when the dose of prednisone is reduced below 5–10 mg/day (steroid dependence). If possible, patients requiring long-term steroid therapy should be weaned onto an alternate-day regime in an attempt to reduce side effects; alternatively, immunosuppressive therapy may allow steroid withdrawal or a lowering of the steroid dose.

In an attempt to develop corticosteroids with fewer systemic side effects, formulations have been designed to be metabolized to inactive agents upon passing through the liver. Budesonide, a first-pass metabolized corticosteroid, designed to be released near the ileum, is one such agent available in Canada. Budesonide 9 mg/day has an efficacy similar or slightly less than prednisone in acute Crohn's disease. While systemic side effects do seem to be less with prednisone, approximately 60% of persons will still have demonstrable suppression of their adrenal axis with 16 weeks of budesonide use. Like prednisone, budesonide is not useful in reducing one-year Crohn's disease relapse rates.

1.8.3.2 Mesalamine (5-aminosalicylic acid mesalazine [5-ASA])
Mesalamine products can be broadly divided into those with predominant therapeutic effect in the colon and those with therapeutic effect in both the small bowel and the colon (Table 8). In Crohn's colitis, all colon-specific mesalamine formulations are equally effective in mild to moderate disease. In Crohn's disease involving the small bowel, the mixed, slow-release and pH-dependent mesalamine (Pentasa®) and the pH-dependent release mesalamine (Mesasal™) appear to be effective in reducing small intestinal inflammation. When used for acute treatment the average daily dose of mesalamine products

TABLE 8.   Comparison of oral mesalamine products

Mesalamine	Average dose for acute therapy	Average dose for maintenance therapy	Approximate cost per month
Predominant colonic delivery			
Salazopyrin®	4 g/d	2 g/d	$ 78 / $45
Asacol®	4 g/d	2 g/d	$183 / $98
Dipentum®	2 g/d	1 g/d	$140 / $76
Salofalk®	4 g/d	2 g/d	$148 / $80
Mesasal™	4 g/d	2 g/d	$160 / $85
Small bowel and colonic delivery			
Pentasa®	4 g/d	2 g/d	$167 / $90

is 4 g/day (except for Dipentum®, which is 2 g/day). When used for maintenance therapy the average dose is 2 g/day (Dipentum® 1 g/day) [6].

1.8.3.3 *Immunosuppressive agents*

Immunosuppressive agents are usually reserved for steroid-dependent or steroid-resistant patients. When combined with steroids, azathioprine (2.0 mg/kg/day), its active metabolite, 6-mercaptopurine (1.5 mg/kg/day), cyclosporine (7.5–15 mg/kg/day), and methotrexate (15–25 mg/week) are useful in cases of both ileal and colonic Crohn's disease. A large number of case reports and open studies have found that immunosuppressive agents will induce remission in steroid-resistant or steroid-dependent patients in approximately 60–70% of cases [7–9]. Methotrexate and cyclosporine appear to work more quickly than 6-mercaptopurine and azathioprine. While cyclosporine can be effective in quickly inducing disease remission, it is expensive, has significant side effects, and is no more effective than placebo in maintaining Crohn's disease in remission. For these reasons, cyclosporine is not generally used, except in the most severe cases of Crohn's disease.

Immunosuppressive agents are usually begun in conjunction with full-dose corticosteroids (e.g., prednisone 40 mg/day), and the corticosteroids are slowly withdrawn by 2.5 mg each week to off. In this way the corticosteroids initiate disease remission during the three- to four-month lag time it takes the immunosuppressive agents to have a clinical effect. The major limiting factor in the use of these immunosuppressive agents is their toxicity. Immunosuppressive agents can cause leukopenia (azathioprine) hepatitis and cirrhosis (methotrexate), pancreatitis (azathioprine), and impaired renal function (cyclosporine), necessitating careful patient and laboratory monitoring during their use. Lymphomas have been described in patients taking these drugs for other diseases, but the magnitude of the risk in Crohn's disease is not yet clear.

1.8.3.4 Specific immunomodulating agents

Immunomodulating agents are being designed to modulate the T-cell immune dysfunction that has been identified in Crohn's disease. Recent advances in reducing the proinflammatory cytokine tumor necrosis factor alpha (TNFα), which is present in the soluble form in the lamina propria of patients with Crohn's disease, with an antibody, have proven effective in inducing remission in approximately 50% of patients who fail all medical management. Unfortunately, the present anti-TNF antibody is a chimeric (mouse/human) antibody, and the development of human chimeric antibodies and delayed hypersensitivity reactions may be a problem with long-term dosing. The administration of interleukin-10, an anti-inflammatory cytokine, by subcutaneous injection is now under investigation to determine whether adding an anti-inflammatory cytokine can ameliorate the unchecked proinflammatory response that occurs in the lamina propria. In the future, agents designed to (1) interfere with neutrophil movement from the circulating bloodstream into the lamina propria, via genetic engineering of the various adhesion molecules, (2) block proinflammatory cytokines, and/or (3) enhance anti-inflammatory cytokines will no doubt revolutionize our management of inflammatory bowel disease.

1.8.3.5 Antimicrobial agents

The role of antibiotic therapy in the treatment of active Crohn's disease remains controversial. Certainly antibiotics have a place in the management of complications such as abscess and perianal disease and in the management of diarrhea caused by bacterial overgrowth in the small bowel. Antibiotics may also be useful in acute severe Crohn's disease requiring hospital admission. In these cases bacteria from the lumen may transmigrate into the bowel wall and further aggravate the ongoing inflammatory process. Nevertheless, controlled trials have not been conducted with the use of antibiotics in this clinical situation.

Metronidazole (250 mg t.i.d.) is as effective as mesalamine in acute colonic disease if the patient has not received prior therapy, in patients whose disease does not respond to mesalamine, and in the treatment of perianal disease. Indeed, the use of metronidazole has been most effective in the treatment of perianal fissures and fistulas. Side effects include metallic taste, nausea and vomiting with ingestion of alcohol, paresthesias and peripheral neuropathy. Most side effects are reversible upon withdrawal of the drugs; however, the peripheral neuropathy may persist. Other antimicrobial agents such as ciprofloxacin, tetracycline and sulfonamides have also been suggested to be effectual in the acute management of Crohn's disease. Nevertheless, large clinical trials will be required to confirm the effectiveness of their use.

1.8.4 MAINTENANCE THERAPY IN CROHN'S DISEASE

1.8.4.1 Corticosteroids
Although some patients require corticosteroids to maintain a state of wellness, not all patients will benefit. Steroid-dependent patients able to taper the corticosteroids off while their disease remains in remission would not prevent relapse by continuing on long-term maintenance corticosteroid therapy. In addition, the multiple complications associated with corticosteroids limit their long-term use.

1.8.4.2 Mesalamine
Several large multicenter trials have demonstrated a potential benefit from mesalamine (2 g/day) as maintenance therapy in preventing relapse of Crohn's disease. While the benefits for mesalamine in maintenance therapy are not very large, the side effects from these drugs are minimal and many physicians have elected to keep patients on mesalamine as maintenance therapy. It would appear that female patients who are immediately post–ileal resection for their Crohn's disease benefit most from mesalamine maintenance therapy.

1.8.4.3 Immunosuppressive agents
Steroid-dependent patients who require immunosuppressive therapy can usually have the corticosteroids withdrawn and remain on the immunosuppressive therapy as "maintenance" therapy. Once the immunosuppressive therapy has been in place for three to four years, it does not appear that continuing it longer has any additional benefit, and it should be stopped at this time. In general, a patient who has remained well for three to four years immunosuppressive will not have relapse of the disease.

1.8.4.4 Antimicrobial agents
There is no clear evidence that antibiotics are useful in maintenance therapy. Nevertheless, the use of metronidazole in the immediate postoperative period may prolong the time to remission.

1.8.5 SURGICAL THERAPY
In view of the high rate of recurrence of Crohn's disease following resection

of diseased bowel, operative therapy should be reserved for complications of the disease or for those cases where the disease unequivocally fails to respond to optimal medical management. Complications requiring surgery are (1) chronic obstruction; (2) symptomatic abscess or fistula formation; (3) enterovesical fistulas; (4) free perforation; and (5) retarded physical or sexual development in children with Crohn's disease. Removal of the diseased segment(s) in a young child will normally allow the child to grow and mature normally until the Crohn's disease recurs. Patients should be forewarned that surgery is not curative but is necessary for the treatment of complications. Patients should also be warned about the common recurrence of Crohn's disease after resection of the small bowel or after colonic disease. The recurrence rate is 40% within 5 years, 60% within 10 years and 85% within 15 years.

2. ULCERATIVE COLITIS

Ulcerative colitis is an inflammatory disease of unknown etiology affecting the colonic mucosa from the rectum to the cecum. It is a chronic disease characterized by rectal bleeding and diarrhea, and given to remissions and exacerbations. Ulcerative colitis differs from Crohn's disease in that it is limited to the colon and is characterized by mucosal inflammation that does not, like Crohn's disease, become transmural.

Ulcerative colitis is not a distinct entity, since most of the histological features of the disease may be seen in other inflammatory states of the colon, such as those caused by bacteria or parasites. The diagnosis of ulcerative colitis, therefore, rests on discovery of a combination of clinical and pathological criteria, investigation of the extent and distribution of lesions, and exclusion of other forms of inflammatory colitis caused by infectious agents.

2.1 Pathophysiology

Ulcerative colitis is an inflammatory state confined to the mucosa, unlike Crohn's disease, which extends into deeper muscle layers of the serosa. Since the inflammatory process involves only the mucosa, sharp localized abdominal pain, perforation and fistula formation are uncommon in ulcerative colitis; this is in contrast to Crohn's disease, where they frequently appear. Under light microscopy, the colonic tissue displays small microabscesses, called crypt abscesses, which involve the crypts of Lieberkühn. Polymorphonuclear cells accumulate in the crypt abscesses, and frank necrosis of the surrounding crypt epithelium occurs; thus the polymorphonuclear infiltrates extend into the colonic epithelium. These microabscesses in the crypts are not visible to the naked eye; however, several crypt abscesses may coalesce to produce a

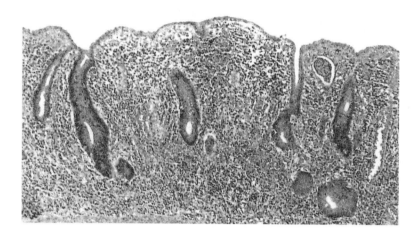

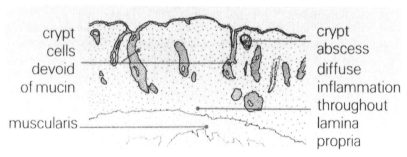

crypt
cells
devoid
of mucin

muscularis

crypt
abscess
diffuse
inflammation
throughout
lamina
propria

FIGURE 7.   Cross-section of colonic mucosa showing typical crypt abscess seen in ulcerative colitis.

shallow ulceration visible on the mucosal surface (Figure 7). Occasionally, lateral extension of crypt abscesses may undermine the mucosa on three sides, and the resulting hanging fragment of mucosa will appear endoscopically and radiographically as a "pseudopolyp." Following this mucosal destruction, highly vascular granulation tissue develops in denuded areas, resulting in friability and bleeding. The two most prominent symptoms of ulcerative colitis – diarrhea and rectal bleeding – are related both to the extensive mucosal damage that renders the colon less capable of absorbing electrolytes and water, and to the highly friable vascular granulation tissue, which bleeds readily.

Radiographically, foreshortening and narrowing of the colon, loss of haustral margins, and stricture formation will often be seen. In contrast to the strictures in Crohn's disease, strictures in ulcerative colitis are often reversible, since they are due to hypertrophy and spasm of the muscularis mucosa and not to fibrosis.

2.2 Clinical Features

Ulcerative colitis typically occurs in patients between 20 and 50 years of age and may present as an early acute fulminating attack or may follow a rather indolent and often chronic course. Approximately 70% of patients will have complete symptomatic remissions between intermittent attacks. Ten percent of patients will have one initial attack and will experience no subsequent attacks, and 15–20% will be troubled by continuous symptoms that occur without remission.

The initial and most common symptom of ulcerative colitis is rectal bleeding. This initial bleeding is often mistaken for bleeding from hemorrhoids. Indeed, this first evidence of blood may follow a bout of constipation, which can sometimes be the presenting complaint. When constipation is the presenting complaint, the colitis is most often associated with disease limited to the rectum, where spasm prevents feces from entering the area involved.

Diarrhea occurs with more extensive colonic involvement, and blood is usually mixed with the feces. The principal mechanism responsible for diarrhea in ulcerative colitis is exudation with resultant secretion of interstitial fluids and loss of mucosal surface area for absorbing water and electrolytes. In addition, involvement of the rectum prevents this segment of the colon from acting as a reservoir for fecal contents prior to defecation. This rectal irritability causes frequent urgent bowel evacuation of minute amounts of blood and mucus, an activity that is termed "urgency."

Since the severity of the disease will affect the therapeutic approach and, indeed, the prognostic implications, it is important for the physician to assess the severity of the disease for every patient. The best indices of severity are clinical signs and symptoms. Large volumes of diarrhea indicate that the colonic mucosa has been involved to the extent that water and electrolyte absorption are significantly impaired. Frequency, however, is an unreliable indicator of severity because frequent bowel movements can indicate either large-volume diarrhea due to extensive disease or rectal irritability due to limited rectal disease. Large quantities of blood in the stools, a fallen hemoglobin concentration, and hypoalbuminemia as a consequence of loss of albumin into the stool are signs of extensive disease. Elevated erythrocyte sedimentation rate, fever, and abdominal pain and tenderness may point to transmural extension of the disease and the development of severe ulcerative colitis.

Ulcerative colitis can be classified according to grade of clinical severity:

1. *Severe.* Diarrhea comprising six or more movements per day, macroscopic blood in the stools, fever, tachycardia greater than 90/min, anemia and an elevated erythrocyte sedimentation rate.

2. *Moderate.* Diarrhea comprising four or fewer movements per day, small amounts of macroscopic blood in stools, no fever, no tachycardia, mild anemia and a minimally elevated erythrocyte sedimentation rate.

3. *Mild.* Diarrhea comprising fewer than four bowel movements per day without anemia, fever, tachycardia, weight loss or hypoalbuminemia.

2.2.1 *SEVERE ULCERATIVE COLITIS*

Severe ulcerative colitis, the least common form of the disease, occurs in 15% of all patients with ulcerative colitis. This form of the disease may be the initial presentation or may represent a progression from a less severe attack. Diarrhea is profuse and rectal bleeding is constant and severe. Fever is marked and sustained, and appetite and weight are both severely diminished. Abdominal cramps are severe and tenderness may be localized, indicating impending perforation. Leukocytes greater than 10,000, severe anemia, and hypoalbuminemia resulting from low protein intake (anorexia) and increased chronic loss of albumin are hallmarks of this form of the disease.

Medical therapy is often ineffective for this type of patient, and colectomy is often required.

2.2.2 *MODERATE ULCERATIVE COLITIS*

Moderate ulcerative colitis affects 25% of all patients with ulcerative colitis. Diarrhea is the major symptom, and it occurs three to four times per day. Invariably, the diarrhea contains macroscopic amounts of blood. Abdominal pain may occur and may awaken the patient at night; usually the cramps are relieved by defecation. Low-grade fever may exist, and the patient may complain of fatigue, anorexia and some mild weight loss.

Generally, moderate ulcerative colitis responds quickly to appropriate therapy. Immediate mortality in this group is low. However, at any time during the moderate attack of ulcerative colitis, the patient may become severely ill, developing a severe colitis characterized by high fever, profuse diarrhea, progressive dilation of the colon (toxic megacolon) and rapid deterioration.

2.2.3 *MILD ULCERATIVE COLITIS*

Mild ulcerative colitis is the most common form of the disease, occurring in 60% of patients. In 80% of those affected with mild disease, the ulcerative colitis will be limited to the distal colon (sigmoid and rectum); in the other 20% the whole colon will be involved. The age, sex and familial incidence of ulcerative colitis are the same for mild disease as for severe disease. As well, the number of patients who have only one attack, intermittent attacks, or continuous disease is the same for both mild and severe ulcerative colitis.

In the case of mild disease limited to the rectal sigmoid, most often the disease will remain in this area; however, in 10% of these patients it will eventually involve the entire colon and bring about the simultaneous development of severe diarrhea and bleeding.

Neither colonic bleeding nor diarrhea is severe in mild ulcerative colitis, and the systemic complications of anorexia, weight loss and fatigue are not seen. Occasionally, the patient may suffer from a few days of crampy lower abdominal pain; however, hospitalization is usually not required and mild ulcerative colitis responds rapidly to therapy.

For patients who have mild ulcerative colitis, particularly proctosigmoiditis, the rate of colonic cancer is similar to that of control populations. Thus, colonic cancer occurs in mild cases of ulcerative colitis only one-fifth as often as in the more severe forms of the disease.

2.3 Diagnosis

The diagnosis of ulcerative colitis is made on the basis of the clinical symptoms listed above, on physical findings, and on the results of laboratory and endoscopic investigations.

2.3.1 PHYSICAL EXAMINATION

Physical examination during mild ulcerative colitis or between attacks may yield completely normal findings. In contrast to Crohn's disease, there are no palpable masses and no specific areas of tenderness, unless serosal involvement, peritoneal irritation or impending perforation (toxic megacolon) exists. Auscultation of the abdomen may reveal increased bowel sounds and audible borborygmi. With toxic megacolon, bowel sounds are quiet or absent.

Rectal examination is usually painful and the anal sphincter is often spastic. The examiner may be able to detect gritty, coarse, granular changes in the rectal mucosa on digital palpation. Pseudopolyps may also be palpated, and a rectal stricture may be detected. In addition, it may be possible to feel a carcinoma. Rectal and perianal complications are far less frequent and destructive than in Crohn's disease and ordinarily consist only of minor fissures.

Examination of the skin and joints may confirm extracolonic complications (uveitis, stomatitis, pyoderma gangrenosum, erythema nodosum, large-joint arthritis, ankylosing spondylitis).

2.3.2 LABORATORY INVESTIGATIONS

There is no single laboratory test that will confirm ulcerative colitis. Anemia, leukocytosis and an elevated erythrocyte sedimentation rate often reflect the severity of the disease. Iron studies reflect iron deficiency anemia (low serum iron, high TIBC, low ferritin). Electrolyte abnormalities including hypokale-

TABLE 9. Endoscopic grading of activity in ulcerative colitis

Activity	Appearance
Quiescent	Distorted or absent mucosal vascular pattern Granularity
Mildly active	Continuous or focal erythema Friability (touch bleeding)
Moderately active	Mucopurulent exudate (mucopus) Single or multiple ulcers (<5 mm); fewer than 10 per 10 cm segment
Severe	Large ulcers (>5 mm); more than 10 per 10 cm segment Spontaneous bleeding

mia, metabolic acidosis, hypocalcemia, hypomagnesemia and/or hypoalbu-minemia may exist in patients with severe diarrhea. Liver function studies may demonstrate an elevated alkaline phosphatase as a manifestation of sclerosing cholangitis. Blood cultures may be positive in patients with toxic megacolon.

Examination of the stool will reveal abundant red and white blood cells as a consequence of denudation of the colonic mucosa and bleeding into the lumen of multiple small submucosal blood vessels. Stool cultures for Shigella, Campylobacter, Salmonella, Clostridium difficile (culture and toxin), E. coli 0157 and Entamoeba histolytica should be done in all cases to exclude the possibility of infectious colitis.

2.3.3 ENDOSCOPIC FINDINGS

The most useful method of establishing a diagnosis of ulcerative colitis is to assess the integrity of the mucosa directly. Since 97% of people with ulcerative colitis have involvement of the rectum, a simple sigmoidoscopy can be used to establish the diagnosis in the majority of cases.

The normal colonic mucosa is a smooth, flat and glistening, pink surface. Seen underneath this smooth surface are the ramifying superficial submucosal blood vessels, which present a prominent vascular pattern. When brushed by a cotton swab, the normal colonic mucosa does not bleed because the mucosa is not friable.

Endoscopic examination of inactive or quiescent ulcerative colitis shows a distorted or absent mucosal vascular pattern with a mild granularity (Table 9). Granularity results when the mucosa becomes edematous and little mounds of swollen tissue surround the crypts, creating an uneven surface. Light from the

TABLE 10.   Inflammatory bowel disease: indications for colonoscopy

---

Differentiating IBD from other diseases and differentiating Crohn's from ulcerative colitis

Establishing the extent of the disease and any complications (fistula, strictures)

Evaluation of abnormalities on radiographs
Strictures
Masses

Evaluation of disease not responsive to standard therapy

Therapeutic applications
Bleeding control
Dilation of strictures
Obtaining biopsies

Screening for malignancy and malignant precursors

---

endoscope reflects off the uneven surface as numerous small spots of light (creating an impression of granularity) rather than large sheets of light (creating a glistening surface). Mildly active disease shows continuous or focal erythema and friability, with the inflamed mucosa bleeding easily when touched with the endoscope or a cotton swab (touch friability). Moderately active disease displays in addition to the findings of mild disease mucopurulent exudate (mucopus) and ulcers less than 5 mm in diameter and fewer than 10 per 10 cm segment. Severe colitis demonstrates ulcers larger than 5 mm and more than 10 per 10 cm segment; these ulcers are often accompanied by spontaneous bleeding.

Although colonoscopy is rarely necessary in diagnosing a new case of ulcerative colitis, some form of endoscopic procedure is essential to distinguish ulcerative proctitis/colitis from other causes of rectal bleeding. The rectal and distal sigmoid mucosa is almost always involved in cases of ulcerative colitis, and a carefully performed sigmoidoscopy with either a rigid or flexible instrument can usually lead to the correct diagnosis. While a limited sigmoidoscopy is generally safe, a full colonoscopy should be very cautiously considered in the case of acute, moderately severe or severe ulcerative colitis because of the risk of perforation during the procedure itself.

Colonoscopy for ulcerative colitis is, therefore, performed for specific indications only. These are (1) to determine the extent and/or activity of the disease; (2) to perform cancer surveillance or diagnosis; and (3) to determine the type of inflammatory disease, whether ulcerative colitis or Crohn's disease (Table 10).

In addition to its role in diagnosis, endoscopy also has an important function in the assessment of disease extent and in defining the severity of inflammation. Endoscopy and biopsy for histologic assessment are much more sensitive then radiographic contrast studies in defining the margins of inflammation, and thus the extent of disease. Knowing the extent of ulcerative colitis is important since both treatment and surveillance strategies will differ depending upon whether the disease is limited to the rectum or to the left side of the colon, or whether it involves the entire colon.

2.3.4 RADIOLOGIC FINDINGS

A plain film of the abdomen should always be obtained, particularly with severe colitis, where the risk of toxic megacolon exists. The plain film may demonstrate foreshortening or loss of haustration; sufficient air in a segment of colon to silhouette the mucosa may reveal irregular mucosa, ulceration and mucosal tags. Patients with toxic megacolon will have mid-transverse colon dilation to a diameter of 6 cm or more.

An air contrast barium enema examination can be used for the same indications as for colonoscopy: to determine disease extent and/or activity, examine for cancer, or differentiate from Crohn's disease. However, it must be remembered that a barium enema is less sensitive than endoscopy and can underestimate disease extent and activity by over 70%. Furthermore, biopsy and histological assessment as critical tools in the diagnosis and differential diagnosis are not possible with the barium enema. During the active disease phase, the colonic preparation, and even the barium enema itself, may precipitate a toxic megacolon. It is therefore prudent to delay the barium enema examination until the disease has been brought under medical control.

Radiologic features vary according to the location and state of the disease. There may be a loss of haustration on the left side of the colon (this can be the normal appearance of the colon in elderly patients) (Figure 8). Additionally, the radiolucent filling defects of pseudopolyps may be seen scattered throughout the colon.

2.4 Differential Diagnosis

The disorder from which ulcerative colitis needs to be distinguished is Crohn's disease of the colon. In addition, a host of other diseases may resemble ulcerative colitis. The possibility of these diseases must also be excluded (Table 11).

Clinical features useful in distinguishing between ulcerative colitis and Crohn's colitis are illustrated in Table 12. It is important to note that, because of the anatomic distribution of ulcerative colitis, proctosigmoidoscopic examination is abnormal in virtually all cases. By contrast, even when Crohn's disease affects the colon, it often does not involve the rectum. In addition, perianal disease is much more characteristic of Crohn's disease. Although diar-

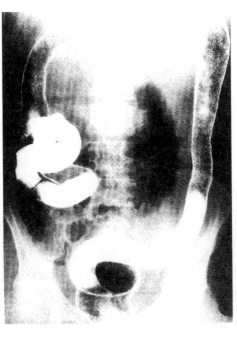

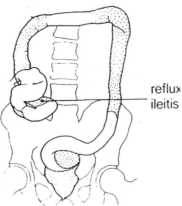

reflux
ileitis

FIGURE 8. "Instant" double-contrast barium enema in total ulcerative colitis. The distal ileum is dilated with a granular surface indicating reflux or "backwash" ileitis.

rhea and weight loss occur with approximately equal frequency in both diseases, abdominal pain is more evident with Crohn's disease. Extraintestinal manifestations occur in about the same proportion with both diseases.

TABLE 11.   Differential diagnosis of ulcerative colitis

Infectious
  Viral
    Cytomegalovirus
    Herpes

  Bacterial
    Salmonella species
    Shigella species
    Yersinia enterocolitica
    Vibrio parahaemolyticus
    Aeromonas hydrophila
    Neisseria gonorrhoeae
    Chlamydia trachomatis
    Syphilis
    Staphylococcus aureus
    Escherichia coli

  Protozoan
    Amebiasis
    Balantidiasis
    Schistosomiasis

  Fungal
    Histoplasmosis
    Candidiasis

  Other
    Clostridium difficile

Radiation colitis

Crohn's colitis

Medication/drugs
    Enemas
    Laxatives
    Nonsteroidal anti-inflammatory drugs
    Penicillamine
    Gold
    Methyldopa

Eosinophilic gastroenteritis

Behçet's syndrome

Colitis in graft-versus-host disease

TABLE 12. Clinical differentiation of ulcerative colitis from Crohn's colitis

Feature	Ulcerative colitis	Crohn's colitis
Clinical features		
Rectal bleeding	Very common – 90%	Uncommon: may be occult
Diarrhea	Early, frequent, small stools	Less prevalent or absent
Abdominal pain	Predefecatory, urgency	Colicky, postprandial
Fever	Uncommon if uncomplicated	Frequent
Palpable mass	Rare	Frequent, right lower quadrant
Recurrence after resection	Never	Frequent
Clinical course	Relapses/remissions 65%	Usually slowly progressive
	Chronic/continuous 20–30%	
	Acute/fulminating 5–8%	
Endoscopic features		
Proctosigmoidoscopy	Diffuse pinpoint ulcerations, continuous lesions	Discrete aphthoid ulcerations, patchy lesions
Radiologic features		
Rectal involvement	Frequent	Infrequent
Distribution	Continuous	Segmental, discontinuous
Mucosa	Fine ulcerations	"Cobblestones"
Strictures	Rare	Frequent
Fistulas	Rare	Frequent
Histologic features		
Distribution	Mucosal	Transmural
Cellular infiltrate	Polymorphs	Lymphocytes
Glands	Mucin depletion	Gland preservation
	Gland destruction	
	Crypt abscesses	
Special features	None	Granulomas, aphthoid ulcers

2.5 Complications

Ulcerative colitis may be complicated by a variety of associated conditions. These are (1) local complications arising in and around the colon, and (2) extraintestinal complications arising at sites distant from the colon (Table 13).

2.5.1 *LOCAL COMPLICATIONS*

2.5.1.1 *Perianal disease*

Perianal disease is much less common in ulcerative colitis then it is in Crohn's disease. Fissures occur more commonly; however, fistula and abscesses are rarely seen.

TABLE 13.   Complications of ulcerative colitis

Local complications	Frequency (%)
Minor	
Hemorrhoids	20
Pseudopolyps	15
Anal fissures	12
Anal fistulas	5
Perianal abscess	5
Rectal prolapse	2
Rectovaginal fistulas	2
Major	
Toxic megacolon	2
Colonic perforation	3
Massive colonic hemorrhage	4
Colonic carcinoma	5
Colonic stricture	5

Extraintestinal complications	Frequency (%)
Hepatic	
Biliary	
Pericholangitis	30
Sclerosing cholangitis	1
Hepatocellular	
Fatty infiltration	30
Chronic active hepatitis	5
Cirrhosis	3
Amyloidosis	1
Hematologic	
Anemia	15
Iron deficiency	5
Autoimmune hemolytic anemia	1
Microangiopathic hemolytic anemia	<1
Heinz-body hemolytic anemia	
(with sulfasalazine therapy)	<1
Thrombocytosis	20
Thromboembolic disease	2
Joint	
Peripheral arthritis, migratory, nondeforming, large-joint,	
seronegative	20
Ankylosing spondylitis, sacroiliitis	20

(cont'd)

TABLE 13.   Complications of ulcerative colitis (cont'd)

Extraintestinal complications	Frequency (%)
Skin	
Erythema nodosum	3
Pyoderma gangrenosum	4
Ocular	
Episcleritis, uveitis	5
Iritis	5

TABLE 14.   Diagnosis of toxic megacolon

Signs of toxicity (three of the following criteria are required)
Fever >38.6°C
Tachycardia >120 beats per minute
Leukocytosis >10,000/mm^3
Anemia <60% of normal
Hypoalbuminemia <3 g/dL

Associated signs (one of the following criteria is required)
Dehydration
Mental confusion
Hypotension
Electrolyte disturbance

Signs of dilation
Colonic diameter >6 cm or progressive distention with abnormal haustral pattern

2.5.1.2 *Toxic megacolon*

Toxic megacolon is characterized by an acute dilation of all or part of the colon to a diameter greater than 6 cm (measured in the mid-transverse colon) and is associated with severe systemic toxicity. Toxic megacolon occurs in 1–2% of patients with ulcerative colitis. Histological examination reveals extensive deep ulcerations and acute inflammation that involves all muscle layers of the colon and often extends to the serosa. This widespread inflammation accounts for toxic megacolon's systemic toxicity (fever, tachycardia, localized abdominal pain and leukocytosis). The loss of colonic muscular tone results in the dilation of the colon.

Though the association between a barium enema and toxic megacolon has not been experimentally proven, there are many reports of toxic megacolon developing after the patient has undergone a barium enema. Thus, a barium enema should not be performed on patients who are acutely ill with ulcerative colitis.

Clinically, the patient with toxic megacolon presents as severely ill with a fever, tachycardia, dehydration, abdominal pain and distention (Table 14). Examination reveals absent bowel sounds, tympany and rebound tenderness. Leukocytosis (greater than 10,000), anemia and hypoalbuminemia are often present. A plain x-ray of the abdomen will reveal dilation of a colonic segment or of the entire colon. On plain supine x-ray, dilation of the transverse colon is most often seen. This distention of the transverse colon does not indicate severity of disease in this segment of the colon; rather, the distention is determined by the anterior position of the transverse colon. Repositioning the patient to a prone position will redistribute the gas to the more posterior descending colon and will dramatically decrease gaseous tension in the transverse colon.

If toxic megacolon is the presenting symptom of ulcerative colitis, diagnosis may be difficult, since a history of rectal bleeding and diarrhea is sometimes obscured by toxic megacolon. Most often, toxic megacolon complicates chronic intermittent ulcerative colitis and the diagnosis is not difficult. Occasionally, however, a patient seriously ill with ulcerative colitis and the resultant profuse bloody diarrhea will experience a sudden decrease in the frequency of bowel motions upon development of toxic megacolon. This decrease in stool frequency represents diminished colonic evacuation rather than improvement in the patient's status. In this instance, a delay in diagnosis could result in perforation and death.

Treatment of toxic megacolon consists of general supportive measures, including replacement of fluid and electrolyte deficits, correction of hypokalemia, transfusions and nasogastric suction. Intravenous steroids (prednisone equivalent 60–80 mg/day) should be utilized for 48 to 72 hours. If there is insufficient response, surgery should be seriously considered. If the systemic symptoms subside and the abdominal signs improve, high-dose steroids should be continued for 10 to 14 days, after which the dose should be gradually tapered off.

Patients whose disease does not respond to appropriate intensive medical therapy within three days have a risk of colonic perforation of 50%. Mortality in the face of recognized or unrecognized perforation is approximately 85%; thus, surgery should be considered at an early stage rather than at a later.

2.5.1.3 *Cancer of the colon*
Carcinoma of the colon afflicts patients with ulcerative colitis 7 to 30 times more frequently than it does the general population. The risk of colon cancer

in ulcerative colitis is related to two factors: (1) duration of the colitis, and (2) extent of colonic involvement. The risk of colon cancer for patients who have had the disease less than 10 years is low, but this risk steadily increases. The cancer risk for patients who have had disease activity for 10 to 20 years is 15 times that of the general population, while a disease duration of more than 20 years is associated with a cancer risk 30 times greater than that of the general population. The extent of colonic involvement in colitis also influences the risk of cancer. The incidence of cancer when ulcerative colitis is limited to the rectum or to the left side of the colon is much lower than when ulcerative colitis involves the entire colon.

The colonic malignancy associated with ulcerative colitis is generally an adenocarcinoma evenly scattered throughout the colon. The adenocarcinoma is often flatter than cancers in the general population and has fewer overhanging margins. It is generally considered extremely aggressive.

Because of this high cumulative risk of cancer, prophylactic diagnostic procedures have been employed in an attempt to detect early malignant changes in the colon of patients with ulcerative colitis. Colonoscopy and biopsy have revealed that colorectal dysplasia is associated with the later development of colonic malignancy. Thus, colonoscopy and biopsies for assessment of dysplasia have become the "gold standard" for surveillance of colon cancer in patients with longstanding ulcerative colitis. Dysplasia is a pathological condition marked by nuclear striation and loss of nuclear and cellular pleomorphism, and appears to be premalignant. However, areas of dysplasia can be missed at the time of biopsy, and the interpretation of dysplasia in the presence of active inflammatory disease is difficult, since regenerative epithelium may exhibit many of the features of dysplasia.

In summary, no test or group of diagnostic tests (not even frequent colonoscopies and biopsies) can absolutely guarantee that the patient with long-term ulcerative colitis is free of focal malignancy.

Patients with ulcerative colitis should have a colonoscopy and multiple biopsies performed after 15 years of disease. If no dysplasia is revealed by multiple colonic biopsies, repeat colonoscopy can be performed every 2 years thereafter. If low-grade dysplasia is persistently found on multiple colonoscopies or if a single colonoscopy reveals high-grade dysplasia, then it is reasonable to approach the patient to discuss a total colectomy as a surgical option.

2.5.1.4 Colonic stricture

Colonic stricture occurs infrequently but may mimic colonic adenocarcinoma clinically and radiologically. If there is any question regarding the diagnosis, surgical removal is advocated.

2.5.2 *EXTRAINTESTINAL COMPLICATIONS*

2.5.2.1 *Hepatocellular disease*

The hepatic complications of ulcerative colitis are uncommon and include fatty liver, chronic active hepatitis and cirrhosis. The biliary tract complications, which are more common, are sclerosing cholangitis and pericholangitis.

Pericholangitis is seen in 30% of patients with ulcerative colitis. It tends to occur more often in patients with pancolitis than in those with ulcerative colitis limited to the distal colon. The diagnosis is made on liver biopsy with the liver lesion characterized by periportal inflammatory infiltrates, degenerative changes in bile ductules, and varying degrees of periportal edema and fibrosis. The lesion of pericholangitis is patchy; therefore, sampling error on needle biopsy of the liver often occurs. Clinical manifestations of pericholangitis or its progression to cirrhosis are exceedingly rare, and many patients are asymptomatic and have only minor abnormalities in serum alkaline phosphatase.

Sclerosing cholangitis develops in 1% of patients with ulcerative colitis. In this disorder, the bile duct becomes severely narrowed and resultant recurrent attacks of jaundice, right upper quadrant pain, fever and leukocytosis occur. Bile duct strictures are a major problem in sclerosing cholangitis. These strictures can occur in both intrahepatic bile ducts (not amenable to endoscopic dilation) and extrahepatic bile ducts (potentially amenable to endoscopic dilation). This lesion must be distinguished from other causes of obstruction of the common bile duct. Sclerosing cholangitis does not respond to any therapy.

Fatty infiltration of the liver is seen in 30% of patients with ulcerative colitis. The etiology of the fat deposition is unknown, but it may be due to malnutrition and protein depletion resulting from diarrhea and protein-losing enteropathy. Liver function studies are normal or only mildly abnormal in patients with fatty infiltration.

2.5.2.2 *Hematologic abnormalities*

The most common hematologic abnormality in ulcerative colitis is iron deficiency anemia secondary to gastrointestinal blood loss. Most often this can be treated with oral ferrous sulfate (300 mg t.i.d.). However, for some patients, gastrointestinal intolerance of ferrous sulfate will necessitate parenteral iron injections (Imferon®).

Heinz-body hemolytic anemia can be seen in patients receiving sulfasalazine. This type of hemolytic anemia is directly related to the sulfasalazine and resolves when the offending agent is withdrawn. Additionally, autoimmune hemolytic anemia and microangiopathic hemolytic anemia, with or without disseminated intravascular coagulation, can occur.

Secondary thrombocytosis may appear. It is not associated with coagulation defects. However, in addition to thrombocytosis, increased levels of factors V and VIII and fibrinogen can be seen, together with reductions in levels of antithrombin III. In rare instances, pulmonary embolism and thrombosis of mesenteric or cranial vessels due to thromboembolic disease can occur. Repeated pulmonary embolisms in spite of adequate anticoagulation therapy or massive colonic hemorrhage during anticoagulation therapy will necessitate a vena cava ligation with colectomy.

2.5.2.3 *Joint manifestations*
The joint manifestations of ulcerative colitis are similar to those of Crohn's disease. The large-joint migratory arthritis tends to occur when the colonic disease is active and responds to the treatment of the colonic inflammation. The inflammatory activity of the sacroiliitis and ankylosing spondylitis does not follow the activity of the bowel disease.

The arthritis of ulcerative colitis may antedate the colonic symptoms. It tends to be migratory and affect the larger joints, is associated with a synovitis and swollen painful joints, and is nondeforming with no involvement of adjacent cartilage or bone. Rheumatoid factors are negative in these patients.

There is a 30-fold increase in the incidence of ankylosing spondylitis in patients with ulcerative colitis. Unlike peripheral arthritis, the ankylosing spondylitis in ulcerative colitis is chronic, progressive, deforming and generalized. It does not respond to corticosteroids and will progress in the face of quiescent colitis. The incidence of sacroiliitis is higher than that of ankylosing spondylitis in patients with ulcerative colitis. However, the sacroiliitis is often asymptomatic and can be identified only through appropriate x-rays of the pelvis.

2.5.2.4 *Skin manifestations*
Erythema nodosum with raised tender erythematous swellings on the extensor surfaces of the legs and arms is less frequent with ulcerative colitis than with Crohn's disease.

Pyoderma gangrenosum complicates severe ulcerative colitis but is rarely seen with mild disease. This skin lesion begins as a small, elevated nodule, which gradually becomes gangrenous, thus resulting in progressive necrosis of the surrounding skin. It tends to ulcerate deeply, involving underlying soft tissue and sometimes bone.

Usually both erythema nodosum and pyoderma gangrenosum will respond to control of the colitis. Occasionally, despite control of the colonic disease, the pyoderma gangrenosum will progress. Persistent severe pyoderma gangrenosum is thus an indication for colectomy.

2.5.2.5 *Ocular manifestations*

Iritis occurs in 5% of patients with ulcerative colitis and presents as blurred vision, eye pain and photophobia. The attack may be followed by atrophy of the iris, anterior and posterior synechiae, and pigment deposits on the lens. Episcleritis is only rarely seen with ulcerative colitis.

2.6 Therapy

2.6.1 *HOSPITALIZATION*

Hospitalization is indicated for the following reasons:

1. Severe illness with anorexia, nausea, vomiting, fever and uncontrollable bloody diarrhea (severe ulcerative colitis). Early hospitalization is critical for such patients so that they may be provided with therapy to control the disease and prevent complications, especially toxic megacolon.
2. Development of local or systemic complications including massive hemorrhage, persistent anemia, severe hypoalbuminemia, and/or cancer. Hospitalization at this time provides for assessment of the need for surgical therapy.

2.6.2 *SUPPORTIVE THERAPY*

Supportive therapy consists of medications that improve the patient's general state of health or alleviate symptoms. Chronic losses of potassium, sodium and water must be replaced with oral and/or intravenous fluids, since uncorrected fluid and electrolyte deficits have been implicated in the development of toxic megacolon and renal calculi. Blood loss due to severe disease should be replaced with transfusions. With mild disease, oral iron replacement is indicated. The use of antidiarrheal agents – e.g., diphenoxylate (Lomotil®) or loperamide (Imodium®) – for patients with ulcerative colitis is generally contraindicated. In severe disease where the colonic mucosa is severely damaged, antidiarrheal agents are generally ineffective, since there is a loss of absorbing capacity. Furthermore, they may contribute to the development of toxic megacolon. Similarly, anticholinergics can also precipitate toxic megacolon and thus should not be prescribed for patients with ulcerative colitis.

2.6.3 *NUTRITIONAL THERAPY*

Neither total parenteral nutrition nor enteral nutrition has yet been shown to have any beneficial effect in inducing remission of ulcerative colitis.

2.6.4 *MEDICAL THERAPY*

2.6.4.1 *Acute ulcerative colitis therapy*

2.6.4.1.1 *Mesalamine derivatives* Mesalamine (5-aminosalicylic acid mesalazine, or 5-ASA) has been shown to be effective in the treatment of acute active mild to moderate disease and in maintenance therapy to prevent relapse.

Mesalamine (5-ASA) rectal preparations During the past several years mesalamine has been developed in the form of rectal enemas and suppositories. Mesalamine enemas have an overall efficacy of about 80% in patients with active left-sided colitis. Side effects occur in less than 2% of ulcerative colitis patients, many of whom would have had previous allergic reactions to sulfasalazine. In comparison studies, mesalamine enemas are as effective as corticosteroid enemas in the treatment of proctitis and proctosigmoiditis [10]. In patients with distal proctitis, mesalamine suppositories (500 mg b.i.d.) are rapidly effective without side effects [11].

The rectum is invariably involved early in the disease and is the last segment to heal. Since the rectum is important as a reservoir, the use of rectal preparations in ulcerative colitis to preferentially heal this area is critical in providing patients with early and rapid symptomatic relief of their urgency and frequency. Thus it is appropriate to combine a rectal mesalamine preparation along with a systemic mesalamine or corticosteroid therapy. The rectal preparation can usually be stopped once the disease is in remission.

Mesalamine (5-ASA) oral preparations Mesalamine is available as sulfasalazine (Salazopyrin®) or as second-generation products that deliver the active ingredient to the colon without the toxic sulfapyridine moiety (Asacol®, Dipentum®, Mesasal™, Pentasa®, Salofalk®) (Table 8).

Sulfasalazine is metabolized by colonic flora, thus releasing sulfapyridine, an absorbable antibiotic, and mesalamine, the active ingredient. The sulfapyridine acts only to carry the mesalamine to the colon and, when released by bacterial metabolism, it is absorbed and is responsible for the dose-related side effects of sulfasalazine. The acetylation rate of sulfapyridine is genetically determined; slow acetylators develop side effects at lower dose levels of sulfasalazine than fast acetylators. The most common dose-related symptoms are anorexia, nausea, dyspepsia and diarrhea. Common hematological complications include impairment of folate absorption (thus supplemental folate therapy is a requirement for all patients on sulfasalazine) and Heinz-body hemolytic anemia. Hypospermia may occur and is reversible through withdrawal of the drug. Hypersensitivity reactions are rare; symptoms include fever, rash, bone marrow suppression, infiltrative lung disease, a lupus-like syndrome, pancreatitis and hepatic toxicity.

The two main pharmacological approaches of the second-generation mesalamine compounds adopted are (1) the creation of azo-derivative compounds similar to sulfasalazine but linked with mesalamine through a diazo-bond with another mesalamine molecule (olsalazine, as in Dipentum®); and (2) the incorporation of mesalamine either into pH-dependent delivery capsules such as Asacol® (pH 7.0) or Mesasal™ and Salofalk® (pH 6.0), or into a mixed slow-release pH-dependent polymer (Pentasa®). These second-generation compounds have shown comparable efficacy to sulfasalazine, with generally fewer side effects [12]. Comparative studies assessing which compound might favor a higher mesalamine release into the colon and thus would be more suitable for patients with colonic inflammation are yet to be finalized. Comparison of mesalamine product dose and cost is presented in Table 8.

For mild to moderate active ulcerative colitis a patient should be started on oral mesalamine 4–6 g/day (along with an enema preparation if urgency is a prominent feature), with the expectation that the disease will gradually come under control within one to two weeks. If the disease has not come under control within this time the addition of an oral corticosteroid will usually be required. Once the disease is under control the corticosteroid is withdrawn as per the tapering protocol in Section 2.6.4.1.2, and the mesalamine is continued at 4–6 g/day for an additional two months before it is changed to its maintenance dose schedule (Section 2.6.4.2).

2.6.4.1.2 *Corticosteroids*   Corticosteroids should be used only to treat acute active moderate to severe ulcerative colitis, as they have no role in maintenance treatment to prevent relapse. The dosage and routes of administration vary with the severity and location of ulcerative colitis.

Rectal corticosteroid preparations   These are available in enema formulations as hydrocortisone 100 mg in a 60 mL aqueous suspension (Cortenema®) and as budenoside (a first-pass metabolized steroid) 2 mg in 100 mL aqueous suspension (Entocort®), in foam formulation as hydrocortisone acetate 80 mg in a propylene glycol gel (Cortifoam®), and in ointment formulation as hydrocortisone acetate 10 mg or 40 mg in an ointment base (Cortiment®). In general, enema preparations will cover a larger surface area of the colon, while the effect of foam and ointment preparations is generally limited to the rectum. With mild disease, especially that of the distal colon, rectal instillation of steroids will induce or maintain remission for a high percentage of patients.

With mild to moderately severe ulcerative proctitis, once-daily rectal steroids combined with systemic therapy will promote remission and more quickly return the rectum to its normal functional reservoir capacity. Patients should instill the solution while in the left lateral decubitus position and then change their position to right decubitus followed by prone for at least 20 minutes after each position, to allow for maximal topical coverage. Studies indicate that up to one-half of rectally administered steroids is absorbed.

Systemic corticosteroid preparations   In active pancolonic disease of mild to moderate severity, prednisone should be started in a dose of 40 mg/day. For patients whose disease responds promptly to oral steroids, withdrawal should be undertaken at 5 mg/week until a dose of 20 mg/day is reached; then the drug should be tapered by 2.5 mg/week to off. In the case of severe ulcerative colitis, the patient requires hospitalization, and intravenous steroids (prednisone 40 mg equivalent/day) should be started. Once the acute colitis is under control with intravenous corticosteroids, the patient can be switched to oral prednisone and the above tapering protocol followed.

Once the disease is in remission, further steroid treatment should be avoided until a subsequent exacerbation occurs. Treatment is then reinstituted at a level appropriate to the severity of exacerbation (steroid enemas for mild to moderate exacerbations of proctosigmoiditis, oral or intravenous steroids for moderate to severe pancolonic relapses). If, however, symptoms recur with the attempted withdrawal of steroids (steroid dependency), then long-term steroid therapy may be necessary until the patient experiences remission. The routine use of steroids as maintainance therapy is not recommended in view of the potential side effects of steroid therapy. If a patient requires more than 10–15 mg of oral prednisone daily for many months in order to keep the colitis in control, elective colectomy should be considered as an alternative means of treatment.

Steroids, particularly steroids in the high doses necessary for severe cases, may "mask" a perforation of the colon and lead to peritoneal soiling and death; therefore, careful monitoring of the patient on such high doses is vitally important.

2.6.4.1.3 *Antibiotics*   Unlike Crohn's disease, ulcerative colitis does not, in general, respond well to the use of antibiotics. While some experts will combine metronidazole with mesalamine, this has not been studied in control trials.

2.6.4.1.4 *Immunosuppressive agents*   Immunosuppressive drugs play a smaller role in the management of ulcerative colitis than in Crohn's disease.

These agents can be used in ulcerative colitis to achieve the same corticosteroid-sparing effects as have been described for Crohn's disease; however, the short- and long-term morbidity of these drugs must be compared with that of a curative colectomy. High doses of intravenous cyclosporine (10–15 mg/kg/day) have been shown effective in improving severe ulcerative colitis that might otherwise have gone to surgery. However, once the cyclosporine is stopped, the vast majority of these patients relapse and end up requiring surgical therapy (colectomy). In this regard, cyclosporine may be useful as a temporary measure in patients who are not psychologically ready for a total colectomy. Since ulcerative colitis is curable with a colectomy, the majority of experts would not use immunosuppressive agents in the treatment of ulcerative colitis over the long term because of their significant side effects.

2.6.4.2 Maintenance therapy

In contrast to Crohn's disease, there is simple and effective maintenance therapy for ulcerative colitis. Once remission has been induced by either corticosteroid or mesalamine therapy, the risk of ulcerative colitis relapse can be reduced from 60% to approximately 20% with maintenance mesalamine therapy at approximately one-half (2 g/day) the acute active disease dose. There is no role for long-term corticosteroids or immunosuppressives in maintenance therapy in ulcerative colitis.

2.6.4.3 Surgical therapy

Twenty to 25% of patients with extensive ulcerative colitis eventually undergo colectomy, usually because their disease has not responded to medical therapy. The decision between surgery and continued medical therapy is often not clear-cut, and in many cases arguments can be made for either course. In ulcerative colitis, colectomy is a "curative" procedure, in contrast to Crohn's disease, in which there is a significant likelihood of recurrence some time after the colectomy. The development of the ileoanal anastomosis, eliminating the need for an ileostomy, has made the thought of colectomy more tolerable for many. In general, patients who require continuous high-dose corticosteroids and/or immunosuppressants to keep their disease under control should be strongly advised to consider colectomy.

The standard operation for ulcerative colitis is a proctocolectomy and Brooke ileostomy. A recent alternative to the Brooke ileostomy has been the development of an operation that establishes an ileoanal anastomosis. In this procedure the colon is removed completely, with the mucosa and submucosa of the rectum dissected from the muscularis. The mucosa and submucosa are removed and the muscularis, including the internal and external sphincters, is left in place. A pouch is then constructed from the terminal 30 cm of ileum. The distal end of the pouch is pulled through the anal canal and the ileal mucosa is sewn to the dentate line to create an ileoanal anastomosis with an ileal pouch. The advantage of this procedure is that the patient has no ostomy and no appliance. For several months after the creation of an ileoanal anastomosis the patient will have numerous bowel motions; however, these gradually decline over time and the majority of patients have continence and fewer than three to four bowel motions daily. The results are relatively better for patients younger than 50 years of age.

REFERENCES

1. Mayer L, Eisenhardt D. Lack of induction of suppressor T-cells by intestinal epithelial cells from patients with inflammatory bowel disease. J Clin Invest 1990; 86:1255–1260.
2. Saxon A, Shanahan F, Landers C, Ganz T, Targan S. A distinct subset of antineutrophil cytoplasmic antibodies is associated with inflammatory bowel disease. J Allergy Clin Immunol 1990; 86:202–210.
3. Gitnick G. Etiology of inflammatory bowel disease: Where have we been? Where are we going? Scand J Gastroenterol 1990; 25(Suppl 175):93–96.
4. Das KM, Vecchi M, Sakamaki S. A shared and unique epitope(s) on human colon, skin, and biliary epithelium detected by a monoclonal antibody. Gastroenterology 1990; 98:464–469.
5. Modigliani R, Mary YJ, Simon JF, et al. Clinical, biological, and endoscopic picture of attacks of Crohn's disease: evolution on prednisolone. Gastroenterology 1990; 98:811–818.
6. International Mesalazine Study Group. Coated oral 5-aminosalicylic acid versus placebo in maintaining remission of inactive Crohn's disease. Aliment Pharmacol Ther 1990; 4:55–64.
7. Present DH. 6-Mercaptopurine and other immunosuppressive agents in the treatment of Crohn's disease and ulcerative colitis. Gastroenterol Clin North Am 1989; 18:57–71.
8. Present DH, Meltzer SJ, Krumholz MP, Wolke A, Korelitz BI. 6-Mercaptopurine in the management of inflammatory bowel disease: short- and long-term toxicity. Ann Intern Med 1989; 111:641–649.
9. Brynskov J, Freund L, Rasmussen SN, et al. A placebo-controlled, double-blind, randomized trial of cyclosporine therapy in active chronic Crohn's disease. N Engl J Med 1989; 321:845–850.
10. Campieri M, De Franchis R, Bianchi Porro G, Ranzi T, Brunetti G, Barbara L. Mesalazine (5-aminosalicylic acid) suppositories in the treatment

of ulcerative proctitis or distal proctosigmoiditis: a randomized controlled trial. Scand J Gastroenterol 1990; 25:663–668.

11. Campieri M, Gionchetti P, Belluzzi A, et al. Topical treatment with 5-aminosalicylic in distal ulcerative colitis by using a new suppository preparation: a double-blind placebo controlled trial. Int J Colorectal Dis 1990; 5:79–81.

12. Riley SA, Turnberg LA. Sulphasalazine and the aminosalicylates in the treatment of inflammatory bowel disease. Q J Med 1990; 75:551–562.

SUGGESTED READING LIST

Calkins BM. A meta-analysis of the role of smoking in inflammatory bowel disease. Dig Dis Sci 1989; 34:1841–1854.

Delpre G, Avidor I, Steinherz R, Kadish U, Ben-Bassat M. Ultrastructural abnormalities in endoscopically and histologically normal and involved colon in ulcerative colitis. Am J Gastroenterol 1989; 84:1038–1046.

Ekbom A, Helmick C, Zack M, Adami HO. Ulcerative colitis and colorectal cancer: a population-based study. N Engl J Med 1990; 323:1228–1233.

Gyde S. Screening for colorectal cancer in ulcerative colitis: dubious benefits and high cost [Editorial]. Gut 1990; 31:1089–1092.

Hamilton PW, Allen DC, Watt PCH. A combination of cytological and architectural morphometry in assessing regenerative hyperplasia and dysplasia in ulcerative colitis. Histopathology 1990; 16:59–68.

Lashner BA, Kane SV, Hanauer SB. Colon cancer surveillance in chronic ulcerative colitis: historical cohort study. Am J Gastroenterol 1990: 85:1083–1087.

Lennard-Jones JE, Melville DM, Morson BC, Ritchie JK, Williams CB. Precancer and cancer in extensive ulcerative colitis: findings among 401 patients over 22 years. Gut 1990; 31:800–806.

11
The Colon
G.K. Turnbull, S.J. Vanner and M. Burnstein

1. INTRODUCTION

This chapter presents an overview of colonic physiology and diseases affecting the colon. It discusses lower gastrointestinal bleeding, infectious diseases affecting the colon and diseases specifically involving the anus. The main inflammatory bowel diseases have been discussed in Chapter 10. Diarrhea and its causes are examined in Chapter 7, "The Small Intestine." Other infections are presented in Chapter 7 and in Chapter 9, "Gastrointestinal Manifestations of Human Immunodeficiency Virus Infection."

2. PHYSIOLOGY OF THE COLON / S.J. Vanner

2.1 Function
The colon contributes to three important functions in the body: (1) concentration of fecal effluent through water and electrolyte absorption, (2) storage and controlled evacuation of fecal material and (3) digestion and absorption of undigested food. Although the colon is not essential for survival, its functions contribute significantly to the overall well-being of humans. The colon can be functionally divided through the transverse colon into two parts, the right and left colon. The right colon (cecum and ascending colon) plays a major role in water and electrolyte absorption and fermentation of undigested sugars, and the left colon (descending colon, sigmoid colon and rectum) is predominantly involved in storage and evacuation of stool.

2.2 Functional Anatomy
The human colon is a muscular organ measuring approximately 125 cm in length in vivo. Its wall consists of the four basic layers found in other GI hol-

low visceral organs – the mucosa, submucosa, circular muscle and longitudinal muscle – but several important differences exist. The mucosa lacks the villous projections found in the small intestine and presents a relatively smooth surface, but numerous crypts extend from its surface. Cell types lining the surface and the crypts resemble those in the small intestine but are composed of significantly greater numbers of goblet cells. These cells secrete mucus into the lumen, and mucus strands can often be identified in association with stool. This observation is misconstrued by some patients as a response to underlying colonic pathology. The haustral folds, which help define the colon on barium x-ray, are not a static anatomical feature of the colon but rather result from circular muscle contractions that remain constant for several hours at a time. The outer or longitudinal muscle is organized in three bands, called taeniae coli, which run from the cecum to the rectum where they fuse together to form a uniform outer muscular layer. These muscular bands and elongated serosal fat saccules, called appendices epiploicae, aid in the identification of the colon in the peritoneal cavity.

The colon is innervated by the complex interaction of intrinsic (enteric nervous system) and extrinsic (autonomic nervous system) nerves (Figure 1). The cell bodies of neurons in the enteric nervous system are organized into ganglia with interconnecting fiber tracts, which form the submucosal and myenteric plexi. These nerves are organized into local neural reflex circuits, which modulate motility (myenteric), secretion, blood flow and probably immune function (submucosal). Release of excitatory neurotransmitters such as acetylcholine, substance P and serotonin (5-HT) serves to activate local circuits such as those innervating muscle contractions. Their receptor subtypes provide pharmacological targets for the development of drugs designed to alter colonic functions such as motility. The major inhibitory neurotransmitter is nitric oxide. The importance of the enteric nervous system is exemplified by Hirschsprung's disease, where there is a congenital absence of nitric oxide – containing inhibitory neurons over variable lengths of the rectum and colon. This results in an inability of the colon to relax in the affected region. Infants typically present with bowel obstruction or severe constipation. Barium x-rays identify the affected region as a constricted segment because the excitatory effects of the neurotransmitter acetylcholine are unopposed as a result of the absence of inhibitory neurotransmitter.

The autonomic nervous system comprises sensory nerves, whose cell bodies are found in the dorsal root ganglia, and motor nerves, the sympathetic and parasympathetic nerves. Parasympathetic nerves innervating the right colon travel in the vagus nerve, and those innervating the left colon originate from the pelvic sacral nerves. Parasympathetic nerves are predominantly excitato-

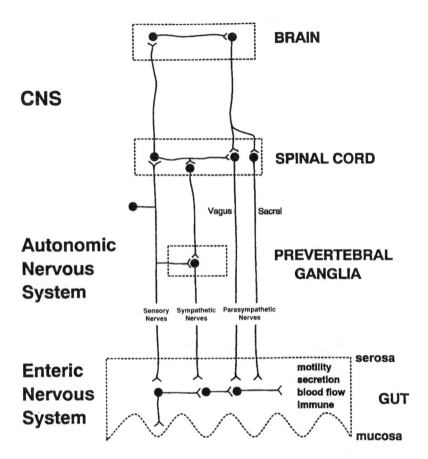

FIGURE 1. Innervation of the colon.

ry, and sympathetic nerves inhibitory. Autonomic nerves modulate the enteric neural circuits within the colon and participate in neural reflexes at the level of the autonomic ganglia, spinal cord and brain. Brain–gut connections are important both for perception of visceral stimuli (sensory) and in modifying colonic function (motor) in response to central stimuli. An example of a central stimulus that can evoke significant changes in colonic activity through this connection is acute stress. This stimulus provokes release of central hormones, such as corticotropin releasing factor. These hormones activate parasympathetic pathways that stimulate motility patterns in the colon and can result in diarrhea.

2.3 Absorption and Secretion

The colon is highly efficient at absorbing water. Under normal physiological conditions, approximately 1.5 L of fluid enters the colon each day, but only about 100–200 mL is excreted in the stool. The maximal absorptive capacity of the colon is up to about 4.5 L per day, so that diarrhea (increased water in stools) will not occur unless the ileocecal flow rate exceeds the absorptive capacity and/or the colonic mucosa itself is secreting. The fundamental feature of colonic electrolyte transport that enables this efficient water absorption is the ability of the colonic mucosa to generate a large osmotic gradient between the lumen and the intercellular space. This osmotic gradient is created by electrogenic sodium transport. This depends upon the energy-dependent Na^+/K^+-ATPase pump on the basolateral membrane, which pumps sodium from inside the cell against a large concentration gradient into the intercellular space (see Figure 6 in Chapter 7, "The Small Intestine"). Luminal sodium in turn enters the apical membrane of the cell through sodium channels, flowing down the concentration gradient created by the pump. In contrast to the small intestine, where sodium in the intercellular space can diffuse back into the lumen and become iso-osmotic, hypertonic solutions are maintained in the intercellular space because the tight junctions are much less permeable to sodium diffusion. The net result is that the hypertonic fluid within the intercellular space draws water passively into the mucosa from the lumen. It also results in highly efficient absorption of sodium. Of the 150 mEq of sodium that enters the colon each day, less than 5 mEq is lost in the stool. The tight junctions are highly permeable to potassium, in contrast to sodium, allowing potassium to move from plasma to the lumen. Potassium pumped into the cell by the Na^+/K^+-ATPase pump can also be secreted into the lumen. Potassium is normally secreted into the lumen unless intraluminal potassium rises above 15 mEq/L. This handling of potassium may account for hypokalemia seen with colonic diarrhea and may play a role in maintaining potassium balance in the late stages of renal failure. Other transport mechanisms, similar to those found in the small intestine (see Chapter 7, Section 5), are also found on colonic enterocytes, which maintain electrical neutrality, intracellular pH and secretion. Nutrient cotransporters, however, are not found in the colon.

The regulation of water and electrolyte transport in the colon also involves the complex interplay between humoral, paracrine and neural regulatory pathways (see Chapter 7). One important difference is the effect of aldosterone, which is absent in the small intestine. This hormone is secreted in response to total body sodium depletion or potassium loading and stimulates sodium absorption and potassium secretion in the colon.

2.4 Motility of the Colon

Much less is known about the motility of the colon compared to other regions of the GI tract. The movement of fecal material from cecum to rectum is a slow process, occurring over days. Functionally, the contraction patterns in the right colon (cecum and ascending colon) cause significant mixing, which facilitates the absorption of water, whereas in the left colon (sigmoid and rectum) they slow the movement of formed stool, forming a reservoir until reflexes activate contractions to advance and evacuate stool.

Several fundamental contractile patterns exist within the colon. Ring contractions are due to circular muscle contraction and can be tonic or rhythmic. Tonic contractions are sustained over hours and form the haustral markings evident on barium x-rays; they appear to play a role in mixing. Rhythmic ring contractions can be intermittent or regular. Regular contractions are non-occlusive, occur over a few seconds, and migrate cephalad (right colon) and caudad (left colon). Presumably, they too play a role in mixing. Intermittent ring contractions occur every few hours, occlude the lumen, and migrate caudad. They result in the mass movement of stool, particularly in the sigmoid colon and rectum. Contractions of the longitudinal muscle appear to produce bulging of the colonic wall between the taeniae coli, but the importance of this action remains poorly understood. The origin of these contractions is also poorly understood but appears to depend on slow-wave properties of the smooth muscle (regular rhythmic contractions) in some cases, and predominantly neural factors (intermittent rhythmic contractions) in others. These in turn are modulated by the interaction of paracrine, humoral and other neural pathways.

The nature of the contractile patterns within the colon depends upon the fed state. This is best exemplified during eating when the "gastrocolic reflex" is activated. Food in the duodenum, particularly fatty foods, evokes reflex intermittment rhythmic contractions within the colon and corresponding mass movement of stool. This action, which is mediated by neural and humoral mechanisms, accounts for the observation by many individuals that eating stimulates the urge to defecate.

Figures 2 and 3 show normal images of the colon at colonoscopy.

2.5 Digestion and Absorption of Undigested Food Products

Greater numbers of bacteria (more anaerobes than aerobes) are found within the colonic lumen than elsewhere in the GI tract. These bacteria digest a number of undigested food products normally found in the effluent delivered to the colon, such as complex sugars contained in dietary fiber.

Complex sugars are fermented by the bacteria, forming the short-chain fatty

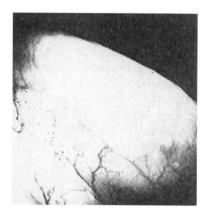

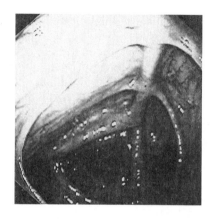

FIGURE 2 (A and B). Normal colon appearance at endoscopy.

FIGURE 2A. Close-up view of the normal submucosal vessels visible through the healthy transparent mucosa overlying the vessels.

FIGURE 2B. Normal transverse colon with the normal triangular appearance to the fold pattern.

acids (SCFAs) butyrate, propionate and acetate. These SCFAs are essential nutrient sources for colonic epithelium, and in addition can provide up to 500 cal/day of overall nutritional needs. They are passively and actively transported into the cell where they become an important energy source for the cell through the β-oxidation pathway. The importance of this role is illustrated by the effects of a "defunctioning" colostomy, which diverts the fecal stream from the distal colon. Examination of this area typically reveals signs of inflammation, termed *diversion colitis*. This inflammation can be successfully treated with the installation of mixtures of short-chain fatty acids into the rectum.

Fermentation of sugars by colonic bacteria is also an important source of colonic gases such as hydrogen, methane and carbon dioxide. These gases, particularly methane, largely account for the tendency of some stools to float in the toilet. Nitrogen gas, which diffuses into the colon from the plasma, is the predominant gas. However, the ingestion of large quantities of undigested complex sugars such as found in beans or the maldigestion of simple sugars such as lactose can result in large increases in production of colonic gas. This can lead to patients' complaints of abdominal bloating and increased flatus.

When bile salts or long-chain fatty acids are malabsorbed in sufficient quantities, their digestion by colonic bacteria generates potent secretagogues.

FIGURE 3 (A, B and C). The ileocecal valve. The three parts of this
figure illustrate examples of the variation in appearance of the ileocecal
valve.

FIGURE 3A. Normal ileocecal
valve.

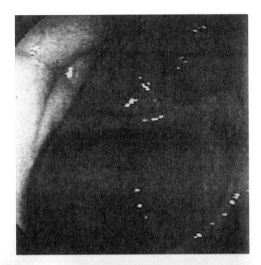

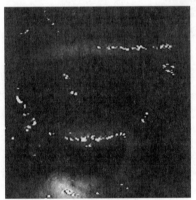

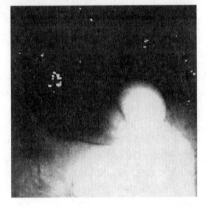

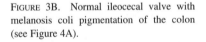

FIGURE 3B. Normal ileocecal valve with
melanosis coli pigmentation of the colon
(see Figure 4A).

FIGURE 3C. A normal variant of the ileocecal valve where fatty infiltration of the valve
makes it appear more prominent; on x-ray it
can be confused with a polyp. The appearance of the mucosa is normal. Biopsy confirms that the mucosa is normal – i.e., not a
polyp.

Bile salt malabsorption causing "choleraic diarrhea" typically occurs following terminal ileum resection, usually for management of Crohn's disease.
When the resection involves segments greater than 100 cm this problem is further complicated by depletion of the bile salt pool, because bile salt produc-

tion cannot compensate for the increased fecal loss. In these circumstances diarrhea also results from fat malabsorption. The proposed mechanisms by which multiple metabolites of bile salts and hydroxylated metabolites of long-chain fatty acids act as secretagogues provide an example of how multiple regulatory systems can interact to control colonic function. These mechanisms include disruption of mucosal permeability, stimulation of Cl⁻ and water secretion by activating enteric secretomotor neurons, enhancement of the paracrine actions of prostaglandins by increasing production, and direct effects on the enterocyte that increase intracelluar calcium.

3. SPECIFIC COLONIC DISEASES / G.K. Turnbull

3.1 Colon Polyps and Cancer

Colon cancer is the second most common cancer (after lung cancer) in men and women combined in Canada. Unlike lung cancer, it has a high survival rate in patients diagnosed before it has spread beyond the confines of the bowel wall. Since it is a very common cancer, has a high survival rate with early curative surgery and is poorly responsive to other forms of cancer therapy, a high index of suspicion must be maintained in approaching patients with symptoms of colonic dysfunction (Table 1), especially if they are over the age of 40, when the incidence of colon cancer begins to rise. Increased colon cancer risk is also seen in patients with ulcerative colitis, a history of female genital or breast cancer, or a family history of colon cancer or adenoma (including familial polyposis syndromes).

The Dukes' classification is used to stage colon cancer after surgical resection. It is based on the pathological extent and invasion of the primary colonic tumor (adenocarcinoma) at the time of resection (Table 2). Dukes' A stage is adenocarcinoma confined to the mucosa and submucosa; the cure rate for this stage of adenocarcinoma with surgery is about 90%. Dukes' B stage has two subdivisions: B1 for adenocarcinomas that have invaded the muscularis propria, and B2 for tumors that have invaded through the longitudinal muscle although regional lymph nodes are free of cancer. Dukes' C stage is adenocarcinoma that has spread to regional lymph nodes, and Dukes' D stage is adenocarcinoma that is metastatic to distant sites, usually the liver and beyond. Cure rates with stage C and D adenocarcinoma of the colon are very low with surgery; as well, both chemotherapy and radiotherapy have limited success, reinforcing the need to make an early diagnosis. Table 2 also describes the newer TNM colorectal adenocarcinoma staging system, which is similar to the Dukes' A–D staging system. The TNM staging system includes stage 0 when the carcinoma is limited to the mucosa and is called "in situ."

TABLE 1.   Presenting features of colon cancer

Abdominal pain, including symptoms of bowel obstruction
Change in bowel habit
Abdominal complaints of recent onset
Abdominal mass
Iron deficiency anemia
Hypokalemia

TABLE 2.   Colorectal adenocarcinoma staging

Dukes' stage	TNM stage	Tumor invasion	5-year survival
	0	Mucosa	100%
A	I	Submucosa No lymph node or distant metastases	90%
B	II	B1: Circular muscle B2: Longitudinal muscle No lymph node or distant metastases	70–75%

C	III	C1: 1–4 lymph nodes
		   positive
		C2: > 4 lymph nodes
		   positive
			45%

D	IV	Distant metastases (e.g., liver)	20% or less

Early recognition is of the utmost importance to try to identify early cancer at a curative stage. Therefore, patients with intermittent symptoms are as important to investigate as patients with persistent symptoms, and the story of occasional blood in the stool in a patient over 40 years of age should not be attributed to local anorectal disease without excluding a more proximal lesion. Many patients may present with no gastrointestinal symptoms, but rather an iron deficiency anemia due to chronic bleeding from the tumor. Patients may not see blood in the stool or note a melena stool, particularly when there is a right-sided colonic lesion. A change in bowel habit, often with constipation alternating with diarrhea, may be the first sign of obstructive symptoms from a colon cancer, and should never be ignored in a patient over 40 years of age with a recent onset of these symptoms. Some patients may present with primarily diarrhea if they have a high output of mucus and fluid from the tumor; in this instance the tumor may be a villous adenoma, and some patients may have hypokalemia due to large amounts of potassium lost with the mucus secretion from the tumor.

Carcinoembryonic antigen (CEA) is a tumor marker that has limited use in diagnosing colon cancer but is often useful in following patients with colon cancer. A high CEA level before surgery often suggests a poor prognosis with probable metastases. CEA that does not fall to normal levels one month after surgery suggests that all the cancer has not been resected. After surgery, regular monitoring of CEA levels can identify patients with early recurrence. Sometimes a search for metastases will discover a solitary lesion in the liver that may be resected with the use of chemotherapy, which may lead to a cure of the cancer.

3.1.1 POLYP–CARCINOMA SEQUENCE

It is now agreed that the majority of colon cancer patients have a colonic adenocarcinoma arising from an adenomatous polyp. Polyps of 2 cm or greater have about 50% incidence of cancer, compared to 1% in adenomas of 1 cm or less. Adenomatous polyps are a premalignant condition, and their identification and removal before becoming malignant prevents the development of colon cancer. These polyps can arise anywhere in the colon, but (as is the case for colon cancer) they are more frequently seen in the left colon. The majority of polyps are completely asymptomatic, but the occurrence of occult bleeding does increase as they grow. Unfortunately, polyps can still be missed, even with occult blood testing of the stool, since the blood loss may be intermittent. Examples of different polyps are seen in Figure 4.

Three histologic types of adenomatous polyps occur: tubular, tubulovillous and villous. The malignant potential is greatest in villous polyps (40%) and lowest in tubular polyps (5%), with an intermediate risk in tubulovillous polyps (22%). The malignant potential may also be described pathologically as the degree of "dysplasia": the more severe the dysplasia, the greater the rate of malignancy. These tubular, tubulovillous and villous polyps can often be completely removed by snare polypectomy at colonoscopy if they are pedunculated on a stalk, but sessile polyps that carpet a wide area of colonic mucosa (often villous polyps) can usually be completely removed only by resection surgery. Since polyps precede cancer and removal of polyps "cures" the cancer, it has been hoped that screening colonoscopy may help reduce the incidence of cancer. Other polyps as well may be present at the initial or index colonoscopy, and polyps and cancer tend to recur. This sets the stage for the rationale for performing follow-up surveillance colonoscopies (colon cancer

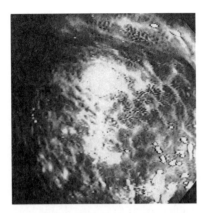

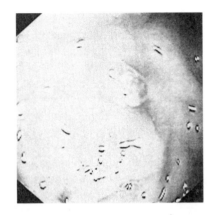

FIGURE 4 (A, B, C and D). Adenomatous polyps of the colon. B, C and D illustrate polyps of different size and morphology. Note in D that although the polyp is rather large, its flat sessile morphology makes it more difficult to see endoscopically.

FIGURE 4B.

FIGURE 4A. A very small adenoma made more obvious in a colon with melanosis coli, a pigment in the mucosa resulting from chronic laxative abuse. See how the adenoma is not pigmented, as its tissue is abnormal and the cells in the polyp divide more rapidly than cells in the "normal" pigmented mucosa.

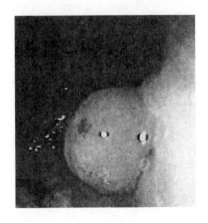

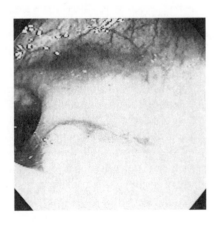

FIGURE 4C.

FIGURE 4D.

surveillance program). The best time interval for this surveillance is probably every three years; longer intervals between surveillance colonoscopies may be safe but have yet to be tested. The cost-effectiveness of screening all patients over the age of 40 has not been proven. If particular subgroups of patients likely to have polyps are identified, then routine colonoscopy screening would be indicated.

Particular conditions have been associated with an increased risk of colon cancer. The polyposis syndromes of familial polyposis and Gardner's syndrome are manifested by early onset (usually before age 30) of innumerable colonic adenomatous polyps that eventually and invariably lead to colon cancer (usually before age 40). Since the colon has too many polyps to remove by endoscopy-guided polypectomy these patients are referred at an early age for total colectomy to remove the risk of colon cancer. After colectomy these patients still need regular gastroscopic surveillance. Biopsies are taken from the ampulla of Vater to look for adenomas that frequently occur in the proximal duodenum around the ampulla, and the stomach is also examined endoscopically for evidence of adenomas of the stomach. An experimental approach at present is to do tests on blood monocytes looking for mutation of the APC gene, which is the cause of this autosomal dominant disease. There are other families (site-specific colorectal cancer, family cancer syndrome) that have a high risk of colon cancer (autosomal dominant inheritance), with more than two first-degree relatives having had colon cancer. This disease is called hereditary nonpolyposis colorectal cancer (HNPCC). It would be prudent to enter such patients into a colon cancer surveillance program of colonoscopy and/or air contrast barium enema if they have colonic polyps when screened at age 40. Female patients with HNPCC also appear to have an increased risk of endometrial and ovarian cancer.

Also at a high risk for colon cancer are patients with chronic ulcerative colitis for more than 10 years; this risk also appears to be present in patients with Crohn's pancolitis. The patients at highest risk are those who have had total colon involvement and those with disease up to and including the hepatic flexure (subtotal colitis); patients with proctosigmoiditis are at least risk – probably not greater than the general population. Curiously, the risk of cancer does not correlate with the degree of disease activity. Therefore, patients with just one bout of proven subtotal ulcerative colitis would have an increased risk of cancer after 10 years of disease, and the younger the patient at the time of onset of his or her disease, the greater the cumulative risk of cancer will be for that patient. Unlike those who experience the "polyp–carcinoma sequence," patients with colitis do not develop adenomatous polyps before they develop cancer; therefore they require colonoscopy about every one to two years, with endoscopic biopsies of the colon performed to identify dysplasia of the

TABLE 3. Complications of diverticulitis

Abdominal abscess/Liver abscess
Colonic obstruction
Fistulas
Colovesical
Colovaginal
Colocutaneous

mucosa. Particular attention should be paid to "elevated" or "flat" lesions seen at colonoscopy where the incidence of early colon cancer is high. If there is dysplasia, either "high grade" or "low grade," colectomy should be recommended to the patient.

3.2 Diverticulosis

In Western societies diverticulosis occurs in at least one person in two over the age of 50 years. The frequency increases with age. Diverticulosis or diverticular disease of the colon is due to pseudodiverticula in that the wall of the diverticulum is not full-thickness colonic wall, but rather outpouchings of colonic mucosa through points of weakness in the colonic wall where the blood vessels penetrate the muscularis propria. These diverticula are prone to infection or "diverticulitis" presumably because they trap feces with bacteria. If the infection spreads beyond the confines of the diverticula in the colonic wall, an abscess is formed. Patients present with increasing left lower quadrant pain and fever, often with constipation and lower abdominal obstructive symptoms such as bloating and distention. Some patients with severe obstructive symptoms may actually describe nausea or vomiting. This can occur with or without abscess formation. Other causes of these symptoms include Crohn's colitis with stricture formation, colonic cancer and ischemic colitis (see Section 4).

On physical examination the patient often has localized tenderness in the left lower quadrant, and with severe infection and an abscess may have rebound tenderness in the left lower quadrant. A palpable mass is often identifiable where the sigmoid colon (the most common site of diverticulitis) is infected. Treatment consists of intravenous fluids and bowel rest by placing the patient on no oral intake or just a clear liquid diet; intravenous antibiotics are administered. Generally broad-spectrum antibiotics are used to cover both gram-negative enteric bacteria and anaerobic bacteria that are normally found in the colon. CT scan may be helpful in outlining the colon and identifying an abscess, and is preferable to barium enema for diagnosis in patients with acute illness.

Many complications can occur in diverticulitis. These are listed in Table 3. Colonic stricture after resolution of diverticulitis is described further in Section 3.3.

Bleeding occurs in less than 5% of diverticulosis patients; it is abrupt in onset, painless, and often massive. A bleeding diverticulum can be from either the left or right colon. The bleeding frequency is approximately equal because of the much higher frequency of left colonic diverticulosis, even though bleeding is more likely to occur in right colonic diverticulosis. It is rare for patients with diverticulosis to have significant bleeding. Over 80% of diverticulosis patients will stop bleeding, but the rest will continue and require investigation and treatment (see Section 5). Segmental colonic resection is reserved for that small group of patients who continue bleeding or have recurrent bleeding. Recent reports recommend that patients under the age of 40 with symptomatic diverticulitis should have surgical resection because this small subgroup is at greater risk of complications.

Figure 5 shows examples of diverticulosis of the sigmoid colon at colonoscopy.

3.3 Colonic Obstruction

Acute colonic obstruction is a surgical emergency that must be recognized early and dealt with expeditiously in order to avoid the high fatality rate due to colonic perforation. The highest risk patients for colonic perforation are those with an intact ileocecal valve that does not allow air to reflux back into the small bowel from the obstructed colon. The cecum is the most frequent site of perforation, because wall tension is highest in the bowel with the largest diameter (Laplace's law).

Patients with colonic obstruction usually have pain as a prominent symptom, with constipation often preceding the complete obstruction. Patients may initially present with diarrhea as the bowel distal to the obstruction empties, but diarrhea may be persistent, especially with a partial obstruction, because of the increased intestinal secretion proximal to the obstruction. The small intestine is the most common site of intestinal obstruction because of the narrower caliber of the bowel, and similarly the left colon is the most common site for colonic obstruction, especially since the stool is more formed in the left colon and unable to pass through a narrowed lumen.

On physical examination the general state of the patient depends upon the duration of the obstruction. With a recent sudden obstruction the patient will be in extreme pain, will often have distention of the abdomen if the ileocecal valve is intact and may describe initially diarrheal stool as the bowel distal to the obstruction is emptied. Abdominal palpation can often discern a mass lesion at the site of the obstruction. Prompt identification of the site of

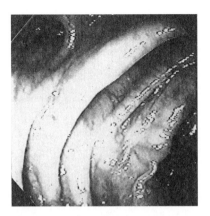

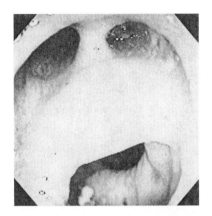

FIGURE 5 (A and B).   Diverticulosis.

FIGURE 5A.   The rounded opening of a single diverticulum is shown at the top left, with the colonic lumen at the bottom right.

FIGURE 5B.   Two diverticulum openings are shown at the top, with the lumen in the lower half of the image. This shows how easy it is to confuse the lumen with a diverticulum opening. With insertion of the colonoscope into a diverticulum, perforation is the result.

obstruction is mandatory, with the use of supine and erect abdominal x-rays. An urgent surgical consultation is required if the rectum is empty of air with dilation of more proximal colon, indicating a complete colonic obstruction.

Many patients present with a more gradual history. If they have had protracted diarrhea up to the point of obstruction, the amount of abdominal pain may be less; they may have abdominal distention, but be less tender on abdominal exam; and they will often show signs of dehydration. Fever and an abdominal mass is particularly common in patients with diverticulitis and a resulting colonic obstruction. A third type of colonic obstruction can be seen that is actually a form of ileus limited to the colon and is sometimes referred to as Ogilvie's syndrome. These patients are most often seen in intensive care units, but the condition can also occur postoperatively (even when no bowel surgery has been performed). As with a "mechanical" bowel obstruction described above, patients with Ogilvie's syndrome may have marked abdominal distention, but frequently they have little abdominal pain and the abdominal x-rays show a picture of dilated colon with impaired movement of air into the distal colon.

Once a diagnosis of colonic obstruction has been made, the site of obstruction should be determined by plain abdominal x-rays and/or with a water-soluble contrast enema (such as iothalamate meglumine) to identify whether

TABLE 4.   Causes of colonic obstruction

Common
Left-sided cancer
Diverticulitis
Ogilvie's syndrome
Others
Hernia
Strictures
Crohn's
Postischemic
Postsurgical
Intussusception
Volvulus
Adhesions

urgent surgery is indicated. Urgent colonoscopy is being done increasingly in this setting, especially if a colonic ileus or Ogilvie's syndrome is suggested, since the excess colonic air can be aspirated via the colonoscope and colonic decompression tubes can be placed in the colon to prevent dangerous reaccumulation of air until the ileus resolves.

Some authorities dispute the safety of colonoscopy in Ogilvie's syndrome and recommend prokinetic drugs instead. A recent study showed promising results where the majority of patients responded to an infusion of neostigmine 2.0 mg IV. Bradycardia may occur with this medication, and all patients must receive cardiac monitoring. This study excluded patients with severe cardiac disease, but the results suggest that this approach may be effective in carefully selected patients. However, the patients not responding to neostigmine were all treated successfully with colonoscopic decompression.

There are many causes of colonic obstruction (Table 4). Colon cancer and diverticulitis are the most common causes. Most colon cancers that obstruct are in the left colon. They cause circumferential disease or "apple-core" lesions (so called because of the irregular mucosal appearance with luminal narrowing seen at x-ray). Diverticulitis commonly occurs in the sigmoid colon, where diverticular disease is most common; the acute abscess formation with swelling of the inflamed diverticulum compresses and obstructs the affected sigmoid colon. Ogilvie's syndrome may initially have been considered to be due to a cancer or diverticulitis, but contrast x-ray or colonoscopy demonstrates a patent lumen and the diagnosis appears to be clear.

Less common causes of colonic obstruction are hernias, in which a loop of colon (usually sigmoid) becomes strangulated and the bowel is acutely obstructed. This is a much more common cause of small bowel obstruction. Strictures in the colon can also be associated with obstruction, especially when they occur in the left colon. These can occur with Crohn's colitis, after a bout of ischemic colitis or at the site of anastomosis following colonic surgery. This latter cause of obstruction should always be visualized endoscopically if possible, since most colonic resections are for cancer and the possibility of a local cancer recurrence can complicate a post-surgical stricture.

Intussusception can occur in the colon, and in adults it almost always occurs at the site of a polyp, which "leads" the intussusception. Typically, this will cause intermittent acute bowel obstruction associated with severe pain and often rectal bleeding from the vascular compromise produced in the intussuscepting bowel. Because of the intermittent nature of the obstruction, a diagnosis may not be made until after repeated attacks. A barium enema should always be considered in this setting, as it identifies the mucosal lesion "leading" the intussusception and can occasionally be used to reduce the intussusception without the need for urgent surgery.

Volvulus of the colon tends to happen in the cecum and/or the sigmoid colon, because the mesentery can be long and redundant in these areas and cause the bowel to rotate upon itself. This can be a surgical emergency, since the affected bowel will strangulate if the volvulus is not relieved quickly. Again, an urgent barium enema may be able to reduce the volvulus, thus allowing a more elective surgical procedure to correct the problem. A sigmoid volvulus will usually be reduced by this approach, and success with colonoscopic decompression of a sigmoid volvulus has been reported. A cecal volvulus may not be easily treatable with either a barium enema or colonoscopic therapy; thus, surgical advice should be sought urgently if cecal volvulus is diagnosed.

Adhesions are often described as a common cause of bowel obstruction, but this is probably true only for small bowel obstruction. Since much of the colon is retroperitoneal or on a limited mesentery, adhesive disease with obstruction of the colon is rare. However, it can occur, particularly in the sigmoid colon if the mesentery is quite long, and particularly after pelvic operations.

3.4 Irritable Bowel Syndrome
Most commonly, patients exhibiting symptoms from the GI tract are suffering from the irritable bowel syndrome. This is a condition that may be a variant of normal function. Causes of irritable bowel are still being evaluated, but the syndrome does sometimes occur after an episode of infectious diarrhea. It appears that patients have no organic disease of the gastrointestinal tract, yet

they experience frequent symptoms from the bowel. Large epidemiologic studies would suggest that the condition occurs in at least 15% of the population.

The commonest symptom that brings a patient to a doctor is abdominal pain. Criteria have been developed to identify with more certainty those patients who have the irritable bowel syndrome. A more positive diagnosis can be made, particularly in women, if the abdominal pain is not localized and tends to have been present for at least three months. The pain is associated with bowel movements and relieved after defecation. Abdominal pain is also associated with increased looseness of stool as well as increased frequency. For a "strict" diagnosis of the irritable bowel syndrome, along with the above criteria it is felt that three of the following symptoms should also be present: (1) patients have difficult defecation; (2) patients complain of abdominal bloating or distention; (3) mucus is present in the stool; (4) there is increased stool frequency; (5) there is increased looseness of the stool at the onset of the abdominal pain.

Patients who have difficulty with defecation can have the following complaints. There can be "urgency," with the sudden urge to pass stool and a fear of incontinence if defecation is not performed immediately. Many patients with this symptom will relate that they always identify where the toilet is when they are away from home. The fear of incontinence can often greatly limit a patient's ability to function normally in society. Other patients with difficult defecation may have to strain – defined as having to hold their breath and push when attempting defecation. Straining is defined as "constipation" when a patient must strain 25% or more of the time when trying to defecate. Finally, some patients describe a feeling of incomplete emptying after passing stool. This symptom has to be asked for specifically, as most patients will not spontaneously report it. Nevertheless, the symptom is commonly reported by patients with an irritable bowel.

The presence of mucus in the stool can be alarming to some patients, since they may interpret this to mean they have "colitis." In the past, some doctors used to refer to irritable bowel as "mucus colitis," which is a misnomer since there is no "colitis" or inflammation of the colon in irritable bowel. Mucus is a normal product of the colon, and only if mucus and blood are seen together should other diagnoses such as "colitis" be considered.

The typical stool pattern described by patients with an irritable bowel is the change in stool character and frequency with the onset of abdominal pain. Typically, patients will pass a normally formed stool (sometimes even a constipated stool) first thing in the morning. Then with the attacks of abdominal pain the stools become more frequent and looser, sometimes becoming just liquid diarrheal stools. Once bowel movements cease the pain is relieved, but it can recur again later in the day, often precipitated by eating high-fat foods or other gut stimulants (e.g., coffee).

There have been reports that in men, the above criteria (called the Manning Criteria) may not be as helpful as they are in women. It is also important to note that the vast majority of people with an irritable bowel have their symptoms begin in young adult life. One should consider other colonic diseases in patients over the age of 40 who develop these symptoms for the first time without previous episodes suggesting irritable bowel. Sometimes later in life patients can develop irritable bowel after severe infectious diarrhea, but in this population as well, further investigations are warranted to ensure no other cause for the change in bowel function.

The irritable bowel syndrome is a disorder affecting the entire gut, and although many of the symptoms appear to arise from the colon, these patients frequently have symptoms from other parts of the GI tract as well as from other organs. Upper GI symptoms are very common in irritable bowel; these consist of increased frequency of esophageal reflux. As well, nonulcer dyspepsia is associated with irritable bowel. Dyspepsia symptoms in general occur more commonly than lower bowel symptoms, but are obviously due to many other causes, including reflux esophagitis, gastritis, peptic ulcer disease and, less commonly, biliary tract and pancreatic disease. When upper GI symptoms are associated with irritable bowel, other underlying diseases must be considered. Other associated symptoms include frequent headaches and urinary symptoms that are similar to bowel symptoms, in that patients can have urgency and frequency of urination. These symptoms are often worse at times when the bowel symptoms are troublesome. In women, irritable bowel symptoms can often be exacerbated or worsened around the time of menstruation. Studies suggest that bowel symptoms associated with menstruation occur in at least 50% of the normal female population.

When assessing a patient complaining of irritable bowel symptoms, remember that only a small proportion of patients with an irritable bowel present to doctors with these symptoms. Recent studies would suggest that patients who see doctors about their symptoms often have psychological problems, with increased levels of distress and depression as common findings. It is important to inquire about these problems, as successful treatment often consists of dealing with the distress and/or depression that accompanies the irritable bowel symptoms. They may often be the reason that the patient has sought medical attention in the first place.

3.4.1 DIFFERENTIAL DIAGNOSIS

The Manning Criteria provide a more positive diagnosis of irritable bowel: abdominal pain with the association of increased frequency and increased looseness of stool, relief of abdominal pain with defecation, abdominal bloating, mucus in the stool and defecation difficulties such as a sensation of incomplete rectal emptying after defecation. However, lactose intolerance is a common cause of change in bowel habit in young adults, particularly if their racial background is not northern European. Therefore, investigating for lactose intolerance in patients who present with increased frequency and looseness of stool is worthwhile, since the ingestion of lactose-containing foods may be the reason for their symptoms. All patients should have a thorough physical examination, looking for evidence of disease in other organ systems such as the thyroid, which can present with a change in bowel habit. Patients with an irritable bowel will often have pain over the colon, particularly the sigmoid colon, on palpation. The identification of an enlarged liver or spleen or other abdominal masses necessitates further investigations. A barium enema is rarely required in a young healthy adult with new onset of irritable bowel symptoms. However, a patient over the age of 40 presenting with symptoms that may be irritable bowel yet of new onset and without previous complaints would warrant at least a barium enema and a sigmoidoscopic examination. The barium enema should also evaluate the terminal ileum if there is pain on palpation in the right lower quadrant. A complete blood count with platelet count should be done, as an elevated platelet count is often a sensitive finding for underlying inflammation and in the presence of bowel symptoms could mean the presence of early inflammatory bowel disease. Crohn's disease is more likely to present this way than irritable bowel. The persistence of the abdominal pain, even though lessened after bowel movements, would suggest possible underlying inflammation of the gut rather than an irritable bowel. Ulcerative colitis usually presents with rectal bleeding. Rectal bleeding is not a symptom of irritable bowel and its cause must always be investigated. Fever, weight loss and symptoms that wake a patient from sleep, as opposed to early waking in the morning, are all symptoms that should be further investigated.

The presence of nocturnal symptoms, particularly with diarrhea waking the patient at night, is almost never due to an irritable bowel. Occasionally patients with depression who have early morning waking report this symptom, but in general further investigations are indicated.

3.4.2 *THERAPY*

The therapeutic approach in irritable bowel is as much reassurance as any specific therapies, as most patients do not have any "disease." It is most important to do a thorough history and physical examination to ensure that the complaints are not due to any underlying disease. Once this has been confirmed, explain to the patient how the bowel can produce these symptoms and that there is no cause for concern. Since patients presenting with irritable bowel symptoms frequently have more distress and tend to be more prone to seek medical attention for other minor medical conditions than other patients (so-called illness behavior), these patients may require considerable reassurance to convince them that they do not have serious disease. Part of this reassurance will be provided by screening blood tests such as a complete blood count with platelet count. Sigmoidoscopic examination will rule out most underlying early inflammatory bowel disease and any rectal pathology, particularly in patients complaining of defecation difficulties or a sensation of being unable to empty the rectum adequately. The stool should be analyzed for pathogens if diarrhea is present. Following these initial screening tests emphasis should be placed on the stresses present in the patient's life. Evaluating the level of stress and taking steps to correct it will often be helpful. Many patients, particularly those who have symptoms of constipation, may be helped with a high-fiber diet (see Section 3.6).

Drug treatment for irritable bowel is generally discouraged. There is no single drug that treats all the varied symptoms in irritable bowel, but occasional patients will continue to have intractable symptomatology. In this situation selected medications for specific symptoms may be helpful. Table 5 outlines some drugs that may be useful for specific symptoms. Drug therapy for irritable bowel should always be restricted to short periods during exacerbation of symptoms, and patients should be taken off medications when well. As irritable bowel is a chronic condition and is probably "normal" for these patients, the chronic use of medications often reinforces the notion that they have a "disease." Reassuring the patient that there is no association between irritable bowel symptoms and the development of more serious bowel disease such as colon cancer or inflammatory bowel disease can often alleviate some of the unreasonable yet very real concerns of many patients who present to doctors with these symptoms.

3.5 Fecal Incontinence

Understanding fecal incontinence requires knowledge of the normal function of the anorectum. Anatomically, it consists of the internal anal sphincter surrounded by the external anal sphincter and puborectalis muscles. The internal anal sphincter consists of smooth muscle and is a continuation of the circular smooth muscle of the rectum. The external anal sphincter is made up of skeletal muscle and surrounds the internal anal sphincter, whereas the puborectalis (also consisting of skeletal muscle) is a large U-shaped muscle that wraps around the upper anal canal at the anorectal junction above the external anal sphincter and loops anteriorly to attach to the pubic bone. This creates an anatomical sling of muscle that pulls the

TABLE 5. Drug therapy in irritable bowel syndrome

Symptom	Drug	Dosage
Abdominal pain	Anticholinergics	
	Hyoscyamine	0.125 mg sl q4h prn
	Dicyclomine	10–20 mg po tid–qid before meals
	Calcium antagonists	
	Pinaverium bromide	50–100 mg po tid before meals
	Antidepressants	
	(e.g.) Amitriptyline	10–25 mg po hs (increase by 10–25 mg increments every 5 to 7 days as tolerated)
	Enteric opioids	
	Trimebutine	100–200 mg po tid before meals
	? Fedotozine	still experimental
Constipation	High-fiber diet	≥ 30 g daily plus 2 L liquid daily
	Osmotic laxatives	
	Milk of magnesia	15–30 mL po bid–tid
	Prokinetic agent	
	Cisapride	20 mg po bid
	Other agents	
	Misoprostol	200 μg po bid–qid before meals
Diarrhea	Binding agent (resin)	
	Cholestyramine	4 g po once to four times daily
	Antimotility agents	
	Loperamide	2–4 mg po prn to a maximum daily dose of 16 mg
	Diphenoxylate	2.5 mg po qid prn
	? 5-HT$_3$ antagonists	
	(alosetron)	still experimental
Abdominal bloating, "gas"	Simethicone	≤ qid prn
	Peppermint oil, enteric coated	1 cap po qid prn
	? motility agents	
	Cisapride	10–20 mg po bid
	Domperidone	10–20 mg po qid

anorectal junction forward when it tightens, thus closing the upper anal canal and creating the anorectal angle that is vital to the maintenance of fecal continence.

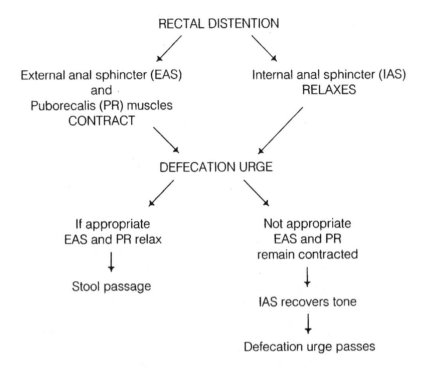

RECTAL DISTENTION

External anal sphincter (EAS) and Puborecalis (PR) muscles CONTRACT

Internal anal sphincter (IAS) RELAXES

DEFECATION URGE

If appropriate EAS and PR relax

Stool passage

Not appropriate EAS and PR remain contracted

IAS recovers tone

Defecation urge passes

FIGURE 6. Physiology of defecation.

When stool (or gas or liquid) enters the rectum or sigmoid colon, a normal rectoanal inhibitory reflex (RAIR) or rectosphincteric reflex is initiated – that is, the internal anal sphincter relaxes and, if voluntary muscle action occurs, the rectum empties through the anal canal (Figure 6). Fecal continence is maintained by contraction under voluntary control of the striated-muscle sphincters – i.e., the external anal sphincter (EAS) and puborectalis (PR) – until the rectal pressure rise decreases and the resting tone of the internal anal sphincter is restored. Thus, the "voluntary" sphincters (i.e., the EAS and PR) have the ability to be maximally contracted for approximately one minute, beyond which fecal continence is lost as a result of fatigue in the muscle if the tone of the internal anal sphincter has not recovered.

The patient with fecal incontinence will often describe the problem as "diarrhea" rather than loss of control of bowel function. All patients with a complaint of diarrhea should be asked if they have lost control of stool, as this may indicate where the problem actually lies. Once fecal incontinence has been noted, it is then necessary to identify the frequency of the incontinence, whether both liquid and solid stool have been leaked and whether the individual has an urge to defecate before the leakage occurs. A history of previous anorectal trauma (surgical or otherwise) is important to note, as is the strength of voluntary anal canal tone on digital rectal exam.

Most patients presenting with fecal incontinence have "idiopathic" fecal incontinence, but recent investigations in females with this complaint indicate they have suffered damage to the pudendal nerves during childbirth and, with time, this has led to gradual striated-muscle anal sphincter weakness. Surgical trauma is the next most common cause of fecal incontinence; it should be remembered that surgery (e.g., a vaginal hysterectomy) can put excess stretch on the pelvic floor nerves and muscles, causing injury that may lead to weakness of the anal sphincters. Another common source of fecal incontinence is disruption of the internal anal sphincter, either during a lateral internal sphincterotomy to treat an anal fissure or, more commonly, with the older "Lord's" procedure of forceful three- or four-finger dilation of the anal sphincter under anesthetic, where the extent of damage to the sphincters is not predictable. The finding of perineal descent can be noted on examination of the perineum when the patient is asked to strain and appears to be associated with weakness of the pelvic floor muscles as well as disruption of the normal anatomy. This gives rise to a mechanical disadvantage affecting the sphincter mechanism. Perineal descent may be associated with a rectocele or, in female patients, with a uterine prolapse. Rectal prolapse can also accompany weakness of the pelvic floor muscles and give rise to fecal incontinence.

Therapy of fecal incontinence has improved over the past decade, primarily because of the introduction of biofeedback training. This technique allows the patient to practice tightening of the striated-muscle portion of the anal sphincter, usually with a surface electromyography (EMG) plug electrode held in the anal canal with audio and visual feedback that the patient can see and hear to encourage maximal contraction of these muscles. Attention should also be given to increasing dietary fiber to help reduce the amount of liquid stool. Other drug therapy is limited, but loperamide has been shown to increase the resting tone of the anal sphincters and is a useful adjunct, especially if the stool frequency is increased (loperamide reduces this contributing factor). Cholestyramine may be useful when the patient has diarrhea or loose stool(s) since cholestyramine can make stool more solid (constipating effect). Surgery is sometimes required and is of greatest benefit in those patients who appear to have a mechanical problem such as rectal prolapse or disruption of the sphincter. Surgery to correct perineal descent is often less helpful, since the problem of muscle weakness that gives rise to the descent is not satisfactorily reversed by any of the surgical procedures currently used, and attempts to "suspend" the pelvic floor muscles cannot strengthen these muscles. Patients should refrain from excess straining if they have significant perineal descent, since this will serve only to worsen the pelvic floor muscle weakness.

3.6 Constipation

In the approach to a patient with constipation, it is first necessary to define what the patient means by the term. Many definitions exist, but the best clinical definition is that over 95% of the North American population has a stool frequency from three times a day to three times a week: therefore, patients who have a bowel frequency less than three times a week would be defined as being constipated. Many patients will describe their stool as "constipated," usually meaning that the stool is hard or in pellets (scybalous), while other patients may have a stool frequency that falls within the "normal" range yet feel that their bowels have not completely emptied. This latter symptom is a frequent complaint of the irritable bowel syndrome, and many patients with this disorder will describe a constipated bowel habit. Those constipated patients who have infrequent stool alternating with occasional diarrheal stool have the most common presentation of irritable bowel syndrome. Yet there are a great many patients, almost all female, who have infrequent stool passage, and this group must be considered as separate from the usual irritable bowel syndrome patient for they may be among those rare patients with a secondary cause of constipation.

In Western culture the most frequent cause of constipation is a lack of dietary fiber. The concept of "fiber" has become quite confusing to many patients with the increased emphasis on "oat fiber" for elevated cholesterol treatment. Many foods that patients consider to be high in fiber (e.g., salads, lettuce, tomatoes and celery) are in fact mainly water, and some vegetables may aggravate their symptoms. Fiber is complex carbohydrates that are incompletely digested by the small bowel and are then "digested" by colonic bacteria, liberating fermentation gases and short-chain fatty acids that may provoke and aggravate many of the associated abdominal symptoms (e.g., abdominal pain, "gas" and bloating). It should be emphasized that cereal grain fibers that have more insoluble fiber (as opposed to soluble oat bran fiber) are best to increase stool frequency, but should be added gradually over 8 to 12 weeks to a daily dose of about 30 g. Other fibers in the form of "bulk laxative" preparations containing psyllium, methylcellulose Sterculia or isphagula may be added to wheat bran fiber to accomplish this level of fiber without completely altering a patient's diet. Many patients who are constipated continue to pass dry, hard stool despite an increase in dietary fiber because they do not increase the water content of their diet. Fiber works in the gut by holding onto water and keeping the stool soft; to achieve this effect, the intake of liquids must be increased. For a 30 g/day fiber diet, it is recommended that patients drink eight 8 oz. glasses (i.e., 2 L) of non–caffeine-containing beverages per day.

Secondary causes of constipation must be excluded. The patient with bowel obstruction can present with constipation, and this possibility should always be considered in a patient with the onset of constipation after the age of 40 years (when the incidence of colon cancer rises). A rarer cause of constipation is hypothyroidism; not infrequently, patients with an underactive thyroid will present with a primary symptom of constipation. Hypercalcemia rarely reaches levels that produce constipation but should always be considered, since it can be a life-threatening disorder; constipation in this setting is always resistant to therapy until the hypercalcemia is treated. Proctitis can present with a complaint of infrequent stool passage due to the functional obstruction caused by the inflammation of the rectum; the colon more proximally continues to produce formed stool, which cannot pass easily through the inflamed rectum. Proctitis will usually be associated with excess mucus production, with or without blood in the stool, and proctosigmoidoscopy will always diagnose this entity.

Another cause of constipation is diabetes mellitus, often as a result of impaired motility; dietary factors may also play a role, along with autonomic neuropathy of the enteric nervous system. A small proportion of these diabetic patients with constipation can go on to develop diarrhea, which again has been linked to the autonomic neuropathy seen with long-standing diabetes mellitus.

Inactivity from whatever cause seems to increase the likelihood of a patient's complaining of a constipated bowel habit. This is presumed to be secondary to reduced colonic activity but could be aggravated by a low fiber intake in many of these patients. Severe cardiopulmonary diseases of whatever cause that limit activity can result in constipation. Neurologic disorders that cause the patient to have a reduced ability to ambulate can have constipation as a feature. Some patients with diseases of the nervous system may have impaired awareness of rectal distention to signal a need to defecate, and nerve dysfunction (both peripheral and central) may impair normal colonic propulsion. Finally, the elderly may develop problems with defecation, and although constipation with fecal impaction occurs they may complain of "diarrhea" or "soiling" due to overflow incontinence of stool from the fecal impaction of the rectum inhibiting the normal resting tone of the anal sphincter. Not surprisingly, many of these patients may respond to laxative therapy after the fecal impaction is removed, since this prevents the recurrence of the fecal impaction with overflow incontinence. Some patients can aggravate long-standing constipation with regular laxative abuse, and some theoretical concerns remain that this practice may indeed damage the normal innervation of the colon, rendering it atonic and nonfunctional.

The physical findings are often minimal in the majority of patients with constipation, but specific secondary causes must be looked for. Signs of hypothyroidism may be present; signs of dehydration should be sought, as this may be an early indicator of hypercalcemia. Thorough cardiopulmonary and neurologic examinations are necessary to pick out associated diseases that may be treated, thereby improving the patient's overall health and thus improving bowel function. On abdominal examination, inspection for evidence of distention or hyperperistalsis or masses may point out the source of the impaired stool passage. Localized tenderness of the abdomen must be noted, along with any evidence of liver, spleen or renal enlargement. A complete rectal examination and proctosigmoidoscopy is required in any patient with constipation so that the presence or absence of a fecal impaction, dilation or enlargement of the rectum or the presence of proctitis can be determined.

3.6.1 *MEGARECTUM*

When the rectum is enlarged, further investigations are required to exclude other causes, particularly Hirschsprung's disease (Section 3.6.2). The majority of patients with constipation and a dilated rectum and/or colon at proctosigmoidoscopy or barium enema have idiopathic or acquired megarectum. A useful guideline for the diagnosis of a "megarectum" is a rectal diameter of greater than 6 cm on a lateral film at the level of the S2 vertebral body. These patients can often present in childhood (many of them presenting with encopresis) and in the elderly with a fecal impaction. The cause of the megarectum is unknown, but if the onset is in childhood it may be the result of chronic stool holding by the child, leading to progressive distention of the rectum and eventual loss of awareness of rectal distention. Once this has occurred the patient can no longer recognize when stool is present in the rectum; the distention of the rectum causes chronic inhibition of the resting tone of the internal anal sphincter. This leads to the loss of control of liquid or semisolid stool that passes by the fecal impaction without the patient being aware of it.

3.6.2 *HIRSCHSPRUNG'S DISEASE*

The majority of patients with this disorder present soon after birth or in early childhood. This is a lesion, present at birth, where variable lengths of distal colon have no myenteric plexus. The distal colon remains contracted and the normal proximal colon dilates as it fills with stool. Most of these patients present early in life with obstipation and colonic obstruction, and require surgery. However, a few patients have a very short segment of denervated distal colon, so that they can overcome the obstruction and force stool out of the rectum. They usually have lifelong constipation; the normal rectum proximal to the denervated segment dilates over time so that the patient presents with constipation and a "megarectum." These patients rarely have fecal incontinence or fecal "soiling" as seen with idiopathic megarectum, since the internal anal sphincter and denervated distal rectum maintain a high resting tone. This condition can be diagnosed by anorectal manometry in that a normal rectoanal inhibitory reflex cannot be identified (Figure 6). However, a definite diagnosis requires deep rectal biopsy from the denervated segment, which will show absence of the myenteric plexus ganglion cells and hypertrophy of nerve fiber bundles. It should be added that an identical condition can be acquired with Chagas' disease from South America, which attacks the myenteric plexus and other autonomic ganglion cells; patients with this condition can also present with achalasia or intestinal pseudo-obstruction as well as cardiac arrhythmias. These patients will also have an absent rectoanal inhibitory reflex if the disease involves the rectal myenteric plexus.

3.6.3 PELVIC FLOOR DYSSYNERGIA
The majority of patients with constipation have a form of irritable bowel syndrome, but there is a small subgroup of patients who may have a specific disorder in colonic and/or anorectal function that produces constipation. These patients are almost all female, may have delayed colonic transit or present with anorectal dysfunction with impaired awareness to rectal distention (without a megarectum), or may demonstrate a phenomenon of rectal outlet obstruction due to inappropriate contraction of the voluntary anal sphincters during defecation. This has been termed pelvic floor dyssynergia or anismus. These patients can present major therapeutic dilemmas and warrant further investigation in specialized coloproctology units involved in the care of such patients.

3.7 Infections of the Colon

3.7.1 SHIGELLA
This infectious diarrhea is the classic cause of "bacillary dysentery." Typical presentation is with fever, abdominal cramping and watery diarrhea that usually becomes bloody within 24 to 48 hours of onset. The incubation period is from 36 to 48 hours. As the disease progresses the symptoms become typical of colonic dysentery, with small, frequent stools and cramping and tenesmus that may lead to rectal prolapse in some individuals with prolonged straining.

The causative organism is a gram-negative bacterium with only humans as its host. The organism is well adapted to causing disease in humans. As few as 200 organisms are needed to cause infection as compared with other enteric infections requiring 10^6 organisms or more. It can persist in food for weeks and on contaminated body surfaces for several hours. Pathogenesis is through production of a cytotoxin called Shiga toxin or similar toxins that are both cytotoxic and neurotoxic, very similar to the toxin produced by E. coli 0157:H7 species. Shigella is a microinvasive bacterium that enters the host via the M cells in the intestine and then spreads laterally through the colonic mucosa to involve the basolateral membrane of the surrounding cells. It is seen mostly in travelers returning from endemic areas (tropical and subtropical). There is also a higher incidence in male homosexuals who practice oral–anal sex.

Treatment depends on the antibiotic resistance of the infecting strain of bacteria. Shigella species quickly develop antibiotic resistance; patients should be encouraged to complete their course of antibiotics to prevent this. Antibiotics shorten the duration of both symptoms and carriage of the organism. Fluoroquinolones are the antibiotics of choice because of the low incidence of resistance at present, but this may change. Ampicillin and trimethoprim-sulfamethoxazole are also effective against sensitive strains. If infection has been acquired overseas, a confirmed Shigella infection is best treated with a fluoroquinolone twice daily for 5 days, but there are reports of a single large dose eradicating infection. Antimotility agents such as loperamide, diphenoxylate or narcotic analgesics are contraindicated with this infection because of the risk of a toxic colon. In general, antimotility agents should never be used in acute infectious diarrhea when bloody stool is present.

3.7.2 SALMONELLA

Infection with nontyphoidal strains of Salmonella results from ingesting foods contaminated with organisms. These bacteria are endemic to poultry and cattle populations. Large epidemics have resulted from undercooked eggs, and these bacteria are also frequently found in reptiles and amphibians. Salmonella contamination of marijuana can be an important infection source in young adults. The usual incubation period is from 8 to 48 hours after ingestion.

S. typhi, which causes typhoid fever, is found only in humans. It will not be discussed further other than to emphasize that all Salmonella species are related and therefore can cause systemic illness of similar severity, especially in patients who are immunocompromised and those at the extremes of age (i.e., those under 2 and the frail elderly).

Salmonella is an invasive bacterium that can cause septicemia after first multiplying in the mesenteric lymph nodes. Resistance to infection is first a result of the presence of gastric acid and then of the integrity of the intestinal flora and of motility. Increased infection is associated with the use of purgatives, antimotility agents and broad-spectrum antibiotics along with acid-suppression therapy. Bowel surgery will also increase the chance of symptomatic infection. Diseases that predispose to infection as a result of impaired host defenses include sickle cell disease, systemic lupus erythematosus (SLE) and AIDS.

Treatment is usually symptomatic. Antibiotics should be used only if the patient is showing signs of bacteremia; antibiotics often increase the development of a chronic carrier state. The antibiotics of choice are ampicillin and trimethoprim-sulfamethoxazole, but recently the fluoroquinolones and the third-generation cephalosporins (especially ceftriaxone with its high biliary excretion) have been shown to be very effective in patients who need antibiotic therapy. Treatment with antibiotics should normally be considered only for patients under the age of 2 years and elderly patients with vascular disease, as well as patients with metal implants in bones, lymphoproliferative disease, sickle cell disease or AIDS. The site of chronic infection is usually the biliary tract. Disease of the biliary tree, especially cholelithiasis, requires surgery to correct the disease followed by a two-week course of therapy, which often leads to resolution of the chronic carrier state.

3.7.3 CLOSTRIDIUM DIFFICILE

This spore-forming anaerobic gram-positive bacterium is the commonest cause of infectious diarrhea in hospitalized patients. The organism is not invasive, but with reduction of the normal colonic bacterial flora it multiplies and produces two toxins, known as toxins A and B. Toxin A causes colitis. Toxin B is a cytotoxin that is often used as a diagnostic test for this infection.

Most commonly, infection is preceded by antibiotic therapy. Outbreaks in hospital frequently occur among the sickest patients, some not receiving antibiotics beforehand. Penicillins, cephalosporins and clindamycin are more likely to be associated with C. difficile infection, but all antibiotics, including metronidazole and vancomycin, have been associated with it. Other risk factors include agents that affect gut motility such as enemas and anti-diarrheal medications, and intensive chemotherapy. Patients with severe illnesses and advanced age are also more prone to manifest disease symptoms.

Diarrhea is the commonest symptom of presentation and is usually non-bloody, but with prolonged diarrhea some blood can result from local anorectal irritation. The typical appearance at endoscopy of the colon and rectum is of "pseudomembranes" or whitish plaques on the surface of the colonic mucosa with intervening areas of mucosa that appear almost normal. For this reason, infection is often called "pseudomembranous colitis" (PMC). Unfortunately, these characteristic changes may not be present in the rectum, so diagnosis is usually confirmed by the presence of cytotoxin in the stool placed on tissue culture. The clinician must be alert to the possibility of this infection in susceptible patients since in some patients, neither culture of C. difficile nor the presence of the cytotoxin in the stool is positive. A careful inventory of any antibiotic therapy in the last three months is crucial in considering this cause for diarrhea, as many patients will have taken the offending antibiotic several days to weeks before symptoms begin.

Metronidazole (Flagyl®) treatment is preferred to vancomycin because both antibiotics show similar efficacy in treating this infection and metronidazole is about one-tenth the cost of vancomycin. Treatment is for 7 to 10 days, usually in a dose of 250 mg p.o. q.i.d. in the studies that have been reported. The vancomycin dosage is 125 mg p.o. q.i.d. but is effective only via the oral route, whereas metronidazole is also effective intravenously in the occasional patient with postoperative ileus. With both regimens there is a high relapse rate of infection, of up to 20%. The best method to prevent relapse is unknown, but relapsing symptoms may respond to retreatment of the infection with either metronidazole or vancomycin.

3.7.4 ENTAMOEBA HISTOLYTICA (AMEBIASIS)

Entamoeba histolytica, the parasite that causes amebiasis infection, appears to be the only ameba that causes disease in humans. Other amebas are often found in the colon as normal commensals. E. histolytica is a cyst-forming parasite, but the cysts do not cause disease. The cysts are ingested and are resistant to destruction by gastric acid; then the trophozoite develops in the colon from the ingested cyst. The cysts spread disease to others, and frequently unaffected carriers spread disease by excreting cysts. The trophozoites, which invade the colonic mucosa, cause disease, but trophozoites passed in the stool of symptomatic individuals cannot survive outside the body and rarely transmit infection. The disease is most prevalent in areas of the tropics where sanitation is poor.

The colon is the usual site of initial disease. Invasion of the mucosa by trophozoites is due to the production of an "amebapore" molecule that causes the lining colonocytes to lyze; the lyzed colonocytes are then ingested by the amebas, leading to ulceration of the colon and dissemination throughout the body. The amebas infect the colon and rarely the ileum, but the cecum is usually involved. E. histolytica is an invasive pathogen and can spread hematogenously to other organs, especially the liver.

Diagnosis is usually made by identification of E. histolytica on microscopic analysis of stool, but can also be made on identification of the ameba on histological diagnosis of colonic biopsies. There is a decreased yield on stool analysis after barium studies and if antibiotics or mineral oil is used prior to collection. At endoscopy the ulcers of the rectum and colon may appear characteristic with undermined edges, and sometimes the intervening mucosa looks normal in contrast to acute bacillary dysentery (see Section 3.7.1) and ulcerative colitis. Diagnosis can also be made by indirect hemagglutination and ELISA tests on serum to detect infection, but if the patient is a carrier with only cyst excretion these tests are often negative. Chronic infection of the cecum leads to a "coned" appearance on x-ray. Other colonic complications include perforation, ameboma (a granulomatous tissue reaction in the colon; the mass effect can lead to obstruction or be mistaken for colonic malignancy), pericolic abscess and fistulas. The liver is the commonest extraintestinal organ infected, but E. histolytica can also spread to the brain, lungs, pericardium and eyes. There is an increased risk of disseminated disease and abscess formation if the patient is on steroids, is pregnant or is immunocompromised.

Treatment is usually metronidazole 400–750 mg t.i.d. × 5–10 days for acute colitis. If the patient has chronic colonic disease with chronic shedding of cysts, diloxanide 500 mg t.i.d. × 10 days is the drug of choice. If this cannot be obtained, then iodoquinol 650 mg t.i.d. × 20 days can be used, but this is the maximal dose because it can cause optic neuritis. Patients with amebic liver abscess should first be treated with metronidazole for 10 days and then be given 10 days of diloxanide. All patients should be reassessed two to three months after treatment to ensure clearance of the parasite and that there is no chronic carrier state with cyst excretion.

3.7.5 BALANTIDIUM COLI

A very large, ciliated protozoan that uncommonly causes an illness similar to amebic dysentery, B. coli is usually easy to identify in stool samples owing to its large size. It is acquired in tropical or subtropical countries from exposure to pigs, which frequently carry this organism without signs of illness. Treatment is with tetracycline 500 mg q.i.d. for 10 days. B. coli is also sensitive to ampicillin and metronidazole.

3.7.6 BLASTOCYSTIS HOMINIS

A yeast frequently found in asymptomatic individuals, recently B. hominis has been suggested as a cause of unexplained diarrhea in some patients found to have large numbers of this protozoan in the stool. Treatment appears to be with either metronidazole 750 mg t.i.d. × 10 days or iodoquinol 650 mg t.i.d. × 20 days. Iodoquinol may be more successful, but the best treatment has not been identified to date.

3.8 Intestinal Nematode Infections

3.8.1 ROUNDWORM (ASCARIS LUMBRICOIDES)
Roundworm or ascaris, one of the more common nematodes found in humans, is most often found in the tropics. Usually eggs are ingested from contaminated foods or dirty hands. The eggs hatch in the intestine and spread by the blood to the liver and then to the lungs. An eosinophilic pneumonitis can develop and then the larvae migrate through the alveoli, up to the trachea and through the larynx where they are swallowed. They develop into adult worms in the small intestine. The adults can cause intestinal obstruction symptoms if large numbers are present, and can cause biliary symptoms if they migrate into the common bile duct.

3.8.2 HOOKWORM (ANCYLOSTOMA DUODENALE; NECATOR AMERICANUS)
Hookworm can infiltrate skin from contaminated earth and is prone to be found in areas with fecal contamination of the soil. A pruritic rash develops at the site of entry into the body. The filarial larvae then travel to the lungs, migrate through the alveoli and then up through the larynx where they are swallowed. After being swallowed, they cause nausea, diarrhea, vomiting, abdominal pain and flatulence. Many patients present with iron deficiency from a daily blood loss of 0.1–0.4 mL with each worm.

3.8.3 WHIPWORM (TRICHURIS TRICHIURA)
Whipworm can also cause iron deficiency if large numbers infect the GI tract. It primarily invades the colon. Bloody diarrhea develops with larger infestations. It is easily diagnosed by stool analysis looking for the typical eggs, but is increasingly diagnosed at colonoscopy during investigation of the bloody diarrhea, where the worms are easily seen if present.

3.8.4 PINWORM (ENTEROBIUS VERMICULARIS)
Pinworm is probably the commonest nematode worldwide. It usually causes pruritus ani, often worse at night when the worms migrate onto the perianal skin and lay their eggs. Pinworm is probably the most common nematode encountered in Canada, especially in children. Diagnosis is by identification of the eggs from the perianal skin, usually collected in the early morning before defecation.

3.8.5 STRONGYLOIDES STERCORALIS (STRONGYLOIDIASIS)
Strongyloides stercoralis is widely found in the tropics. It is the only nematode that can multiply and reproduce its entire life cycle within the human

host, thus causing persistent reinfection over many years after the original infection. Larvae can penetrate intact skin or the eggs can be ingested. Filariform larvae that penetrate the skin travel hematogenously to the lungs and then, as with the other worms, travel into the airways and are swallowed. In the intestine the larvae become adult worms. When the eggs are ingested, they become filariform larvae in the intestine; then the larvae invade the blood vessels, thus reinfecting the host.

Symptoms of strongyloidiasis vary and may include abdominal pain, diarrhea, nausea and vomiting. With mostly intestinal involvement diarrhea can develop; especially in children, a syndrome similar to celiac disease with protein-losing enteropathy can develop. The majority of adult infections are asymptomatic or are only intermittently symptomatic. Recurrent urticaria can develop where the worms infiltrate the skin, particularly the perianal skin and gluteal areas.

Diagnosis can be confirmed by stool analysis but can be negative in up to 25% of cases, even after repeated stool analysis. The larvae look similar to hookworm. An ELISA test is useful for diagnosis, but there may be overlap with the presence of Filaria species. Eosinophilia is often present, even in asymptomatic individuals.

Thiabendazole is usually used to treat, 25 mg/kg twice daily to a maximum of 3 g daily for two days, or five days for disseminated disease. Albendazole or ivermectin may be used if the patient is unable to tolerate thiabendazole, but these drugs appear to be less effective against S. stercoralis. With the hyperinfection syndrome, when large numbers of the worms are present (often in association with immune suppression, as with steroid therapy), antibiotics are often needed to treat the septicemia that results if the intestinal damage allows secondary bacterial invasion.

3.9 Microscopic Colitis

A rare condition has been recognized increasingly in which the patient presents with usually painless diarrhea. Investigations often find signs of inflammation, but the colon appears normal on both radioscopic and colonoscopic examination. This condition is sometimes called "lymphocytic colitis" and may also be part of a spectrum of colitis conditions that include "collagenous colitis." The natural history of these diseases is unclear at present, and no infective agent has been found. These disorders can be diagnosed only by colonoscopic biopsy. The colonic mucosa appears normal, yet on histological examination there is an increase in the inflammatory infiltrate of the lamina propria. In collagenous colitis the basement membrane of the colonic mucosa is thickened by a band of collagen. In most patients the disease appears to follow a benign course, but about half of patients continue to have significant diarrhea for more than two years. The disease is controlled by antimotility agents such as loperamide or by use of 5-aminosalicylic acid–based therapies directed at the colon (see Chapter 10, "Inflammatory Bowel Disease"), which often help to lessen the diarrhea. Glucocorticoids also control the diarrhea, but in view of the benign course of this illness in most patients, steroid therapy should be used only in severely symptomatic patients who cannot be controlled by other therapy.

3.10 Eosinophilic Colitis
Eosinophilic gastroenteritis is an uncommon inflammatory condition that affects primarily the upper GI tract and small intestine (see Chapters 5, 6 and 7). However, there have been recent reports of an apparently separate condition called "eosinophilic colitis" in which patients with connective tissue disease present with diarrhea of uncertain cause with negative stool investigations. These patients have all been diagnosed at colonoscopy by biopsy of essentially normal-looking mucosa, yet with increased eosinophils in the lamina propria. All patients respond to steroids, but it would appear that not all patients resolve over time and some may need prolonged steroid therapy.

4. THE ANAL CANAL / M. Burnstein

4.1 Functional Anatomy of the Anal Canal and Anorectal Spaces

4.1.1 THE ANAL CANAL
The anal canal begins where the terminal portion of the large bowel passes through the pelvic floor muscles, and it ends at the anal verge. It measures roughly 4 cm in length. The wall of the anal canal is formed by a continuation of the circular muscle of the rectal wall; the smooth muscle is thickened in this area to form the internal anal sphincter. This smooth-muscle sphincter is wrapped by skeletal muscle, the external anal sphincter. The top of the external anal sphincter is formed by the U-shaped puborectalis muscle, which loops around the anus, arising and inserting on the pubis. This is felt posteriorly and laterally as the anorectal ring on digital examination. The longitudinal muscle coat of the rectum descends in the plane between the sphincters as the conjoined longitudinal muscle, and it sends fibers across the lower part of the external anal sphincter to insert on the skin (corrugator cutis ani, responsible for the anocutaneous reflex or "anal wink"). These fibers also traverse the internal anal sphincter to insert on the submucosa ("mucosal suspensory ligament").

In approximately the mid-anus there is a rolling line of demarcation called the dentate line. Above the line is columnar epithelium; below it is squamous epithelium without appendages (the anoderm). The demarcation does not really occur at a line, but at a transitional zone of 0.5–1 cm in length.

As the rectum narrows into the anal canal, the mucosa develops 6 to 14 longitudinal folds, Morgagni's columns. Between the distal ends of the columns are small crypts. Anal glands open into the crypts. There are 4 to 10 glands, and they are lined by stratified columnar epithelium. About half of these tubular glands end in the intersphincteric plane.

Blood is supplied to the anus via the inferior rectal artery, a branch of the internal pudendal artery. The inferior rectal artery crosses the ischiorectal fossa. The superior rectal vein drains the upper part of the anal canal via the inferior mesenteric vein to the portal vein. The middle and inferior rectal veins drain the upper and lower anal canal into the systemic circulation via the internal iliac and internal pudendal veins, respectively.

Lymphatic drainage above the dentate line is via the superior rectal lymphatics (accompanying the superior rectal vessels) to the inferior mesenteric nodes, and laterally along the middle and inferior rectal vessels to the internal iliac nodes. Lymphatic drainage from the anal canal below the dentate line may be in a cephalad or lateral direction, but is primarily to the inguinal nodes.

Motor innervation of the external anal sphincter is via the inferior rectal branch of the pudendal nerve and the perineal branch of the fourth sacral nerve. The internal anal sphincter has sympathetic (motor) and parasympathetic (inhibitory) innervation. Parasympathetic supply is from the nervi erigentes (S2, S3, S4). Sympathetic innervation is from the first three lumbar segments via the preaortic plexus. Fibers from the preaortic plexus ultimately join the nervi erigentes to form the pelvic plexuses. Sensation below the dentate line (and for up to 1.5 cm above the dentate line) is carried by the inferior rectal nerve. Above the level of the inferior rectal nerve sensory distribution, there are only dull perceptions, mediated by parasympathetic fibers.

4.1.2 ANORECTAL SPACES

Around the anorectum are a number of potential spaces filled with fat or connective tissue. These may become the sites of abscess formation. The perianal space is at the anal verge, and is continuous with the intersphincteric space. The pyramid-shaped ischiorectal (ischioanal) fossa is medially bounded by the external anal sphincter and the levator ani muscles. The lateral wall is the obturator internus muscle and fascia. The inferior boundary is the skin of the perineum, and the apex is the origin of the levator ani from the obturator fascia. Posteriorly is the gluteus maximus muscle, and anteriorly the transverse perinei muscles. On the obturator fascia is Alcock's canal, containing the internal pudendal vessels and pudendal nerve. The fossa is filled with fat and also contains the inferior rectal nerve and vessels, and the fourth sacral nerve. The two ischiorectal spaces communicate with one another behind the anal canal.

4.2 Evaluation of Anorectal Complaints

This section will review the symptoms associated with anorectal pathology and the techniques of anorectal examination.

4.2.1 *HISTORY*

As in most of medicine, taking a careful history is the most productive step in leading to a diagnosis. In the evaluation of the patient with anorectal complaints, there are a limited number of questions to be asked:

4.2.1.1 *Pain*

There are three common lesions that cause anorectal pain: fissure in ano, anal abscess and thrombosed external hemorrhoid. If the pain is sharp and occurs during, and for a short time following, bowel movements, a fissure is likely. Continuous pain associated with a perianal swelling probably stems from thrombosis of perianal vessels, especially when there is an antecedent history of straining, either at stool or with physical exertion. An anal abscess will also produce a continuous, often throbbing pain, which may be aggravated by the patient's coughing or sneezing. Anorectal abscesses are generally associated with local signs of inflammation. The absence of an inflammatory mass in the setting of severe local pain and tenderness is typical of an intersphincteric abscess; the degree of tenderness usually prevents adequate examination, and evaluation under anesthesia is necessary to confirm the diagnosis and to drain the pus.

Anal pain of any etiology may be aggravated by bowel movements. Tenesmus, an uncomfortable desire to defecate, is frequently associated with inflammatory conditions of the anorectum. Although anal neoplasms rarely produce pain, invasion of the sphincter mechanism may also result in tenesmus. Tenesmus with urgency of evacuation suggests proctitis.

Transient, deep-seated pain that is unrelated to defecation may be due to levator spasm ("proctalgia fugax").

Anorectal pain is so frequently, and erroneously, attributed to hemorrhoids, that this point bears special mention: pain is *not* a symptom of uncomplicated hemorrhoids. If a perianal vein of the inferior rectal plexus undergoes thrombosis, or ruptures, an acutely painful and tender subcutaneous lump will appear. This is the "thrombosed external hemorrhoid." Internal hemorrhoids may prolapse and become strangulated to produce an acute problem of anorectal pain, tenderness, and mucous, bloody discharge. Gangrene and secondary infection may ensue.

4.2.1.2 Bleeding

The nature of the rectal bleeding will help determine the underlying cause. However, the clinician must remember that the historical features of the bleeding cannot be relied upon to define the problem with certainty. Bright red blood on the toilet paper or on the outside of the stool, or dripping into the bowl, suggests a local anal source, such as a fissure or internal hemorrhoids. Blood that is mixed in with the stool, or that is dark and clotted, suggests sources proximal to the anus. Melena is always due to more proximal pathology.

The associated symptoms are very helpful. A history of local anal bleeding, as described above, associated with painful defecation, suggests a fissure. The same bleeding pattern without pain suggests internal hemorrhoids; this may be associated with some degree of hemorrhoidal prolapse. Bleeding and diarrhea may occur with inflammatory bowel disease. When bleeding is associated with a painful lump and is not exclusively related to defecation, a thrombosed external hemorrhoid is likely. Bleeding associated with a mucopurulent discharge and tenesmus may be seen with proctitis, or possibly with a rectal neoplasm.

Bleeding per rectum is an important symptom of colorectal cancer, and although this is not the most common cause of hematochezia, it is the most serious and must always be considered. This does not mean that every patient who passes blood must have contrast radiography of the colon or total colonoscopy. If the bleeding has an obvious anal source, it may be prudent not to proceed with a total colon examination, especially in a patient at low risk for colorectal neoplasms (i.e., age under 50 years; no history of Crohn's or ulcerative colitis; no family history of colon cancer; and no personal history of colorectal neoplasms). However, if bleeding persists after treatment of the anal pathology, more ominous lesions have to be excluded.

4.2.1.3 Prolapse

In evaluating protrusion from the anal opening, there are several relevant questions: Is the prolapse spontaneous or exclusively with defecation? Spontaneous prolapse is less characteristic of internal hemorrhoids than of hypertrophied anal papillae or complete rectal prolapse. Does the prolapsing tissue reduce spontaneously (as may be the case with second-degree internal hemorrhoids) or does it require manual reduction (as with third-degree internal hemorrhoids or complete rectal prolapse)? The patient may be able to describe the size of the prolapsing tissue, and this may suggest the diagnosis.

Complete rectal prolapse (procidentia) must be distinguished from mucosal prolapse or prolapsing internal hemorrhoids. Procidentia occurs mainly in women (female:male = 6:1), with a peak incidence in the seventh decade. Procidentia is often associated with fecal incontinence. In later stages, protrusion occurs even with slight exertion such as coughing or sneezing. The extruded rectum becomes excoriated, leading to tenesmus, mucus discharge and bleeding. (Examination of the patient with procidentia usually reveals poor anal tone, and with the tissue in a prolapsed state, the mucosal folds are seen to be concentric, whereas with prolapsed hemorrhoids there are radial folds.) Rarely, a large polypoid tumor of the rectum may prolapse through the anal canal.

4.2.1.4 *Perianal mass*
A painful perianal lump may be an abscess or a thrombosed external hemorrhoid. Knowing whether there has been a discharge of blood or pus may be helpful. An intermittent mass suggests a prolapsing lesion.

External or "skin" tags are very common deformities of the anal margin. They may be the result of previous or active fissure disease, or the sequelae of a thrombosed external hemorrhoid. Condylomata acuminata – or venereal warts – are caused by a sexually transmitted virus. The perianal skin is frequently affected, and the condition occurs with greatest frequency in gay men.

The differential diagnosis also includes benign and malignant neoplasms.

4.2.1.5 *Pruritus*
Itching is a common associated feature of many anorectal conditions, especially during the healing phase or if there is a discharge. But pruritus ani may also be an isolated symptom or the patient's primary complaint. As a chief complaint, pruritus may be caused by infections (e.g., pinworms, condylomata, Candida) or skin conditions (e.g., contact dermatitis, psoriasis). More commonly, no specific underlying pathology is identified, and the problem is idiopathic.

Idiopathic pruritus ani is more common in men, and is typically worse at night. When chronic, the characteristic changes of hypertrophy and lichenification, nodularity, scarring and fissuring of the skin become apparent.

4.2.1.6 *Discharge*
Although mucus is a normal product of the colorectal mucosa, it is not normally seen in the stool. Increased mucus may be the result of proctocolitis or

a colorectal neoplasm, especially a villous adenoma of the rectum. Both inflammatory and neoplastic conditions may present with mucus and blood. Phosphate enemas are irritating and often elicit copious mucus production. Patients with the irritable bowel syndrome may complain of mucous stools.

Mucus staining of the underclothes may be associated with prolapsing tissue. When the staining has a fecal component, or when there is associated inability to control gas or to discriminate gas from solids within the rectum, a disturbance of the continence mechanism exists. A history of "accidents," or the need to wear pads during the day or night, will help indicate the magnitude of the problem. The discharge may arise from an obvious external lesion – e.g., blood from a thrombosed external hemorrhoid, or pus from an abscess, from the external opening of a fistula, from a pilonidal process or from perianal hidradenitis suppurativa.

Other issues that will prove helpful in coming to a diagnosis of anorectal pathology include bowel habits, associated medical conditions and medications, sexual practices, travel history and family history.

4.2.2 EXAMINATION

The patient about to undergo examination of the anorectum may not only be embarrassed, but also afraid of impending pain and discomfort. Explanation of the examinations to be performed, and reassurance, will lessen the patient's anxiety and contribute greatly to patient cooperation.

The four steps in anorectal evaluation are inspection, palpation, anoscopy and proctosigmoidoscopy.

4.2.2.1 Positioning

The patient is placed either in the left lateral position or (preferably) in the prone-jackknife position. The prone-jackknife position requires a special table that tilts the head down and raises the anorectal region, with the buttocks tending to fall apart. This provides the best and easiest access for the examiner, although patient comfort may be less.

The left lateral (Sims') position has the advantages of patient comfort and of being suitable for any examining table, bed or stretcher. The patient's buttocks are allowed to protrude over the edge of the table, with hips flexed and knees slightly extended. The examiner may sit or stand.

The patient is unable to see "what's going on back there," and it is important to continually explain what you are doing and what can be expected.

4.2.2.2 Inspection

Looking at the anal area may reveal obvious external pathology. The resting anal aperture should be observed: a patulous opening may be seen with procidentia, sphincter injury or neurologic abnormality. Straining and squeezing by the patient may provide information about anorectal function.

Gentle spreading of the buttocks may elicit pain in a patient who has an anal fissure. Asking the patient to strain down may provide information: internal hemorrhoids may protrude or procidentia may be seen. However, if procidentia is suspected, it should be sought with the patient squatting or sitting at the toilet.

4.2.2.3 Palpation

A disposable plastic glove and water-soluble lubricant are required. The patient is told that a finger will be gently placed into the rectum. While one hand separates the buttocks, the index finger is placed on the anal verge, and with the patient bearing down, thereby relaxing the anus, the digit is advanced into the anal canal.

A methodical approach is best. Palpation anteriorly checks the prostate in males, and the cervix in females. The finger then sweeps backward and forward to palpate the rest of the circumference of the anorectum. This may be the only part of the examination that identifies submucosal lesions, which may easily go undetected by endoscopy. Resting tone and ability to squeeze should also be assessed. The location of tenderness or a palpable abnormality should be precisely recorded.

4.2.2.4 Anoscopy

The anoscope is the optimal instrument for examining lesions of the anal canal. It is not a substitute for proctosigmoidoscopy, and the proctosigmoidoscope does not provide as satisfactory a view of the canal as does the anoscope. Many anoscopes are available; the best instrument is end-viewing, with an attached fiberoptic light source.

4.2.2.5 Proctosigmoidoscopy

The rigid 25 cm sigmoidoscope (or proctoscope) is the best instrument for examining the rectum. A barium enema, because of the balloon-tipped catheter used in administering the contrast material, does not adequately evaluate the rectal ampulla and is never a sufficient workup of a lower GI complaint.

A variety of rigid sigmoidoscopes are available: disposable or reusable, in a range of diameters (1.1 cm, 1.9 cm, 2.7 cm) and with proximal or distal lighting. The 1.9 cm instrument provides good visibility with minimal patient discomfort. The instrument includes a 25 cm tube, a magnifying lens, a light source, and a bulb attachment for air insufflation. Long swabs may be helpful in maintaining visibility, but suction is best.

A single Fleet® enema provides excellent preparation of the distal bowel and should be used just before the examination. The Fleet® enema may produce transient mucosal changes, and if inflammatory bowel disease is suspected, it should be avoided.

The digital examination has set the stage for instrumentation by permitting the sphincter to relax. With the tip well lubricated, the sigmoidoscope is inserted and passed quickly up the rectum. As always, the patient is informed of what is being done, and is reassured that the sensation of impending evacuation is caused by the instrument, and that the bowels are not about to move.

Air insufflation should be kept to a minimum, as it may cause discomfort, but it is of value both on entry and on withdrawal in demonstrating the mucosa and lumen and in assessing rectal compliance and the presence of normal sensation of rectal distention. Advancement should occur only with the lumen clearly in sight. When the lumen is "lost," withdraw and redirect to regain it.

As the rectosigmoid is reached (approximately 15 cm along), the patient should be warned of possible cramping discomfort that will disappear as the scope is removed. Frequently, even with experience, the rectosigmoid angle cannot be negotiated, and the examination should be terminated. Most importantly, the patient should not be hurt or caused significant discomfort. The scope should be withdrawn making large circular motions, carefully inspecting the circumference of the bowel wall, flattening the mucosal folds and valves of Houston. The posterior rectal wall in the sacral hollow must be specifically sought out, or it will be missed.

In most large studies, the average depth of insertion is 18–20 cm; the full length of the instrument is inserted in less than half the patients.

Perforation of the normal rectum by the sigmoidoscope is extremely rare (1 in 50,000 or less). However, advancing the instrument or insufflating air may be hazardous in settings such as inflammatory bowel disease, radiation proctitis, diverticulitis and cancer. Of course, biopsy and electrocoagulation have to be performed with care and with knowledge of the technique and equipment.

The incidence and significance of bacteremia following anorectal manipulations is controversial, and has been reported in 0–25% of proctoscopies. Prophylactic antibiotics should be considered in patients with prosthetic heart valves.

4.3 Specific Anorectal Problems
This section will briefly review some of the more common anorectal problems.

4.3.1 *HEMORRHOIDS*

4.3.1.1 *Background*
The upper anal canal has three sites of thickened submucosa containing arteri-

oles, venules and arteriovenous communications. These three vascular "cushions" are in the left lateral, right anterior and right posterior positions. Minor cushions may lie between the three main ones. The cushions are held in the upper anal canal by muscular fibers from the conjoined longitudinal muscle of the intersphincteric plane.

Hemorrhoids exist when the anal cushions prolapse after disruption of their suspensory mechanism, or when there is dilation of the veins and arteriovenous anastomoses within the cushions. Various theories can be put forward for the development of internal hemorrhoidal disease: raised intra-abdominal pressure, pressure on the hemorrhoidal veins by an enlarging uterus, poor venous drainage secondary to an overactive internal anal sphincter, straining at stool with a resultant downward displacement of the cushions, etc.

Skin tags are projections of skin at the anal verge. They may be the result of previous thrombosed external hemorrhoids, fissure in ano, or inflammatory bowel disease.

External hemorrhoids are dilated veins of the inferior hemorrhoidal (rectal) plexus. This plexus lies just below the dentate line and is covered by squamous epithelium.

Internal hemorrhoids are the symptomatic, enlarged submucosal vascular cushions of the anal canal. The cushions are located above the dentate line and are covered by columnar and transitional epithelium. The patient's history allows internal hemorrhoids to be subdivided. First-degree hemorrhoids produce painless bleeding but do not protrude from the anal canal; at anoscopy, they are seen to bulge into the lumen. Second-degree hemorrhoids protrude with bowel movements, but reduce themselves spontaneously. Third-degree hemorrhoids prolapse outside the anal canal, either spontaneously or with bowel movements, but require digital reduction. Fourth-degree hemorrhoids are always prolapsed, and cannot be reduced.

4.3.1.2 *Diagnosis and treatment*

4.3.1.2.1 *Thrombosed external hemorrhoids* As a rule, external hemorrhoids are asymptomatic until the complication of thrombosis (intravascular clot) or rupture (perianal hematoma) supervenes. In either case, the presentation is severe pain with a perianal lump, often after straining. The natural history is one of continued pain for 4 to 5 days, then slow resolution over 10 to 14 days. The treatment depends on the severity of the pain and the timing of presentation. A patient who presents within 24 to 48 hours and with severe pain is best dealt with operatively. Under local anesthesia, the involved perianal vessel and clot are excised. The wound may be left open or may be closed. Simple evacuation of the thrombus is less effective. A patient presenting later, after 3 to 4 days, is advised to take frequent warm baths, a bulk laxative, a surface-active wetting agent, and oral analgesics. This regimen is also prescribed post-excision.

4.3.1.2.2 Internal hemorrhoids Painless, bright red rectal bleeding (usually with or following bowel movements) is the most common symptom of this condition. Blood appears on the toilet paper or on the outside of the stool, or drips into the bowl. It is very rare for the volume of blood lost from internal hemorrhoids to be sufficient to explain iron deficiency anemia; further workup is always indicated.

Prolapse with defecation or other straining activities is also a common symptom of internal hemorrhoids. Chronic prolapse is associated with mucus discharge, fecal staining of the underclothes and pruritus.

Anal sphincter spasm may result in thrombosis and strangulation of prolapsed hemorrhoids. This presents as an acute problem of a painful, discharging, edematous mass of hemorrhoids.

Inspection will identify the later stages of the disease, especially when the patient is asked to bear down. Digital examination can rule out other pathology, as well as assess the sphincters. A palpable abnormality suggests some other process. Anoscopy provides a diagnosis in first- and second-degree disease. With the anoscope in place, the patient is once again asked to strain, and the degree of prolapse observed. Proctosigmoidoscopy should always be performed to exclude other diseases, particularly rectal neoplasms and inflammatory bowel disease.

If the symptoms are at all atypical, or the physical findings leave any doubt about the source of blood, a colon-clearing examination (either colonoscopy or barium enema) should be performed.

In patients over the age of 50, it is reasonable to take the opportunity to screen (or to practice "case-finding") for colorectal cancer by performing sigmoidoscopy with the 60 cm flexible instrument. If risk factors for colorectal neoplasia are present, then colonoscopy or barium enema should certainly be performed.

Occasional bleeding, especially if it is related to hard stools or straining, should be managed by improving bowel habits using high-fiber diet and bulk agents (e.g., psyllium). If bleeding persists or is frequent, intervention is indicated, and in most cases should take the form of rubber-band ligation. Prolapsing hemorrhoids that reduce spontaneously, or can be easily reduced, are also nicely treated by rubber-band ligation. If prolapsing tissue is not easily reduced, or if there is a significant external component, surgical hemorrhoidectomy offers the best cure. Similarly, prolapsed, thrombosed internal hemorrhoids should be surgically excised.

4.3.1.2.3 Rubber-band ligation In this technique, strangulating rubber bands are placed at the cephalad aspect of the internal hemorrhoids. The absence of somatic pain fibers above the dentate line renders this a relatively painless procedure, as long as the rings are properly positioned. The banded tissue infarcts and sloughs over the next week, resulting in reduction of hemorrhoidal tissue, as well as fixation of the residual hemorrhoid in the upper anal canal. It is a simple office procedure requiring an anoscope and ligator. In general, only one or two areas are banded at a time, so that several treatments are often required. Long-term success is expected in approximately 75% of patients with second-degree hemorrhoids. Pain, bleeding and infection are rare complications.

4.3.1.2.4 Hemorrhoidectomy Since the popularization of rubber-band ligation, excisional hemorrhoidectomy has been much less frequently performed. The important principles of all excisional procedures are removal of all external and internal hemorrhoids, protection of the internal anal sphincter from injury, and maintenance of the anoderm, so as to avoid anal stenosis.

4.3.2 FISSURE IN ANO
This is a linear crack in the lining of the anal canal, extending from the dentate line to the anal verge. It is seen equally in men and women, and at all ages, but is a common entity in young adults. It is encountered mainly in the posterior midline, but also occasionally in the anterior midline. If a fissure persists, secondary changes occur. These include the "sentinel pile" at the distal end of the fissure and the "hypertrophied anal papilla" at the proximal end. They are due to edema and low-grade infection.

4.3.2.1 Pathogenesis
Fissure in ano is probably the result of trauma during the passage of hard stool, but not all patients with fissure in ano give a history of "constipation." While most fissures will readily heal with an appropriate change in bowel habits, some will persist. This may be due to continued trauma or to spasm of the internal anal sphincter.

There is an association between fissures and inflammatory bowel disease, particularly Crohn's disease, and this should be kept in mind.

4.3.2.2 Diagnosis
Pain with defecation is the chief complaint. The pain may persist for minutes to hours. Bright red blood is often seen on the toilet paper and on the stool. The patient with an edematous, tender skin tag (sentinel pile) may complain of a painful hemorrhoid. The patient may be constipated in response to painful defecation.

With gentle separation of the buttocks, most fissures will be visible. The sentinel pile of a chronic fissure may be the initial finding. With acute fissures, digital and anoscopic examination are usually not possible because of local tenderness. However, these examinations should be performed later to rule out other pathology. With chronic fissures, anoscopy reveals the defect in the ano-derm, with exposed muscle fibers of the internal anal sphincter at the fissure base. The hypertrophied anal papilla may be seen.

Fissures off the midline should raise the possibility of other diseases. Crohn's disease may be associated with atypical-looking fissures that are off the midline and have atypical symptoms. Anal and rectal carcinoma should be palpably different from fissures, but if any doubt exists, a biopsy should be done. A syphilitic chancre may occasionally look like an idiopathic fissure.

4.3.2.3 Treatment

The mainstay of therapy for acute fissures is to achieve daily soft bowel movements. This will prevent further tearing and relieve the anal spasm, allowing most acute fissures to heal within one to two weeks. Warm tub baths are soothing and cleansing, and may also reduce spasm. A high-fiber diet supplemented with bulk agents and surface-active wetting agents will accomplish the desired effect.

If the history is longer than a few weeks and the physical findings suggest chronicity (i.e., exposed sphincter fibers, hypertrophied papilla, sentinel pile and palpable induration), this conservative therapy may not help. If symptoms warrant, such a fissure should be treated operatively, generally by lateral internal sphincterotomy. This relieves the internal anal sphincter spasm and allows the fissure to heal in over 90% of cases. Minor disturbances of continence, especially for flatus, may complicate a sphincterotomy in 5–10% of patients.

4.3.3 FISTULA-ABSCESS DISEASE

Anorectal abscess and fistula are the acute and chronic phases, respectively, of the same disease. The disease begins as an infection in the anal glands and initially presents as an abscess. When the abscess is surgically drained, or drains spontaneously, a communication (i.e., a fistula) exists between the gland of origin and the perianal skin.

The infection begins in the intersphincteric plane, where many of the anal glands terminate. The infectious process may remain in this plane as an intersphincteric abscess, or, more commonly, it may track downward in the intersphincteric plane to present as a perianal abscess. Similarly, infection may penetrate the external sphincter to enter the ischiorectal fossa. Many complex variations are seen, determined by the direction of spread and sometimes by inappropriate intervention. The infection may track circumferentially from one side of the anal canal to the other to cause a "horseshoe" abscess. Perianal and ischiorectal abscesses account for at least three-quarters of anorectal abscesses.

The classical signs of inflammation are generally present, although with an intersphincteric abscess there may be nothing to see. In the case of intersphincteric abscess, the patient will be too tender for adequate examination, and examination under anesthesia will be necessary.

Management of the abscess consists of incision and drainage, and this can usually be accomplished under local anesthesia. To ensure adequate drainage, a cruciate or elliptical incision is made. For the one-half to two-thirds of patients who go on to develop a fistula in ano, a fistulotomy, or laying-open, with curettage of the track is required. The wound heals secondarily. Nonhealing or recurrence of the fistula usually indicates a failure to destroy the gland of origin. In performing fistulotomy, the utmost attention must be paid to the anatomic relationship between the fistula track and the sphincter mechanism. Excessive division of muscle contained within the fistula can lead to partial or complete fecal incontinence.

4.3.4 PILONIDAL DISEASE

This is an acquired condition in which body hair is drilled into the skin of the natal cleft by the back-and-forth motion of the buttocks. This produces a primary midline opening or track, from which abscesses and secondary tracks and openings may form.

The disease is mainly seen in young, hirsute males. It commonly presents as an acute abscess, but may also present as a chronic "sinus," usually with multiple openings.

The abscess stage is treated by incision and drainage, usually under local anesthesia. After the abscess has healed, some of these patients will require definitive surgery to deal with the primary and secondary tracks. The preferred treatment consists of opening the anterior wall of the tracks and suturing the edge of the track to the skin edge. This technique is called "marsupialization."

4.4 Sexually Transmitted Diseases of the Anorectum

There is an increasing incidence of venereal infections of the anorectal region, mainly accounted for by sexual practices among gay men. Many of these diseases may mimic nonvenereal conditions of the anorectum, and multiple venereal infections may coexist.

While immunocompetent gay men are subject to infection with the usual venereal pathogens, AIDS patients may additionally suffer from opportunistic infections of the gut.

The common anorectal venereal infections seen in North America are discussed here.

Condylomata acuminata, or venereal warts, are seen in the perianal region and anal canal, as well as the vulva, vagina and penis. They are most often seen in male homosexuals. The causative agent is believed to be a papilloma virus with an incubation period of one to six months. Symptoms are generally minor – itching, and occasionally bleeding. Perianal warts are frequently accompanied by warts within the anal canal, and these must be looked for at anoscopy.

Many treatments exist. None has a better than 70% chance of eradicating the disease by a single application. For perianal and anal canal warts, electrocoagulation or laser destruction is preferred. For extensive persistent disease, immunotherapy with an autologous vaccine has been very successful.

Squamous cancer has been seen to arise in condylomata acuminata.

Neisseria gonorrhoeae may produce proctitis. The incubation period of *gonococcal proctitis* is five to seven days. Gonococcal proctitis is most often asymptomatic; symptoms may include mucopurulent discharge and tenesmus. Proctoscopy reveals a thick, purulent discharge on a background of mild, non-ulcerative inflammation of the distal rectum. Gram's stain is unreliable, but culture of the pus confirms the diagnosis. Serologic testing for syphilis should be carried out. Treatment for homosexual men is ceftriaxone, 250 mg IM once.

Syphilis can affect the anal region. The incubation period ranges from 9 to 90 days. The primary lesion is a chancre, and because it is painful, it may be mistaken for a fissure. However, chancres are off the midline, are often multiple, and have an atypical appearance. Bilateral inguinal lymphadenopathy may be present. The chancre regresses over 6 weeks. Treponema pallidum is demonstrated from the primary lesion by darkfield microscopy. Serologic testing will be positive within a few weeks of the appearance of the chancre. If untreated, the secondary stage of syphilis may involve the anal area 6 to 8 weeks after healing of the chancre. This takes the form of a rash or of condylomata lata – flat, wart-like lesions teeming with Treponema pallidum. Treatment of primary and secondary syphilis is with benzathine penicillin G, 2.4 million units IM once. Sexual contacts should be treated prophylactically.

Herpes simplex 2 may infect the anorectum. The incubation period is 4 to 21 days. Constitutional symptoms are followed by severe anorectal pain. Small vesicles and aphthous ulcers are seen perianally and in the anal canal and lower rectum. Examination may reveal tender inguinal lymphadenopathy. Viral cultures of the vesicular fluid will be positive and rectal biopsy has a characteristic appearance. Spontaneous resolution occurs over several weeks. Recurrences are frequent but less severe. Immunosuppressed patients may develop a severe, destructive process. Treatment is with tub baths and analgesics. Topical acyclovir q8h × 5 days shortens the symptomatic period and the duration of viral shedding. Intravenous acyclovir is used when there is proctitis in addition to anal and perianal disease. In the AIDS patient, acyclovir is used intravenously in the acute phase, followed by oral acyclovir for 6 months.

Chlamydia proctitis with non-LGV (lymphogranuloma venereum) serotypes is almost identical to gonococcal proctitis. However, the LGV serotypes are invasive and produce a severe proctocolitis with pain, tenesmus, discharge and diarrhea. Chlamydia is isolated from the rectum. Treatment is with tetracycline.

5. LOWER GASTROINTESTINAL BLEEDING / S.J. Vanner

Lower GI bleeding often presents as a medical emergency. Like other medical emergencies, optimum patient care requires careful assessment and resuscitation. The history and physical findings provide important clues to the etiology and are critical for determining the severity and location of the bleeding site.

Lower GI bleeding can be classified arbitrarily as major or minor. Patients presenting with the passage of significant amounts of bright red blood per rectum and hemodynamic compromise have major GI blood loss and are at risk of life-threatening hypovolemia. Be wary of the patient who may have stabilized temporarily or received intravenous fluids prior to a full clinical assessment. Historical clues to a major bleed include the occurrence of syncope or presyncope prior to seeking medical care. The vital signs, with particular attention paid to postural changes, are crucial to assessing severity. *The passage of bright red blood per rectum almost always orginates from the colon. However, it is important to remember that brisk bleeding from a site in the upper GI tract may masquerade as a major lower GI bleed.* In contrast to the patient with major lower GI bleeding is the patient who describes the passage of bright red blood per rectum as blood on the tissue paper or on the outside of formed stool in the absence of other symptoms. Such patients, whose general physical examination is normal, usually have a minor lower GI bleed. Most often this is due to local perianal pathology.

5.1 Determining the Site of Bleeding (Upper or Lower GI Tract)
In the clinical setting of a major lower GI bleed with the passage of bright red blood per rectum and hemodynamic compromise, there are a number of

important clues that may raise the suspicion of an upper GI source. These include a past history or symptoms of peptic ulcer disease, NSAID use, prior abdominal aneurysm repair, alcohol abuse and coexisting liver disease. Unfortunately, the lack of upper GI symptoms does not exclude peptic ulcer disease, as a number of duodenal ulcers present as major GI bleeds without a previous typical ulcer history. On physical examination, the finding of hypovolemic shock, particularly in a young person, should trigger immediate consideration of a proximal source of bleeding. Features of chronic liver disease and portal hypertension suggest varices as a possible cause. Most major upper GI bleeding, even in a young person, is accompanied by a transient rise in the BUN (blood urea nitrogen), whereas this is not typical in a lower GI bleed unless there is renal comorbidity.

When an upper GI source is considered, several actions are necessary. A nasogastric tube returning bloody gastric aspirate positively identifies a proximal source of bleeding, but a negative aspirate may not. A negative aspirate will exclude significant bleeding from the esophagus or stomach but may fail to identify bleeding from the duodenum. Even aspirates with bile staining and no blood may fail to identify 5–10% of bleeding duodenal ulcers. When an upper GI source cannot be excluded with confidence, urgent upper endoscopy is required.

Another potentially confusing scenario involves the patient presenting with melena. Melena results from the digestion of blood as it travels through the GI tract, and almost always originates from the upper GI tract. However, occasionally transit of blood from a bleeding right colon is sufficiently slow that stool can appear as melena or melena mixed with dark red blood.

Positive fecal occult blood tests are another clue to lower gastrointestinal bleeding. Many results prove to be false positives; testing should be done with patients on a controlled diet (no red meat, vitamin C or aspirin) to minimize this possibility. Occult positive stools can result from bleeding sites in either the upper or lower GI tract.

5.2 Major Lower GI Bleeding

Angiodysplasia and diverticular bleeding are the two most common causes of major lower GI bleeding, accounting for up to 60–70% of cases.

Angiodysplastic lesions result from dilation and tortuosity of submucosal veins associated with small arteriovenous communication with submucosal arterioles. These lesions are typically multiple, less than 5 mm in diameter, and are most commonly found in the right colon and cecum. The pathogenesis of these lesions is unknown but they occur most commonly in elderly patients and differ from congenital vascular lesions. Diverticula are located predominantly in the left colon, but angiographic studies have shown that

TABLE 6.   Causes of major lower GI bleed

Very common
Diverticular disease
Angiodysplasia
Less common
Ischemia
Neoplasia
Inflammatory bowel disease
Hemobilia
Perianal disease
Aortoenteric fistula
Solitary rectal ulcer

those in the right colon bleed more frequently. The pathophysiology underlying diverticular bleeding is also uncertain but is thought to result from rupture of arteries that penetrate the dome of the diverticulum.

A number of other possible but less common causes exist (Table 6), but many of these more typically present with minor lower GI bleeding and a clinical picture dominated by other features such as diarrhea. Angiodysplasia, unlike diverticular bleeding, can also present with minor chronic GI bleeding, and may even present as chronic anemia secondary to microscopic blood loss. In contrast to angiodysplasia and diverticular bleeding, which are relatively painless, bleeding secondary to colonic ischemia is typically preceded by minutes to hours of significant abdominal pain. Abdominal x-rays may demonstrate "thumb-printing," but this finding is neither specific nor sensitive.

Most major lower GI bleeding will stop without intervention and can be investigated electively, but up to 25% will continue to bleed and require immediate investigation and treatment (Figure 7). After resuscitation, the next priority is to identify the site of bleeding. Radionuclide scanning using technetium-labeled red blood cells is least invasive and readily available in most centers, but interpretation is fraught with false negative and positive results. Although angiography is less available and more invasive, it is more accurate and has the advantage of therapeutic intervention with embolization of the arteriole feeding the bleeding lesion. Colonoscopy can also be attempted to identify the bleeding lesion, and if angiodysplasia is evident it can be treated with electrocautery. However, unless the rate of bleeding is relatively slow, ongoing bleeding usually obscures the lumen, making it difficult to identify the responsible lesion and technically difficult to advance the colonoscope to the site of bleeding. In some cases, continuing bleeding (requiring transfusions of 6–10 units of blood) requires

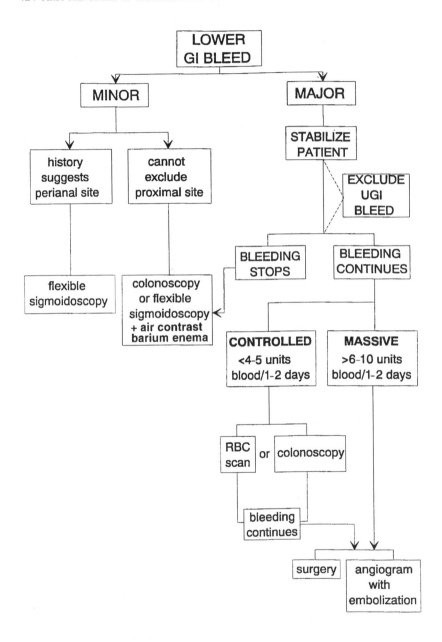

FIGURE 7.   Flowchart for investigation of lower GI bleed.

TABLE 7.   Causes of minor lower GI bleed

Very common
Hemorrhoids
Fissures
Other perianal disease
Proctitis

Less common
Neoplasia
Inflammatory bowel disease
Infectious colitis
Radiation colitis
Angiodysplasia
Ischemia
Rectal ulcer

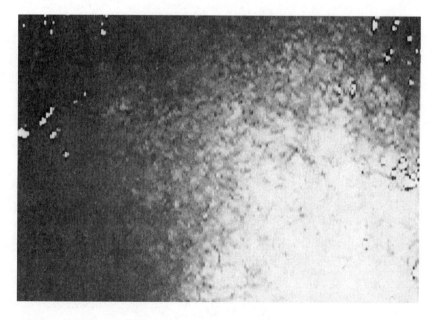

Figure 8.   Endoscopic appearance of colitis. Note the diffuse reddening of the mucosa, which will bleed if touched. This patient had moderately active ulcerative colitis, but infection and other causes of colitis (e.g., ischemia) can look identical.

either urgent angiography with embolization or surgical resection with a subtotal colectomy.

5.3 Minor Lower GI Bleeding

Minor bleeding from the lower GI tract is a common complaint and requires a careful approach (Figure 7) to differentiate minor pathology such as hemorrhoids and fissures from serious problems such as colonic tumors. Patients may notice blood only on the outside of formed stool or on the tissue paper, suggesting that the blood originates from the anal canal or the rectosigmoid region. Alternatively, some patients notice that the blood is mixed in the stool, suggesting that bleeding is more proximal within the colon.

Hemorrhoids are the commonest cause of minor bleeding (Table 7), but even when the history is very suggestive, proctoscopic or sigmoidoscopic assessment should be carried out to ensure that a rectal lesion such as proctitis (Figure 8) or a tumor is not mimicking this presentation. Patients with ulcerative proctitis often have frequent bowel movements but pass only bright red blood and mucus on many occasions. Radiation proctitis can present shortly after radiotherapy treatment but is often delayed by many months or years. This condition results from chronic inflammation within the blood vessels, called endarteritis obliterans, and this indolent process underlies the delayed presentation.

SUGGESTED READING LIST

Benson JT (ed.). Female pelvic floor disorders. New York: WW Norton, 1992.

Cash R. Inappropriate treatment for dysentery. Br Med J 1996; 313:181–182.

Farthing MJG. Intestinal parasites. Clin Gastroenterol 1993; 7:333–364.

Feldman M, Scharschmidt BF, Sleisenger MH (eds.). Sleisenger and Fordtran's gastrointestinal and liver disease: pathophysiology/diagnosis/management. 6th ed. Philadelphia: WB Saunders, 1997.

Griffiths JK, Gorbach SL. Other bacterial diarrhoeas. Clin Gastroenterol 1993; 7:263–305.

Jensen DM, Machicado GA. Diagnosis and treatment of severe hematochezia. Gastroenterology 1988; 95:1569–1574.

Konvolinka CW. Acute diverticulitis under age forty. Am J Surg 1994; 167:562–565.

Mayer RJ. Gastrointestinal Cancer. In: Scientific American medicine. New York: Scientific American, 1996.

Phillips SF, Pemberton JH, Shorter RG (eds.). The large intestine: physiology, pathophysiology and disease. New York: Raven Press, 1991.

Quinolones in acute non-travellers' diarrhoea [Editorial]. Lancet 1991; 335:282.

Reinus JF, Brandt LJ. Vascular ectasias and diverticulosis. Gastroenterol Clin North Am 1994; 23:1–20.

Rubin RH, O'Hanley P. Infections due to gram-negative bacilli. In: Scientific American medicine. New York: Scientific American, 1995.

OBJECTIVES

The student should be able to discuss the following with regard to colonic and anorectal function and disease.

Physiology
1. The role of the colon in the intestinal transport of fluid and electrolytes.
2. The mechanism of defecation.
3. The different motility patterns in the right and left colon and how they determine colonic function.
4. The coordination of colonic motility with eating and the innervation of the colon and its relationship with the central nervous system.
5. The role of the colon in digestion.

Carcinoma of the Colon
1. The epidemiology of colonic carcinoma and the predisposing causes to colon cancer.
2. The use of CEA in diagnosis and follow-up of patients with colon cancer.
3. The Dukes' classification of carcinoma of the colon and the percentage survival after five years for each group in the classification.
4. The role of diet in the etiology of colon cancer.
5. The role of chemotherapy and radiation therapy in carcinoma of the colon.
6. Classification of colonic polyps and how to determine their malignant potential.
7. How polyposis syndrome differs from other conditions associated with polyps.

Diverticular Disease
1. The pathophysiology of diverticular disease.
2. The complications and management of diverticular disease.

Colonic Obstruction
1. The symptoms and signs of colonic obstruction.
2. The causes of colonic obstruction in adults and children.
3. The diagnostic approach to a patient with presumed large bowel obstruction.

4. The x-ray findings of partial large bowel obstruction.

Irritable Bowel Syndrome

1. The Manning criteria and how to make a positive diagnosis of an irritable bowel.
2. The symptoms that are not associated with an irritable bowel.
3. When a patient with an irritable bowel should have further investigations to confirm the diagnosis and the appropriate screening tests to rule out other diseases.
4. The factors that influence patients with an irritable bowel seeking medical attention.
5. The treatment of irritable bowel and the approach to differential diagnosis.

Fecal Incontinence

1. The pathophysiology of fecal incontinence.
2. The mechanism by which the anal sphincter maintains continence.
3. The investigation and management of fecal incontinence.

Constipation

1. The etiological classification of constipation.
2. The investigation and differential diagnosis of constipation.
3. The management of constipation.
4. The identification of "laxative abuse."
5. The causes of solitary rectal ulceration.

Colonic Ischemia

1. The colonic blood supply and the areas of the colon at greatest risk for ischemia.
2. The symptoms and signs of colonic ischemia.
3. The diagnosis and management of ischemia.

Infectious Diarrhea

1. The common causes of dysentery in the tropics.
2. The treatment of common bacterial infections of the colon and choice of the most appropriate antibiotic.
3. The infectious causes of persistent diarrhea.
4. The nematode infections that cause diarrhea and the presentation of nematode intestinal infections.

Perianal Disease
1. The proper techniques of examining the perineum and doing a complete rectal examination (students should be able to demonstrate these techniques).
2. The symptoms of hemorrhoids and their management.
3. The difference between internal and external hemorrhoids.
4. The symptoms and management of fissure in ano.

12
The Pancreas
F. Habal

1. ANATOMY

The pancreas is located retroperitoneally in the upper abdomen overlying the spine and adjacent structures, including the inferior vena cava, aorta and portal vein and parts of their major tributaries. Its retroperitoneal location makes the pancreas relatively inaccessible to palpation. The head and uncinate process lie within the curvature of the duodenum, while the body and tail extend to the hilus of the spleen. The arterial supply of the pancreas is from the major branches of the celiac artery, including the splenic and gastroduodenal arteries, and the superior mesenteric artery, as well as an arborization of smaller branches (i.e., the superior and inferior pancreaticoduodenal arteries) arising from these main arterial trunks. Venous supply comes from the superior mesenteric and splenic veins, which join together to become the portal vein (Figure 1). The pancreas does not have a capsule, and therefore pancreatic cancer often invades vascular structures, particularly the superior mesenteric vessels located directly posterior to the angle between the head and body of the pancreas. Nervous supply comes from parasympathetic branches of the vagus nerve, which provide a major secretory stimulus, and the sympathetic branches of the intermediolateral column of the thoracic spinal cord. Pain fibers are believed to accompany these sympathetic branches, which overlap those supplying the posterior abdominal wall structures, and which thereby account for the back pain experienced with pancreatic diseases.

The exocrine pancreas is drained by two duct systems. The major duct (duct of Wirsung) originates from the embryonic ventral pancreas and tra-

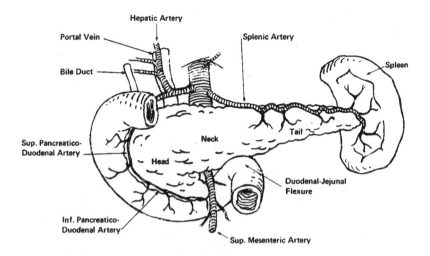

FIGURE 1. Relationships and blood supply of pancreas.

verses the pancreas from the head of the pancreas to the tail. At the head it turns downward and backward to approach the infraduodenal portion of the common bile duct at the ampulla of Vater. The ampulla's opening is regulated by the sphincter of Oddi. The minor duct (duct of Santorini) originates from the embryonic dorsal pancreas, which supplies part of the anterior head, and enters the duodenum as a separate minor ampulla several centimeters above the ampulla of Vater. The minor duct fuses with the major duct in >90% of people, but in the minority, a lack of fusion of these two ducts results in the drainage of the head and body of the pancreas into the minor duct at the smaller ampulla, causing relative outflow obstruction. This anatomical variation, called pancreas divisum, is believed by some to be a cause of pancreatitis.

The pancreatic tissue consists of endocrine and exocrine portions. The islets of Langerhans are islands of cells scattered throughout the pancreas. The majority of the islet cells are beta cells, which secrete insulin, whereas the non-beta cells secrete glucagon, pancreatic polypeptide and somatostatin. The exocrine portion (Figure 2) accounts for over 80% of the pancreatic mass, and is composed of acinar cells that secrete digestive enzymes, and centroacinar and ductal cells that secrete fluid and electrolytes, particularly bicarbonate.

Pancreatic Lobule

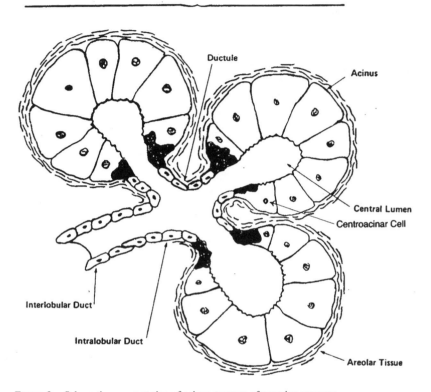

FIGURE 2.   Schematic representation of acinar structure of exocrine pancreas.

2. PHYSIOLOGY

Pancreatic acinar and ductal secretions are regulated by neural and endocrine stimuli. The major peptide hormones stimulating acini and ductal cells, respectively, are cholecystokinin (CCK) and secretin. Some peptide hormones, including somatostatin and pancreatic polypeptide, inhibit secretion.

2.1 Enzyme Secretion

The acinar cells secrete about 20 digestive enzymes, the vast majority of which are in their inactive forms. These enzymes become activated in the intestinal lumen to digest ingested proteins, carbohydrates and fat. The pancreas has a great capacity to secrete these enzymes, such that at least 90% of the gland has to be destroyed before clinically significant maldigestion of nutrients leading to malnutrition would be observed.

The pancreatic acinar cell secretes mainly enzymes whose purpose is to digest proteins, carbohydrates and lipids. Other secretory products include ribonucleases, antiproteases and glycoprotein-2 (GP-2). All the digestive enzymes are packaged in zymogen granules within the acinar cell in their inactive proenzyme forms, except for amylase and lipase. The digestive enzymes synthesized in the rough endoplasmic reticulum are packaged within the Golgi apparatus and specifically targeted into the zymogen granules, which undergo a series of maturation steps involving condensation of the protein contents and shedding of excess membranes of the secretory vesicle. Each zymogen granule becomes very densely packed with digestive enzymes (they are called "dense core granules") and lodges at the apical pole of the acinar cell, waiting for a stimulus to induce exocytotic fusion at the apical plasma membrane, which releases the granule's contents. These vesicular transport processes could be blocked in a manner that causes fusion of the zymogen granule with lysosomes, allowing lysosomal hydrolytic enzymes to activate the digestive enzymes, or alternatively, causes pathologic fusion of the zymogen granule with the lateral side of the acinar cell. These pathologic processes result in intracellular and interstitial digestion, respectively, resulting in cellular damage and cellular death — i.e., pancreatitis. This is currently believed to be the earliest initiating cellular process causing clinical acute pancreatitis.

Glycoprotein-2 (GP-2), which plays a role in stabilizing the zymogens, has the tendency of forming protein plugs when excreted in excess into the ducts. These protein plugs serve as a nidus for calcium deposition and result in pancreatic ductal obstruction and smoldering inflammation leading to fibrosis and atrophy. This mechanism has been implicated in alcohol-induced chronic pancreatitis. A recently discovered relationship between ductal bicarbonate secretion and acinar GP-2 secretion also implicates GP-2 in chronic pancreatitis of patients with cystic fibrosis.

Upon release of the digestive proenzymes into the intestinal lumen, trypsinogen is activated by enterokinase to active trypsin, which in turn activates all the other enzymes (Figure 3). Appropriate conditions, most importantly an alkaline pH brought about by the ductal bicarbonate secretion, should be present for the digestive enzymes to be active. The optimal pH of these digestive enzymes ranges from 7 to 10. The proteases break down specific peptide bonds in the middle of the protein, called endopeptidases (trypsin and chymotrypsin), or at the carboxyl end (carboxypeptidases A and B). Amylase hydrolyzes starch to maltose, maltotrioses and dextrins.

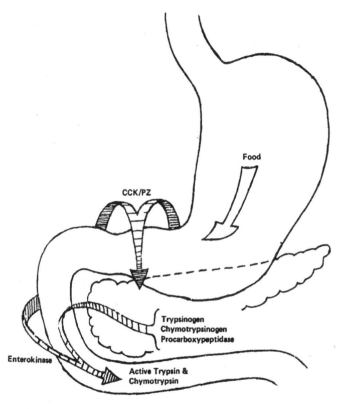

FIGURE 3.   Role of cholecystokinin/pancreozymin and of enterokinase activation in pancreatic secretion.

The effective action of lipase is more complex than the proteases and amylase. This complexity accounts for the relatively low survival of lipase among the digestive enzymes. In fact, in pancreatic exocrine insufficiency, frequently only fat maldigestion is evident. Among these enzymes, lipase has the highest optimal pH (>8) requirement, is most susceptible to inactivation by low pH, and requires a cofactor, called colipase, for its optimal activity. Lipase acts at the oil–water interface of fat droplets. Its action results from emulsification of the food bolus, which is effected by the churning motion of the stomach and the action of bile acids. The bile salts then solubilize the fat into micelles. Colipase binds to lipase to stabilize the lipase in a manner that prevents lipase from being inhibited and removed from the oil–water interface by bile salts. Perturbation of any of these processes will adversely affect the action of lipase on fats.

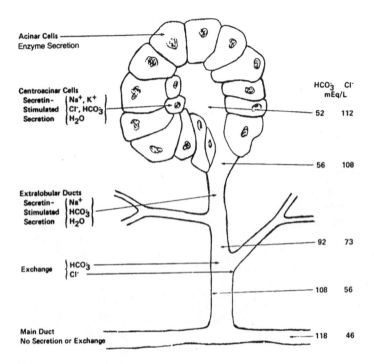

FIGURE 4. Secretion by centroacinar cells and by cells of the extralobular ducts of the pancreas. Chloride concentrations (right) were determined on fluid collected by micropuncture, and the bicarbonate concentrations were inferred from the fact that the fluid is isotonic. These data are for the cat pancreas, but other species seem to be similar.

SOURCE: Adapted from Lightwood R, Reber HA. Micropuncture study of pancreatic secretion in the cat. Gastroenterology 1977; 72:61.

2.2 Bicarbonate Secretion

The ductal and centroacinar cells secrete about 1–2 L of pancreatic juice per day. The pancreatic juice is isotonic with a pH of 8–9. The anion concentration exceeds 150 mEq/L, consisting of Cl^- and HCO_3^- (Figure 4). At high flow rates such as after a meal, HCO_3^- secretion predominates over Cl^- secretion, and the reverse is true at low flow rates. This change in HCO_3^- / Cl^- ratio is effected by a ductal plasma membrane HCO_3^-/ Cl^- exchanger, which is activated by secretin-mediated cAMP pathways. The HCO_3^- is necessary to neutralize the acidic (pH < 2) gastric chyme entering the duodenum to a pH level (>6) that is optimal for enzymatic digestion.

2.3 Regulation of Pancreatic Secretion

There are two patterns of pancreatic secretion. The first pattern is *basal secretion*, which is punctuated every 1 or 2 hours by bursts of increased bicarbonate and enzyme secretion that last 10 to 15 minutes. The second pattern is the *postprandial stage*, which results from a complex interaction of neural and hormonal mechanisms. The postprandial stage is divided into three phases. The *cephalic phase* occurs in response to the sight, smell and taste of food and is mediated by the vagus cholinergic nerves. Cholinergic stimulation has a primary stimulatory effect on acinar enzyme secretion, and a secondary potentiating effect on secretin-mediated ductal HCO_3^- secretion. The *gastric phase* occurs in response to distention of the stomach, which affects vagovagal neural reflexes and stimulates the release of gastrin. Both vagal reflexes and gastrin stimulate pancreatic enzyme secretion and gastric parietal cell acid secretion. The *intestinal phase*, which is initiated in the duodenum, accounts for the major stimulation of both enzyme and bicarbonate secretion. The presence of products of fat and protein digestion in the duodenum stimulates the release of CCK, which in turn stimulates acinar enzyme secretion. When gastric acid entering the duodenum decreases the duodenal pH to <4.5, secretin is released, which stimulates ductal bicarbonate secretion. CCK acting via calcium pathways and secretin acting via cAMP pathways potentiate each other's effects on enzyme and bicarbonate secretion. Vasoactive intestinal polypeptide (VIP), like secretin, also acts on cAMP pathways to stimulate bicarbonate secretion, and is present and released at vagal nerve endings.

As the chyme reaches further into the small intestine, a number of hormones are released which are capable of inhibiting both basal and stimulated pancreatic secretion, and therefore serve as feedback inhibitory mechanisms on enzyme and bicarbonate secretion. These hormones are released not only by the small intestine, but also by the stomach and pancreatic islets, which therefore indicate the complexity of feedback inhibitory pathways. These hormones include pancreatic polypeptide (PP), peptide YY, glucagon, somatostatin and other hormones.

3. PANCREATIC FUNCTION TESTS

The diagnosis of pancreatic insufficiency is quite evident in the presence of the clinical triad of pancreatic calcification, steatorrhea and, less commonly, diabetes. Pancreatic calcification along with other structural abnormalities of the pancreas, including pancreatic atrophy and ductal dilation, can be diag-

TABLE 1.   Exocrine pancreatic function

Direct invasive intubation tests
CCK/secretin stimulation
Lundh meal
ERCP and pancreatic aspiration
Indirect noninvasive tests
Stool fats and nitrogen
Stool trypsin and chymotrypsin
Breath tests
Oral function tests (bentiromide test and pancreolauryl test)
Blood determination
Trypsinogen
Lipase
Pancreatic amylase

nosed by radiological imaging (plain x-ray, ultrasound and computerized tomography [CT scan]) or endoscopic retrograde cholangiopancreatography (ERCP). These radiological tests demonstrating structural abnormalities of the pancreas are largely sufficient to diagnose pancreatic diseases, particularly chronic pancreatitis, which makes it unnecessary in the vast majority of cases to proceed to functional testing. Steatorrhea resulting from fat malabsorption has typical clinical features (foul-smelling floating stools, oil droplets) and appears earlier than protein malabsorption (azotorrhea) in pancreatic exocrine insufficiency, because of the low survival of lipase. Nonetheless, development of steatorrhea and azotorrhea requires the destruction of at least 90% of the pancreas. Diabetes is less common in pancreatic diseases, since the islets are remarkably resistant to damage during the inflammatory process. However, when diabetes is present, it follows a more brittle course, since the nonbeta cells producing the counter-regulatory hormones glucagon and somatostatin are also affected.

Over the years, pancreatic function tests have been devised not only as a diagnostic tool, but more frequently as research tools. These pancreatic function tests may be divided into two main groups: direct (duodenal intubation) and indirect (Table 1).

3.1 Direct Tube Tests

Tube tests require an oroduodenal tube positioned at the level of the ampulla of Vater to aspirate pancreatic secretion in response to stimuli, including a specific (Lundh) meal or intravenous administration of secretin, with or without CCK. These tests are based on the principle that as pancreatic flow increases with stimulation, there is a progressive increase in bicarbonate concentration (>80 mEq/L) and a corresponding decrease in chloride concentration. When CCK is infused in conjunction with these tests, trypsin secretion can also be measured. This hormonal stimulation (secretin-CCK) test is believed to be the most sensitive (>90%) pancreatic function test. The Lundh test meal, although slightly less sensitive, is more physiologic since it also assesses the normal release of CCK and secretin in response to a meal containing protein, fat and carbohydrates. However, the accuracy of the Lundh test is affected by small bowel mucosal disease, rate of gastric emptying and surgical interruption of the gastroduodenal anatomy. Neither test is frequently used because of their disadvantages, including the prolonged (2–3 hours) and unpleasant intubation, and the difficulty of accurate tube positioning. They are therefore not widely available.

Cannulation of the pancreatic duct during ERCP has been combined with direct stimulation of the pancreas. This technique allows the measurement of pure pancreatic juice uncontaminated by biliary or intestinal secretions, but this method is possibly no more sensitive than other tests in the diagnosis of pancreatic diseases.

3.2 Indirect Pancreatic Function (Tubeless) Tests

The standard indirect pancreatic function test is the 72-hour fecal fat determination. The patient is placed on a 100 g/day fat diet and the stool is collected daily for three days. Individuals with normal pancreatic function excrete less than 7% of the total amount of fat ingested, whereas those with pancreatic exocrine insufficiency excrete more than 20%. Only a few other conditions could cause such a degree of fat malabsorption, such as very extensive small bowel mucosal disease and short bowel syndrome. The major drawbacks to stool fat estimations are the lack of specificity and the inconvenience of collecting and analyzing the specimens. Measurements of stool nitrogen and stool chymotrypsin have not proved superior to fecal fat determinations. Attempts to screen for steatorrhea with less offensive tests (such as urine oxalate levels, ^{14}C-triolein/^{3}H-oleic acid assimilation test tripalmitate or palmitic acid breath tests) are promising but not generally accepted. After a rice-flour challenge, breath hydrogen is negligible in normal subjects but is dramatically reduced in those with pancreatic insufficiency; this abnormality is reversed when the test is given with pancreatic enzymes.

Two oral function tests are available for assessing pancreatic functions: the bentiromide test and the pancreolauryl test. The bentiromide test is a urinary test that indirectly determines pancreatic chymotrypsin secretion.

Bentiromide (N-benzoyl-L-tyrosyl-p-aminobenzoic acid [PABA]) is given orally, and hydrolyzed by chymotrypsin to release PABA. PABA is absorbed by the intestinal mucosa, conjugated by the liver, and excreted in the urine. Fifty percent of the PABA ingested should be recovered in the urine during a six-hour urine collection in normal subjects; less than this indicates pancreatic exocrine insufficiency. Intestinal mucosal, liver and kidney diseases understandably adversely affect the accuracy of the bentiromide test. Measuring plasma levels of PABA could circumvent the problem. A number of medicines can also interfere with urine measurement of free PABA, including acetaminophen, sulfonamides and thiazide diuretics.

The pancreolauryl test, using fluorescein dilaurate, has been extensively evaluated in Europe. However, it can detect only severe pancreatic insufficiency and is therefore rarely used.

Chronic pancreatitis may give rise to an abnormal Schilling test, but rarely causes clinical B_{12} deficiency. Vitamin B_{12} is initially bound to an R factor present in saliva, which stabilizes B_{12} in acidic gastric pH. Pancreatic enzymes release the R factor from B_{12} to allow B_{12} to bind to the intrinsic factor secreted by the stomach, which is required for B_{12} absorption at the terminal ileum.

3.3 Miscellaneous Tests

Differentiating pancreatic carcinoma from chronic pancreatitis can at times be difficult; many tests have been described to aid diagnosis, but none are of proven value. Assay of carcinoembryonic antigen (CEA) in serum or from pure pancreatic juice obtained during ERCP has not proved to be a useful discriminator. The pancreatic oncofetal antigen has proved to be of uncertain significance. Serum galactosyl II transferase activity has recently been shown to be a reasonably specific indicator of pancreatic carcinoma in some patients. A sophisticated assay, it is unlikely to be suited to widespread use.

Trypsinogen, a proteolytic proenzyme, is exclusively produced in the pancreas. This enzyme can be detected by radioimmunoassay. It is elevated during an attack of pancreatitis and in renal failure, and is decreased in severe pancreatic insufficiency, cystic fibrosis and insulin-dependent diabetes without exocrine insufficiency. The levels of trypsinogen in cystic fibrosis decrease with age if the pancreas is involved. Low levels are found in about 60% of patients with pancreatic insufficiency. Patients with pancreatic insufficiency who have ongoing inflammation may have normal or raised levels. This fact, in addition to low levels in non–insulin-dependent diabetes, casts some doubt on the usefulness of this test in diagnosing pancreatic insufficiency. It may be useful in patients with steatorrhea that is due to nonpancreatic causes.

TABLE 2. Conditions associated with hyperamylasemia

Pancreatic amylase
(Pancreatic pancreatitis/carcinoma/trauma, including surgical
and post-ERCP complications of pancreatitis)
Intra-abdominal
Drugs
Diabetic ketoacidosis

Salivary amylase
Malignant neoplasms
Pulmonary diseases/pneumonia/tuberculosis/carcinoma
Diabetic ketoacidosis/ruptured ectopic pregnancy/ovarian cyst

Mixed or unknown
Renal insufficiency
Thermal burns
Macroamylasemia

3.4 Tests Suggestive of Active Disease

When faced with a patient with hyperamylasemia, it is necessary to exclude disease involving many organs other than just the pancreas (Table 2).

Amylase is produced and released from a variety of tissues, including the salivary glands, intestine and genitourinary tract. Normal serum contains three types of isoamylases as identified by isoelectric focusing. The pancreatic gland secretes one amylase at an isoelectric point of 7.0 that constitutes 33% of the total normal serum amylase. The parotid secretes several isoamylases with isoelectric points of about 6.4 and 6.0. Electrophoresis on polyacrylamide gel can separate five isoamylases on the basis of electrode mobility. Amylases originating in the fallopian tubes, tears, mucus and sweat have the same mobility as salivary amylase. All amylases have similar molecular weight and amino acid composition, but vary in terms of their glycosylation or deamination.

Amylase is filtered through the glomerular membrane and is reabsorbed in the proximal tubule. In healthy individuals, the amylase clearance parallels creatinine clearance. During acute pancreatitis, there is an increase in amylase clearance as opposed to creatinine clearance. Although this ratio was once thought to be specific to acute pancreatitis, other conditions that produce hyperamylasemia (such as diabetic ketoacidosis, burns, renal failure and perforated duodenal ulcer) may demonstrate a similar elevation. Occasionally, the serum amylase may be markedly increased in the absence of pancreatic or salivary diseases, whereas the urinary amylase is normal. In this instance, one must suspect either renal disease or macroamylasemia. In the latter condition normal serum amylase is bound by an immunoglobulin A (IgA), forming a complex that is too large to be filtered by the glomerulus. Affected individuals have an elevated serum amylase and a low to normal urinary excretion rate. Frequently physicians are faced with a patient who has no overt salivary gland disease but has hyperamylasemia and no specific abdominal findings. As a rule, the level of amylase in pancreatitis usually is elevated to greater than 3 times the upper limit of normal and returns to normal within 2 to 10 days. If the amylase continues to be elevated in the absence of pancreatic complications, other causes (such as malignancy and macroamylasemia) should be investigated.

A rapid rise and fall in serum amylase in a patient with abdominal pain suggests the passage of a stone through the ampulla of Vater. When the serum amylase remains elevated for several days, the gallstone disease is usually complicated by pancreatitis.

Marked hyperamylasemia has been observed in patients with metastatic disease with ovarian cysts and tumors, and ruptured ectopic pregnancy. Isoamylase analysis reveals that the amylase has the same electrophoretic mobility as salivary-type isoenzyme. Macroamylase consists mostly of salivary amylase complexed with globulins, being therefore too large to be filtered at the glomerulus. Therefore these individuals have elevated serum amylase and low urinary amylase, with a low amylase-to-creatinine clearance ratio.

While the amylase levels in serum and urine are usually used as a measure of acute pancreatitis, measurements of lipase may be more specific and sensitive than total serum amylase. The assay of lipase is as accurate as the pancreatic isoamylase assay, and is likely to replace the amylase assay. Measuring both offers no advantage. Amylase and lipase measurements are readily available clinically, whereas radioimmunoassays are still being developed for other pancreatic enzymes (such as trypsin, chymotrypsin and elastase). Their role in the diagnosis of pancreatic disease needs to be established.

A recent urinary test for trypsinogen-2, which can be done with a urinary dipstick, appears to be quite promising in detecting patients with acute pancreatitis. It has a sensitivity of 94% and a specificity of 95%, as compared to serum amylase assay which has a sensitivity of 85% and a specificity of 91%. A negative test rules out acute pancreatitis with a high probability. A positive result usually identifies patients in need of further evaluation.

4. PANCREATITIS

4.1 Etiology and Pathogenesis

Inflammatory disease of the pancreas is a common problem in North America, with gallstones and alcohol being the major causes (Table 3). Pancreatitis

TABLE 3.   Causes of acute pancreatitis

Alcoholism

Gallstones

Postoperative (post–coronary bypass)

Traumatic
Abdominal trauma
Iatrogenic intraoperative, post-ERCP, diagnostic and therapeutic

Penetrating duodenal ulcer

Metabolic
Hyperlipoproteinemia, especially types 1, 4 and 5
Hypercalcemia
Renal failure
Acute fatty liver of pregnancy

Viral infections
Mumps
HIV (AIDS)
Varicella
Viral hepatitis
CMV
Epstein-Barr virus

Parasitic infections
Ascariasis

Drug-associated
Diuretics (e.g., thiazides, furosemide)
Tetracycline
Sulfonamides
Estrogens
Azathioprine and mercaptopurine
Pentamidine
Valproic acid
Salicylates
Steroids

(cont'd)

---

tends to present with abdominal pain, which may improve with no sequelae or may run a more severe course that can lead to death. When the pancreas is continuously injured, such as with alcohol, a chronic condition results in obstruction and fibrosis of the gland, which leads to pancreatic insufficiency and chronic pain. Even one attack of pancreatitis from alcohol use can lead to some residual pancreatic damage.

Pancreatitis results from an autodigestive process. Pancreatic digestive enzymes, vasoactive materials and other toxic materials extravasate out of the

TABLE 3.   Causes of acute pancreatitis (cont'd)

Toxins
  Ethyl alcohol
  Methyl alcohol
  Scorpion venom
  Organophosphorous insecticides
  Amanita (toxin in some mushrooms)
Miscellaneous
  Hereditary
  Regional enteritis
  Connective tissue disorders with vasculitis
  Systemic lupus erythematosus (SLE)
  Polyarteritis
  Thrombotic thrombocytopenic purpura (TTP)
  Duodenal diverticulum
Undetermined

---

pancreas into the surrounding areas, leading to a widespread chemical irritation resulting in simple edema to severe hemorrhage and necrosis. Serious complications include hypovolemia and hypotension. Trypsin and chymotrypsin are the initiating enzymes; their release can in turn result in the release and activation of other proenzymes (including proelastase, procollagenase and phospholipases). Trypsin damages endothelial cells and mast cells, resulting in the release of histamine. This major inflammatory mediator enhances vascular permeability, leading to edema, hemorrhage and the activation of the kallikrein system, which in turn results in the production of vasoactive peptides or kinins. The latter are thought to cause pain and further aggravate the inflammatory response. The other released enzymes destroy the supporting matrix of the gland and the plasma membrane of the acinar cell, precipitating further release of digestive enzymes, which in turn leads to further damage. Lysolecithin, which is released by the action of phospholipase on lecithin (a phospholipid found in bile), has also been implicated in pancreatic damage, because of its cytotoxic and hemolytic properties. When the pancreas is inflamed but remains viable, the condition is termed *interstitial pancreatitis*; this may occur in up to 80% of cases. In the remaining cases, there is a significant pancreatic necrosis resulting from disruption of the microcirculation, destruction of the pancreatic parenchyma and peripancreatic necrosis. Although the action of these enzymes results in pancreatic damage, the triggering mechanism is not well known. In the case of gallstones, the major theories include (1) reflux of bile into the pancreatic duct; (2) reflux of duodenal contents into the pancreatic duct; and (3) distal obstruction of the pan-

TABLE 4. Poor prognostic indicators in acute pancreatitis (Ranson's criteria, 1978, modified by Hollander et al., 1983)

First 24 hours
Age > 55
Leucocytosis > 16,000
Hyperglycemia, serum glucose > 200 mg/dL
LDH > 350 units/L

After 24 hours
Decrease in hematocrit by > 10%
Hypocalcemia (< 2.0 mmol/L)
Hypoxemia pO_2 < 60 mm Hg
Hypovolemia
Base deficit > 4.0 mmol/L
Amylase > 1,000

creatic duct, with continued pancreatic secretion leading to increased ductal pressure and resulting in pancreatitis.

Although alcohol has been implicated as a major cause of acute pancreatitis, there is no evidence that an occasional bout of excessive alcohol intake can lead to an acute attack. It is suggested that chronic ingestion may lead to chronic damage and sensitization, which may lead to acute pain even with small amounts of alcohol. Alcohol can cause direct damage to acinar cells in a manner similar to that in which it damages liver cells.

Hyperlipoproteinemia types 1, 4 and 5 are associated with the majority of lipid-associated cases of pancreatitis. The incidence of pancreatitis varies from 15–40% of patients. Hyperlipidemia has been suggested to be the cause of pancreatitis; however, recent evidence suggests that mild to moderate elevation of serum triglyceride levels is likely to be an epiphenomenon of the pancreatitis rather than the primary etiology. Hypercalcemia and hyperparathyroidism may also induce pancreatitis. Although the incidence of pancreatitis in patients with hyperparathyroidism was at one time shown to vary from 7–19%, recent findings suggest this variation to be closer to 1.5%. This discrepancy can be accounted for by the difference in the degree or duration of the hyperparathyroidism and by the earlier treatment of hypercalcemia. Other causes of pancreatitis are shown in Table 3.

4.2 Acute Pancreatitis

4.2.1 CLINICAL MANIFESTATIONS

The clinical spectrum of acute pancreatitis ranges from mild, self-limiting disease to fulminant lethal disease. Up to 80% of patients will have an uneventful recovery; the remainder will have serious complications with a high mortality rate. Objective measurements such as Ranson's criteria (Table 4) show a good correlation with the risk of major complications and death. The overall mortality rate of acute pancreatitis ranges from 7–20%. The mortality rate correlates well with complications such as shock and hemorrhage.

4.2.2 SYMPTOMS

Pain from acute pancreatitis is a knife-like, steady, sharp pain that starts suddenly and reaches its zenith rapidly. It is commonly localized to the epigastric area and may radiate directly to the back. It improves on leaning forward and is frequently associated with nausea or vomiting. Depending on the location of the inflammation, the pain may be referred to either the left upper quadrant or the right upper quadrant. When the pancreatitis is severe, it may result in shock and may lead to death. Frequently the pain is dyspeptic in quality and aggravated by food. This is due partially to the fact that eating stimulates secretion. Classically the pain lasts between three and four days. When the pancreatitis is severe, it may result in peripheral circulatory failure; under these conditions, the mortality rate approaches 60%.

Recurrent nausea and vomiting may be due to a reflex mechanism secondary to pain and occurs in over 90% of the cases. Other causes include pseudo-obstruction secondary to ileus and distention or obstruction secondary to a pancreatic mass or pseudocyst. Since the common bile duct traverses the pancreatic head before entering the duodenum, jaundice may occur, often transiently.

4.2.3 SIGNS

Depending on the severity of pancreatitis, the patient may appear in distress or be in shock. Jaundice may be caused by edema of the head of the pancreas or by an obstructing stone. Tachycardia could be secondary to pain, volume depletion or the inflammatory process. Low-grade fever could be secondary to the inflammation in the pancreas or result from such complications as abscess formation.

Abdominal examination may reveal epigastric and abdominal tenderness with guarding or rigidity. Bluish discoloration of the flanks (Grey Turner's sign) or of the periumbilical area (Cullen's sign) indicates that blood from hemorrhagic pancreatitis has entered the fascial planes. The signs are not specific and may occur in any condition that causes retroperitoneal hemorrhage.

TABLE 5. Systemic complications of pancreatitis

Metabolic
 Hypocalcemia, hyperglycemia, hypertriglyceridemia, acidosis

Respiratory
 Hypoxemia, atelectasis, effusion, pneumonitis
 Acute respiratory distress syndrome (ARDS)

Renal
 Renal artery or vein thrombosis
 Renal failure

Circulatory
 Arrhythmias
 Hypovolemia and shock; myocardial infarct
 Pericardial effusion, vascular thrombosis

Gastrointestinal
 Ileus
 Gastrointestinal hemorrhage from stress ulceration; gastric
  varices (secondary to splenic vein thrombosis)
 Gastrointestinal obstruction

Hepatobiliary
 Jaundice
 Portal vein thrombosis

Neurologic
 Psychosis or encephalopathy (confusion, delusion and coma)
 Cerebral emboli
 Blindness (angiopathic retinopathy with hemorrhage)

Hematologic
 Anemia
 DIC (disseminated intravascular coagulopathy)
 Leucocytosis

Dermatologic
 Painful subcutaneous fat necrosis

Tender red and painful nodules that mimic erythema nodosum may appear over the extremities. These are often due to circulating lipases.

4.2.4 COMPLICATIONS

Since the signs and symptoms of acute pancreatitis may mimic those of surgically correctable intra-abdominal disorders, the diagnosis of acute pancreatitis is often one of exclusion. Other diseases to be considered are a perforated peptic ulcer, mesenteric thrombosis, intestinal obstruction, dissecting aneurysm, peritonitis, acute cholecystitis and appendicitis. The diagnostic process is complicated by the fact that hyperamylasemia can occur in disorders other than pancreatic inflammation (such as ectopic pregnancy, parotiditis, carcinoma of the lung, posterior penetrating ulcer, ruptured aortic aneurysm and opiate administration). Although amylase values greater than 1,000 units have been said to occur principally in conditions requiring surgery (e.g., biliary tract disease), this distinction is not absolute.

Local involvement of pancreatitis includes phlegmon (18%), pancreatic pseudocyst (10%), pancreatic abscess (3%) and thrombosis of the central portal system. Phlegmon is an area of edema, inflammation and necrosis without a definite structure (unlike an abscess). A phlegmon results from acute intrapancreatic inflammation with fat necrosis and pancreatic parenchymal and peripancreatic necrosis. This arises from the ischemic insult caused by decreased tissue perfusion and release of the digestive enzymes. When this damage is not cleared, further inflammation ensues, declaring itself by increased pain, fever and tenderness. In severe cases a secondary infection ensues, a process termed *infected necrosis of the pancreas*, which occurs within the first one to two weeks of the illness and carries a high mortality. This diagnosis can be made by CT and percutaneous aspiration of the area with subsequent bacterial staining and appropriate cultures. In 3% of acute pancreatitis cases an abscess develops, usually several weeks into the illness. An abscess is a well-defined collection of pus occurring after the acute inflammation has subsided.

A pseudocyst develops as a result of pancreatic necrosis and the escape of activated pancreatic secretions through pancreatic ducts. It contains blood and debris. This fluid coalesces and becomes encapsulated by an inflammatory reaction and fibrosis. These patients usually have pain and hyperamylasemia, but may be asymptomatic. They may present with an abdominal mass, causing compressive symptoms.

Systemic complications of acute pancreatitis are numerous (Table 5) and correlate well with the severity of the inflammatory process. They may be manifested by shock (circulatory collapse secondary to sequestration of retroperitoneal fluid or hemorrhage), respiratory and renal failure and profound metabolic disturbances.

Although acute pancreatitis may run a mild self-limiting course, severe pancreatitis occurs in up to 25% of acute attacks, with a mortality approaching 10%. The majority of deaths occur within the first week of hospital admission and are caused by local and systemic complications, including sepsis and respiratory failure. Most clinical studies in the adults cite pancreatic infection as the most common cause of death, accounting for 70–80% of deaths.

4.2.5 DIAGNOSTIC EVALUATION
The diagnosis of acute pancreatitis is based on a combination of clinical findings and the use of laboratory and radiographic techniques. Elevation of

serum amylase in acute pancreatitis is short-lived. Amylase is rapidly cleared by the renal tubules and may return to normal within 24 hours from the time of onset. Although amylase-to-creatinine clearance was used in the past to diagnose pancreatitis, it is now rarely used. Lipase levels appear to be a more sensitive and specific method of diagnosing acute pancreatitis and may remain elevated for several days following the onset of pain. Immunologic assays for trypsinogen or immunolipase are experimental and do not add any more information than the serum lipase.

4.2.6 RADIOLOGIC EVALUATION

A plain film of the abdomen is very helpful. It may reveal calcification of the pancreas (indicative of a chronic process) or it may reveal gallstones (if calcified). The presence of free air suggests perforation, whereas the presence of thumb-printing in the intestinal wall may indicate a mesenteric ischemic process. A localizing ileus of the stomach, duodenum or proximal jejunum (all of which are adjacent to the pancreas) is highly suggestive of pancreatic inflammation. Similarly, when the transverse colon is also involved, air filling the transverse colon but not the descending colon (colon "cut-off" sign) may be seen. The chest x-ray can show atelectasis or an effusion, more often involving the left lower lobe.

Although clinical, biochemical and simple radiographic evaluation suffice for the diagnosis of pancreatitis, ultrasonographic and computerized tomography imaging are essential. These confirm the diagnosis, provide an early assessment regarding the course of the disease and detect complications such as phlegmon, pseudocyst and abscess formation. A pseudocyst or an abscess may also be drained percutaneously under CT or ultrasound guidance.

The most common ultrasonographic and CT finding in patients with acute pancreatitis is diffuse glandular enlargement. Ultrasonographically there is a decrease in echogenicity of the organ; on CT scan there is decreased attenuation from edema of the tissues. Frequently intravenous contrast is given, and this may demonstrate a uniform enhancement in the pancreatic parenchyma. A normal examination does not rule out the presence of acute disease. In up to 30% of uncomplicated cases of acute pancreatitis CT scan may be normal; these patients usually have a mild form of pancreatitis. When a stone or an obstruction of the distal common bile duct is present, the common bile duct and the intrahepatic biliary tree may be dilated.

ERCP involves the cannulation of the ampulla of Vater and then injection of contrast material into the pancreatic duct and the biliary tree. This procedure is usually contraindicated during the acute phase, except when the pancreatitis is caused by an impacted common bile duct stone. Under those conditions, a sphincterotomy and stone removal may be performed. If performed as early as 24 hours following admission, this procedure may result in significant improvement in morbidity and mortality.

4.2.7 TREATMENT

The aims of therapy of acute pancreatitis are (1) hemodynamic stabilization, (2) alleviation of pain, (3) stopping the progression of the damage, and (4) treatment of local and systemic complications. As yet there are no specific medical therapies capable of reducing or reversing the pancreatic inflammation. Hence therapeutic interventions are aimed at the complications of the disease.

Once the diagnosis is established with certainty, the patient's intravascular volume is replenished, and electrolytes, calcium, magnesium and blood sugar are closely monitored. Depending on the severity of the attack, an indwelling urinary catheter and close monitoring of urinary output may be necessary. Analgesics such as meperidine should be administered regularly during the first several days of the attack. This may alleviate the pain, decrease the patient's apprehension and improve respiration, thus preventing pulmonary complications such as atelectasis. The risk of narcotic addiction is minimal during the first days; most patients settle within 72 hours. The patient is kept off oral feeding; nasogastric suctioning is maintained if the disease is severe and complicated by vomiting and ileus. Mild cases with minimal symptoms may be managed without suctioning. The rationale behind nasogastric suctioning is to place the pancreas at rest by removing the acidic gastric juices. This suppresses secretin release and decreases pancreatic stimulation. The validity of this postulate has not been substantiated. Similarly, the use of acid-suppressive medications such as cimetidine has failed to show benefit in the treatment of acute pancreatitis. The use of enzyme inhibitors such as soybean trypsin inhibitor to prevent further damage is controversial, as is the use of prostaglandins and corticosteroids.

The routine administration of antibiotics does not improve the course of mild to moderate disease. However, when the development of pancreatic abscess is suspected from an increase in fever and abdominal pain, antibiotic therapy should be instituted.

Respiratory insufficiency may occur in up to 40% of the cases, usually in patients with severe or recurrent pancreatitis. In such patients, arterial oxygen saturation should be monitored and corrected. Fluid overload should be avoided. Intubation and ventilation may be required.

Peritoneal lavage has been advocated in patients with severe disease, such as those with marked hypovolemia or hypotension or those who continue to deteriorate despite appropriate medical therapy. Although this technique reduces the circulatory and renal complications, it does not seem to alter the local complications.

Intravenous hyperalimentation has been advocated in patients who continue to have pain and whose symptoms are aggravated postprandially. If during a trial of six weeks or longer, complications develop (such as an abscess or an enlargement of phlegmon), a surgical debridement may be warranted, albeit as a last resort. Several studies have documented equally effective results with enteral alimentation.

4.3 Chronic Pancreatitis

Chronic pancreatitis is defined as a continued inflammation characterized by irreversible morphologic changes. These changes include fibrosis, ductal abnormality, calcification and cellular atrophy. Alcohol is the major etiologic factor, accounting for about 75% of the cases. Repeated attacks of gallstone-related pancreatitis rarely if ever result in chronic pancreatitis. Other causes include diabetes, protein-calorie malnutrition, hereditary pancreatitis, cystic fibrosis and idiopathic causes.

Recent evidence suggests the possibility that some patients with chronic pancreatitis have a mutation of the CFTR gene (see Section 8) that predisposes them to this complication. This may explain some of the cases of idiopathic or familial pancreatitis.

Alcohol presumably causes pancreatic injury by the intraductal formation of protein plugs secondary to increased protein concentration and precipitation, with or without calcification. These plugs lead to obstruction and secondary pancreatic damage caused by autodigestion. In developed countries chronic pancreatitis occurs after a long history (6 to 17 years) of alcohol ingestion of 150 to 170 g per day. Alcoholic pancreatitis is known to occur with much less consumption of alcohol, as low as 50 g per day. The mean age of a patient with new onset of disease is around 32 years, with a male predominance. Despite heavy drinking only a small number of alcoholics develop chronic pancreatitis, suggesting other factors that potentiate the injurious side effects of alcohol, including high-protein diet with either very high or very low fat content.

4.3.1 *CLINICAL MANIFESTATIONS*

Chronic pancreatitis is characterized by irreversible injury to the pancreas and clinically by intractable abdominal pain and loss of exocrine and endocrine pancreatic function. The pain is localized to the upper abdomen, with radiation to subcostal regions and to the back. The pain is aggravated by meals and improves with fasting.

When more than 90% of exocrine pancreatic function is lost, maldigestion and malabsorption ensue. This is manifested by steatorrhea (fat malabsorption) associated with diarrhea and bloating, azotorrhea (protein malabsorption) and progressive weight loss. These patients frequently present with loss of adipose tissue, judged by hanging skin folds, and more objectively by demonstrating that the skin fold at the mid-triceps is less then 8 mm in males and less than 12 mm in females. In addition, they manifest muscle wasting and edema, indicating protein deficiency. Latent fat-soluble vitamin deficiency (vitamins A, D, E and K) in addition to deficiencies of magnesium, calcium and essential fatty acids may occur and are closely related to dysfunction of fat digestion. Endocrine insufficiency presenting as diabetes mellitus may present at the same time as exocrine insufficiency or a few years later.

4.3.2 COMPLICATIONS

4.3.2.1 Pancreatic pseudocyst
Pancreatic pseudocyst is localized fluid collection occurring within a pancreatic mass or in the peripancreatic spaces following acute or chronic pancreatitis (Figure 5). The pseudocyst is usually surrounded by a non-epithelial-lined fibrous wall of granulation tissues. Its frequency varies from 10–50% of patients experiencing severe pancreatitis. When a pseudocyst is present for less than six weeks, it is considered acute; after that it becomes chronic. The pseudocyst may be asymptomatic or may present as an acute exacerbation of pancreatitis, with abdominal pain, nausea, vomiting and weight loss. These pseudocysts may obstruct intra-abdominal viscera, cause pancreatic ascites, rupture into viscera or the abdominal cavity, hemorrhage or become infected. Spontaneous resolution occurs in 20% of the cases within the first six weeks of the pseudocyst's development. Chronic pseudocysts or pseudocysts greater than 5 cm rarely improve. Asymptomatic patients with persistent pseudocysts should be observed and intervention may be considered if symptoms appear. Successful percutaneous catheter drainage may be accomplished by CT- or ultrasound-guided drainage techniques. The catheter may be required for up to six weeks and is frequently associated with infections. Surgical drainage is sometimes necessary for failed percutaneous drainage or for complicated pseudocysts. If the pseudocyst is in the head of the pancreas, drainage can be done via ERCP.

4.3.2.2 Pancreatic ascites
Pancreatic ascites results from the leakage of pancreatic juices into the peritoneal cavity through a fistula or a ruptured pseudocyst. It presents with gradually increasing massive ascites, with high levels of amylase, abdominal pain and weight loss. Painful areas of subcutaneous fat necrosis result from the high levels of circulating pancreatic lipase.

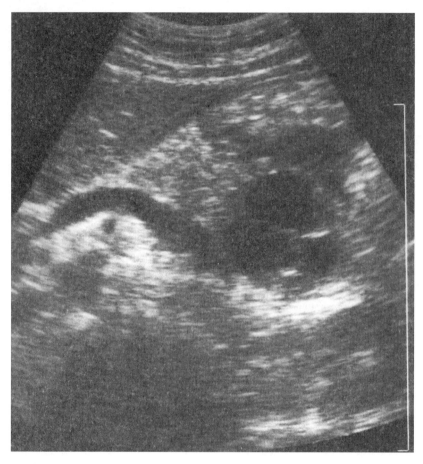

FIGURE 5. Pancreatic foil pseudocyst. Transverse sonogram showing a cystic septated well-defined mass in the pancreatic tail. It is touching and compressing the line of the splenic vein.

4.3.2.3 Common bile duct stricture

Common bile duct compression is another manifestation of chronic pancreatitis, but it rarely results in significant obstruction. As the distal common bile duct traverses the head of the pancreas, it may be narrowed secondary to inflammation, with edema or fibrosis of the gland.

Although pancreatic carcinoma was formerly thought to be increased in chronic pancreatitis, the incidence is now believed to be the same as in the general population. Pancreatic carcinoma may present as pancreatitis.

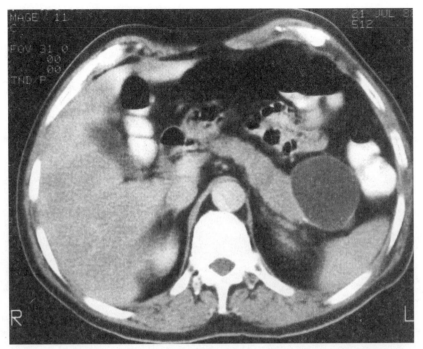

FIGURE 6.   Computerized tomography of a pancreatic pseudocyst in the tail of the pancreas.

4.3.3 *DIAGNOSTIC AND RADIOGRAPHIC EVALUATION*

The diagnosis of chronic pancreatitis is straightforward in patients with advanced pancreatic disease. This can be demonstrated by the presence of calcification seen exclusively in the ductal system on plain radiographic abdominal films, by ultrasonography or on computerized tomography. The radiologic evidence may be seen in up to 30% of patients with chronic pancreatitis.

Although ultrasonography may demonstrate pancreatic enlargement, ductal dilatation or pseudocysts, these findings may be better seen on computerized tomography (Figure 6). Abnormalities of the ducts associated with chronic pancreatitis can also be demonstrated by ERCP. In mild to moderate disease these findings may be subtle and even normal. In more severe disease there is narrowing and dilation of the ducts, stenosis and filling of side ductules. Examination may reveal a tortuous main duct containing stones or protein plugs, or obstruction of the common bile duct (Figure 7). These changes may not be closely related to the degree of pancreatic insufficiency; hence the need for pancreatic function studies.

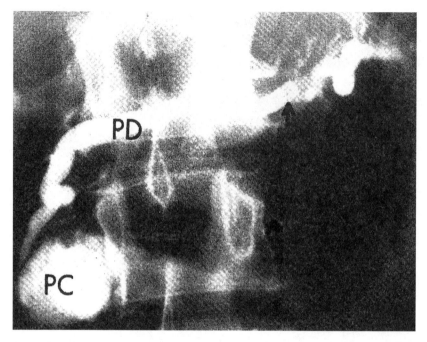

FIGURE 7. ERCP of a patient with chronic pancreatitis demonstrating dilation of the duct (PD) with filling of side branches in the tail. This is complicated by pancreatic pseudocyst.

The only tests that appear to accurately measure pancreatic function in chronic pancreatitis are the direct tube tests that measure the response of the pancreas to various stimuli. The commonest manifestation is a decreased bicarbonate concentration (<50 mEq/L) and decreased volume of secretion.

4.3.4 *TREATMENT*
The ultimate goals of treatment in chronic pancreatitis are to alleviate pain, maintain adequate nutritional status, and reduce symptoms associated with steatorrhea such as abdominal pain, bloating and diarrhea.

The mechanism of pain in chronic pancreatitis is not known. Abstinence from alcohol may decrease the frequency and severity of painful attacks in patients with alcoholic pancreatitis. Large meals with foods rich in fat should be avoided. Analgesics should be given prior to meals, since the pain is maximal postprandially. The continuous use of narcotics often leads to drug addiction, which makes the management of pain more difficult. Large doses of pancreatic extracts may reduce the frequency and severity of the pain in patients with no demonstrable duct obstruction. These enzymes appear to suppress pancreatic exocrine output, thus putting the pancreas at rest and resulting in pain relief. Pancreatic replacement is given with meals and at bedtime. Patients who respond to this therapeutic regimen tend to be middle-aged women with idiopathic pancreatitis who suffer from mild or moderate disease. These patients tend to have a bicarbonate output greater than 55 mEq/L and normal fat absorption. Patients with more severe disease, whose peak bicarbonate output is less than 50 mEq/L, tend not to respond to this regimen.

Patients with intractable pain who fail to respond to medical therapy may benefit from surgical intervention. When there is a dilated pancreatic duct with obstructive areas, longitudinal pancreatojejunostomy (modified Pustow operation) may induce immediate pain relief. When the duct is small, partial surgical resection of the pancreas may control the pain in a certain percentage of patients. Although pain alleviation with surgery may be achieved in certain patients, its long-term benefit is limited since pain recurs in the majority of patients. An alternative to surgical drainage may be achieved by endoscopic insertion of an endoprosthesis (stent) into the pancreatic duct. Although this approach is promising, its long-term benefit has not been proven.

Octreotide, a long-acting somatostatin analogue, appears to decrease the pain of chronic pancreatitis. Its action is mediated by suppressing pancreatic secretion, hence resting the pancreas. The role of octreotide remains uncertain.

Administration of high-potency, enteric-coated pancreatic enzymes remains the main therapy for the treatment of steatorrhea in the majority of patients with idiopathic and alcoholic pancreatitis. This will improve fat digestion, increase absorption and allow weight gain, although it will not correct the steatorrhea completely. Azotorrhea is more easily reversed than steatorrhea, since trypsin is more resistant to acid inactivation than lipases. It seems that the most important barrier preventing correction of steatorrhea is the destruction of enzymes in the stomach, which prevents the delivery of enough active enzyme into the duodenum.

Replacement pancreatic enzymes are made from hog pancreas and contain a mixture of proteases, lipase and amylase, along with a variety of enzymes normally present in pancreatic secretions. Different preparations vary in the amount of lipase activity and the method of enzyme delivery (e.g., tablets, capsules or enteric-coated microspheres). Treatment with these enzymes is lifelong. Pancreatic enzymes are inactivated by pH 4 or below; hence, enteric-coated preparations such as Pancrease® or Cotazym® may be appropriate. In patients who do not respond well, the use of histamine H_2-receptor antagonists (cimetidine, ranitidine or famotidine) or antacids with meals may overcome the detrimental effect of acid on the enzymes. The causes of failure to respond to pancreatic enzyme supplementation are shown in Table 6.

TABLE 6.   Causes of failure of pancreatic replacement

Incorrect diagnosis (nonpancreatic causes of steatorrhea, such as sprue, bacterial overgrowth)
Poor compliance

Incorrect timing of the medications (should be given with meals)

Variability in the enzyme content of the pancreatic replacement or loss of potency of the
enzyme (inadequate amount of enzymes)

Inactivation of the enzymes by gastric juices or by sunlight

Hypersensitivity to pancreatic enzymes has been reported in patients who have hypersensitivity to pork proteins. Hyperuricosuria may occur in patients receiving high doses of pancreatic extracts, although recent reports have questioned this relationship. There appears to be a relationship between urinary urate concentration and the severity of pancreatitis. It appears that oral pancreatic enzymes may bind to folic acid, thereby impairing its absorption, but the clinical significance of this is not clear. Fat-soluble vitamins (e.g., vitamins A and E) are poorly absorbed when steatorrhea exceeds 20 g of fat loss per day. Vitamin D and calcium malabsorption leads to osteopenia and tetany. Vitamin K is also malabsorbed, but bleeding is rare. Malabsorption of vitamin B_{12} occurs in up to 40% of patients with chronic pancreatitis, although vitamin B_{12} deficiency is rare. This malabsorption is thought to be due to the failure of R factor to cleave from the vitamin B_{12}–intrinsic factor complex, resulting in failure to absorb vitamin B_{12}.

5. CARCINOMA OF THE PANCREAS

The incidence of cancer of the pancreas has increased steadily over the past 25 years. In males it is the fourth commonest cancer causing death, exceeded only by cancers of the lung, colon and rectum, and prostate. In females it is the fifth commonest cause of death, with only cancers of the breast, colorectum, lung, and ovary/uterus being more frequent. The incidence is higher in males, with a sex ratio of two males to each female; peak incidence occurs in the fifth through seventh decade.

The overall five-year survival rate is less than 3%, and most patients who develop carcinoma of the pancreas die within six months of diagnosis. The poor prognosis in this condition is secondary to the inability to diagnose the carcinoma at an early stage. When symptoms present, the tumor is far advanced and often has metastasized to regional lymph nodes and to adjacent and distant organs, as shown in Table 7.

TABLE 7. Commonest sites of metastases from pancreatic carcinoma

Local nodes
Liver
Peritoneum
Adrenal glands
Lung
Kidneys
Spleen
Bone

TABLE 8. Putative causes of pancreatic cancer

Tobacco smoking
    Tobacco-specific nitrosamines
Alcoholic beverages
    Common in drinkers of whisky and beer, which may contain nitrosamines in higher concen-
    tration than other alcoholic beverages
Coffee
    Consumption of more than five cups per day
Diet
    High consumption of total and saturated fats, higher protein intake with lower intake of total
    carbohydrates such as those in vegetables and fruit
    High levels of total energy intake and high total carbohydrate intake
Obesity
Diabetes
Exposure to DDT
Genetic defects

Ductal cell adenocarcinoma accounts for 90% of pancreatic tumors. Approximately 5% of pancreatic carcinomas are of islet cell origin; the rest consist of cystadenocarcinoma, giant cell carcinoma and epidermoid carcinoma. The head of the pancreas is the commonest site of involvement, accounting for 70% of the cases, whereas the body and tail account for 20% and 10% of the cases, respectively. Hereditary pancreatitis appears to carry a 40-fold increased risk of developing pancreatic cancer by 70 years of age; the risk seems to be associated with a paternal mode of inheritance.

Several etiological agents have been invoked in the pathogenesis of pancreatic carcinoma (Table 8), although most of the studies have not yielded consistent results. Epidemiologically, long-term cigarette smoking is a well-established risk factor. Two tobacco-specific nitrosamines have been proposed as causative agents in the pathogenesis of carcinoma. Little is known of the role of the pancreas in the metabolism of carcinogens involved in exocrine pancreatic carcinoma. High-fat or high-protein diets tend to stimulate CCK release from the duodenum, which in turn can cause pancreatic hypertrophy and may predispose to carcinoma, although the evidence is not convincing. Diabetics are at twice the risk of developing carcinoma of the pancreas as the general population. The mechanism of this is not known. There is no evidence to suggest that alcoholic chronic pancreatitis predisposes to carcinoma. A recent study has shown a four- to five-fold increase in pancreatic carcinoma in individuals exposed to DDT (dichlorodiphenyltrichloroethane). Some epidemiological studies have suggested an increased rate of pancreatic carcinoma in patients who drank chlorinated water; this remains to be proven.

Genetic defects such as K-ras oncogene, and tumor-suppressor genes including p16, DPC4 and p53 have been proposed to be involved in the pathogenesis of pancreatic carcinoma. Attempts to use the presence of these gene mutations in the diagnosis of occult pancreatic carcinoma seem to be vulnerable to a high false-positive rate.

5.1 Clinical Manifestations

The major symptoms of pancreatic carcinoma include pain, jaundice and weight loss.

Rapid and progressive weight loss is probably the commonest symptom of carcinoma of the pancreas, and is not related to the location or to the extent of the tumor.

Most (up to 90%) of the patients suffer from pain during the course of the disease. The pain frequently is a dull aching or boring. Located in the epigastrium, it radiates to the back and increases in severity at night. Depending on the site of the tumor, the pain may radiate to the right or left upper quadrant. Unrelenting pain results from retroperitoneal extension, with invasion of the neural plexuses around the celiac axis.

Jaundice may be the presenting symptom in up to 30% of the patients, and the incidence increases as the disease progresses. It may be associated with pain and pruritus. Jaundice is more common when the head of the pancreas is involved, but obstruction or jaundice can occur secondary to spread to the liver or to lymph nodes around the bile duct. Other nonspecific symptoms include bloating, nausea and vomiting, weakness and fatigue, and diarrhea.

5.2 Signs

The commonest finding in carcinoma of the head of the pancreas is jaundice, with abdominal tenderness and an enlarged liver. Less common signs include a palpable gallbladder, an abdominal mass and edema. Thrombophlebitis occurs in less than 10% of the patients.

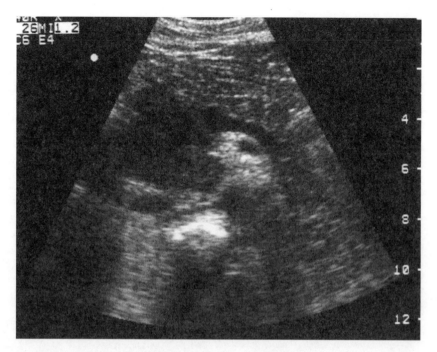

FIGURE 8. Pancreatic head carcinoma. Transverse sonogram shows the confluence of splenic vein and portal vein. The pancreatic body and tail are normal. The head is enlarged and bulbous with an abnormal texture, appearing hypoechoic on the image.

The development of diabetes in a middle-aged man or elderly patient with no family history of diabetes should suggest pancreatic carcinoma, especially when this is associated with abdominal pain or weight loss.

5.3 Diagnostic Evaluation

Laboratory tests are often normal or nonspecific. Serum alkaline phosphatase and bilirubin are evaluated when the bile duct is obstructed or there are hepatic metastases. Serum amylase may be moderately elevated but also may be normal. Pancreatic secretory studies are not often helpful, since findings overlap with chronic pancreatitis.

Several tumor markers have been detected in the sera of patients with pancreatic carcinoma. CA19-9 is the most widely studied pancreatic tumor marker. Its importance and significance in the management of pancreatic cancer are unclear. This marker may be useful as an adjunct in the diagnosis, selection of therapy and postoperative follow-up of patients with pancreatic cancer. Other serum markers include pancreatic oncofetal antigen (POA), α-fetoprotein

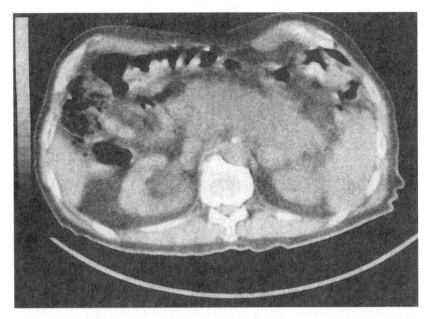

FIGURE 9.   Computerized tomography showing a cancer in the head and body of the pancreas. The tumor is overlapping the superior mesenteric artery posteriorly.

(AFP), carcinoembryonic antigen (CEA), and pancreatic cancer–associated antigen. These tests are nonspecific and not sensitive enough for screening purposes. Cytologic specimens can be obtained by percutaneous needle aspiration under ultrasound or CT guidance and by aspiration of duodenal or pancreatic juices at ERCP. Positive cytology may guide further management; on the other hand, negative cytology does not rule out the disease.

Ultrasonography is the procedure of choice for detecting pancreatic cancer (Figure 8). Its usefulness is dependent on the examiner's expertise. Examination may be less than optimal in the presence of increased bowel gas. The sensitivity of this test in pancreatic cancer is reported to be 76–94%, with a specificity of 96%. Once a lesion is detected, a guided biopsy may be helpful in establishing the diagnosis. When obstructive jaundice is present, ultrasound may reveal the presence of hepatic lesions or obstruction of the biliary tree. This procedure is simple and involves no radiation exposure.

CT is more accurate and gives more information than ultrasonography for diagnosis and staging pancreatic carcinoma (Figure 9). In contrast to ultrasonography, with this technique bowel gas does not interfere with the resolution. Unfortunately, CT has limitations in detecting early small cancer and

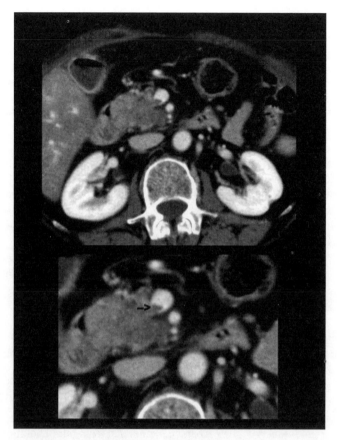

FIGURE 10. Pancreatic adenocarcinoma in the head with direct invasion into the superior mesenteric vein. (Courtesy of Dr. A. Hanbidge.)

small metastases to lymph nodes, liver and peritoneum. Helical CT scan, a newer diagnostic modality, has the capability of producing precise images of the major pancreatic vessels (celiac, superior mesenteric arteries and their branches, and the superior mesenteric veins and their tributaries). This technique detects vascular involvement with great accuracy, hence predicting tumor resectability and retroperitoneal invasion (Figure 10). A guided biopsy of the lesion is also possible. Endoscopic ultrasonography (EUS) in combination with guided fine-needle aspiration may become a useful tool in the evaluation of focal pancreatic lesions. Its overall accuracy in detecting parenchymal lesions and lymph node involvement is about 84%.

When there is a clinical suspicion of a pancreatic lesion and the ultrasound or CT scan is normal, an ERCP is helpful. It has the advantage of combining gastroduodenoscopy, cholangiography and pancreatography. The papilla may also be examined and cytologic sampling may be obtained. When obstruction is present, therapeutic drainage via stents may be attempted. Angiography is no longer used for diagnosing pancreatic carcinoma, but is still useful to evaluate patients who have known carcinoma for resectability, outlining vascular anatomy. Newer diagnostic tools such as endoscopic ultrasound may further improve selection of patients who might benefit from curative surgery. Magnetic resonance imaging has no apparent advantage over CT.

5.4 Treatment

For localized cancers, surgical resection alone, such as pancreatectomy or pancreatoduodenal resection, offers the potential for long-term survival. Unfortunately, at the time of presentation, 75–80% of patients have an unresectable tumor. Despite this intervention, the disease carries a poor long-term prognosis, with a survival rate of 3% at five years. Factors that lead to a poor prognosis in pancreatic carcinomas include the presence of tumor in the lymph nodes and neural tissues, vascular invasion, tumor encasement of celiac or superior mesenteric artery, tumor size greater than 2.5 cm and histologically poorly differentiated tumor. Pancreatic surgery should be done only in specialized centers where such an operation is performed by a small number of highly trained surgeons. In such centers the mortality rate approaches 6%, as compared to nonspecialized centers where the mortality rate reaches 28%. The five-year survival rate in some recent studies appears encouraging.

Complications can occur in up to 20% of patients following pancreatoduodenectomy. These include delayed gastric emptying (20%), pancreatic fistula (14%), wound infection (10%), pancreaticojejunal leak, intra-abdominal sepsis, biliary anastomotic leak, gastrointestinal bleeding and other intra-abdominal hemorrhage. Factors favoring longer survival include jaundice at presentation, a small tumor mass, early tumor stage and a well-differentiated tumor. Palliative operations for unresectable tumor, such as alleviating biliary or duodenal obstruction, offer some relief. Surgery is frequently associated with high morbidity and mortality; hence, nonsurgical intervention may be preferable. Biliary obstruction can be relieved by percutaneous drainage or by endoscopic stenting of the bile duct. Unfortunately these stents tend to occlude and may require frequent changes.

Adjuvant chemotherapy in combination with radiotherapy, such as with 5-fluorouracil (5-FU), has shown minimal effect in long-term survival. Recently a new chemotherapeutic agent, gemcitabine, has shown similar results to 5-FU in terms of response rate and survival, with more tolerable side effects. Irradiation therapy has been advocated in treating larger tumors; it may offer local control and pain management, although its benefit in long-term survival has not been proven.

6. PANCREATIC ISLET CELL TUMORS

Pancreatic islet cell tumors are divided into two types: (1) an endocrine type that elaborates excessive gastrointestinal tract hormones, causing specific clinical syndromes, and (2) a nonfunctioning type that is characterized by symptoms related to the size, location and invasion of the tumor mass. Patients with multiple endocrine neoplasm type 1 and von Hippel-Lindau disease (VHL) are predisposed to develop pancreatic endocrine tumors. Pancreatic islet cell tumors have a better prognosis than those associated with ductal cell adenocarcinoma. They may be diagnosed by the classic clinical manifestation, by the detection of hormones in the serum and by dynamic CT scan with intravenous and oral contrasts.

Several pancreatic islet cell tumors have been identified. These tumors tend to elaborate a variety of biologically active peptides, resulting in a variety of clinical presentations. These peptides include glucagon, insulin, gastrin, vasoactive intestinal peptide (VIP), somatostatin and pancreatic polypeptide (PP).

Insulinoma is the most common neoplasm of the endocrine pancreas. The insulinoma syndrome is associated with Whipple's triad, which includes symptoms of (1) fasting hypoglycemia (confusion, seizures, personality changes, in addition to palpitation, tremulousness and diaphoresis), with (2) a low serum glucose level, and (3) a relief of symptoms by the administration of glucose. The diagnosis can be made by the demonstration of high serum insulin and low blood sugar, and an elevation in the insulin-to-glucose ratio (IG). The tumor may be localized by dynamic CT scan. Treatment includes surgery to remove the tumor if it is well localized or amenable to surgery, and a combination chemotherapy including streptozocine, doxorubicin and 5-fluorouracil.

Glucagon-secreting tumors (*glucagonomas*) arise from the alpha cells of the pancreas. Patients commonly present with mild diabetes, dermatitis, delayed gastric emptying, stomatitis, ileus and constipation. The dermatitis is manifested by a skin rash termed necrolytic migratory erythema, commonly appearing over the lower extremities. The diagnosis is established by the demonstration of elevated plasma glucagon levels that increase, paradoxically, with challenge by intravenous tolbutamide. Glucagonoma tends to present with large tumors and can be demonstrated by dynamic CT scan.

Gastrin-secreting tumors (*gastrinomas*; Zollinger-Ellison syndrome) arise from nonbeta islet cells. They are frequently malignant and tend to be multiple. They commonly present with recurrent severe peptic ulceration accompanied by marked gastric acid hypersecretion and occasionally diarrhea. The diagnosis is established by the demonstration of marked fasting hypergastrinemia and marked gastric acid hypersecretion. In patients who have borderline increases in gastrin, provocative testing with secretin is indicated. Following secretin stimulation, gastrin levels increase in patients with gastrinoma, whereas in patients with common duodenal ulcer, gastrin levels may show a minimal increase, a decrease or no change. High levels of gastrin may be present in a condition known as G-cell hyperplasia. This can be distinguished from gastrinoma by the sharp rise in gastrin level (> 200%) in response to meals. Patients with gastrinoma show minimal or no rise in gastrin level.

Vasoactive intestinal peptide–secreting tumors (*VIPoma*; Werner-Morrison syndrome) produce the pancreatic cholera syndrome, which is characterized by severe diarrhea, hypokalemia and hypochlorhydria or achlorhydria. Fluid secretion may exceed 3–5 L, with a loss of 200–300 mEq of potassium daily. Although the diagnosis is established by the demonstration of high levels of VIP, other substances, such as prostaglandins and secretin-like substances, may contribute to this syndrome.

Somatostatin-producing tumors (*somatostatinomas*) are the least common of pancreatic islet cell tumors, so by the time of diagnosis they tend to be malignant and have usually metastasized. They commonly present with mild diabetes mellitus, gallstones with a dilated gallbladder, anemia, hypochlorhydria and malabsorption. The diagnosis is established by the demonstration of high serum levels of somatostatin.

Pancreatic polypeptide–producing tumors have not been shown to produce any clinically defined syndrome.

6.1 Treatment

Pancreatic endocrine tumors are ideally treated by resection. Unfortunately, despite all our available techniques, up to 40% of these tumors tend to escape localization. These tumors tend to be single or multiple and may be located in any portion of the pancreas or ectopically in the duodenum or any other part of the gastrointestinal tract. It appears that endoscopic ultrasonography may play an important role in tumor localization, but this technique is operator dependent and is not widely used.

Recently octreotide scintigraphy has shown promise in detecting endocrine islet cell tumors, which appear to have somatostatin receptors. Radiolabeled somatostatin analogues bind to these receptors and can be demonstrated by gamma camera scintigraphy. This test offers some hope in differentiating endocrine versus ductal cell tumors. It may assist the surgeon in delineating and removing the tumor and possibly the metastatic lesions.

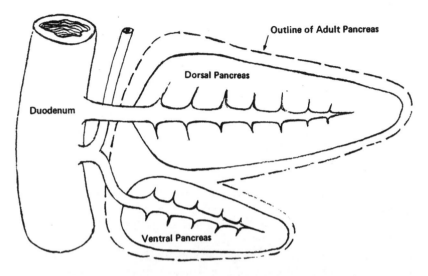

FIGURE 11. Pancreas at approximately 7 weeks fetal life.

7. PANCREAS DIVISUM

Pancreas divisum is the most common variant of human pancreas, occurring in nearly 10% of the population. This anomaly results from the failure of fusion of the dorsal and ventral pancreatic ducts, which usually occurs in the second month of fetal life. This results in the drainage of the main pancreatic duct (including the superior-anterior aspect of the head, the body and the tail) into the dorsal duct via the accessory papilla. The ventral duct, which drains the posterior-inferior aspect, joins the common bile duct and empties into the major papilla (Figure 11). The diagnosis of this condition is made by ERCP.

Most patients having this anomaly are symptom-free, although some reports have suggested a high incidence of abdominal pain and pancreatitis. It has been suggested that the relative stenosis of the accessory papillary orifice, the major outflow tract for pancreatic secretions, is the cause of problems.

Endoscopic sphincterotomy or transduodenal sphincteroplasty has been advocated as the operation of choice in these individuals. The results obtained with this intervention have been controversial. Some studies have reported a success rate of 90% in patients with pancreas divisum pancreatitis after two years, whereas other reports did not support such findings. From the available literature, surgical intervention in pancreas divisum is as controversial as its causative relationship in abdominal pain and pancreatitis.

8. CYSTIC FIBROSIS IN THE ADULT

Cystic fibrosis (CF) is no longer solely a pediatric disease. CF is the most common potentially lethal genetic disease affecting Caucasians. Its incidence shows regional variations, but overall incidence in Caucasians is approximately 1 per 2,500 live births; it is inherited as an autosomal recessive trait. CF is also the most common cause of chronic lung disease and pancreatic insufficiency in patients under the age of 20. It is practically unknown among North Americans of African origin, with an incidence of less than 1 in 99,000 among orientals.

Over the past decade the fundamental biochemical defect in CF has been identified. The gene has been cloned and up to 300 alleles have been discovered. The gene product is a protein called the cystic fibrosis transmembrane conductance regulator (CFTR) and is present on the long arm of chromosome 7. This regulator, the main chloride transport system, is defective in individuals with CF. The regulator is synthesized within the epithelial cell, then transported to the apical cell membrane of the epithelial duct cells of the proximal pancreatic duct. The commonest mutation in CF is that of a three-nucleotide base pair deletion that results in a missing phenylalanine at position 508 in the first nucleotide binding fold. This mutation is often referred to as delta F508. Its main function is to act as a chloride channel that is activated through cAMP-mediated phosphorylation, thus allowing secretion of chloride ions into the pancreatic duct or to the skin through the sweat glands. In addition to CFTR, these cells contain Cl^-/HCO_3^- exchangers, which are responsible for bicarbonate secretion and are dependent on luminal chloride, which is supplied by cAMP-activated chloride channels. Thus, in CF, altered chloride secretion results in decreased bicarbonate production and ultimately failure to adequately hydrate and alkalinize the concentrated protein secretions of the acinar cells. This proteinaceous material becomes inspissated, resulting in ductal obstruction and ultimately acinar cell destruction, fibrosis and malabsorption. The decrease in bicarbonate secretion also results in failure to neutralize duodenal acid, thus leading to further malabsorption by decreasing lipase activity and altering the bioavailability of enteric-coated enzyme supplement.

The "classic" picture of a chronically malnourished child with progressive lung disease and pancreatic dysfunction culminating in early death is an oversimplification. CF should now be regarded as a syndrome with a heterogeneous assortment of presentations involving variable degrees of organ dysfunction and damage. Pulmonary disease and its complications still dominate the clinical picture in most patients, and are the primary determinants of overall morbidity and mortality. However, as many as 20% of CF patients are not diagnosed until after the age of 15 because they have atypical presentations (e.g., recurrent sinusitis, nasal polyps, chronic bronchitis, recurrent abdominal pain, loose, foul-smelling stools, cirrhosis and infertility).

The advent of vigorous physiotherapy, more effective antibiotics, improved pancreatic extracts and continuing care in specialized CF clinics has resulted in a median survival of at least 18 years. Indeed, in many CF centers, half the patients survive 26 years, and up to 90% of patients may live more than 18 years after the diagnosis has been made. With such increased survival, gastrointestinal complications are becoming increasingly common.

Abnormalities have been identified in glycoproteins, mucus secretions, circulating proteases and cell transport mechanisms. Liver and biliary tract disease may occur in individuals with CF. The incidence of biliary cirrhosis reaches 14% during the second decade of life in these who have pancreatic insufficiency. In these individuals subclinical hepatic involvement, manifested as biochemical or ultrasound abnormalities of the liver, is common. High losses of sodium and chloride through sweating during periods of heat in the summer months can lead to sodium depletion, dehydration, cardiovascular collapse and death. The abnormally thick mucus produced obstructs ductules and tubules, and results in distal organ damage, which leads to chronic obstructive lung disease, pancreatic insufficiency, hepatic fibrosis and intestinal obstruction. The mucosal and submucosal glands of the small intestine are dilated, with acidophilic concretions. Steatorrhea and enteral protein loss result from exocrine pancreatic failure, low duodenal pH and perhaps also impaired absorption of fatty acids. These patients require supplementation with fat-soluble vitamins A, D, E and K.

Abdominal pain is common in CF patients. It may be related to steatorrhea, constipation, meconium ileus equivalent, intussusception, cholelithiasis, duodenal ulcer or pancreatitis. In contrast to infants and children, adults are less affected by malabsorption, although close questioning may reveal that they experience cramps, flatulence and frequent, greasy, foul-smelling, bulky stools.

8.1 Complications

There are a number of nonpulmonary gastrointestinal complications of CF in adults (Table 9). Most CF patients have height and weight levels that are less than the mean for their age and sex. Although during adulthood nutritional status declines progressively with advancing age, not all patients are malnourished at the time of diagnosis or in early adulthood. In early adulthood, some 10% of patients are above the 90th percentile, while others are even overweight.

There is no correlation between the patient's nutritional status and the severity of the steatorrhea or gastrointestinal symptoms, or age at diagnosis.

TABLE 9.   Gastrointestinal complications of cystic fibrosis

Gastroesophageal reflux
  Caused by complications of the disease such as coughing and wheezing, and by its treatment,
  including medications that lower LES pressure
Rectal prolapse and constipation
  Associated with injudicious pancreatic enzyme replacement resulting in the passage of large,
  bulky stool
Meconium ileus and intestinal obstruction
  Obstruction occurring at the distal terminal ileum with resultant complications including
  obstruction and vomiting
Fibrosing colonopathy presenting with symptoms suggestive of distal large bowel obstruction
  Patients may present with bloody diarrhea suggestive of colitis. The condition is associated
  with high intake of pancreatic enzymes, and frequently resolves by decreasing the dose

---

The height and weight attained seem to correlate only with the severity of the pulmonary disease; those individuals with the least pancreatic insufficiency tend to have better preservation of pulmonary function.

Pancreatic insufficiency markedly overshadows the other complications of CF. In spite of the clinical impression of a voracious appetite, overall energy intake in the CF patient is usually inadequate. Maldigestion and malabsorption, along with the increased energy requirements associated with pulmonary disease, further compound the energy problem.

CF patients also show biochemical evidence of essential fatty acid deficiency. Improvement may be achieved with oral linoleic acid monoglyceride or with total parenteral nutrition. Essential fatty acid deficiency is associated with impaired intracellular oxygenation, decreased membrane fluidity and impaired transport mechanisms. It has not yet been established, however, what benefit will be derived by treating and preventing essential fatty acid deficiency.

In addition to the problems of essential fatty acid and energy deficiency, there is a third major problem in the nutrition of the CF patient: deficiency of fat-soluble vitamins. Even with a standard supplementation of vitamin A 4,000 IU/day, vitamin A levels, retinol binding protein levels and serum carotene may remain low. Approximately 25% of patients have evidence of vitamin D deficiency.

The management of pancreatic insufficiency in adults with CF is similar to the management of pancreatic insufficiency due to other conditions. About half of the adults with CF show some degree of glucose intolerance. Diabetes mellitus is easy to control with insulin; because glucagon levels are decreased, ketoacidosis is extremely uncommon. The presumed pathogenesis of the pancreatic islet cell dysfunction is fibrosis-induced islet cell disarray and strangulation.

Meconium ileus is seen in approximately 10% of neonates with CF and is primarily related to the secretion of abnormal mucinous (glycoprotein) material by the intestinal glands. Children, adolescents and adults have a counterpart, termed *meconium ileus equivalent*, that is characterized by recurrent episodes of intestinal obstruction. Typically, there is colicky abdominal pain, a palpable, indentable right lower quadrant mass and evidence of mechanical obstruction. Constipation is considered a milder form of this disorder, and must be differentiated from intussusception, which occurs in a small number of CF patients. There is usually a history of precipitating cause, such as immobilization, use of antidiarrheal agents, dietary indiscretions, or reduction or abrupt discontinuation of oral enzyme therapy.

The diagnosis of meconium ileus equivalent is suggested by the presentation. Plain abdominal radiographs may show an empty colon with bubbly granular material proximally, and ileal distention with air fluid levels. It is necessary to confirm the diagnosis by early Gastrografin® enema studies because of the high mortality of this condition and the need to rule out intussusception. Nasogastric suction and correction of electrolyte imbalance result in resolution of the obstruction in 80% of cases. Decompressive surgery may be necessary if medical management fails.

Pancreatitis is relatively uncommon in CF patients, but tends to occur in those patients (some 15%) whose pancreatic function is initially normal. The pathophysiology of the pancreatitis is presumably related to precipitation of abnormal secretions in the tubules, with subsequent damage. Biliary tract disease and alcohol are other possible causes of pancreatitis in these patients.

An increase in the incidence of duodenal ulcer might be expected in CF patients because of the loss of pancreatic bicarbonate buffer, but in fact duodenal ulcer is uncommon.

Patients with untreated pancreatic insufficiency commonly have profound malabsorption of bile acids in the terminal ileum and fecal losses of bile acids. This interrupts the normal enterohepatic circulation of bile acids. The etiology of bile acid wastage is unknown, but it probably relates to the presence of steatorrhea, with bile acid binding to undigested fat, fiber and other intraluminal contents. As a result of the excessive fecal bile acid loss, there is a decrease in the total bile acid pool; the bile becomes saturated with cholesterol. Up to 60% of adolescents and adults with CF have gallbladder abnormalities (e.g., cholelithiasis, nonvisualization, microgallbladder, and marginal filling defects or septation). There is a high incidence of both gallbladder abnormalities and abdominal pain in these patients, but there is not necessarily a cause–effect relationship between the cholelithiasis or gallbladder abnormalities and the clinical symptoms. The hazards of surgery must be weighed against the hazards of nonoperative intervention. The structure and function of the gallbladder may be evaluated by ultrasonography and oral cholecystography.

Treatment of pancreatic insufficiency with oral enzymes will decrease bile acid loss, thus correcting the lithogenic nature of the bile. However, the abnormal glycine:taurine ratio and the preponderance of cholic and chenodeoxycholic acid persist despite enzyme replacement. Ursodeoxycholic acid therapy remains experimental.

With increased age and survival, liver disease is becoming increasingly prevalent in CF patients. The most common hepatic lesion in CF is steatosis, secondary to decreased circulating lipoprotein levels and decreased hepatic triglyceride clearance. Other hepatic lesions seen include nonspecific portal changes, excessive biliary ductal mucus, mild ductal proliferation and focal biliary cirrhosis. A small number of these patients will develop multilobular biliary cirrhosis, the progression remaining clinically silent until portal hypertension supervenes with classical presentation of ascites, hypersplenism or variceal bleeding. Hepatic decompensation and portosystemic encephalopathy are extremely uncommon because of the relative hepatic parenchymal integrity and the overall focal nature of the pathology. The only clinical clue is the development of a hard, knobby liver, while liver biochemical tests remain relatively normal. The results of therapeutic portacaval anastomoses are encouraging, with no development of portosystemic encephalopathy.

8.2 Diagnosis

Classical CF in infants and children is easy to diagnose. However, diagnosis of CF is more difficult in adults and in mild or atypical cases. The cornerstone of diagnosis is the quantitative pilocarpine iontophoresis sweat chloride test. This should be performed on two separate occasions, using a sample of 100 mg of sweat or more. Chloride levels that are continually above 60 mEq/L are virtually diagnostic. Such levels are not found with other chronic pulmonary or gastrointestinal tract diseases. Sweat chlorides may, however, occasionally reach 60 mEq/L or more in a variety of other disorders, including untreated adrenal insufficiency, hereditary nephrogenic diabetes insipidus, hypothyroidism, and a variety of genetic mucopolysaccharide disorders.

Sweat chloride testing should be performed in infants and children with chronic pulmonary disease, meconium ileus, steatorrhea, rectal prolapse, failure to thrive, heat prostration or pansinusitis, and in siblings of affected individuals. In addition, children, adolescents and young adults should be screened if they have any type of chronic liver disease, long-standing gastrointestinal complaints, childhood or cryptogenic cirrhosis, aspermia or malabsorption.

8.3 Treatment

Pancreatic enzyme replacement is the mainstay of treatment in patients with CF who suffer from pancreatic insufficiency. Enteric-coated enzymes ideally should be used, since they are not inactivated by gastric acids. Ultimately these enzymes could be used in combination with an H_2 blocker. At least 30,000 USP units of lipase should be administered and taken together with food.

Hyperuricosuria may occur in these patients secondary to the large purine content in the enzyme preparation. This complication can be controlled by decreasing the dose of the enzymes.

OBJECTIVES

Pancreatitis

1. Classify pancreatitis on the basis of the severity of injury to the organ.
2. List four etiologies of pancreatitis.
3. Discuss at least five potential early complications of acute pancreatitis.
4. Discuss four potential adverse outcomes of chronic pancreatitis.
5. Describe the clinical presentation of a patient with acute pancreatitis.
6. Outline the appropriate diagnostic approach for a patient with acute pancreatitis, emphasizing the timing, interpretation and reliability of various studies.
7. Discuss the management of acute pancreatitis, including the specific medical management of the initial phase and indications for surgical intervention.
8. Discuss the criteria used to predict the prognosis for acute pancreatitis.

Pancreatic Pseudocysts

1. Discuss the mechanism of pseudocyst formation with respect to the role of the pancreatic duct.
2. List and discuss five symptoms and physical signs of pseudocysts.
3. Given a patient with a pancreatic mass suspected to be a pseudocyst, discuss the indications for and sequence of diagnostic methods, including laboratory, radiological and invasive studies.
4. Discuss the natural history of an untreated pancreatic pseudocyst.
5. Describe the medical and surgical treatment of a pancreatic pseudocyst.

Carcinoma of the Pancreas

1. List four pancreatic neoplasms; describe the pathology of each with reference to cell type and function.

2. Describe the symptoms and physical signs of pancreatic cancer on the basis of the location of the tumor in the pancreas.
3. Outline the diagnostic approach for pancreatic masses, including laboratory, radiological and invasive methods.
4. List the laboratory tests that would be expected to be abnormal in a patient with a large cancer of the head of the pancreas.
5. Describe the surgical treatment for pancreatic neoplasms.
6. On the basis of pathology and cell type, discuss the long-term prognosis for pancreatic cancers.

Skills
1. Demonstrate the ability to perform a complete abdominal examination of a patient with an upper abdominal mass.
2. Given a patient with suspected pancreatitis, interpret a plain abdominal x-ray and identify pertinent positive and negative findings.
3. Given a patient with obstructive jaundice and a mass in the head of the pancreas, accurately interpret the transhepatic cholangiogram.

13
The Biliary System
E.A. Shaffer and A.N.G. Barkun

1. GALLSTONE DISEASE

Gallstones (cholelithiasis) are the most common cause of biliary tract disease in adults, afflicting 20–30 million persons in North America. Approximately one-fifth of men and one-third of women will eventually develop cholelithiasis (Table 1). In Canada, calculous disease of the biliary tract is also a major health hazard, accounting for over 100,000 cholecystectomies annually. Cholecystectomy is the second most common operation in Canada and the United States, having increased significantly over the past few years with the advent of laparoscopic cholecystectomy. This appears to reflect an overuse of this new technology, as less than 20% of people with gallstones ever develop gallstone-related symptoms.

1.1 Classification of Gallbladder and Bile Duct Stones
Two major types of gallstones exist (Table 2).

1. *Cholesterol stones* are hard, crystalline stones that contain more than 50% cholesterol plus varying amounts of protein and calcium salts. They predominate (>85%) in the Western world.
2. *Pigment stones* consist of several insoluble calcium salts that are not normal constituents of bile.

Pigment stones can be further divided into (a) black pigment stones, which consist of a linear polymer of bilirubin, large amounts of calcium salts such as phosphates and carbonates (making 50% of these radiopaque) and only trace amounts of cholesterol; and (b) brown pigment stones, which are predomi-

TABLE 1. Frequency of gallstone disease in different countries

Very common (30–70%)	Common (10–30%)	Intermediate (<10%)	Rare (≈0%)
American Indians	United States (whites)	United States (blacks)	East Africa
Sweden	Canada (whites)	Japan	Canada (Inuit)
Chile	Russia	Southeast Asia	Indonesia
Czechoslovakia	United Kingdom	Northern India	West Africa
United States	Australia	Greece	Southern India
(Hispanics)	Italy	Portugal	
	Germany		

TABLE 2. Classification of gallstones

		Pigment	
	Cholesterol	Black	Brown
Composition	Cholesterol	Pigment polymer Calcium salts (phosphates, carbonates)	Calcium bilirubinate Calcium soaps (palmitate, stearate)
Consistency	Crystalline	Hard	Soft, greasy
Location	Gallbladder +/– common duct	Gallbladder Bile ducts	Common duct
Radiodensity	Lucent (85%)	Opaque (50%)	Lucent (100%)
Clinical associations	Metabolic	Hemolysis Cirrhosis	Infection Inflammation Infestation

nantly calcium bilirubinate (an amorphous polymer) and calcium salts of fatty acids – hence their earthy friability.

1.2 Basis for Gallstone Formation

1.2.1 *CHOLESTEROL STONES*
Cholesterol gallstones form in three stages (Figure 1). Both genetic (e.g., presence of apolipoprotein E4) and environmental (e.g., obesity, low-fiber diet) causes are involved.

1.2.1.1 *Chemical stage*
Bile secreted by the liver becomes supersaturated with cholesterol. Such abnormal bile contains an excess of cholesterol relative to the solubilizing

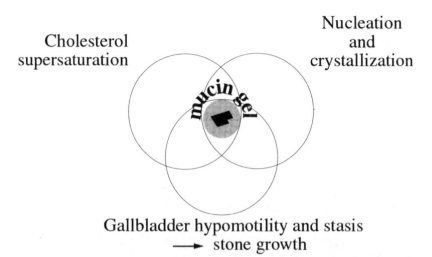

Cholesterol
supersaturation

Nucleation
and
crystallization

Gallbladder hypomotility and stasis
⟶ stone growth

FIGURE 1. Key events in cholesterol gallstone formation, expressed as a Venn diagram. Excess cholesterol secretion causes bile to become supersaturated. This results in the production of pronucleating proteins (including mucins), which precipitate cholesterol microcrystals (shown as a notched rhomboid). Excessive bile cholesterol also becomes incorporated into the sarcolemma of smooth muscle cells, lessening gallbladder contractility. The resultant stasis traps the microcrystals of cholesterol in a mucin gel, allowing them to agglomerate, attract other insoluble components of bile (such as bile pigment and calcium), become biliary sludge and grow into overt gallstones.

agents, bile salts and the phospholipid, lecithin. This stage may develop as early as puberty and is often associated with obesity. The liver, perhaps as a result of genetic programming, produces supersaturated bile by a decreased secretion of bile salts, an increased secretion of cholesterol, or both. Obesity is associated with excess cholesterol production. With ileal disease or loss, bile salt malabsorption breaks the enterohepatic circulation, decreasing its hepatic return and thus decreasing secretion. Reduced bile salt flux through the liver produces lithogenic bile with excess cholesterol. Enterohepatic cycling through the intestine is impaired, resulting in greater bacterial metabolism to secondary bile salts, which in turn may adversely increase the hepatic secretion of cholesterol.

1.2.1.2 Physical stage
The excess cholesterol precipitates out of solution as solid microcrystals. A nucleating factor (e.g., mucin) secreted in bile hastens this relatively rapid precipitation. Conversely, there may be a deficiency of antinucleating factors.

1.2.1.3 *Gallstone growth*

The cholesterol microcrystals precipitate from bile, are retained, aggregate and grow into macroscopic stones. Retention occurs in the gallbladder because the epithelium in stone-formers secretes excess mucus (consisting of mucin, a glycoprotein). This mucus gel forms a colloidal shell that entraps cholesterol microcrystals, preventing them from being ejected from the gallbladder. Mucin also creates a scaffold for the addition of more crystals. A defect in the contractile function of the gallbladder smooth muscle results in failure to properly evacuate the solid material.

"Biliary sludge" consists of calcium bilirubinate, cholesterol microcrystals and mucin. On ultrasound, biliary sludge is echogenic material that layers but does not cast an acoustic shadow (unlike gallstones). Sludge develops in association with conditions causing gallbladder stasis, such as pregnancy or total parenteral nutrition. Though frequently asymptomatic and prone to disappear, sludge in the gallbladder can produce biliary-type pain and progress to overt gallstones or precipitate pancreatitis.

1.2.2 *PIGMENT STONES*

In North America, black pigment stones constitute about 15% of gallstones found at surgery (cholecystectomy). They are frequently associated with hemolysis or alcoholic cirrhosis (Table 3). The basis for their formation is excessive bilirubin excretion in bile. Curiously, this also occurs with bile salt malabsorption. When ileal disease or loss causes bile salt malabsorption, bile salts reach the colon in large quantities. Here, the excess bile salts solubilize bilirubin, increase its absorption and so enhance enterohepatic cycling and thus bilirubin secretion into bile. Brown pigment stones are associated with stagnation and infection (often from a stricture) or infestation (e.g., liver flukes) of the biliary tract. Such conditions predispose to chronic cholangitis and eventually cholangiocarcinoma. Infection and inflammation increase β-glucuronidase, an enzyme that deconjugates bilirubin; the resultant free bilirubin then polymerizes and complexes with calcium, forming calcium bilirubinate in the bile duct system.

1.3 **Natural History of Gallstone Disease**

Gallstones grow at about 1–2 mm per year over a 5- to 20-year period before symptoms develop. They frequently are clinically "silent," being incidentally detected on routine ultrasound performed for another purpose. Most patients (80%) with gallstones never develop symptoms. Problems, if they do occur, usually arise in the form of biliary pain during the first 5 to 10 years. Complications are from stones obstructing

TABLE 3.   Risk factors for gallstone formation

Factor	Pigment stone	Cholesterol stone
Demography		
Race	Asian	American Indian
Female sex	?	++
Age	+	++
Familial	Hemoglobinopathies	++
Diet	+	Obesity (high calorie)
		Weight reduction
		High animal fats
		Low fiber
Gallbladder stasis	+	++
	Total parenteral nutrition	Reduced meal frequency
		Vagotomy
		Pregnancy
Female sex hormones		
Parity/fertility	—	Early menarche
Oral contraceptives	—	+
Estrogens	—	+
Associated disease	Cirrhosis	Cystic fibrosis
	Hemolytic anemia	Ileal disease or loss
	Biliary infections	Diabetes mellitus
Drugs	Clofibrate	

++ = definite; + = probable; ? = questionable; — = unknown

1. the cystic duct, leading to cholecystitis: this begins as a chemical inflammation and later may become complicated by bacterial invasion; or
2. the common duct, causing biliary obstruction (cholestasis), sometimes accompanied by bacterial infection in the ductal system (cholangitis), and at other times by pancreatitis or, infrequently, fistulous tracts (Figure 2).

1.4 Clinical Features

Biliary colic pain ensues when an obstructing stone causes sudden distention of the gallbladder and/or the biliary tract. "Colic" is a poor term, as biliary pain typically does not increase and decrease spasmodically. Rather, abdominal pain onsets suddenly, quickly becomes severe, remains steady for at least 30 minutes, persists for up to 12 hours and then gradually disappears over 30

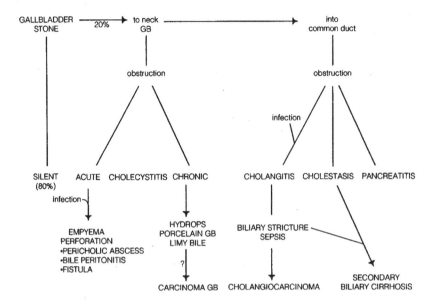

FIGURE 2. Potential complications of cholelithiasis. Migration of the stone in the gallbladder to impact in the neck of the gallbladder or the bile duct can cause obstruction and result in complications. Cystic duct obstruction results in cholecystitis. Chronic calculous cholecystitis may be associated with carcinoma of the gallbladder, but causality is unproven. Common duct obstruction leads to cholangitis, cholestatic jaundice and/or pancreatitis. Chronic cholestasis results in malabsorption. Stricture formation and recurrent cholangitis on occasion can lead to secondary biliary cirrhosis. Chronic duct obstruction and injury may lead to cholangiocarcinoma.

to 90 minutes, leaving a vague ache. Although biliary-type pain can follow a fatty or spicy meal, such "fatty food intolerance" is not specific for biliary tract disease. Its location usually is the epigastrium or right upper quadrant. Mediated by splanchnic nerves, biliary pain may radiate like angina to the back, right scapula or shoulder tip, down the arm or into the neck. The pain may also be confined to the back. Analgesics are usually required for relief. Episodes of pain occur irregularly, being separated by pain-free periods lasting from days to years. The severity of pain also varies. Being a visceral pain, biliary colic is not aggravated by movement but is deep-seated. The patient is usually restless and may exhibit vasomotor features such as sweating and pallor. Nausea and vomiting often accompany a severe attack. Fever and rigors are absent unless infection supervenes.

Findings consist of right upper quadrant or epigastric tenderness, perhaps with some guarding. During an attack or often soon after one, the tenderness disappears. There are no peritoneal signs. Often the examination is completely normal.

TABLE 4. Comparison of biliary colic to acute cholecystitis

	Biliary colic	Acute cholecystitis
Pain	Constant	Constant
Duration	Hours	Hours to days
Vomiting	Yes	Yes
Onset	Rapid	Variable
Jaundice	No	Later (20%)
Tenderness	RUQ	RUQ
Fever	No	Yes
Leukocytosis	Minimal	Marked
Resolution	Spontaneous	Spontaneous ($\approx$66%)

Laboratory tests are usually normal. In 10–20% of cases, there may be a slight elevation of serum bilirubin, alkaline phosphatase, aminotransferases (AST and ALT) or γ-glutamyl transpeptidase (GGT), especially if the attack is associated with common duct stones. Between attacks the patient feels well. Liver biochemistry is normal. Over long periods the activity of the disease remains fairly constant. If having frequent episodes of biliary pain, the patient will probably continue to experience this pattern.

Pain lasting more than 6 to 12 hours, especially if accompanied by persistent vomiting or fever, suggests another process such as cholecystitis or pancreatitis (Table 4). Conversely, abdominal pain and bloating relieved by defecation suggests the irritable bowel syndrome.

1.5 Diagnosis

Diagnosis of the gallstones (but not symptomatic disease) is radiological. Plain abdominal x-ray will identify the 10–15% with a high calcium content as radiopaque densities in the right upper quadrant. Transabdominal ultrasonography is the most sensitive and specific method for detecting gallstones (appearing as echogenic objects that cast an acoustic shadow) or a thickened gallbladder wall (indicating inflammation). Endoscopic ultrasound is quite good at detecting small gallstones < 3 mm. In suspected cases of acute cholecystitis, cholescintigraphy will assist the diagnosis by failing to visualize the gallbladder because of a stone obstructing the cystic duct.

1.6 Management

1.6.1 *EXPECTANT MANAGEMENT*

Management should be expectant in asymptomatic adults with gallstones, as most will never develop problems. The risk associated with cholecystectomy is greater than the likelihood of a major complication. In minimally symptomatic patients without major complications or those unfit for or unwilling to undergo surgery, medical therapy offers techniques for dissolving, fragmenting or extracting stones.

1.6.2 MEDICAL THERAPY

1.6.2.1 Bile acids[1]

The bile acid ursodeoxycholic acid, administered orally, reduces the cholesterol saturation of bile and dissolves cholesterol gallstones. The stones must be radiolucent and hence presumably composed of cholesterol, while the gallbladder must function (i.e., fill and empty through a patent cystic duct) for the unsaturated bile to bathe the stones. Gallbladder function can be assessed by visualization on either oral cholecystography or cholescintigraphy, or by change in gallbladder size on fatty meal ultrasonography. The reported success rate for ursodeoxycholic acid therapy (8–10 mg/kg/day) taken for one to two years varies from 13–80%. Gallstone size largely determines the success rate. Stones must be less than 1.5 cm in diameter. Small stones with a relatively great surface area have the best result. Ideal cases have tiny (< 0.5 cm) gallstones that float on oral cholecystography (floating indicates a low calcium content). In such patients, dissolution occurs in 80% by six months. Large stones in obese individuals have much less favorable results. Ursodeoxycholic acid (8–10 mg/kg/day) reduces the frequency of episodes of biliary colic, but can result in calcification of gallstones, negating dissolution. About 15–20% of patients are candidates for ursodeoxycholic acid therapy. Even after successful dissolution, 50% will experience gallstone recurrence, limiting its utility. Prevention of gallstone formation is possible in those at high risk, such as obese people undergoing rapid weight loss either after gastric bypass surgery or while on a very restrictive caloric diet.

1.6.2.2 Shock-wave lithotripsy

Because the surface area of gallstones is so critical to successful dissolution, stone fragmentation has been undertaken with shock-wave lithotripsy. Shock-wave fragmentation has a low complication rate: 1% develop pancreatitis and 40% develop biliary pain. Bile acid therapy then follows to dissolve the residual fragments, producing successful clearance dissolution of the remaining debris in 60–80% of patients within a year. The best results occur in patients with a single, small (< 2 cm) gallstone in a functioning gallbladder. Unfortunately, only about 20% of patients overall are eligible. Furthermore, gallstones

---

[1] Bile acid and bile salt are used as synonyms in this chapter, despite some physiochemical differences.

recur in 50–75% by five to seven years. These medical therapies are thus significantly limited by modest efficacy and a high recurrence rate. This is why they have not gained wide acceptance, especially since the advent of laparascopic cholecystectomy.

1.6.3 CHOLECYSTECTOMY

1.6.3.1 Open cholecystectomy

The term "open" connotes the need for an incision to open the abdominal cavity for direct visualization and operation. In contrast, the laparoscopic technique uses endoscopy and tiny incisions. Cholecystectomy is the "gold standard" for treating gallstone disease. The operation is relatively safe, with mortality less than 0.5% when selectively performed for biliary colic. Mortality reaches 3% for emergency surgery in acute cholecystitis or for common duct procedures, and is higher in the elderly.

1.6.3.2 Laparoscopic cholecystectomy

This technique views the abdominal contents through a laparoscope (with the peritoneal cavity insufflated with gas) and uses instruments inserted through three trocars in the abdominal wall to perform surgical manipulation. In 5% of cases the procedure must be converted to an open cholecystectomy because of technical problems. There is overwhelming enthusiasm for this procedure. It leaves the patient with less postoperative pain and only tiny scars, and allows for an outpatient procedure or a one-day hospital stay, with a return to work within 7 to 10 days. The disadvantages are a somewhat higher complication rate, particularly from common bile duct injury and retained stones, and the potential for overuse. Laparoscopic cholecystectomy is now the standard for elective surgery and for most cases of acute cholecystitis.

Surgery is indicated in those with significant symptoms (e.g., repeated visits to the emergency room for narcotic relief) or with complications. Prophylactic cholecystectomy is not warranted except for rare cases suspected of developing/harboring carcinoma of the gallbladder (e.g., very large stones >3 cm, gallbladder polyp > 2 cm or a calcified gallbladder wall). It otherwise should not be done on asymptomatic patients with gallstones.

2. CHOLECYSTITIS

2.1 Chronic Calculous Cholecystitis

Chronic inflammation of the gallbladder is the most common pathologic process in this organ. Some degree of chronic inflammation inevitably accompanies gallstones, but the stones will have developed first. Even transient obstruction of the cystic duct can produce biliary colic. Yet there is little correlation between the severity and frequency of such biliary episodes and the pathology found in the gallbladder. There may be only modest round cell infiltration with marked symptoms. Conversely, symptoms may be minimal while gallbladder scarring is marked. Prolonged obstruction can lead to acute cholecystitis (Figure 2). Chronic inflammation may follow acute cholecystitis or evolve insidiously. The inflammatory process is chemical in origin.

2.1.1 CLINICAL FEATURES
The clinical features are those of either biliary colic or a previous episode of acute cholecystitis that has resolved, leaving the gallbladder chronically inflamed. Some may have no further symptoms. Others develop recurrent biliary-type pain, characteristically a constant dull ache in the right hypochondrium and epigastrium, and sometimes in the right shoulder or back. Nausea is frequent. There may be local tenderness in the right upper quadrant of the abdomen. Flatulence, fatty food intolerance and dyspepsia occur, but are equally frequent in patients without gallstone disease. Fever or leukocytosis suggests acute cholecystitis or another entity.

2.1.2 DIAGNOSIS
Diagnosis largely depends upon detecting gallstones by plain film of the abdomen (10–15% are calcified), ultrasound or oral cholecystogram. The latter two are more than 95% accurate. Abdominal ultrasonography is most cost-effective to detect stones in the gallbladder, although it is insensitive (like oral cholecystography) to common duct stones. If the gallbladder is fibrotic and shrunken, visualization may be difficult. This is considered a positive finding, given the accuracy of these tests. Merely identifying calculi in the gallbladder confirms biliary tract disease but does not necessarily mean that gallstones were responsible for the symptoms. Nuclear medicine scanning sometimes helps. Cholescintigraphy normally demonstrates filling of a healthy gallbladder. Nonvisualization (with radioactivity present in the common duct and duodenum) is diagnostic in suspected cases of acute cholecystitis. The test is much less sensitive for chronic cholecystitis, in which the gallbladder commonly fills. If no filling occurs, then biliary tract disease is likely. Failure of the gallbladder to fill can occur with use of narcotics or after a prolonged fast.

2.1.3 MANAGEMENT
Once symptoms begin, they are likely to recur. Symptomatic gallstone disease warrants laparoscopic cholecystectomy unless significantly co-morbid condi-

tions are present (e.g., age, obesity, diabetes). Cholecystectomy provides definitive treatment, removing the stones and the gallbladder.

2.2 Acute Cholecystitis

Here the gallbladder becomes acutely inflamed. In most, a stone obstructs the cystic duct, resulting in a vicious cycle of increased secretion of fluid, causing distention, mucosal damage and the release of chemical mediators of the inflammatory process. Inflammatory damage results from agents such as lysolecithin, derived from the hydrolysis of lecithin by phospholipase, and prostaglandins whose synthesis increases. Any role that bile salts and regurgitated pancreatic enzymes may have is unclear. Bacterial infection is a late complication.

Obstruction of the cystic duct results in the gallbladder becoming distended with bile, an inflammatory exudate or even pus. The gallbladder wall can go on to necrosis and perforation. If resolution occurs, the mucosal surface heals and the wall becomes scarred, but the gallbladder may not function (i.e., fill with contrast agent) on oral cholecystography.

2.2.1 CLINICAL FEATURES

Acute cholecystitis onsets like biliary colic (Table 4). The abdominal pain rises to a plateau and remains constant. Its location is usually the right upper quadrant or epigastrium, sometimes radiating to the back or the right shoulder. There may be a previous history of biliary pain. Pain in acute cholecystitis, unlike biliary colic, persists for more than 6 to 12 hours. As the gallbladder becomes inflamed, the visceral pain is replaced by parietal pain that is aggravated by movement. Anorexia and vomiting are common. Fever is usually low-grade. If rigors occur, suspect bacterial invasion.

Abdominal examination characteristically shows tenderness in the right upper quadrant. During palpation of the right upper quadrant, a deep breath during the inspiratory effort worsens the pain; inspiration suddenly ceases (Murphy's sign). Severe cases exhibit peritoneal signs: guarding and local rebound tenderness. A reflex paralytic ileus may be present. Patients appear unwell and are reluctant to move with such parietal pain. An enlarged gallbladder is sometimes palpable, particularly with the first attack.

2.2.2 DIAGNOSIS

Jaundice with mild hyperbilirubinemia and elevated liver enzymes occurs in about 20% of cases, even in the absence of common duct stones. The higher the bilirubin level, the more likely is a common duct stone. High levels of aminotransferase and of amylase or lipase suggest a common duct stone. Leukocytosis is common. If the patient is febrile, blood cultures may be positive. Cholangitis suggests an associated common duct stone.

Diagnosis is best confirmed by ultrasound, which detects the stone(s) and a thickened gallbladder wall. The gallbladder may be distended and fluid may be present around the gallbladder bed. In doing the procedure, the radiologist may elicit tenderness ultrasonographically when pressing over the gallbladder (the ultrasonographic Murphy's sign). A plain film may reveal calcification of the stone(s). Cholescintigraphy typically fails to visualize the gallbladder at one hour, a feature highly accurate for acute cholecystitis. Conversely, a normal scan filling the gallbladder virtually eliminates acute cholecystitis, but cannot detect gallstones. Late visualization (after one hour) sometimes occurs in chronic cholecystitis.

2.2.3 MANAGEMENT

Treatment is surgical and is performed in hospital. General measures include rehydration, observation, analgesia and antibiotics. In mild cases of acute cholecystitis that resolve, cholecystectomy can be delayed for up to six weeks. Because of the risk of recurrent cholecystitis, surgery should be performed early, once the patient has been stabilized during the current admission.

2.2.4 COMPLICATIONS

Acute cholecystitis normally resolves spontaneously, usually within three days. Inflammation may progress to necrosis, empyemas or perforation in about one-third of cases. These complications will be heralded by (1) a continuation of the pain, along with tachycardia, fever, peritoneal signs and leukocytosis; (2) features of a secondary infection, such as empyema or cholangitis; or (3) a suspected perforation. Urgent surgery then becomes mandatory.

Empyema is suppurative cholecystitis with an intraluminal abscess (i.e., an inflamed gallbladder containing pus). It develops from continued obstruction of the cystic duct leading to secondary infection. The abdominal findings of acute cholecystitis are accompanied by systemic features of bacteremia, with a hectic fever and rigors. Treatment consists of antibiotics and surgery.

Perforation of the gallbladder occurs when unresolved inflammation leads to necrosis, often in the fundus, a part of the gallbladder that is relatively avascular. Gallstones also may erode through a gangrenous wall. If localized, the perforation spawns an abscess, clinically evident as a palpable, tender mass in the right upper quadrant. Free perforation with bile peritonitis is uncommon, fortunately, as the mortality reaches 30%. With perforation the gallbladder, if enlarged, suddenly disappears. The pain and temperature may also transiently resolve, only to be replaced by acute peritonitis. Both localized and free perforations demand surgical drainage of the abscess. Rupture into adjacent viscera (e.g., the small intestine) creates an internal biliary fistula. Large stones can produce a mechanical small intestine obstruction (*gallstone ileus*). Obstruction usually occurs at the terminal ileum, rarely at the duodenal bulb or the duodenojejunal junction. This is a rather common cause of distal small bowel obstruction in the elderly. Radiologic diagnosis comes from finding air in the biliary system, a small bowel obstruction and perhaps a calcified gallstone ectopically located. Urgent surgery with appropriate antibiotic coverage is imperative.

Hydrops of the gallbladder occurs when the inflammation subsides but the cystic duct remains obstructed. The lumen becomes distended with clear mucoid fluid. The hydropic gallbladder is evident as a right upper quadrant mass that is not tender. Treatment is cholecystectomy.

Limy bile occurs when prolonged gallbladder obstruction causes loss of the pigment material from bile and the residual calcium salts precipitate. The hydropic, obstructed gallbladder secretes calcium into the lumen. Calcium can also accumulate in the wall of the gallbladder, producing a *porcelain gallbladder*. The mural calcifications are easily identified on plain films of the abdomen. Although presumably there has been at least one episode of acute cholecystitis in the past, most patients with a porcelain gallbladder are asymptomatic. One-quarter will develop carcinoma of the gallbladder, making prophylactic cholecystectomy necessary.

2.3 Choledocholithiasis (Common Duct Stones)

Stones in the common duct are classified according to their site of origin: *primary stones* are formed in the bile ducts; *secondary stones* originate in the gallbladder and then migrate into the common duct. In North America, virtually all cholesterol stones and most pigment stones are considered secondary when the gallbladder is intact. Thus, more than 85% of patients with common duct stones also have stones in the gallbladder. Conversely, up to 10% of patients with symptomatic gallstones have associated common duct stones. *Residual stones* are those missed at the time of cholecystectomy; *recurrent stones* develop in the ductal system more than three years after surgery.

The composition of stones also varies with their site of origin. Stones are predominantly (approximately 80%) cholesterol when situated in the gallbladder and in the common duct. After cholecystectomy, the proportion of ductal stones that are pigment rises with time: most recurrent ones (more than three years after surgery) are pigment stones. These brown stones result from stasis (e.g., a postoperative stricture) and infection. Bacteria and inflamed tissues release β-glucuronidase, an enzyme that deconjugates bilirubin. The result is calcium bilirubinate, which polymerizes and precipitates along with calcium soaps. Biofilm, a glycoprotein produced by bacteria as its glycocalyx, then agglomerates this pigment material, leading to brown stones.

2.3.1 *CLINICAL FEATURES*

Common duct stones may be asymptomatic, but usually cause biliary colic, obstructive jaundice, cholangitis or pancreatitis (Figure 2). Biliary colic results from sudden obstruction of the common duct, which increases biliary pressure. The abdominal pain is steady, located in the right upper quadrant or epigastrium, and often bores through to the back.

Acute cholangitis results when duct obstruction leads to infection. Obstruction and ductal damage permit bacteria to regurgitate across the ductal epithelium into the hepatic venous blood, causing a bacteremia with chills and a spiking fever. The raised intrabiliary pressure also initiates abdominal pain. The classical "Charcot's triad" consists of jaundice, upper abdominal pain and a hectic fever. Jaundice results from the mechanical obstruction of the ducts plus a component of intrahepatic cholestasis due to sepsis (endotoxin, for example, impairs hepatic bile formation). Pain and fever are common, though jaundice is often less apparent on presentation. Most patients are toxic. There is abdominal tenderness and a large, tender liver (often containing liver abscesses). Hypotension, confusion and a septic picture predominate in critical cases.

2.3.2 *DIAGNOSIS*

Leukocytosis and abnormal liver biochemistry are common. Urine may be positive for bilirubin. Blood cultures reveal the causal microorganisms, which are usually enteric (e.g., E. coli or Klebsiella) in origin. Imaging the biliary tract is key. Abdominal ultrasound is the best first step in determining the presence of biliary tract obstruction, as evidenced by dilated intra- and/or extrahepatic bile ducts, depending upon the level of obstruction; transabdominal ultrasound, however, will not reliably detect biliary stones. Advanced cases may have liver abscesses.

New imaging techniques have improved noninvasive visualization of the biliary tree. Endoscopic ultrasound, in which an ultrasound probe mounted on an endoscope is passed through the upper GI tract, provides excellent images of the pancreas and can detect large and small stones in the gallbladder and in the distal common bile duct. Magnetic resonance cholangiopancreatography (MRCP) produces choliographic images using MR technology that rival endoscopic retrograde cholangiopancreatography (ERCP), but without the attendant risk. Computerized tomographic (CT) scanning visualizes the liver and pancreas, revealing dilated ducts, but is better at detecting space-occupying lesions (tumors or abscesses) than stones. CT cholangiography also appears promising, and is used to better visualize the biliary tree in a non-invasive way (like MRCP). Cholangiography (by endoscopy [ERCP] from below or via percutaneous transhepatic catheterization [PTC] from above) is necessary to locate the site and cause, and treat the obstruction. Such direct cholangiographic methods, however, also carry risks of bleeding, pancreatitis, perforation and bile leaks.

2.3.3 *MANAGEMENT*

The presence of cholangitis necessitates urgent decompression of the biliary system. In the past, laparotomy was the only recourse. Now, endoscopic surgery (using the ERCP procedure) is routinely performed under antibiotic coverage (for enteric gram-negative organisms, enterococci and anaerobes). ERCP is not only diagnostic but at the same setting allows sphincterotomy followed by extraction of the stone and, if needed, placement of a stent through a stricture. Large common duct stones may need fragmentation, either by mechanical means using a basket for crushing, or by energy delivered as shock or laser waves. This can relieve a biliary obstruction due to a stone. Cholecystectomy can then be undertaken selectively. Another option is open cholecystectomy with common duct exploration, removing the gallbladder and all stones. In very high risk patients for cholecystectomy, sphincterotomy alone is quite reasonable.

Pancreatitis can result from gallstones impacting at the ampulla of Vater. Acute biliary pancreatitis does not differ clinically from other forms of acute pancreatitis. Biliary pancreatitis tends to be more commonly associated with jaundice and higher serum levels of bilirubin, alkaline phosphatase and aminotransferase than alcohol-induced pancreatitis, but there is significant overlap. Ultrasound should detect any gallstones and may visualize the inflamed pancreas. In patients with severe pancreatis thought to be of gallstone origin, early ERCP with papillotomy is indicated within 48 hours of presentation, but its definitive role is controversial. Most will come to early elective cholecystectomy to prevent recurrent pancreatitis. Unlike alcoholic pancreatitis, gallstone-related disease does not progress to chronic pancreatitis.

3. NONCALCULOUS GALLBLADDER DISEASE

3.1 Congenital Anomalies

Congenital abnormalities of the gallbladder and biliary system result from embryonic maldevelopment and are most interesting for the surgeon attempting to identify biliary anatomy at cholecystectomy. Agenesis of the gallbladder is rare. Curiously, it is associated with common duct stones.

3.2 Acalculous Cholecystitis

3.2.1 *ACUTE ACALCULOUS CHOLECYSTITIS*

Inflammation of the gallbladder can occur in the absence of gallstones. Though uncommon in adults, acute acalculous cholecystitis may appear associated with AIDS, pregnancy, trauma, burns or sepsis, or following major surgery. In young children, acute cholecystitis frequently occurs without gallstones and follows a febrile illness, although no definite infectious agent is identified. Biliary stagnation sometimes accompanied by sludge appears to be a factor. Impaired blood flow to the gallbladder, coagulation factors and prostaglandin may also have roles. Cytomegalovirus or Cryptosporidia can cause gangrenous cholecystitis in AIDS.

Clinical presentation is identical to that of acute cholecystitis, with pain, fever and abdominal tenderness in the right upper quadrant. These features are often obscured by the patient's underlying critical condition. Diagnosis is then revealed at laparotomy, but sometimes can be determined preoperatively by nonvisualization of the gallbladder on cholescintigraphy (although nonvisualization is less sensitive here because of the prolonged fast many are on) or by ultrasonographic evidence of a dilated gallbladder with a thickened wall. Perforation, gangrene and empyema are all too frequent complications. The best treatment is prompt cholecystectomy. Percutaneous "mini" cholecystectomy may be considered for patients at very high risk for surgery. Prevention is possible in some patients on complete TPN (no oral intake) following major surgery, trauma or burns. Daily injections of cholecystokinin (CCK) can prevent sludge formation and its complication, cholecystitis.

3.2.2 CHRONIC ACALCULOUS CHOLECYSTITIS

Recurrent biliary-type pain in the absence of gallstones has been associated with rather modest inflammation. The basis is presumed to be a motility disorder, impaired gallbladder evacuation; hence the alternative term "biliary dyskinesia." Relief can follow cholecystectomy. Difficulties arise in attempting to make this diagnosis: the symptoms are often not clear-cut (sometimes having features of the irritable bowel syndrome or nonulcer dyspepsia), and there are no gallstones to detect. Abnormal gallbladder evacuation in response to CCK may be evident on cholescintigraphy. Sensitivity and specificity of these tests remain unclear. CCK infusion alone can reproduce the biliary pain, but the value of this provocative test is uncertain. The entity remains poorly defined. In some, the origin of the problem is dysfunction of the sphincter of Oddi. In many, it may represent one facet of the irritable bowel syndrome.

3.3 Cholecystoses

Cholesterolosis consists of deposits of cholesterol esters and triglycerides within the gallbladder wall. These submucosal deposits produce a fine yellow reticular pattern on a red background of mildly inflamed mucosa, providing an appearance like a strawberry: hence the term "strawberry gallbladder." Some of the cholesterol deposits protrude like polyps and can be detected on ultrasound. There is no well-defined symptom complex linked to this entity. Although frequently an incidental finding at post mortem, it is sometimes associated with vague dyspeptic complaints, the irritable bowel syndrome or recurrent right upper quadrant abdominal pain. The importance of CCK provocative tests to reproduce the pain or demonstrate reduced gallbladder emptying on quantitative cholescintigraphy in response to CCK is unclear.

Adenomyosis is characterized by hyperplasia of the gallbladder mucosa and by deep clefts. The meaning of any biliary-type symptoms is moot.

3.4 Postcholecystectomy Syndrome

Cholecystectomy relieves the symptoms of most, but definitely not all, patients with biliary calculi. The occasional patient will experience diarrhea following cholecystectomy, perhaps the result of unmasking a malabsorption of bile acids, which leads to a cholerrheic (bile acid–induced) diarrhea. Symptoms persist or recur in 5–50%, depending upon selection bias. Most often the original complaint was not true biliary pain, but rather reflux esophagitis, peptic ulcer disease or the irritable bowel syndrome. There may be recurrent biliary tract problems such as a biliary stricture, retained common duct stone or even pancreatic disease. In suspected cases, ERCP is indicated. Occasionally, narrowing (papillary stenosis) or increased tone in the sphincter of Oddi (sphincter dysfunction) will produce recurrent biliary-type pain, often with abnormal liver biochemistry tests or increased serum amylase or lipase. Nuclear medicine scanning (cholescintigraphy) and sphincter of Oddi pressure and pancreatic duct measurements (manometry) provide diagnostic clues. Endoscopic sphincterotomy relieves pain in selected patients.

3.5 Neoplasms of the Gallbladder

Carcinoma of the gallbladder is fortunately uncommon, as its prognosis is extremely poor. Adenocarcinoma is generally cured only when incidentally discovered at cholecystectomy for cholelithiasis. Gallstones are present in most (75%) cases, probably as innocent bystanders rather than as causal agents (Figure 2). Any risk is too low to advocate prophylactic cholecystectomy in the many people with asymptomatic gallstones. A porcelain gallbladder with calcifications in the wall predisposes to adenocarcinoma and calls for cholecystectomy, as does a large gallbladder polyp. Large gallstones (>3 cm) are also a risk factor for carcinoma.

The clinical features of gallbladder carcinoma consist of pain, a hard mass in the right epigastrium, jaundice, pruritus and weight loss. Ultrasound and CT scan help define the mass and metastases. Prognosis is grim, as it is common for the cancer to spread. The five-year survival is less than 5%. Therapy is palliative; most are not resectable unless removed incidentally at the time of cholecystectomy.

Benign tumors of the gallbladder are uncommon. Adenomas are asymptomatic, being detected on ultrasound or found incidentally at surgery. Small masses in the wall of the gallbladder, however, are relatively common findings on ultrasound; when multiple they usually represent cholesterol polyps or adherent gallstones. Polypoidal masses warrant a repeat ultrasound in six months. If these are larger than 1 cm, surgery is necessary to exclude a carcinoma.

4. DISEASES OF THE BILE DUCTS

4.1 Congenital

Caroli's disease (congenital intrahepatic biliary dilation) is a rare condition in which saccular, dilated segments of the intrahepatic bile ducts lead to stone formation, recurrent cholangitis and hepatic abscesses with sepsis. Episodes of abdominal pain, fever and jaundice may onset at any age, most commonly in childhood or young adult life.

Cholangiography reveals the irregularly dilated segments of the intrahepatic bile ducts that connect with the main ducts. The common duct is normal, unless associated with a choledochal cyst. Endoscopy (or surgery) can remove some stones but does little for the process that affects small bile ducts in the liver. If involvement is unilateral, partial hepatectomy can be curative. Otherwise, management is conservative, using antibiotics for infectious complications of the duct system. These recurrent episodes of cholangitis sometimes progress to secondary biliary cirrhosis, portal hypertension and eventually cholangiocarcinoma. Partial hepatectomy of an affected segment sometimes is feasible. Liver transplantation may become necessary in other cases.

Congenital hepatic fibrosis frequently accompanies Caroli's disease (perhaps reflecting a developmental defect of the small interlobular ducts). It clinically presents as portal hypertension with esophageal varices in children. Liver biopsy is diagnostic, revealing broad bands of fibrous tissue entrapping bile ducts but no cirrhosis (i.e., no regeneration). Liver transplantation may be necessary in complicated cases.

Choledochal cyst is a congenital dilation of a portion of the common bile duct, which may form a diverticulum in the intraduodenal segment. This congenital cystic anomaly can be associated with Caroli's disease: both represent a spectrum of defective budding and cannulation from the primitive foregut. Presentation may be as cholestasis in infants, or intermittent jaundice, pain and fever (cholangitis) later in young adults. Complications include chronic obstruction leading to biliary cirrhosis and the development of ductal carcinoma. Chronic pancreatitis also may develop. Diagnosis is provided by ultrasound or CT scan and verified by endoscopic cholangiography. Surgery involves excising the cyst and re-establishing biliary drainage with a biliary-enteric anastomosis.

Alagille's syndrome is a marked reduction in intrahepatic (actually inter-lobular) bile ducts. Although it is believed to be congenital, being inherited in an autosomal dominant pattern, presentation may be as a neonatal jaundice or as cholestasis in older children. There are associated triangular facies, cardio-vascular anomalies (e.g., pulmonary artery stenosis) and vertebral body abnormalities. Outcome is variable, depending upon the attendant anomalies and the severity of the liver disease.

Biliary atresia is a common cause of neonatal cholestatic jaundice. Although congenital (appearing at birth), it is not inherited. Complete absence of the extrahepatic bile ducts reflects either an arrest in remodeling of the duc-tal plate in utero or, more probably, an inflammatory destruction of the formed bile ducts during the postpartum period. The latter process is evident by an inflammatory infiltrate in the portal tracts and, in some, features of neonatal hepatitis, perhaps initiated by a viral infection. Large duct obstruction then leads to small duct injury within the liver and hence secondary biliary cirrho-sis. Severe cholestasis develops in the neonatal period. The stools are pale and the urine is dark and devoid of urobilinogen. Cholestatic features predomi-nate, with the development of steatorrhea, skin xanthoma, bone disease and failure to thrive. Surgery is usually necessary to confirm the diagnosis and attempt some form of biliary drainage. In some, existence of a patent hepatic duct or dilated hilar ducts potentially allows correction of the obstruction by anastomosis to the small intestine (e.g., a Roux-en-Y choledochojejunosto-my). Much more common is an absence of patent ducts; dense fibrous tissue encases the perihilar area and precludes conventional surgery. Such oblitera-tion of the proximal extrahepatic biliary system requires the Kasai procedure. A conduit for biliary drainage is fashioned by resecting the fibrous remnant of the biliary tree and anastomosing the porta hepatis to a Roux-en-Y loop of jejunum. With either surgery, most children eventually develop chronic cholangitis, hepatic fibrosis/cirrhosis and portal hypertension. When the child is larger, hepatic transplantation dramatically improves the prognosis.

4.2 Inflammatory

4.2.1 *CHOLANGITIS*

Cholangitis is any inflammatory process involving the bile ducts, but common usage implies a bacterial infection, usually above an obstructive site. The presence of bacteria in the biliary tree plus increased pressure within the sys-tem results in severe clinical features of cholangitis (*suppurative cholangitis*). Any condition producing bile duct obstruction is liable to cause bacterial infection of bile. Most commonly, such obstruction results from a common duct stone (Section 2.3), a benign biliary stricture (trauma from biliary surgery, ischemia following liver transplantation or sclerosing cholangitis), stasis in a congenital biliary cyst (Section 4.1), a parasite residing in the ducts (Clonorchis sinensis, Opisthorchis viverrini or Fasciola hepatica), an occluded biliary stent or extrinsic compression from a diseased papilla or pancreas. A less likely cause of infection is neoplastic obstruction. The difference relates to the high-grade, fixed obstruction of neoplasms versus the intermittent blockage with a stone or an inflammatory stricture. Such intermittent blockage allows retrograde ascent of bacteria; the stone may act as a nidus for infection. The bacteria are commonly thought to ascend the biliary tree (hence the term "ascending cholangitis"), but may enter from above via the portal vein or from periductular lymphatics.

In acute bacterial cholangitis, particularly if severe, the classical Charcot's triad of intermittent fever and chills, jaundice and abdominal pain may be followed by septic shock. Most cases are less severe and life-threatening; jaundice may be absent. Mild cases may respond to antibiotics and conservative measures. Investigation and decompression of the biliary system are mandatory in all patients, whether by ERCP, percutaneous transhepatic cholangiography or surgery.

4.2.2 SCLEROSING CHOLANGITIS
Primary sclerosing cholangitis is a chronic cholestatic syndrome of unknown etiology characterized by progressive inflammation of the intra- and extra-hepatic bile ducts. The entity may appear either alone or in association with inflammatory bowel disease, particularly ulcerative colitis. Primary sclerosing cholangitis may precede inflammatory bowel disease and runs a separate course, not being cured by colectomy. The patchy scarring (sclerosis) leads to fibrotic narrowing and eventually obliteration of the bile ducts. Like other organs, the biliary tract exhibits a limited number of responses to injury: here it responds with diffuse strictures and segmental dilations. Periductal inflammation and fibrosis in the portal areas, termed "pericholangitis," probably represents the intrahepatic extension of this process. The basis may be an infectious agent, an enterohepatic toxin, ischemia or an immunological attack on the biliary epithelium.

Diffuse stricturing also occurs in *secondary sclerosing cholangitis*, which may complicate a biliary obstruction from a common duct stone, biliary stricture or cholangiocarcinoma, or some AIDS-related infections.

The presentation in primary sclerosing cholangitis is insidious in most cases, with fatigue, pruritus or just an elevated alkaline phosphatase level. In others, acute cholangitis develops with obstructive jaundice, pruritus, abdominal pain and fever. Biliary stagnation leads to pigment stones. Eventually, secondary biliary cirrhosis supervenes with portal hypertension, pronounced cholestasis and progressive liver failure. Antimitochondrial antibody is negative. ERCP provides the diagnosis, showing thickened bile ducts with narrowed, beaded lumens.

Therapeutic trials of corticosteroids and immunosuppressive agents (for the presumed immunologically mediated inflammatory process), penicillamine (to mobilize copper, because this potentially toxic material accumulates in cholestasis) and proctocolectomy in patients with inflammatory bowel disease have all failed. As some patients may be asymptomatic for a decade, only careful observation is warranted early on. Recurrent bacterial cholangitis requires antibiotics. Predominantly large-duct strictures respond to endoscopic or transhepatic dilation and stent placement. Evaluation of ursodeoxycholic acid (which helps the pruritus but may not change the disease process), cyclosporine, methotrexate and colchicine awaits good clinical trials. Some 10–15% of patients develop cholangiocarcinoma, creating a diagnostic challenge. Primary sclerosing cholangitis is a frequent indication for liver transplantation that has a good outcome.

4.3 Neoplasia (Including Cholangiocarcinoma)

Benign tumors (adenomas, papillomas, cystadenomas) are rare causes of mechanical biliary obstruction.

Adenocarcinoma, the most common malignancy, is uncommon in the Western world. Predisposing factors are chronic parasitic infestations of the biliary tract (e.g., a liver fluke, such as Clonorchis sinensis or Opisthorchis viverrini), congenital ectatic lesions (Caroli's disease, choledochal cyst) and primary sclerosing cholangitis.

Jaundice and pruritus are common, but the presentation is varied. Cholestasis and weight loss eventually develop. There may be a deep-seated, vague pain localized in the right upper quadrant of the abdomen, in contrast to the severe pain of biliary colic and the septic picture of cholangitis. Indeed, cholangitis is not a feature if no biliary manipulations have been performed, such as an ERCP-placed stent. Hepatomegaly is frequent. A distended, nontender gallbladder may occasionally be palpated, feeling like a small rubber ball, if the common duct is obstructed below the entry of the cystic duct ("Courvoisier's sign"). Obstruction produces dilation of the biliary tree that can be readily detected on ultrasound or CT scan. Cholangiography with cytology and biopsy, usually by ERCP, should reveal the diagnosis. This slow-growing tumor presents late. The terminal event is usually hepatocellular failure. Palliation using biliary stents placed across strictures sometimes helps. Occasionally, a distal common duct lesion is amenable to curative surgery. Transplantation does not provide a good outcome.

OBJECTIVES

1. Recognize the normal anatomy of the biliary tree.
2. Discuss the mechanisms for the stimulation of bile secretion and the hormonal mediators of this response.
3. Describe the physicochemical characteristics of normal bile and its production, and the physiologic mechanism of bile salt reabsorption.

Acute and Chronic Gallbladder Disease, Carcinomas of the Biliary Tract

1. Identify the common types of gallstones and describe the pathophysiology involved in their formation.
2. Recognize the mechanisms by which risk factors predispose to gallstone formation.
3. List the tests commonly used in the diagnosis of calculous biliary tract disease. Describe the indications for, limitations of and potential complications of each.
4. Describe the probable natural history of a young patient with asymptomatic gallstones.
5. Know the complications that can occur from biliary calculi and describe the history, physical examination and laboratory findings for each.
6. Outline the management of a patient with acute cholecystitis.
7. Describe the symptoms and signs of choledocholithiasis; construct the management of this problem.
8. Outline a diagnostic and management plan for a patient with acute right upper quadrant pain.
9. Describe the diagnostic evaluation and management of a patient with fever, chills and jaundice.
10. Describe the following:
    a. Murphy's sign
    b. Courvoisier's sign
    c. Gallstone ileus
11. Contrast carcinomas of the gallbladder, bile duct and ampulla of Vater with regard to presenting features and survival.

Diagnostic Studies in Biliary Tract Disease

1. Contrast the liver enzyme abnormalities in cholestasis and viral hepatitis.
2. Identify the most common bacteria found in cholecystitis and cholangitis.
3. Describe the indications for and risks of oral cholecystogram, transhepatic cholangiogram and ERCP.

4. Accurately interpret an abnormal ultrasonogram of the gallbladder, oral cholecystogram, transhepatic cholangiogram and ERCP.

Skills
1. Given a patient with acute cholecystitis, demonstrate the right upper quadrant physical findings that indicate this diagnosis.

14
The Liver

L.J. Worobetz, R.J. Hilsden, E.A. Shaffer,
J.B. Simon, P. Paré, V.G. Bain, M. Ma, F. Wong,
N. Girgrah, P. Adams, J. Heathcote, S.S. Lee,
L.B. Lilly, G. Malkan and G.A. Levy

1. LIVER STRUCTURE AND FUNCTION / R.J. Hilsden and E.A. Shaffer

1.1 Liver Morphology

The liver is the largest and most metabolically complex organ in the body. Anatomically, it consists of two main lobes, right and left, divided by the round ligament and falciform ligament, plus two smaller lobes, the caudate lobe located on the posterior surface and the quadrate lobe on the inferior surface. The liver is functionally divided into eight segments based on the distribution of the portal and hepatic veins. Each segment receives a pedicle of the portal vein and is an independent functional unit. The caudate lobe (segment 1) differs from other segments in that it receives blood from both the right and left branches of the portal vein and drains directly into the inferior vena cava.

At a microscopic level, the liver consists of a myriad of individual functional units, traditionally called lobules. Each lobule is bounded by four to five portal triads (supplied from the portal vein and hepatic artery) and has a central terminal hepatic venule (central vein). A more physiologically sound concept is the unit termed the acinus. At the center is the portal triad, while the terminal hepatic venules are at the periphery. The acinus is divided into three zones based upon the distance from the feeding vessels (Figure 1).

The liver receives a dual blood supply. The portal vein drains the splanchnic circulation and provides 75% of the total blood flow (1,500 mL/min). The hepatic artery provides the remaining 25%. Small branches of each blood vessel (the terminal portal venule and the terminal hepatic arteriole) enter the acinus at the portal triad (zone 1). Blood then flows through sinusoids between plates of hepatocytes toward the terminal hepatic venule (zone 3), where blood from several adjacent acini merges. The terminal hepatic venules coa-

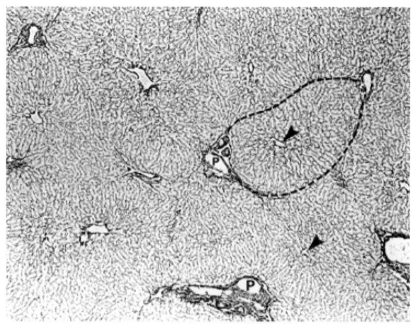

FIGURE 1.   Normal liver. This liver biopsy shows the orderly arrangement of the liver cell plates, central veins (arrowheads) and portal tracts (P). A hepatic lobule is outlined. (Retic. stain, original magnification × 370)

lesce to form the hepatic vein, which carries all efferent blood to the inferior vena cava. A rich supply of lymphatic vessels also drains the liver.

Hepatocytes make up the bulk of the organ. They are arranged in plates that radiate from each portal triad toward adjacent central veins. Those hepatocytes surrounding the portal tract, which form an interface between the connective tissue of the portal tract and the hepatic parenchyma, are termed the limiting plate.

The bile canaliculus is formed by grooves on the contact surface of adjacent liver cells. Bile forms in these canaliculi and progressively flows into ductules, interlobular bile ducts and then larger hepatic ducts. Outside the porta hepatis, the hepatic duct joins the cystic duct from the gallbladder to form the common bile duct, which drains into the duodenum.

Sinusoidal lining cells comprise at least four distinct populations: endothelial cells, Kupffer's cells, perisinusoidal fat-storing cells and pit cells. Endothelial cells differ from the vascular endothelium elsewhere in the body in that they lack a basement membrane and contain numerous fenestrae. The porous nature of the sinusoidal lining allows nutrients and macromolecules to gain access to the hepatocytes across the intervening space of Disse. Endothelial cells are also responsible for endocytosis of molecules and particles, and play a role in lipoprotein metabolism.

Spindle-shaped Kupffer's cells are tissue macrophages. They form an important part of the body's reticuloendothelial system. Their major functions include phagocytosis of foreign particles, removal of endotoxins and other noxious substances, and modulation of the immune response through the release of mediators and cytotoxic agents.

Perisinusoidal fat-storing cells (Ito cells) store vitamin A. They transform into fibroblasts in response to hepatic injury, contributing to hepatic fibrosis.

Pit cells, the least common sinusoidal lining cells, are large, granular lymphocytes, which function as natural killer cells.

The extracellular matrix of the liver includes its reticulin framework and several molecular forms of collagen, laminin, fibronectin and other extracellular glycoproteins.

1.2 Hepatobiliary Function

1.2.1 *METABOLISM*

The liver plays a central role in carbohydrate, protein and fat metabolism. It stabilizes glucose level by taking up and storing glucose as glycogen (glycogenesis), breaking this down to glucose (glycogenolysis) when needed, and forming glucose from noncarbohydrate sources such as amino acids (gluconeogenesis). Hypoglycemia occurs only late in the course of severe liver disease because the liver has a large functional reserve; glucose homeostasis can be maintained with only 20% of the liver functioning. The liver synthesizes the majority of proteins that circulate in the plasma, including albumin and most of the globulins other than gamma globulins. Albumin provides most of the oncotic pressure of plasma and is a carrier for drugs and endogenous hydrophobic compounds such as unconjugated bilirubin. Globulins include the coagulation factors: fibrinogen, prothrombin (factor II), and factors V, VII, IX and X. Factors II, VII, IX and X are vitamin K–dependent. Availability of vitamin K, a fat-soluble vitamin, requires adequate bile salts for the vitamin's absorption. These factors decrease with fat malabsorption (as with prolonged cholestasis) and with the reduced synthetic function of hepatocellular disease. (In hepatocellular diseases, deficiency of these coagulation factors is not corrected by parenteral vitamin K administration.) The liver is also the site of most amino acid interconversions and catabolism. Amino acids are catabolized to urea. During this process ammonia, a product of nitrogen metabolism and a possible neurotoxin, is utilized and therefore detoxified. Fatty acids are taken up by the liver and esterified to triglycerides. The liver packages triglycerides with cholesterol, phospholipids and an apoprotein into a lipoprotein. The lipoprotein enters blood for utilization or storage in adipocytes. Most cholesterol synthesis takes place in the liver. Bile salts are the major product of cholesterol catabolism.

1.2.2 *DRUG DISPOSITION*
The liver's rich enzyme system allows the metabolism of many drugs, including alcohol. The liver detoxifies noxious substances arriving from the splanchnic circulation, preventing them from entering the systemic circulation. This makes the liver particularly susceptible to drug-induced injury. The liver converts some lipophilic compounds into more water-soluble agents, which are then easily excreted in the urine or bile. Others are metabolized to less active agents.

1.2.3 *BILE FORMATION*
Bile provides the main excretory pathway for toxic metabolites, cholesterol and lipid waste products. Bile is also necessary for the efficient digestion and absorption of dietary fats. Bile salts are synthesized exclusively in the liver from cholesterol and are the driving force behind bile formation. After secretion by the liver, bile is stored in the gallbladder during periods of fasting.

Cholecystokinin (CCK), released from the small intestine during digestion by fatty acids and amino acids, stimulates gallbladder evacuation. When the bile reaches the duodenum it aids in fat absorption by acting as a biologic detergent. Bile salts are reabsorbed predominantly in the ileum and return to the liver via the portal vein to be taken up and secreted once again. This is the enterohepatic circulation (intestine-to-liver).

2. APPROACH TO THE PATIENT WITH LIVER DISEASE / J.B. Simon

Because of the liver's complexity, liver disease is often reflected by abnormalities of different hepatic "systems" – i.e., hepatocytes (hepatocellular dysfunction), the biliary excretory apparatus (cholestasis) and the vascular system (portal hypertension). In addition, the liver often is involved in systemic disease by virtue of its rich metabolic and reticuloendothelial activity and its large blood supply.

Patterns of disproportionate involvement often provide an important clue to the underlying disorder. For example, viral hepatitis characteristically produces predominantly hepatocellular dysfunction; primary biliary cirrhosis, predominantly cholestasis; cryptogenic cirrhosis, predominantly portal hypertension; and alcoholic liver disease, variable dysfunction of any of these three systems. The clinician can usually take advantage of these general patterns to help establish a diagnosis, though overlap and exceptions are frequent.

TABLE 1.   Major clinical manifestations of liver disease

Systemic
   Anorexia, malaise, fatigue
   Fever
   *General deterioration, weight loss, "cirrhotic habitus"
   Cholestasis: pruritus, *xanthelasma/xanthomas, *malabsorption problems

Jaundice

Hepatomegaly ± pain

Portal hypertension

Fluid derangements
   *Ascites ± edema
   Electrolyte disturbances
   Functional renal failure ("hepatorenal syndrome")

Hepatic encephalopathy (portosystemic encephalopathy)

*Cutaneous and endocrine changes
   Spider nevi, palmar erythema, Dupuytren's contractures
   Gynecomastia, testicular atrophy, impotence
   Amenorrhea
   Parotid enlargement

Coagulopathy
   Hypoprothrombinemia
   Thrombocytopenia
   Dysfibrinogenemia

Circulatory changes
   Hyperdynamic circulation
   *Arterial desaturation, clubbing

---

*asterisk implies chronicity

2.1 Clinical Features of Liver Disease

Table 1 lists the most important clinical manifestations of liver disease. Most can be seen in both acute and chronic hepatic disorders. Features denoting chronicity can be of diagnostic value at the bedside. For example, a clinical diagnosis of acute hepatitis should be reconsidered if physical examination reveals spider nevi and palmar erythema.

2.1.1 SYSTEMIC FEATURES

Nondescript anorexia, malaise and fatigue are common manifestations of both acute and chronic liver disease. An abrupt onset often reflects acute viral or drug-induced hepatitis, whereas an insidious development typifies alcoholic liver disease, autoimmune hepatitis and other chronic disorders.

Fever is another nonspecific feature of some liver conditions, especially the prodromal phase of acute viral hepatitis, severe alcoholic hepatitis and occasionally malignancy. However, frank rigors and chills are rare in these conditions, and instead strongly suggest acute cholangitis, usually secondary to common duct stone, or more rarely a liver abcess.

Patients with advanced chronic liver disease, especially alcoholic cirrhosis, often develop deterioration of general health, weight loss and a characteristic "cirrhotic habitus" in which wasted extremities and shoulder girdle contrast with a bloated belly from ascites.

Generalized pruritus is a hallmark of cholestatic disorders, especially if chronic. When cholestasis is prolonged – for example, in primary biliary cirrhosis – this may be accompanied by cutaneous lipid deposits (xanthelasma, xanthomas) and by features of malabsorption.

2.1.2 JAUNDICE

This cardinal feature of liver disease indicates hyperbilirubinemia. Bilirubin arises primarily from the physiologic breakdown of senescent red blood cells, with a minor contribution from other heme sources. It is not water-soluble and is therefore transported in plasma attached to albumin. This form of the pigment is called *unconjugated* or *free bilirubin*. The molecule is then taken up by hepatocytes and conjugated in microsomes with glucuronic acid to form bilirubin diglucuronide; the reaction is catalyzed by the enzyme glucuronyl transferase. Other minor conjugates are also formed; their clinical significance is unknown.

Transformed bilirubin is then secreted into the bile canaliculus along with the other constituents of bile. A small amount normally enters the blood as *conjugated bilirubin*. In contrast to unconjugated bilirubin, this form of the pigment is water-soluble and is therefore excreted into urine. Standard assays for bilirubin provide only the total, unconjugated plus conjugated. The "direct" component is conjugated bilirubin. The difference represents the unconjugated component.

After reaching the gut through the biliary tree, bilirubin is transformed by intestinal bacteria into pigmented breakdown products collectively called urobilinogen; these impart the normal brown color to stool. With impairment of biliary secretion (cholestasis) the stools are therefore often pale, but this is a relatively crude and unreliable diagnostic feature. Some urobilinogen is absorbed from the intestine and recycled through the liver (the enterohepatic circulation), with a portion escaping into the urine.

Various derangements in the above metabolic steps can result in jaundice. An increased bilirubin load from hemolysis may overwhelm the liver's conjugating capacity, resulting in unconjugated hyperbilirubinemia. This is invariably mild, unless there is also concomitant hepatic dysfunction. Isolated unconjugated hyperbilirubinemia also occurs in some specific defects of bilirubin metabolism, though these are rare except for Gilbert's syndrome (see Section 3 below).

In the vast majority of cases, jaundice is due to either hepatocellular disease or biliary obstruction. Both produce multiple defects in the pathway of bilirubin metabolism, including impaired hepatocellular uptake and transport, defective conjugation, decreased canalicular secretion, and "leakage" of conjugated bilirubin into the circulation. The resultant hyperbilirubinemia is a mixture of unconjugated and conjugated pigment; usually the latter predominates, but the exact proportion varies widely and has no specific diagnostic value.

Clinically, mild jaundice can usually be detected when serum bilirubin is about twice the upper limit of normal, and is best diagnosed by inspecting the patient's sclerae in natural daylight. More advanced cases are often apparent at a glance. Patients with severe long-standing jaundice sometimes have a generalized muddy-yellow appearance.

2.1.3 HEPATOMEGALY WITH OR WITHOUT PAIN

A readily palpable liver is not necessarily enlarged, for it may merely be low-lying – as, for example, in emphysema. Thus the upper border should be percussed when the edge is palpable.

The "quality" or feel of the liver is at least as important diagnostically as its size. For example, the liver usually retains its rubbery, relatively sharp edge when enlargement is due to fatty infiltration, acute hepatitis or passive congestion, whereas chronic fibrosis typically produces a blunt, indurated edge. Individual cirrhotic nodules are rarely detectable clinically. Palpable lumpiness instead favors malignant infiltration. It is important to remember that major liver disease – including a high proportion of cirrhosis – may not be associated with hepatomegaly.

Abdominal pain is common in biliary or pancreatic disease that might secondarily affect the liver – for example, common duct stone or pancreatic carcinoma – but pain is relatively uncommon in primary hepatic disorders. True hepatic pain is usually due to distention of the liver capsule, typically felt as a deep-seated right upper quadrant ache. This is often accompanied by hepatic tenderness on physical examination, best elicited by compression of the rib cage or fist percussion over the liver. The commonest causes are acute hepatitis, passive congestion from cardiac failure, and malignancy. Pain from malignancy is sometimes pleuritic in character and may be accompanied by a hepatic friction rub or bruit on auscultation. Some individuals claim some discomfort when the liver edge is palpated; this has no special significance and should not be interpreted as hepatic tenderness.

2.1.4 CUTANEOUS AND ENDOCRINE CHANGES
These findings as listed in Table 1 are important clues to chronic liver disease. Their pathogenesis is still poorly understood, but altered metabolism of sex hormones by the diseased liver appears important. The abnormalities may be seen in any chronic hepatic disorder, but are especially prevalent in alcoholic liver disease; this probably relates in part to a direct toxic effect of ethanol on gonadal function.

2.1.5 COAGULATION DISTURBANCES
The liver synthesizes most clotting factors, including vitamin K–dependent factors II, VII, IX and X. Severe hepatocellular dysfunction is therefore often accompanied by an enhanced bruising and bleeding tendency and by abnormal coagulation studies, particularly an increased INR/prothrombin time. Malabsorption of the fat-soluble vitamin K in prolonged cholestasis can also produce an abnormal INR/prothrombin time.

Thrombocytopenia is common in patients with cirrhosis, primarily as a result of hypersplenism from portal hypertension, but usually the platelet counts are not low enough to induce clinical bleeding. In patients with alcoholic liver disease, thrombocytopenia may also be due to direct marrow suppression by alcohol and/or nutritional folate deficiency.

Dysfibrinogenemia can also contribute to the coagulopathy from severe hepatic dysfunction.

2.1.6 CIRCULATORY CHANGES
A hyperdynamic circulation and relatively low blood pressure are sometimes seen in patients with severe liver disease, especially fulminant hepatitis and advanced cirrhosis. The mechanism may relate to increased synthesis of nitric oxide and accumulation of other vasoactive agents that reduce tone and are normally cleared by the liver. Occasional patients with cirrhosis develop intrapulmonary A–V shunting, with resultant arterial desaturation and (rarely) clubbing (hepatopulmonary syndrome).

A number of topics will be discussed in later sections, including portal hypertension (Section 11), fluid derangements (Sections 12 and 14) and hepatic encephalopathy (Section 13).

2.2 Laboratory, Radiologic and Histologic Evaluations
No single test can assess overall hepatic function, as the liver is a complex

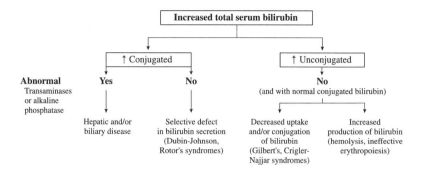

FIGURE 2.   Diagnostic approach to hyperbilirubinemia.

organ with interdependent metabolic, excretory and defense functions. Thus a number of laboratory tests are usually combined to detect hepatobiliary abnormalities and to assess their severity, follow the course of the disease, and help establish an etiology. Diagnosis is often based on patterns of abnormality that help distinguish hepatocellular dysfunction from excretory impairment (cholestasis), though overlap is great. In only a minority of cases does a specific laboratory test establish the diagnosis.

Radiologic imaging techniques and liver biopsy often provide essential diagnostic information, but their use should be tailored to the specific clinical circumstances.

2.2.1 SERUM BIOCHEMICAL TESTS

2.2.1.1 Bilirubin
Although this is a relatively insensitive test of liver function, an elevated level of bilirubin is responsible for jaundice and is therefore a classic indicator of hepatic or biliary disease. The degree of bilirubin elevation often correlates poorly with clinical severity, but serial values are useful for following the course of the illness. Fractionation into direct versus indirect bilirubin is *not* of diagnostic value in most cases of jaundice, and cannot distinguish hepatocellular disease from biliary obstruction. Measuring the fraction of unconjugated hyperbilirubinemia is useful only in cases of mild, isolated bilirubin elevation to corroborate hemolysis or Gilbert's syndrome (Figure 2).

Urine bilirubin has little diagnostic value except in early hepatitis, when bilirubinuria precedes clinical jaundice, and in isolated unconjugated hyperbilirubinemia, when bilirubinuria is absent despite jaundice (unconjugated bilirubin is not cleared into urine). Otherwise bilirubinuria is commonly present in hepatobiliary jaundice of any cause.

2.2.1.2 Aminotransferases (transaminases)

These liver enzymes include alanine aminotransferase (ALT), found primarily in liver cytosol, and aspartate aminotransferase (AST), also found in several other tissues, most notably skeletal and cardiac muscle. Both are exquisitely sensitive indicators of hepatocellular injury and provide the best guide to hepatocellular necrosis/inflammation.

The magnitude of elevation covers a very wide range. Levels <100 IU are common and nonspecific, and often have no clinical significance; levels of 100–300 IU are seen in numerous mild/moderate inflammatory processes. In acute viral or drug hepatitis aminotransferase levels are typically in the 500–1,500 IU range, but in alcoholic hepatitis they are usually <300 IU, even if the disease is severe. Values >3,000 IU usually are seen only in acute toxic necrosis or severe hypoxia ("shock liver," "ischemic hepatitis"); in both disorders levels typically plummet within two to three days, whereas values fall more slowly in viral hepatitis. Aminotransferase levels are variable in biliary obstruction but usually remain <200 IU, except with acute passage of common duct stone, characterized by a sudden rise to hepatitic levels and a rapid fall over the next one to two days.

The AST to ALT ratio is usually <1 in most circumstances, but is typically >1.5 in alcoholic liver disease; though not absolute, this is diagnostically helpful for alcoholic injury. Alcohol consumption lessens the ALT rise as a result of deficiency of a coenzyme needed for ALT synthesis.

2.2.1.3 Alkaline phosphatase (ALP)

The level of this bile canalicular enzyme is disproportionately increased in impaired bile excretion. Therefore, an elevated ALP is a hallmark of cholestasis. High levels are due to enhanced synthesis rather than hepatocytic leakage; thus, the level usually rises slowly over days or weeks rather than abruptly. A disproportionately elevated ALP is also common in infiltrative disorders, especially malignancy.

ALP isoenzymes also are present in bone and placenta. If the source of an isolated increase in ALP is not clinically clear, a concomitant elevation of γ-glutamyl transpeptidase (GGT) indicates a hepatobiliary origin. A form of ALP specific to the liver is 5'-nucleotidase.

2.2.1.4 Gamma-glutamyl transpeptidase (GGT)

Levels of GGT usually parallel ALP, but this microsomal enzyme is also easily inducible – for example, by ethanol and numerous drugs. Thus, GGT is often disproportionately elevated in alcoholic liver disease, although this is too nonspecific for diagnostic reliability.

2.2.1.5 *Proteins*

2.2.1.5.1 *Albumin* Synthesized by the liver, albumin is the major contributor to oncotic pressure in the serum. Decreased levels usually develop only in severe hepatic dysfunction – most often in advanced cirrhosis – and therefore imply a relatively poor prognosis. Albumin usually remains normal in acute hepatitis; falling values in this setting imply an unusually severe course.

2.2.1.5.2 *Globulins* A nonspecific diffuse elevation is common in chronic liver disease, and of no consequence. Sometimes there is disproportionate elevation of IgG in autoimmune hepatitis, of IgM in primary biliary cirrhosis, and of IgA in alcoholic liver disease.

2.2.1.6 *International Normalized Ratio (INR) and prothrombin time (PT)*
The INR/prothrombin time is a valuable index of the liver's ability to synthesize vitamin K–dependent clotting factors – a true "function" test. Increasing INR/PT implies relatively severe dysfunction, analogous to low serum albumin, and is especially worrisome in acute hepatitis. An abnormal value may be found in chronic cholestasis due to vitamin K malabsorption rather than impaired hepatic synthesis of clotting factors. Improvement after parenteral administration of vitamin K therefore favors a diagnosis of cholestasis over hepatocellular failure, but there are too many exceptions for diagnostic reliability.

2.2.1.7 *Lipids*
Complex lipoprotein derangements are common in liver disease, though usually not routinely studied. Cholesterol is often low in acute or chronic liver failure, whereas hypercholesterolemia is associated with prolonged cholestasis. Striking triglyceride elevations occasionally occur in alcoholic liver disease ("alcoholic lipemia").

2.2.2 *SERUM IMMUNOLOGIC TESTS*

2.2.2.1 *Hepatitis serology*
Serology is crucial for the specific diagnosis of hepatitis A, B, C and D. See Section 4 for details.

2.2.2.2 *Antimitochondrial antibody*
This is actually a complex series of antibodies directed against dehydrogenase

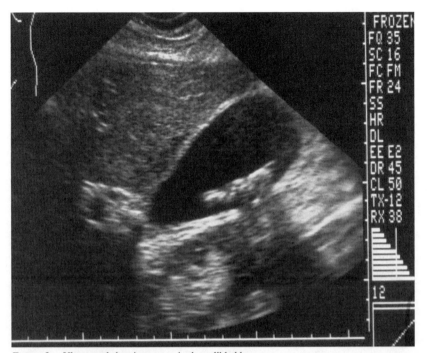

FIGURE 3.   Ultrasound showing stones in the gallbladder.

enzymes in mitochondrial membranes, especially pyruvate dehydrogenase. It serves as a valuable marker for primary biliary cirrhosis, as it is present in >90% of cases. Its role in the pathogenesis of the disease is unclear. Antimitochondrial antibody is uncommon in other disorders, though there is some overlap with autoimmune hepatitis.

2.2.2.3 Antinuclear factor and antismooth muscle antibody
Such nonspecific immune markers are seen relatively commonly in autoimmune hepatitis; they are infrequent in other hepatic diseases.

2.2.2.4 Alpha-fetoprotein
This normal hepatic fetal protein disappears soon after birth. Detection therefore reflects hepatic dedifferentiation. Levels >250 ng/mL serve as a relatively specific marker for hepatocellular carcinoma, though they are also seen occasionally in other tumors, especially testicular. Values <100 ng/mL are nonspecifically seen in hepatic regeneration – e.g., recovering from hepatitis.

2.2.3 IMAGING PROCEDURES

In general, radiologic imaging is essential for the accurate diagnosis of biliary disease, important for focal liver disease (e.g., tumor), but overused and of relatively little value for diffuse hepatocellular disease (e.g., hepatitis, cirrhosis).

2.2.3.1 Ultrasonography (US)

Ultrasound is now the most widely used imaging procedure. Highly reliable for diagnosis of gallstones (>95% sensitivity), it has replaced oral cholecystography (Figure 3). US is less accurate in detecting common bile duct stones (<40% sensitivity), but reliably establishes the presence of a dilated biliary tree, which implies mechanical obstruction. It is therefore the primary initial tool to distinguish intrahepatic from extrahepatic cholestasis. It also detects focal hepatic lesions (e.g., tumor, cysts), sometimes with characteristic diagnostic features. It is less useful in diffuse hepatocellular disease, as features are usually nonspecific. Abdominal ultrasound can be useful in the detection of fatty liver (steatosis), which results in a diffuse increase in echogenicity.

Ultrasonography can also provide important ancillary information relevant to hepatobiliary disease – e.g., splenomegaly or pancreatic mass. Doppler US is valuable in establishing the patency of hepatic vessels, especially the portal vein. Endoscopic US can detect calculi of the biliary tract and pancreatic masses.

2.2.3.2 Computerized tomography (CT)

A more expensive alternative to US, CT sometimes provides additional hepatic information, especially in focal lesions (Figure 4). Generally less valuable than US for biliary disease, CT is often more helpful in assessing the pancreas.

2.2.3.3 Direct biliary visualization

2.2.3.3.1 Endoscopic retrograde cholangiopancreatography (ERCP) Upper endoscopy allows direct cannulation of the common bile duct and/or pancreatic duct; the injection of contrast agent yields excellent definition of ductal anatomy. ERCP permits definitive visualization of the biliary tree for common duct stone, sclerosing cholangitis and other conditions. It also allows therapeutic intervention – e.g., removal of common duct stones via endoscopic papillotomy or stenting a stricture.

2.2.3.3.2 Percutaneous transhepatic cholangiography (PTC) In PTC, direct contrast visualization of the biliary tree is obtained via percutaneous needle puncture of the liver. This is done less often than ERCP, but is especially use-

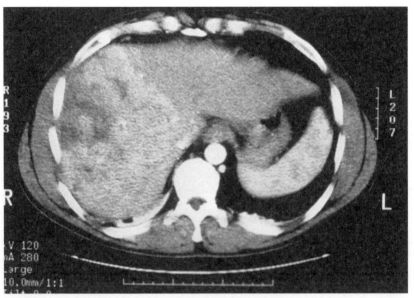

FIGURE 4.   CT scan showing extensive metastatic tumor in the liver.

ful if there is high biliary obstruction – e.g., a tumor at the bifurcation of the hepatic ducts. It also permits therapeutic intervention such as stent insertion to bypass a ductal malignancy.

ERCP and PTC require considerable technical expertise and have significant risks. They should not be undertaken lightly, but are highly valuable in selected cholestatic situations and often obviate laparotomy.

2.2.3.4 Radionuclide scanning

A liver–spleen scan using 99mTc-sulfur colloid can reveal space-occupying lesions and diffuse parenchymal disease. Such scans are much less sensitive than US or CT and their use has rapidly waned. A 99mTc-labeled RBC scan can visualize suspected vascular lesions, especially hemangiomas. Cholescintigraphy using 99mTc-iminodiacetic acid derivatives (termed HIDA scan) can reveal cystic duct obstruction, especially in acute cholecystitis. The HIDA scan also assesses biliary excretion/patency, but results often are less than ideal or misleading. Occasionally 67Ga-citrate scans are used to help detect liver abscess or tumor.

2.2.3.5 MRI and MRCP

Nuclear magnetic resonance imaging (MRI) is an expensive but valuable imag-

TABLE 2.   Indications for liver biopsy

Unexplained liver enzyme abnormalities
Hepatosplenomegaly of unknown cause
Diagnosis and staging of alcoholic liver disease
Cirrhosis – diagnosis and etiology
Chronic hepatitis
Unexplained intrahepatic cholestasis
Acute necrosis, if cause unclear
Suspected infiltrative disorder, especially malignancy
Unexplained systemic illness – fever of unknown origin, suspected granulomatous disease, etc.

ing technique that is becoming widely available. It can detect some lesions poorly seen by US or CT and sometimes can better clarify the nature of focal defects (e.g., hemangiomas). Magnetic resonance cholangiopancreatography (MRCP) can visualize the biliary tree, but in less detail than ERCP. MRCP may be a noninvasive alternative to ERCP to evaluate possible biliary obstruction.

2.2.4 *LIVER BIOPSY*
Percutaneous liver biopsy provides important diagnostic information at relatively low risk, but is needed in only a minority of cases of hepatic dysfunction. A small core of liver tissue is obtained at the bedside by needle aspiration under local anesthesia. This usually provides a surprisingly reliable reflection of the underlying disorder, though sampling error can occur in focal disease and some cases of cirrhosis.

The major indications for liver biopsy are shown in Table 2. Transient right upper quadrant pain is not uncommon after biopsy, but significant hemorrhage, bile peritonitis or other major complications are rare if cases are properly selected.

Relative contraindications include a clinical bleeding tendency, INR > 1.5 or prothrombin time more than three seconds greater than control, severe thrombocytopenia, marked ascites, and high-grade biliary tract obstruction. A transjugular approach can be used with relative safety in cases of coagulopathy or severe ascites.

Fine-needle aspiration of specific hepatic lesions can be obtained under US or CT guidance. This provides a cytologic sample, but is usually inadequate for full histologic assessment. Ultrasound guidance can also be used to obtain a core biopsy from the liver.

2.3 Clinical Approach
When faced with a patient with known or suspected liver disease, the physician should attempt to answer several central questions: (1) Is the disorder

acute or chronic? (2) Is it primarily a hepatocellular problem (e.g., hepatitis), a disorder of hepatobiliary secretion (cholestasis) or a vascular problem (e.g., portal hypertension)? (3) If hepatocellular, is alcohol, a virus or a drug responsible? If cholestatic, is it an intrahepatic problem or due to mechanical biliary obstruction? If vascular, is it due to cirrhosis or to a less common cause? (4) Is this actually a systemic disorder involving the liver rather than a primary hepatic problem? (5) Are there complications that require specific treatment? These and other pertinent questions are approached by bedside clinical judgment coupled with ancillary tests.

Broadly speaking, the most important diagnostic tool is a complete history and physical examination. Laboratory tests, imaging techniques and liver biopsy are valuable and sometimes essential for diagnosis, but in most cases clinical acumen provides the most important diagnostic information. Moreover, clinical judgment determines what additional studies should be undertaken and how to interpret the results. *Diagnostic errors most often arise from an inadequate history and physical examination with undue reliance on ancillary tests.*

The clinical assessment should emphasize aspects discussed above in Section 2.1. Inquire about ethanol, drugs (prescribed, over-the-counter and illicit) and epidemiologic factors relevant to viral hepatitis, especially in cases of suspected hepatocellular injury. In addition, pursuit of systemic illness is often necessary. A positive family history may also be obtained from patients with certain metabolic diseases such as Wilson's disease, α_1-antitrypsin deficiency and hemochromatosis. If a cholestatic disorder is suspected, clues to a possible extrahepatic cause should also be sought – e.g., biliary or pancreatic pain, rigors and chills or weight loss. The physical examination may provide valuable information on the size and nature of the liver, presence or absence of signs of chronic liver injury, and complications such as portal hypertension, fluid retention or encephalopathy (see Section 2.1).

The extent and nature of laboratory investigations are guided by the initial clinical evaluation. Broadly speaking, a minimal initial study will include CBC plus bilirubin, AST and/or ALT, and ALP. These few simple tests usually clarify whether the problem is primarily a hepatocellular injury (disproportionate aminotransferase elevations) or an excretory problem (predominant ALP elevation). If the former is clinically apparent but the etiology is not, viral hepatitis markers may help. A high AST:ALT ratio > 2 plus a disproportionate elevation of GGT often signals alcoholic injury. A low serum albumin level and high INR usually indicates relatively advanced hepatocellular dysfunction. If a cholestatic problem seems most likely, early US (or CT) should help distinguish intrahepatic from extrahepatic causation. If US indicates extrahepatic obstruction, direct biliary visualization by ERCP (or PTC)

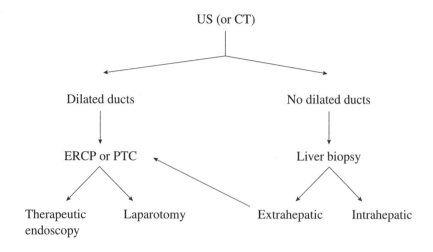

FIGURE 5.   A pragmatic approach to the investigation of cholestatic jaundice.

should be considered, whereas liver biopsy may be warranted if the process appears intrahepatic (Figure 5).

As yet there is no reliable biochemical marker of liver fibrosis. Thus laboratory indicators of hepatic dysfunction are often normal or only mildly deranged in cases of inactive cirrhosis; this is a common circumstance. It is well to remember that alcoholic liver disease is the commonest cause of chronic hepatocellular injury, even in patients who initially deny heavy ingestion.

With appropriate evaluation, a diagnosis can readily be established in the majority of patients with hepatobiliary dysfunction. In many circumstances, especially if the hepatic abnormalities are minor, the wisest approach is simply to follow the patient's progress with periodic clinical and laboratory assessments.

3. CONGENITAL HYPERBILIRUBINEMIAS / P. Paré

The importance of recognizing congenital hyperbilirubinemia lies mainly in distinguishing it from other, more serious hepatobiliary disease: congenital conjugated hyperbilirubinemia or hepatobiliary diseases. Except for Crigler-Najjar syndrome, congenital hyperbilirubinemias do not impair either the quality of life or the life expectancy of affected subjects. By definition, patients with familial hyperbilirubinemia have normal standard liver tests. The

TABLE 3. Congenital syndromes of hyperbilirubinemia

	Gilbert's	Crigler-Najjar type 1	Crigler-Najjar type 2	Dubin-Johnson	Rotor's
Prevalence	7% of population	Very rare	Uncommon	Uncommon	Rare
Inheritance (all autosomal)	Dominant	Recessive	Dominant	Recessive	Recessive
Serum bilirubin concentration (μmol/L)	< 100 (all unconjugated)	> 400 (all unconjugated)	< 400 (all unconjugated)	< 100 (about half conjugated)	< 100 (about half conjugated)
Diagnostic features	Bilirubin concentration ↓↑ with fasting ↓ with phenobarbital	No response to phenobarbital	Bilirubin concentration ↓ with phenobarbital	Characteristic urinary coproporphyrin excretion (>80% isomer 1) Pigment in centro-lobular hepatocytes	Normal gallbladder visualization at oral chole-cystography
Prognosis	Normal	Early death from kernicterus	Usually normal	Normal	Normal
Treatment	None needed	Liver graft	Phenobarbital	Avoid estrogens	None available

liver histology is also normal (except for the pigment accumulation in Dubin-Johnson syndrome). With the exception of Gilbert's syndrome, these syndromes are distinctly uncommon and are divided into two groups on the basis of the type of the serum hyperbilirubinemia (Table 3).

3.1 Unconjugated Hyperbilirubinemia

3.1.1 *GILBERT'S SYNDROME*

Gilbert's syndrome is the most common congenital hyperbilirubinemia syndrome, occurring in about 5% of Caucasians. It is probably transmitted through an autosomal dominant mode. Its pathogenesis is related to a partial deficiency in hepatic UDP-glucuronyl transferase, the enzyme responsible for the glucuronidation of bilirubin. In addition, some patients have reduced bilirubin uptake by the hepatocytes, as observed with diagnostic substances (BSP, indocyanine green) and drugs (tolbutamide). The syndrome is usually detected in adolescents and young adults, most commonly in males. Such a sex difference may be explained by testosterone inhibiting whereas estrogen and progesterone augment the action of UDP-glucuronyl transferase. Complaints leading to the diagnosis are various (fatigue, nausea, vague abdominal discomfort) and unrelated to the condition. Scleral icterus may be present and fluctuating, but the physical examination is otherwise normal. Liver tests and hemogram (to exclude hemolysis) are normal except for unconjugated serum bilirubin, which is elevated between 20 and 100 μmol/L, whereas conjugated bilirubin is often unrecordably low. Diagnostic tests are available but usually not necessary: fasting for two days or intravenous administration of nicotinic acid significantly increases serum unconjugated bilirubin, while phenobarbital significantly decreases it. No treatment is warranted. Prognosis is excellent.

3.1.2 *CRIGLER-NAJJAR SYNDROME*

This syndrome may present in two types. Type 1 is a very rare and serious disease characterized by unconjugated hyperbilirubinemia often greater than 400–500 μmol/L. It is due to an absolute deficiency of UDP-glucuronyl transferase. Jaundice occurs almost immediately after birth and may lead to kernicterus with consequent neurologic damage and mental retardation. Kernicterus involves damage to the basal ganglia and cerebral cortex because unconjugated bilirubin is able to penetrate the immature blood–brain barrier of infants. The syndrome is inherited in an autosomal recessive fashion, often with a family history of consanguinity. Phenobarbital treatment is ineffective in inducing UDP-glucuronyl transferase activity; death occurs early. The treatment of choice appears to be hepatic transplantation.

Crigler-Najjar syndrome type 2 is a much more benign condition in which the unconjugated hyperbilirubinemia usually does not exceed 400 μmol/L. Kernicterus rarely develops in these patients (except with prolonged fasting, in which bilirubin can rise). Hepatic UDP-glucuronyl transferase activity is very low or undetectable, but phenobarbital therapy reduces serum bilirubin levels. (Phenobarbital presumably induces even the low levels of this enzyme.) Prognosis is quite good despite a lifelong persistent unconjugated hyperbilirubinemia.

3.2 Conjugated Hyperbilirubinemia

Two conditions characterized by congenital conjugated hyperbilirubinemia without cholestasis have been described. Both syndromes are inherited as autosomal recessive traits. Both are uncommon disorders believed to result from specific defects in the hepatobiliary excretion of bilirubin. These conditions are benign, and their accurate diagnosis provides reassurance to the patient. Plasma bilirubin levels are usually in the range of 35–85 μmol/L, although occasionally levels may be as high as 400 μmol/L. Plasma bilirubin may further increase in both conditions during intercurrent infection, pregnancy or use of oral contraceptives. Pruritus is absent and serum bile acid levels are normal, as are routine biochemical liver tests, except for the serum bilirubin concentration. Bilirubinuria is usually present. No treatment is necessary.

Some distinctive features allow differential diagnosis between the two syndromes.

3.2.1 *DUBIN-JOHNSON SYNDROME*

Patients with the Dubin-Johnson syndrome have a black liver, which results from the accumulation of a melanin-like pigment in lysosomes. Visualization of the gallbladder during oral cholecystography is usually delayed or absent. Urinary excretion of total coproporphyrin is normal, whereas the proportion of isomer 1 is higher than in normal controls (>80%). Finally, the BSP plasma retention test is normal in its initial phase, but there is a secondary rise in plasma BSP concentration at 90 minutes due to reflux of BSP from the hepatocyte to the plasma.

3.2.2 *ROTOR'S SYNDROME*

In patients with Rotor's syndrome, the appearance and histology of the liver are normal. Oral cholecystography usually visualizes the gallbladder. Total coproporphyrin excretion is greater than normal, as in other hepatobiliary disorders, and isomer 1 makes a smaller proportion (<80%) than in Dubin-Johnson patients. The plasma disappearance of injected BSP is delayed, with no secondary rise.

TABLE 4.   Causes of acute hepatitis

Viruses
Hepatitis A
Hepatitis B
Hepatitis C
Hepatitis D
Hepatitis E
Herpes simplex
Cytomegalovirus
Epstein-Barr
Adenoviruses
Exotic viruses
Drugs
Toxins
Alcohol
Ischemia
Wilson's disease
Other

4. ACUTE VIRAL HEPATITIS / V.G. Bain and M. Ma

The term *hepatitis* refers to any inflammatory process of the liver. The most common etiology of acute hepatitis is viral infection (Table 4). In North America, hepatitis A, hepatitis B and hepatitis C are the commonest causes of viral hepatitis. Viral hepatitis occurs less commonly with infections such as Epstein-Barr virus, cytomegalovirus, adenovirus, herpes simplex and Cox-sackie virus. In these cases, the clinical picture is usually dominated not by the hepatitis but by other features of the viral illness.

The clinical course of acute hepatitis varies from mild symptoms requiring no treatment to fulminant liver failure requiring liver transplantation. In the last decade, the treatment of acute viral hepatitis has not progressed as rapidly as our understanding of these hepatitis viruses' epidemiology and molecular biology. The mainstay of treatment is still supportive care, because the inflammation is self-limited in most cases. Postexposure prophylaxis is possible for some of the hepatitis viruses.

4.1 The Hepatitis Viruses and Their Epidemiology

4.1.1 *HEPATITIS A VIRUS (HAV)*
Previously termed "infectious hepatitis," hepatitis A virus (HAV) is an RNA virus that belongs to the enterovirus family. It is present in the stool of patients

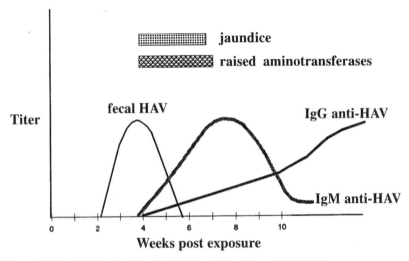

FIGURE 6.   Typical clinical and serologic features of acute hepatitis A infection.

during the prodrome or pre-icteric phase until about two weeks after the onset of jaundice. Both IgM and IgG antibodies to the virus (anti-HAV) can be detected, the more helpful of these being the demonstration of an elevated IgM antibody, indicating recent infection (Figure 6).

HAV infection is common. The anti-HAV IgG can be detected in 30–40% of the population in developed countries and 90% of the population in developing countries. HAV is usually transmitted by the fecal–oral route. Thus, food or water contamination may lead to epidemic outbreaks. Several outbreaks have been associated with ingestion of raw clams and oysters from polluted water. Person-to-person spread results in sporadic cases. Parenteral transmission is also possible, especially in intravenous drug users, but is much less common.

Infection can occur at any age but is most common in younger age groups. Infection can present as a gastrointestinal illness and therefore diagnosis can be missed. In countries with good water supplies and sanitation, more symptomatic hepatitis A is seen in older age groups, since fewer adults are exposed to hepatitis A as children. The incubation period is about one month, and rarely is longer than 40 days. The mortality rate – usually from fulminant hepatitis – is very low (0.1%). There is no evidence for a chronic carrier state or the development of chronic liver disease.

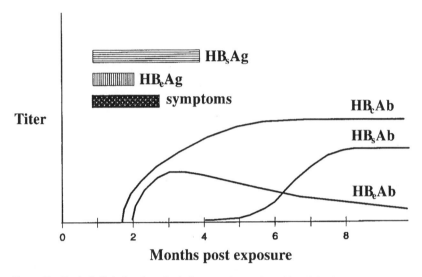

FIGURE 7. Typical clinical and serologic features of acute hepatitis B infection.

4.1.2 *HEPATITIS B VIRUS (HBV)*

In 1965, an antibody in a hemophiliac patient was found to react with an antigen in the serum from an Australian aborigine; this antigen was subsequently found in patients with viral hepatitis. This antigen was termed the Australian antigen and is now known to be the surface coat of the hepatitis B virion, now called the hepatitis B surface antigen (HB_sAg).

HBV is a unique DNA virus that replicates through reverse transcription of its mRNA. It behaves more like a retrovirus than a DNA virus. HBV consists of a 28 nm central core containing the genome (a single molecule of partially double-stranded DNA) and a specific DNA polymerase with a surrounding core protein shell. The core is commonly found in the nuclei of infected hepatocytes, with the outer HB_sAg coat being acquired from the cytoplasm of the hepatocyte. The core antigen is antigenically distinct from the HB_sAg. This allows separate detection of core antibody (anti-HB_c) and surface antibody (anti-HB_s). A further viral antigen, termed HB_eAg, can be detected in the serum, together with DNA polymerase. HB_eAg is a subunit of HB_cAg. HB_eAg positivity implies viral replication and is an indicator of high infectivity. Mutants that do not produce HB_eAg exist; these "pre-core mutants" can cause severe hepatitis.

The typical course of HBV infection, appearance of the viral antigens and host immune response are shown in Figure 7. The significance of HBV markers and their importance in interpretation is summarized in Table 5.

TABLE 5.   Interpretation of hepatitis B markers

Marker	Interpretation
HB$_s$Ag	HBV infection; may be acute or chronic
HB$_s$Ab	Immune to HBV; may be natural immunity or following vaccination
HB$_c$Ab-IgM	Acute HBV infection (newer and more sensitive assays may also be positive during reactivation of chronic infections)
HB$_e$Ag	High infectivity, active viral replication
HB$_e$Ab	Low or no infectivity; need only be measured in chronic HBV
HBV-DNA	Direct measure of infectivity or replicative state; becoming increasingly available

TABLE 6.   Risk factors associated with reported cases of acute HBV in the U.S.

Risk factors	%
Heterosexual activity	48
IV drug use	11
Homosexual activity	7
Health-care employment	2
Household contact	1
Transfusion, dialysis	1
Unknown	30

SOURCE: Data from Centers for Disease Control and Prevention, 1992.

In North America, HBV infection occurs primarily in adolescents and adults. High-risk groups for HBV infection are summarized in Table 6. The transmission may be sexual, vertical or parenteral (most commonly through inoculation by contaminated needles in intravenous drug users). Hepatitis B infection from transfusion has been almost completely eliminated by routine screening and by the use of volunteer blood donors. Vertical transmission is common in developing countries, passing from a mother who is a chronic hepatitis B carrier to a fetus or newborn; the infection is acquired at the time of birth or shortly thereafter. This vertical transmission of HBV results in the vast majority of chronic carriers worldwide.

4.1.3 HEPATITIS C VIRUS (HCV)

Hepatitis C virus is a recently discovered single-stranded RNA virus of less than 80 nm in diameter that has been classified as a member of the flavivirus family. The virus itself has not been isolated or visualized, although the majority of its genome has been cloned and sequenced. It is worldwide in distribution. The prevalence of HCV infection in the general population is approximately 1%. However, prevalence is highly variable among different risk groups. Hemophilia patients who have received concentrated factor have a prevalence rate as high as 90%, whereas health-care workers have a prevalence rate of 1%.

The principal mode of HCV transmission is parenteral exposure, but a significant percentage of patients do not have identifiable risk factors. Transfusion-related cases make up only 10% of the total hepatitis C cases. Intravenous drug use is the main cause of hepatitis C infection, but interestingly, the exposure may predate clinical hepatitis by decades. HCV also accounts for 12–25% of cases of sporadic hepatitis.

The incubation period is 5 to 10 weeks (mean 7 weeks), with the acute phase being clinically mild and the majority of cases being anicteric. The elevated aminotransferase pattern may be monophasic or multiphasic. The latter suggests chronicity, which develops in over 80% of cases. Histologically, it is not possible to distinguish between progressive and nonprogressive forms of hepatitis C. Liver biopsy is not recommended in the acute phase.

Serologic testing for this virus has developed rapidly following its discovery in 1989. The third-generation ELISA (enzyme-linked immunosorbent assay) and RIBA (recombinant immunoblot assay) identify antibodies to the nonstructural as well as structural epitopes of the virus. The ELISA test is very sensitive but less specific, and therefore all positives must be confirmed with the highly specific RIBA, a different ELISA assay, or an HCV-RNA determination. From Red Cross blood donor data, about 50% of individuals who have normal liver enzymes and are anti-HCV positive by ELISA will be negative on subsequent RIBA testing. Hypergammaglobulinemia is a common reason for a false-positive ELISA test. An additional problem with the ELISA test for anti-HCV is that the antibody cannot be detected in the circulation for several weeks following the onset of acute hepatitis C. Moreover, not all patients with acute HCV infection will develop anti-HCV ELISA positivity.

Studies measuring HCV-RNA to detect the virus, using a highly sensitive polymerase chain reaction assay, have shown that 80% of antibody-positive individuals have viremia and are potentially infectious. In contrast to hepatitis B, sexual and vertical transmission is uncommon. HCV infection from contaminated needles in health-care workers occurs in less than 5%.

4.1.4 HEPATITIS D VIRUS (HDV)

HDV is a defective RNA virus that requires the presence of hepatitis B sur-face antigen for its expression. HDV utilizes the HB$_s$Ag protein as its external coat to attach to and enter hepatocytes. It is found worldwide, but Italy, East-ern Europe, the Middle East, the South Pacific, South America and Africa have the highest incidence. In North America, less than 1% of HB$_s$Ag-positive patients have evidence of HDV infection, whereas in parts of Italy 14–50% of HB$_s$Ag-positive patients are co-infected with HDV. In the United States and Canada, HDV infection is found almost exclusively among intra-venous drug abusers and their sexual partners.

Hepatitis D infection may originate as a co-infection with hepatitis B or as a superinfection in a patient who is already a chronic HBV carrier. Co-infection produces a more severe acute hepatitis than that caused by hepatitis B alone, but it is usually self-limited. Superinfection often results in more severe chronic hepatitis than hepatitis B alone. The delta virus circulates in association with the delta antigen, but until more sensitive assays are devel-oped, this antigen can be detected only during the early phases of infection. The serologic marker for acute and chronic hepatitis D infection is the anti-body to delta antigen (anti-HDV). It often appears late in the course of acute delta hepatitis, leading to an erroneous diagnosis of acute hepatitis B.

4.1.5 HEPATITIS E VIRUS (HEV)

Hepatitis E (epidemic hepatitis) is caused by a single-stranded RNA virus of 27–34 nm in size. It shares many similarities with hepatitis A. Although HEV was previously included in the group labeled non-A non-B hepatitis, it has now been classified as an enteric virus transmitted by contaminated water supplies or by the fecal–oral route. Cases of HEV infection may be part of an epidemic or may be isolated, sporadic cases. HEV is the leading cause of acute viral hepatitis in young to middle-aged adults in many developing countries. It is associated with a high mortality rate (approaching 20%) in infected pregnant women in the third trimester. It is seen only rarely in North America and almost exclusively in travelers returning from endemic regions. The incubation period is 10–50 days. There are no distinctive clinical fea-tures. Secondary cases are rare. Chronic infection does not develop. Testing for anti-HEV is available at reference laboratories.

4.1.6 HEPATITIS F VIRUS (HFV)

An as yet unidentified virus is believed to be associated with some cases of fulminant hepatitis that are negative for all other viral serology. Most such cases are fatal without a liver transplant. Some of these cases are associated with the development of aplastic anemia.

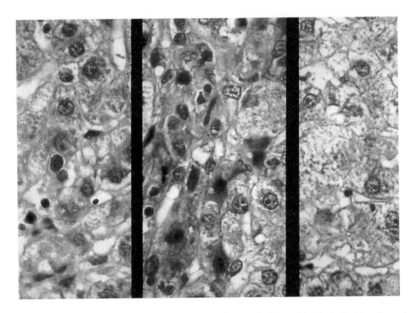

FIGURE 8.   This composite shows patterns of necrosis in viral hepatitis. In the left-hand panel, two apoptotic bodies are seen. The central panel shows eosinophilic degeneration that probably represents an earlier stage of apoptosis. Lytic or ballooning degeneration is quantitatively the major form of hepatocellular damage in viral hepatitis and is seen in the right-hand panel.

4.1.7 HEPATITIS G VIRUS (HGV)

In 1995, a new virus that was believed to cause hepatitis was cloned. It is known as the GB agent, so named after the initials of a surgeon who contracted this infection. It is similar to flaviviruses and shares 25% homology with hepatitis C. Very little is known about this new virus or group of viruses. The most recent studies suggest that it does not cause hepatitis, so "hepatitis G" may be a misnomer.

4.2 Pathology

Acute viral hepatitis causes inflammation of the liver involving primarily the parenchyma. There is evidence of hepatocellular degeneration (ballooning, acidophilic bodies, spotty necrosis), inflammation (lobular and portal mononuclear infiltrate) and hepatocyte regeneration (Figures 8 and 9). More severe cases demonstrate bridging necrosis between central veins and portal tracts (Figures 10 and 11). Because there is usually preservation of the retic-

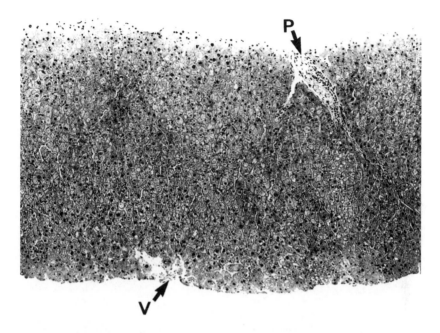

FIGURE 9. Mild hepatitis. There is some increase in inflammatory cells but no obvious hepato-cellular necrosis. P, portal tract; V, central vein. (H & E, original magnification × 92.5)

ular framework, the liver completely restores itself with hepatocyte regeneration. Liver biopsy is not generally helpful in distinguishing between the different types of acute hepatitis, as the histology is quite similar.

4.3 Clinical Features

Most viral hepatitis infections are asymptomatic, especially in younger individuals. When symptomatic, initial symptoms are nonspecific, beginning with malaise, nausea, vomiting, fatigue and a low-grade fever. More characteristic are severe anorexia, an aversion to smoking, and the passing of dark urine. Right upper quadrant discomfort is common in acute hepatitis, but severe abdominal pain is not a feature. After several days, jaundice appears, often preceded by dark urine and light-colored stool. The convalescent stage is usually 7 to 10 days, with the total illness lasting 2 to 6 weeks. Physical findings are usually minimal, aside from jaundice and a tender, enlarged liver. Alcoholic hepatitis (see Table 13 in Section 5.4) can usually be differentiated from acute viral hepatitis by a longer history of illness (months vs weeks).

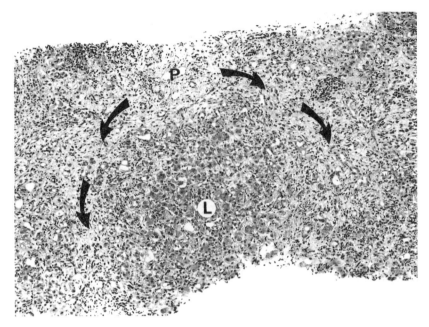

FIGURE 10. Severe hepatitis. Marked inflammation has resulted in confluent hepatocellular necrosis, termed bridging necrosis (curved arrows), along the portal tracts (P) that surround a residual hepatic lobule (L). (HPS, original magnification × 92.5)

4.4 Diagnosis

Acute viral hepatitis can be suspected by the presence of viral prodrome symptoms, which often precede the more classical symptoms (including jaundice, dark urine and pruritus). Of diagnostic importance are a history of exposure to jaundiced persons, recent intravenous drug use or transfusions, sexual orientation and safe sex practices, travel history, drug or toxin exposure (including herbs) and the absence of significant abdominal pain.

If viral hepatitis is suspected clinically, laboratory evaluation will help confirm the presence of acute liver injury, may define the etiology and may help monitor the course and prognosis of hepatitis. Characteristically, the serum aminotransferase level is significantly elevated, often to levels >1,000 IU/L (normal is 10–40 IU/L), with the alkaline phosphatase only mildly to moderately elevated. The serum bilirubin is mainly conjugated and reflects the severity of the hepatitis. The INR/prothrombin time defines the extent of liver injury in the acute stage. An increasing INR/PT implies a poor prognosis and

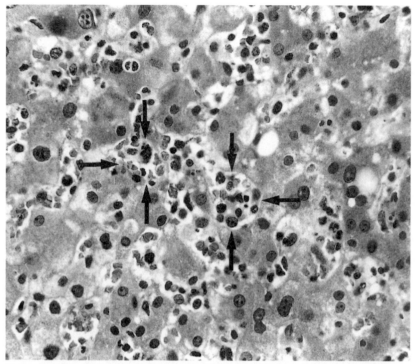

FIGURE 11.   Severe hepatitis. High power shows numerous inflammatory cells within the sinu-soids as well as foci of hepatocellular necrosis (arrows). Reactive changes, including binucleation and prominent nucleoli, are seen in the viable hepatocytes. (Gomori, original magnification ✕ 370)

the need for referral to a regional liver center. Initial serologic testing should include only HAV-IgM and HB$_s$Ag. Anti-HCV should be done at the onset only if specific risk factors are present (especially intravenous drug use) or subsequently if the HAV and HBV serology is negative.

The differential diagnosis includes other viral infections (such as infectious mononucleosis or cytomegalovirus infection), drug-induced liver disease, autoimmune hepatitis and Wilson's disease. Biliary tract disease (including cholecystitis and cholangitis) is distinguished by the presence of fever and significant abdominal pain. If doubt exists as to the diagnosis of hepatitis, abdominal ultrasound to investigate extrahepatic biliary obstruction and even liver biopsy may be necessary. In general, liver biopsy is rarely required in patients with acute hepatitis.

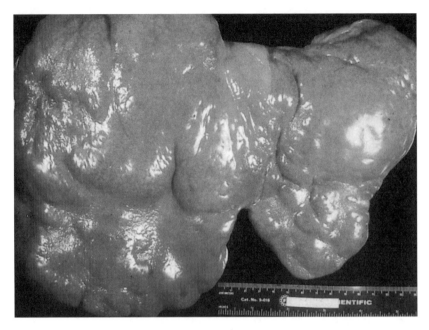

FIGURE 12.   This gross specimen shows the characteristic loss of hepatic substance with collapse and wrinkling of the capsule. Such an appearance is seen in massive hepatic necrosis of any etiology.

4.5 Complications

Most patients with viral hepatitis recover completely. The most important complication is the development of chronicity, which may follow hepatitis B, C and D. Most other complications are fortunately rare.

4.5.1 FULMINANT HEPATITIS

This is defined as the development of acute liver cell injury proceeding to liver failure and hepatic encephalopathy within eight weeks in a patient without any known previous liver disease. Clinically, the patient deteriorates with development of deep jaundice, confusion and drowsiness. The encephalopathy can progress into deep coma. Because of massive liver necrosis, there is deficiency of clotting factors, and hence the INR/PT is always increased. At this stage, mortality is greater than 50% unless a liver transplant can be performed. Death may occur from infection, hypoglycemia, increased intracranial pressure with cerebral edema, or renal failure. Massive hepatic necrosis leads to shrinkage of the liver (Figure 12) and architectural collapse is seen histologically (Figures 13 and 14). Despite this, if regeneration occurs, histo-

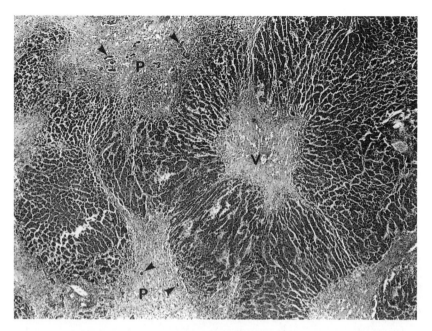

FIGURE 13.   Submassive necrosis. Extensive hepatocellular necrosis is seen, leaving large areas of connective tissue around the central vein (V) and widening of the portal tracts (P), which have become confluent. Residual bile ducts (arrowheads) are seen in the portal tracts. (HPS, original magnification × 370)

logic recovery is the rule. Usually a liver biopsy is not required; the procedure is associated with considerable bleeding risk unless done by the transjugular route.

4.5.2 CHOLESTASIS
Occasionally acute viral hepatitis exhibits a cholestatic phase, in which the patient becomes intensely pruritic and jaundiced, and the enzyme pattern changes with a fall in the aminotransferase but with an increased alkaline phosphatase value. Biliary tract disease and drug toxicity should be ruled out. Resolution within a few weeks is the usual course. This occurs most commonly in hepatitis A.

4.5.3 RELAPSING (BIPHASIC) HEPATITIS
Clinically, these patients are improving, only to have a recurrence of the signs and symptoms of their hepatitis. Resolution is almost always complete. This pattern is most characteristic of hepatitis A. In some cases of hepatitis B, the second phase is due to acute hepatitis D. Hepatitis C is characterized by

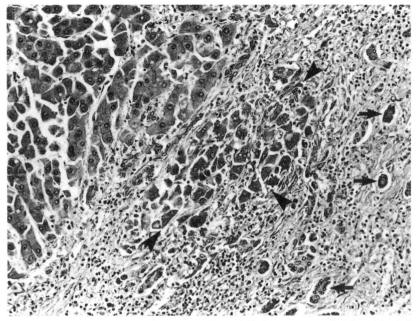

FIGURE 14.   Submassive necrosis. High power shows viable hepatocytes on the left, an island of degenerating cells centrally (arrowheads) and residual bile ducts (arrows) in the widened portal tract. (HPS, original magnification × 185)

repeated and wide fluctuations in liver aminotransferase values, but a biphasic clinical course is uncommon.

4.5.4 IMMUNE COMPLEX DISEASE

In hepatitis B, about 5–10% of cases initially develop a serum-sickness–like syndrome characterized by skin rash, angioedema and arthritis, which is due to circulating immune complexes of viral proteins and antibody with complement activation. Other immunologic manifestations include pericarditis, aplastic anemia or neurologic abnormalities such as Guillain-Barré syndrome. Chronic hepatitis B may have persisting circulating immune complex disease that leads to such diseases as membranous glomerulonephritis with nephrotic syndrome or polyarteritis nodosa. Chronic hepatitis C can cause cryoglobulinemia secondary to viral protein and antibody interaction. Clinical features of cryoglobulinemia include glomerulonephritis, vasculitic skin rash and arthritis.

4.5.5 *CHRONIC HEPATITIS*

Chronic hepatitis represents continued disease activity beyond six months. This complicates acute hepatitis B infrequently in adults but occurs in acute hepatitis C in over 80% of cases. It does not occur in hepatitis A or E. Chronic hepatitis can be suspected if there are persistent symptoms or persistent elevation of serum aminotransferase levels after six months.

4.6 Treatment

Most cases of acute viral hepatitis resolve spontaneously and require no specific treatment. Strict bed rest is not necessary. The patient may undertake any activity that does not exacerbate symptoms. Diet can be liberal, encouraging a high calorie intake but excluding alcohol. Fatty foods are poorly tolerated and are best avoided. Hospitalization is not necessary. All drugs, especially tranquilizers and sedatives, should be avoided. Corticosteroids do not alter the degree of hepatitis or rate of healing and should be avoided to allow a normal immunologic response, which then can eliminate the virus. Indeed, their use in acute viral hepatitis may increase the risk of a chronic carrier state. Interferon-α may be useful in acute hepatitis C.

Return to work and activity should be guided by the patient's symptoms. Patient education will help alleviate anxiety. Specialist referral is not usually required. Prophylaxis and prevention of secondary spread is perhaps the most important aspect of treatment.

4.7 Prophylaxis

The control of hepatitis A is dependent on good sanitation and hygiene, because the virus is excreted in the stool early in the course of the infection. An attack of hepatitis A confers lifelong immunity. An effective vaccine has been developed for use by high-risk individuals such as those traveling to endemic areas, day-care workers, armed forces personnel or those living in institutions. Serum immunoglobulin (ISG) is also available. This should be provided to all household contacts, and is optimally given within one week of exposure at a dose of 0.02 mL/kg IM. Casual school or work contacts are not usually treated prophylactically unless an epidemic is identified.

A specific globulin preparation and a vaccine are available for HBV. Hepatitis B immunoglobulin (HBIG) should be given when there has been a clear-cut exposure such as inadvertent "needlestick" or sexual contact. It also should be given, along with hepatitis B vaccine, within 24 to 48 hours to the neonates of mothers with acute or chronic hepatitis B. Hepatitis B vaccine, originally manufactured from pooled donor sera, is now synthesized from recombinant DNA. Side effects are minimal with both forms. Vaccination targeted against high-risk groups such as homosexuals, health-care workers,

TABLE 7. Overview of viral hepatitis

Virus type		Transmission	Incubation (days)	Serologic diagnosis	Chronicity
HAV	RNA	Fecal–oral	20–35	HAV-IgM	No
HBV	DNA	Percutaneous, venereal	60–110	HB_sAg	Adults <5% Preschoolers 25% Neonates >90%
HCV	RNA	Percutaneous	35–70	anti-HCV	>80%
HDV	RNA	Percutaneous, venereal	60–110	anti-HDV	Usual in superinfection; rare in co-infection
HEV	RNA	Fecal–oral	10–50	anti-HEV	No
HFV	?	?	?	?	No
HGV	RNA	Percutaneous	?	(Research only; HGV-RNA)	Yes

IV drug users, family contacts of chronic carriers, chronic transfusion recipients and dialysis patients has surprisingly failed to affect the incidence of hepatitis B. Universal vaccination is therefore advocated and has been initiated in some provinces. Vaccination for hepatitis B is also protective against hepatitis D.

There is no vaccine or specific immunoglobulin available for hepatitis C. Following a high-risk exposure such as a needlestick from a known case of hepatitis C, an individual should be closely followed and tested for liver enzymes and HCV-RNA. If the latter becomes positive, prompt treatment should be considered with interferon-α and ribavirin.

4.8 Summary

Table 7 summarizes the important features of the different types of viral hepatitis. Acute viral hepatitis is a self-limited disease and requires supportive care only. For the few patients who develop fulminant liver failure, liver transplantation may be required. Chronic infection can develop in patients with HBV, HCV, HDV and HGV infection.

5. CHRONIC HEPATITIS / V.G. Bain and M. Ma

The term *chronic hepatitis* means active, ongoing inflammation of the liver persisting for more than six months that is detectable by biochemical and his-

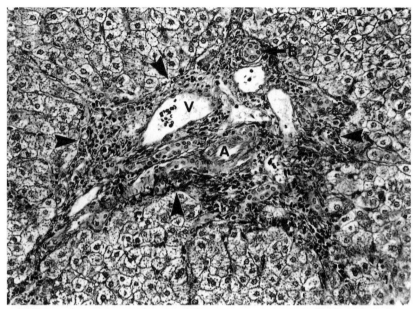

FIGURE 15. Mild chronic hepatitis. This portal tract contains a chronic inflammatory infiltrate that is confined to the portal triad and does not extend past the limiting plate (arrowheads). V, vein; A, artery; B, bile duct. (Masson, original magnification × 185)

tologic means. It does not imply an etiology. The biochemical hallmark of chronic hepatitis is an increased serum aminotransferase (AST and ALT) with minimal elevation of alkaline phosphatase. When the inflammation is severe and/or prolonged, hepatic dysfunction may become apparent with an increase in serum bilirubin and INR/prothrombin time, and a decrease in serum albumin. Typically, biochemical tests are used to identify and follow patients with chronic hepatitis, while liver biopsies serve to more precisely define the nature of the chronic hepatitis and provide useful information regarding the extent of damage and prognosis.

Histologically, chronic hepatitis is characterized by infiltration of the portal tracts by inflammatory cells. These cells are predominantly mononuclear cells including lymphocytes, monocytes and plasma cells. Chronic hepatitis is designated as mild when the infiltrate is confined to the portal triad (Figure 15). It is designated as moderately severe chronic hepatitis (Figure 16) when the infiltrate extends into the parenchyma (piecemeal necrosis) and when it extends to adjacent portal triads (bridging necrosis). The inflammatory process can also "bridge" from the portal tract to the central vein. Severe chronic hepatitis is associated with multilobular or confluent necrosis and is

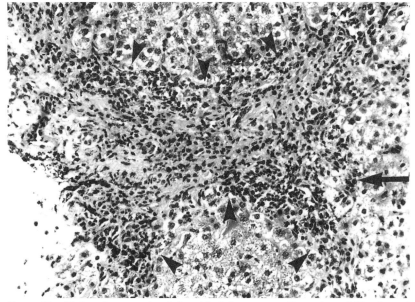

FIGURE 16.   Moderately severe chronic hepatitis. Inflammatory cells are shown infiltrating and destroying the periportal hepatocytes (arrow) and disrupting the limiting plate (piecemeal necrosis) (arrowheads). (HPS, original magnification × 185)

much more likely to progress to cirrhosis. The newer terms *mild*, *moderate* and *severe chronic hepatitis* replace the older terminology including *chronic persistent hepatitis* and *chronic active hepatitis*, which are still frequently mentioned in older textbooks. The amount of fibrosis is staged separately, from mild fibrosis to cirrhosis.

By far, the commonest cause of chronic hepatitis is viral infections of the liver. Other causes include autoimmune hepatitis, drug-induced hepatitis, Wilson's disease, α_1-antitrypsin deficiency and steatohepatitis. Primary biliary cirrhosis and primary sclerosing cholangitis may occasionally mimic chronic hepatitis, but are not usually classified as such. An approach to help determine the etiology of chronic hepatitis is summarized in Table 8.

5.1 Chronic Viral Hepatitis

5.1.1 *GENERAL CONSIDERATIONS*
Of the known viral infections of the liver, HBV, HCV, HDV and HGV can cause chronic liver disease; HBV and HCV make up the vast majority of these

TABLE 8. Role of history in diagnosis of chronic hepatitis

Etiology	Key points in the history	Useful lab tests
Hepatitis B	Sexual history (homosexuality, use of prostitute services, promiscuity), family history, country of origin, IV drug use	HB_sAg – if positive, measure HB_eAg, HB_eAb and HBV-DNA (if available)
Hepatitis C	Blood transfusions (pre-1990), IV drug use (even once), tattoos, ear or body piercing, sexual promiscuity, HCV-positive partner, incarceration	anti-HCV HCV-RNA
Autoimmune hepatitis	Usually young or middle-aged females, often chronic symptoms – especially fatigue (but may present acutely), other autoimmune disease (e.g., thyroid)	Quantitative immuno-globulins Antinuclear antibodies Smooth-muscle antibody Anti-LKM
Drug-induced hepatitis	Careful history of all drugs and herbs: common offenders include isoniazid, nitrofurantoin, NSAIDs, sulfa drugs	None
Wilson's disease	Family history, neurologic or psychiatric symptoms in children or young adults	Serum ceruloplasmin 24-hr urinary copper Liver biopsy
α_1-antitrypsin deficiency	Family history of liver or lung disease (emphysema)	α_1-antitrypsin levels and Pi typing
Nonalcoholic steatohepatitis (NASH)	Obesity – especially recent weight gain, diabetes mellitus, corticosteroids, intestinal by-pass surgery	Glucose Hgb Al_c Abdominal ultrasound

cases. A careful history is most helpful in determining the cause of chronic hepatitis (Table 8). In most cases, selected laboratory tests will provide the confirmation of diagnosis. Sometimes liver biopsy is required to identify the cause of chronic hepatitis. The liver biopsy will also provide important information about the extent of damage and current activity.

TABLE 9. Seromarkers of HBV infection and vaccination

	Acute infection*	Chronic infection		Previous infection	Vaccination
		Inactive	Active		
HB$_s$Ag	+	+	+	–	–
HB$_s$Ab	–	–	–	+	+
HB$_e$Ag	+	–	+/–**	–	–
HB$_e$Ab	–/+	–/+	–	+	–
HBV-DNA	+	–	+	–	–

* Core IgM (+)
** HB$_e$Ag is negative in pre-core mutant

5.1.2 HEPATITIS B VIRUS

5.1.2.1 Evolution to chronic liver disease
A number of factors determine whether an individual will clear an acute HBV infection or progress to a chronic carrier state. Of these, the age at infection is most important, with carrier rates of greater than 90% occurring in vertically infected newborns as compared to less than 5% in adults. The immunologic status of the host is also important, with immunocompromised individuals (e.g., HIV, renal failure, post-transplant) being more likely to become chronic carriers. The severity of the acute disease has also been correlated with outcome. In general, the milder the acute illness the more likely that progression to chronic liver disease will occur. Presumably, individuals with mild acute disease are those with a suboptimal immunologic response to the virus, whereas patients with more severe acute disease are manifesting a prompt and effective immunologic attack on hepatocytes harboring HBV.

5.1.2.2 Presentation
The majority of patients with chronic type B hepatitis are asymptomatic or have mild fatigue only. The patients might give a history of risk-taking behavior or a family history of hepatitis B infection. Liver enzyme abnormalities discovered incidentally will frequently alert the physician to the possibility of underlying viral infection. Screening of family and sexual contacts of known cases will often discover additional cases.

5.1.2.3 Diagnosis
By the strictest definition, a patient is not a chronic HBV carrier until the HB$_s$Ag test is found to be positive for six months, but the diagnosis is often suspected much earlier.

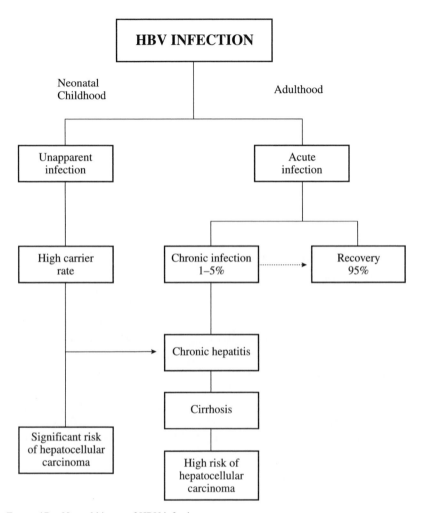

FIGURE 17.   Natural history of HBV infection.

It is important not to be confused by other viral markers of previous hepatitis B exposure (Table 9). Antibodies to HB$_s$Ag (anti-HB$_s$) indicate immunity against HBV and may be acquired either after vaccination or after clearance of HBV infection. On the other hand, the presence of HB$_e$Ag and HBV-DNA indicates active HBV replication. The level of HBV-DNA correlates with the amount of virus present in the circulation. When HBV-DNA is strongly positive, there is a high viral load, which indicates a high degree of infectivity (all

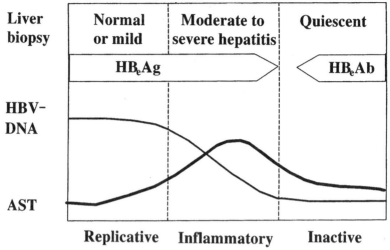

FIGURE 18.   Phases of chronic hepatitis B.

physiologic fluids are potentially infectious). A negative HBV-DNA indicates very low or absent infectivity. Unfortunately, serum HBV-DNA testing is not widely available. If HB_eAg is negative there is usually lower infectivity. Positive antibodies to the core antigen (anti-HB_c) indicate exposure to the virus. The presence of IgM anti-HB_c suggests recent HBV exposure. In chronic HBV infection the anti-HB_c is positive but the IgM anti-HB_c is negative because exposure took place more than six months previously. The exception is in patients with reactivation of chronic hepatitis B who may also be IgM anti-HB_c positive, which reduces the usefulness of this test in diagnosing acute HBV infection.

5.1.2.4 *Natural history*
The natural history of chronic HBV infection has been well defined (Figure 17). The first six months of the illness represent the acute hepatitis phase of the infection. This acute phase is not often seen in chronically infected patients who have contracted the virus at birth or in early childhood. Chronic hepatitis has three phases, termed the replicative, inflammatory and inactive phases (Figure 18). During the replicative phase, HB_eAg is positive as is HBV-DNA, indicating high levels of viral replication. Despite this, the aminotransferases are normal or near normal and the liver biopsy is relatively inactive. For unknown reasons, patients may then enter the inflammatory phase in which their immune system now recognizes those hepatocytes har-

TABLE 10. Factors predictive of a response to interferon treatment in HBV infection

HBV: Characteristics of responders to interferon treatment
Immunocompetency
Adult-acquired infection
Active liver disease
Low HBV-DNA level
Female
Absence of HDV infection

boring virus and begins to attack them. Accordingly, the aminotransferase becomes elevated and the biopsy shows chronic hepatitis, often of a severe degree The level of viral replication as measured by the HBV-DNA will decline. If the patient has successfully cleared viral replication, he or she will enter an inactive phase characterized by normalization of the aminotransferases and relative inactivity on the liver biopsy. HB_eAg will be cleared and anti-HB_e will form (seroconversion).

It is the severity and duration of the inflammatory phase that determine whether a patient will develop cirrhosis. This progression of chronic hepatitis to cirrhosis occurs in 20–30% of all chronic hepatitis B patients. Those with cirrhosis are at highest risk for developing hepatocellular carcinoma. Even patients who successfully enter the inactive phase are still at risk of hepatocellular carcinoma (relative risk greater than 100 vs the general population). Screening for hepatocellular carcinoma has been recommended in chronic carriers by performing a serum α-fetoprotein and an abdominal ultrasound each 6 to 12 months; more recently, however, the efficacy and cost benefit of this approach have been questioned. The problem is that even cases discovered by screening are often beyond cure by resection or liver transplantation.

5.1.2.5 *Treatment*
There are few therapeutic options for the treatment of patients with chronic hepatitis B, although different agents have been tried. Of these agents, only interferon-α has been licensed for use. In most studies, 30–40% of chronic hepatitis B patients successfully respond to interferon treatment with a loss of serologic markers of viral replication (HB_eAg and HBV-DNA). A minority of responders will also lose all evidence of infection (clear HB_sAg) during treatment. The relapse rate following discontinuation of therapy is less than 15%.

Since the majority of patients do not respond to interferon, an important question is, which patients warrant a trial of therapy? Those most likely to respond include patients who acquired their infection during adulthood,

TABLE 11. HBV vaccination

Candidates for HBV vaccination
Sexually active people
People with occupational risks of blood or body fluid contact
   (health-care workers, police officers, firefighters)
IV drug users
Inmates of prisons and institutions
Hemophiliac patients
Hemodialysis patients
Travelers to HBV-endemic areas

---

females, patients with elevated ALT and low HBV-DNA levels, those with active hepatic inflammation on biopsy, patients who are HIV antibody negative and those who are anti-HDV negative. Stated another way, patients in the inflammatory phase are most likely to benefit from interferon (Table 10).

A number of new medications are being tested for efficacy against HBV. Lamivudine is a new nucleoside analogue with very potent antiviral effect against HBV. It can suppress viral replication to undetectable levels. A small number of patients will clear HB_eAg and develop anti-HB_e after one year of therapy. Most patients will have recurrence of HBV infection when lamivudine is stopped. A lamivudine-resistant mutant can appear during treatment. However, it appears to be a less aggressive virus.

5.1.2.6 *Prevention*
Active immunization is important to prevent transmission of HBV infection from a chronic carrier to sexual and family contacts. The safety of the vaccine is well established. It should be given to all high-risk groups (Table 11), but ultimately the goal is universal vaccination. As universal vaccination becomes a reality, prophylaxis with hyperimmune hepatitis B globulins for HBV contacts will become unnecessary.

5.1.3 *HEPATITIS C VIRUS*
Chronic hepatitis C virus has become the commonest type of chronic viral hepatitis in most developed countries. The identified cases may represent only the tip of the iceberg, with most being undiagnosed. Many cases are identified after investigation of raised liver enzymes in asymptomatic individuals or during screening of blood donors and those at higher risk such as IV drug users. Other patients present to physicians with fatigue, malaise and abnormal liver enzymes.

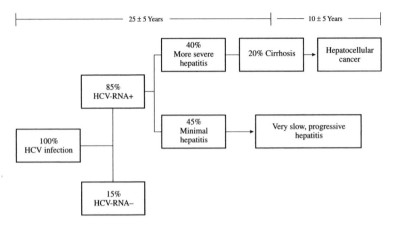

FIGURE 19.   Natural history of HCV infection in immunocompetent hosts.

5.1.3.1 *Epidemiology*

Although HCV infection can be transmitted by the same routes as HBV infection, the majority of cases are related to intravenous drug abuse (60–70%). Ten percent of patients with chronic HCV infection will have had a previous blood transfusion. Nasal cocaine use, body piercing and tattoos are also associated with HCV transmission. In the remaining patients, one cannot identify a possible source of infection. Nonparenteral transmission through sexual or intimate contact and maternal–infant exposure can occur with HCV infection, but much less often than with HBV infection.

5.1.3.2 *Natural history*

The natural history of HCV infection has been better defined with the availability of anti-HCV serologic testing. Widespread application of this test has revealed that more than 85% of patients with acute HCV infection will remain chronically infected. Of the patients with chronic hepatitis, 20% either have or will go on to develop cirrhosis by 25 years (Figure 19). Thereafter, an additional 1% per year develop cirrhosis. Of much concern is the fact that recent data document a strong association between chronic HCV infection and hepatocellular carcinoma. The exact relative risk has yet to be determined but appears to be as high as or higher than that with HBV. Other disorders that have been described in association with chronic HCV infection include cryoglobulinemia, porphyria cutanea tarda and membranoproliferative glomerulonephritis.

TABLE 12.   Predictors of sustained response to interferon treatment in HCV infection

HCV: Interferon response predictors
1. Young patients
2. Short duration of infection
3. Absence of cirrhosis
4. Low level of HCV-RNA
5. Non genotype 1b
6. Abnormal aminotransferases

5.1.3.3 *Treatment*

Interferon-α is the only therapy available for chronic HCV infection. Numerous studies have identified a 40–50% response rate (normalization of ALT abnormalities). However, at least 50% of these responders will relapse, with the majority of relapses occurring within three months following discontinuation of therapy. Therefore, only about 10–20% of treated patients enjoy a sustained response, or presumed cure (clearance of HCV-RNA). The most recent clinical trials have utilized 12 to 24 months of therapy instead of the standard 6 months. Sustained response rates in excess of 30% have been reported. Factors that predict a favorable response to interferon include recent infection, minimally elevated ALT, absence of cirrhosis, low titer of virus in serum and certain hepatitis C genotypes or genetic variants (Table 12).

Ribavirin is a guanosine nucleoside analogue that independently is not effective against chronic HCV infection. However, in combination with interferon-α, sustained response rates after one year of therapy approach 45%. Thus, the combination therapy of interferon-α and ribavirin is now the treatment of choice in previously untreated patients.

A vaccine for HCV has not been developed, but is an active area of research. There are currently insufficient data to advocate the use of immune serum globulin for the prevention of HCV infection. HCV-infected individuals must avoid sharing razors, dental products and anything else that might be contaminated with their blood. Condoms should be used during the acute phase of the illness and indefinitely for patients who are immunocompromised. Couples in whom one is chronically infected with hepatitis C must make their own decision in regard to condom use after being advised of the risks; the risk of spread to regular sexual partners is 2–5%. Vertical transmission from a normal mother to her newborn is rare; however, the risk of HCV vertical transmission is much higher if the mother is co-infected by HIV.

5.1.4 *HEPATITIS D VIRUS*

Chronic hepatitis D usually results from HDV superinfection of an HBV carrier. Less commonly, acute HBV/HDV co-infection leads to chronic infection. Either way, chronic hepatitis D is usually aggressive and severe with rapid progression to cirrhosis.

The diagnosis is made by testing for anti-HDV in the serum of HBV carriers with risk factors for HDV infection. HDV antigen and HDV-RNA in serum or liver can also be measured, but only in a limited number of laboratories. In North America this virus is most often transmitted by intravenous drug abuse. In Mediterranean countries nonparenteral transmission may also occur. Treatment with interferon for HDV infection has been disappointing. Because of the dependency of HDV on HBV, prevention of HBV infection with vaccine can prevent HDV infection also.

5.2 Drug-Induced Chronic Hepatitis

Many drugs can cause chronic hepatitis. The decision to discontinue an implicated drug depends to some extent on whether the drug is merely causing persistent enzyme abnormalities or hepatic dysfunction with severe histologic abnormalities. In severe cases, fibrosis, cirrhosis and death from liver failure or complications of portal hypertension can result. Examples of drugs that are capable of causing chronic hepatitis that may progress to liver failure and portal hypertension are diclofenac, amiodarone, isoniazid, nitrofurantoin, alpha methyldopa and dantrolene. On the other hand, if a drug is essential to the health of the patient and there are no unrelated agents that can be substituted, it is reasonable to continue therapy under close clinical supervision providing the enzyme abnormalities are mild and not associated with symptoms or functional derangements (i.e., serum bilirubin, albumin and INR/PT remain normal). Liver biopsy may be helpful in defining the severity of liver injury.

5.3 Autoimmune Hepatitis

Autoimmune hepatitis is an immunologically mediated disorder of the liver that often affects young females with a personal or family history of autoimmune disease. The etiology is unknown. The onset may be insidious or acute. The hepatic presentation can be that of sudden hepatic failure, chronic hepatitis or inactive cirrhosis. Common complaints include fatigue, amenorrhea, symptoms associated with an accompanying rheumatological disorder such as arthritis, or those from thyroid disease. Physical findings include jaundice (in severe cases), spider nevi, palmar erythema and hepatosplenomegaly. Laboratory investigations reveal hypergammaglobulinemia with pronounced elevation of IgG levels, reduced serum albumin, positive antinuclear factor and smooth-muscle antibody. A proposed subclassification includes type 1 and

TABLE 13.   Differentiating viral and alcoholic hepatitis

	Viral hepatitis	Alcoholic hepatitis
History	Risk factors	Significant alcoholic intake
Physical examination	Mild hepatomegaly, extrahepatic stigmata not prominent	Moderate to marked hepatomegaly, florid stigmata
Laboratory examination	AST variable ALT > AST	AST <300 AST > ALT (often 2:1 or more)
Liver biopsy	Mononuclear cells Portal tract centered Ground glass cells (HBV) Special stains (HBV)	Polymorphs Pericentral, diffuse Mallory's hyaline Fat

type 2 autoimmune hepatitis, with the latter demonstrating antibodies to liver/kidney microsome (anti-LKM 1 hepatitis). Liver biopsy is essential to establish the diagnosis and severity of the underlying disease as well as to exclude other liver disease. Cirrhosis is present in over 50% of autoimmune hepatitis on initial biopsy.

Treatment is initiated with high-dose corticosteroids (prednisone 40–60 mg/day) for 4–6 weeks. The dose is then tapered to a maintenance level (e.g., 5–10 mg/day) just sufficient to keep the liver enzymes within normal values. Often azathioprine is used for its steroid-sparing effect. Following discontinuation of treatment, most patients will relapse, requiring reinitiation of therapy. Untreated autoimmune hepatitis progresses rapidly to cirrhosis (three to five years). Although corticosteroids may not prevent cirrhosis, they are clearly lifesaving in this otherwise fatal condition. With careful titration of their medication, most patients remain in stable condition for years. In the remaining minority, liver transplantation is highly successful.

5.4 Alcoholic Hepatitis
The condition is usually readily diagnosed on clinical grounds with a good medical history and laboratory investigations (see Table 13). There is no specific therapy for alcoholic hepatitis. Avoidance of alcohol, good nutrition and supportive medical therapy are essential to allow the liver to recover.

5.5 Fatty Liver
The accumulation of fat, sometimes accompanied by inflammation and hepatic necrosis, is a common disorder, even in the absence of alcoholism. It is usually asymptomatic, found most commonly in patients who are obese, diabetic

and, occasionally, hyperlipidemic. Mild right upper quadrant pain may be present with aminotransferase levels typically <3–4 times normal. The diagnosis can be established by ultrasound (or CT) examination of the liver or by liver biopsy showing macrovesicular fat. The treatment is that of the underlying condition, including weight loss and therapy of diabetes and hyperlipidemia. Most cases of fatty liver are not associated with inflammation and hepatocellular necrosis. Between 10 and 20% have nonalcoholic steatohepatitis (NASH) with inflammation and some necrosis. These have the potential to progress to fibrosis and cirrhosis.

6. ALCOHOLIC LIVER DISEASE / N. Girgrah and F. Wong

Liver disease is the fourth commonest cause of death in adults between the ages of 20 and 70 years in Canada. Alcohol is still the commonest cause of chronic liver disease in this country, but not all those who abuse alcohol develop liver damage. The incidence of cirrhosis among alcoholics is approximately 10–20%. The mechanism by which certain people are predisposed to develop cirrhosis is still unknown. The quantity of alcohol ingested has been shown in epidemiological studies to be the most important factor in determining the development of cirrhosis. Males drinking in excess of 80 g and females in excess of 40 g of alcohol per day for 10 years are at a high risk of developing cirrhosis. The alcohol content rather than the type of beverage is important. Binge drinking is less injurious to the liver than continued daily drinking.

Women are more susceptible to liver damage than men. They are likely to develop cirrhosis at an earlier age, present at a later stage and have more severe liver disease with more complications. Genetics may play a role in the development of alcoholic liver disease. Patterns of alcohol drinking behavior are inherited. Alcohol is metabolized to acetaldehyde by alcohol dehydrogenase and then to acetate by acetaldehyde dehydrogenase. Genetic pleomorphism of the enzyme systems that metabolize alcohol can lead to different rates of alcohol elimination and contribute to the individual's susceptibility to alcohol damage. Some studies have reported an increased frequency of the gene that encodes for dehydrogenase in patients with alcoholic liver disease, leading to increased production of acetaldehyde. Alcoholics with decreased acetaldehyde dehydrogenase activity also develop alcoholic liver disease at a lower cumulative intake of alcohol than others.

Alcohol has a direct hepatotoxic effect and does not require pre-existing malnutrition, but malnutrition may play a permissive role in producing alcohol hepatotoxicity. There is a threshold of alcohol toxicity beyond which no dietary supplements can offer protection. Obesity may also be an independent

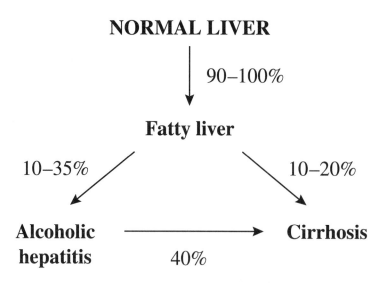

FIGURE 20. Schematic representation of the progression of the different stages of alcoholic liver disease.

risk factor for the development of alcoholic liver disease. Finally, hepatitis C infection appears to play a role in the development of advanced alcoholic liver disease. Patients with alcoholic liver disease and hepatitis C infection tend to develop their disease at a younger age and have more severe histological features and decreased survival. In addition, the presence of hepatitis C is a major risk factor for the development of hepatocellular carcinoma in patients with alcoholic cirrhosis.

The spectrum of liver disease ranges from relatively benign steatosis to potentially fatal alcoholic hepatitis and cirrhosis (Figure 20).

6.1 Alcoholic Fatty Liver

Fatty liver is the most frequent hepatic abnormality found in alcoholics. It is a toxic manifestation of ethanol ingestion, appearing within three to seven days of excess alcohol intake. Fat accumulates with ethanol ingestion because of increased triglyceride synthesis, decreased lipid oxidation and impaired fat mobilization by the liver. This results in the accumulation of triglycerides in the hepatocytes, mainly in the terminal hepatic venular zone. In more severe cases, the fatty change may be diffuse. The fat may be macrovesicular (large droplets) or microvesicular (small droplets), which represents more active lipid synthesis by the hepatocyte. Fatty liver may occur alone or be part of the picture of alcoholic hepatitis or cirrhosis.

Clinically, the patient is usually asymptomatic, and examination reveals a firm, smooth, enlarged liver. Occasionally the fatty liver may be so severe that the patient is anorexic and nauseated and has right upper quadrant pain or discomfort. This usually follows a prolonged heavy alcoholic binge. Liver function tests including bilirubin, albumin and INR are frequently normal, although the γ-glutamyl transpeptidase (GGT) is invariably elevated while the aminotransferases and alkaline phosphatase may be slightly increased. A fatty liver can be detected by ultrasound. Liver biopsy is required to make a definitive diagnosis. When fatty liver is not associated with alcoholic hepatitis, its prognosis is excellent. Complete abstinence from alcohol and a nutritious diet will lead to disappearance of the fat over four to six weeks.

6.2 Alcoholic Hepatitis

Alcoholic hepatitis may occur separately or in combination with cirrhosis. There are all grades of severity. It is a condition characterized by liver cell necrosis and inflammatory reaction. Histologically, hepatocytes are swollen owing to an increase in intracellular water secondary to increase in cytosolic proteins. Steatosis, often of the macrovesicular type, is present. Alcoholic hyaline (or Mallory) bodies are purplish red intracytoplasmic inclusions consisting of clumped organelles and intermediate microfilaments. Polymorphs are seen surrounding Mallory-containing cells and also within damaged hepatocytes. Collagen deposition is usually present. It is maximal in the zone 3 and extends in a perisinusoidal pattern to enclose hepatocytes, giving it a "chicken wiring" effect. Changes in the portal triad are inconspicuous. Marked portal inflammation suggests an associated viral hepatitis such as hepatitis C, whereas fibrosis suggests complicating chronic hepatitis. When the acute inflammation settles, a varying degree of fibrosis is seen, which may eventually lead to cirrhosis.

Clinically, mild cases of alcoholic hepatitis are recognized only on liver biopsy in patients who present with a history of alcohol abuse and abnormal liver enzymes. In the moderately severe case, the patient is usually malnourished and presents with a two- to three-week prodrome of fatigue, anorexia, nausea and weight loss. Clinical signs include a fever of <40°C, jaundice and tender hepatomegaly. In the most severe case, which usually follows a period of heavy drinking without eating, the patient is gravely ill with fever, marked jaundice, ascites, and evidence of a hyperdynamic circulation such as systemic hypotension and tachycardia. Florid palmar erythema and spider nevi are present, with or without gynecomastia. Hepatic decompensation can be precipitated by vomiting, diarrhea or intercurrent infection leading to encephalopathy. Hypoglycemia occurs often and can precipitate coma. Gastrointestinal bleeding is common, usually from gastritis or a peptic ulcer, aggravated by any bleeding tendency. Signs of malnutrition and vitamin deficiencies are common. Acetaminophen is a hepatotoxin when taken in large quantities. Alcohol increases the patient's susceptibility to liver damage by acetaminophen owing to induction of metabolizing enzymes. Smaller doses of acetaminophen in an alcoholic may precipitate liver failure.

Laboratory abnormalities include elevations of the aminotransferases, bilirubin, alkaline phosphatase and GGT. The aminotransferase levels rarely exceed 300 IU/L, except in association with acetaminophen ingestion; the AST/ALT ratio is usually >2. Hyperbilirubinemia can be quite marked, with levels reaching 300 to 500 μmol/L, and is a reflection of the severity of the illness. The increase in GGT is proportionally greater than that of alkaline phosphatase. There is also leukocytosis of up to 20–25 × 10^9/L and a prolongation of the INR/prothrombin time, which does not respond to vitamin K. The serum albumin falls. Serum IgA is markedly increased, with IgG and IgM raised to a lesser extent.

Patients with acute alcoholic hepatitis often deteriorate during the first few weeks in hospital, with a mortality rate of 20–50%. Bad prognostic indicators include spontaneous encephalopathy, markedly prolonged INR/PT unresponsive to vitamin K and severe hyperbilirubinemia of greater than 350 μmol/L. The condition may take one to six months to resolve, even with complete abstinence. Alcoholic hepatitis progresses to cirrhosis in 40% of clinical episodes.

6.3 Alcoholic Cirrhosis

Established cirrhosis is usually a disease of middle age after the patient has had many years of drinking. Although there may be a history of alcoholic hepatitis, cirrhosis can develop in apparently well-nourished, asymptomatic patients. Occasionally the patient may present with end-stage liver disease with malnutrition, ascites, encephalopathy and a bleeding tendency. A history of alcohol abuse usually points to the etiology. Clinically, the patient is wasted. There may be bilateral parotid enlargement, palmar erythema, spider nevi and Dupuytren's contracture. Males develop gynecomastia and small testes. Hepatomegaly is often present, affecting predominantly the left lobe as a result of marked hypertrophy. There may be signs of portal hypertension, which include splenomegaly, ascites and distended abdominal wall veins. At the late stage, the liver may become shrunken and impalpable. There may be signs of alcohol damage in other organ systems, such as peripheral neuropathy and memory loss from cerebral atrophy. Alcoholic cirrhosis is also associated with several renal problems. These include IgA nephropathy, renal tubular acidosis and the development of hepatorenal syndrome. There is an association between hepatitis B and C and alcoholic cirrhosis.

Histologically, the cirrhosis is micronodular. The degree of steatosis is variable and alcoholic hepatitis may or may not be present. Pericellular fibrosis around hepatocytes is widespread. Portal fibrosis contributes to the development of portal hypertension. There may be increased parenchymal iron deposition. When this is marked, genetic hemochromatosis has to be excluded. With continued cell necrosis and regeneration, the cirrhosis may progress to a macronodular pattern.

Biochemical abnormalities include a low serum albumin with elevated bilirubin and aminotransferases. AST and ALT levels rarely exceed 300 IU/L and the AST/ALT ratio usually exceeds 2. GGT is disproportionately raised with recent alcohol ingestion and is a widely used screening test for alcohol abuse. With severe disease, the INR/PT may be prolonged. Portal hypertension results in hypersplenism leading to thrombocytopenia, anemia and leukopenia. Other nonspecific serum changes in acute and chronic alcoholics include elevations in uric acid, lactate and triglyceride, and reductions in glucose, magnesium, potassium and phosphate.

The prognosis of alcoholic cirrhosis depends on whether the patient can abstain from alcohol. This in turn is related to family support, financial resources and socioeconomic state. The presence of hepatitis also influences prognosis. Patients who abstain have a five-year survival rate of 60–70%, which falls to 40% in those who continue to drink. Women have a shorter survival rate than men. Bad prognostic indicators include a low serum albumin, prolonged INR/PT, low hemoglobin, encephalopathy, persistent jaundice and azotemia. Zone 3 fibrosis and perivenular sclerosis are also unfavorable features. Complete abstinence may not improve prognosis when portal hypertension is severe, although at the earlier stages of cirrhosis, the portal pressure may actually fall with abstinence. Hepatocellular carcinoma occurs in 10% of stable cirrhotics, and the incidence is higher in patients who also have hepatitis C infection. It usually develops after a period of abstinence and when macronodular cirrhosis is present. Treatment strategies can be instituted if it is detected early. Therefore, long-term follow-up and periodic screening are advisable.

6.4 Management
Early recognition of alcoholism is important. Physicians should have a high index of suspicion when a patient presents with anorexia, nausea, diarrhea, right upper quadrant tenderness and an elevated GGT. The most important therapeutic measure is total abstinence from alcohol. Support groups and regular follow-up can reinforce the need for abstinence. Withdrawal symptoms should be treated with chlordiazepoxide or diazepam. A nutritious, well-

balanced diet with vitamin supplements should be instituted.

Alcoholic fatty liver responds to alcohol withdrawal and a nutritious diet. Patients with severe alcoholic hepatitis should be admitted to hospital and complications of liver failure treated appropriately. These patients usually have significant metabolic abnormalities that have to be corrected. Specific treatments for alcoholic hepatitis include the use of corticosteroids. A recent meta-analysis of 12 controlled trials showed a significant benefit of steroids for patients with severe alcoholic hepatitis complicated by encephalopathy. A discriminant function of >32 is a predictor of poor prognosis and favorable response to corticosteroid therapy.

Discriminant function =

$4.6 \times (PT - control\ PT) + serum\ bilirubin\ in\ \mu mol/L \div 17$

Propylthiouracil has been used to dampen the hepatic hypermetabolic state in alcoholic hepatitis, and in a recent long-term controlled trial significantly reduced the two-year mortality in patients who continued to drink moderately. Those who were abstinent from alcohol did not derive any additional benefits. Testosterone and anabolic androgenic steroids have been tried with conflicting results. Intravenous amino acid supplements have been given to the severely protein malnourished with varying degrees of success. Oral supplementation is the preferred route if the patient can tolerate a diet.

Cirrhosis is an irreversible process, and therapy is directed at the complications of liver failure and portal hypertension, although colchicine has been used as an antifibrotic agent without much success. Patients need to be assessed for the presence of esophageal varices, and in those with significant varices, consideration should be given to prophylactic sclerotherapy or β-blocker therapy. The transjugular intrahepatic portosystemic stent shunt (TIPS) has replaced a surgical portacaval shunt as the treatment of choice for uncontrolled bleeding esophageal varices. Hepatic encephalopathy remains a complication, but usually can be controlled with prophylactic laculose. TIPS stenosis is usually managed with angioplasty dilation or the placement of a parallel TIPS. Ascites is managed with a low-sodium diet and diuretic therapy. TIPS has also been shown to be effective in the management of refractory ascites and should be considered in these patients. Every effort should be made to exclude spontaneous bacterial peritonitis and prevent hepatorenal syndrome, two life-threatening complications of ascites. Periodic screening for the presence of hepatoma should be done, since early detection allows surgical resection in the stable compensated cirrhotic patient and local ablative therapy such as intralesional alcohol injection in the patient with decompensation. Hepatic transplantation is a treatment option for patients with end-stage alcoholic cirrhosis, and this is the treatment of choice in the patient with a small hepatoma and decompensated liver cirrhosis. Ethical issues surrounding the use of such a scarce resource for a self-inflicted disease still need to be settled. In the centers that transplant in cases of alcohol cirrhosis, the results are comparable to those in patients with other forms of cirrhosis.

7. DRUG-INDUCED LIVER DISEASE / J.B. Simon

Drugs are an important and common cause of hepatic injury. This is not surprising, as the liver is the predominant site of drug clearance, biotransformation and excretion. Abnormalities cover a wide spectrum from minor nonspecific derangements to fulminant hepatic necrosis. The two most common, however, are acute inflammation and cholestasis, which can closely mimic viral hepatitis and biliary obstruction, respectively. Various other acute and chronic disease patterns also occur (as noted below). Thus drug-induced liver disease is complex, has protean manifestations, and can simulate a wide variety of other hepatic disorders.

The pathogenesis varies with the offending agent, and in most cases is poorly understood. Sometimes the drug or one of its metabolites exerts a direct toxic effect on liver membranes. This type of injury is predictable and dose-related, but is relatively infrequent. Much more commonly, the injury occurs unpredictably in only a tiny fraction of individuals receiving the drug and is independent of dosage. In some such instances genetic predisposition or idiosyncratic metabolism of the drug may be responsible. Immune hypersensitivity is often invoked, but only a minority of cases have concomitant evidence of an allergic reaction such as a rash, arthralgias or eosinophilia. Many instances of putative hypersensitivity may actually be due to toxic intermediate drug metabolites in rarely susceptible individuals. In most situations the reasons for individual susceptibility are unknown, and the precise pathogenesis of the hepatic injury is equally obscure.

Diagnosis requires first and foremost a careful history of drug ingestion, including over-the-counter and illicit agents as well as prescribed medications. A temporal association is also important in cases of acute dysfunction: injury typically develops within days or a few weeks of starting the drug. Other reactions involve chronic insidious injury and therefore require prolonged drug exposure – e.g., methotrexate fibrosis and oral contraceptive–induced adenomas. Liver biopsy sometimes provides an important clue to certain drug injuries, but more commonly the histologic pattern is nonspecific and/or mimics other primary liver disorders. Thus in many cases the diagnosis of drug injury remains uncertain or unproven even after appropriate patient assessment.

TABLE 14. Drug-induced liver disease

Type and example	Pathogenesis
Acute hepatocellular injury Toxic necrosis (e.g., CCl₄, acetaminophen)	Membrane damage, some via toxic metabolite; dose-related, predictable
Hepatitis-like (e.g., isoniazid, methyldopa)	Idiosyncrasy; ? immune, ? metabolic; unpredictable, not dose-related
Cholestasis Inflammatory (e.g., chlorpromazine)	Unknown; unpredictable; periportal inflammation and cholestasis
Pure (e.g., oral contraceptives)	Exaggeration of normal hormonal effect on bile transport; ? genetic idiosyncrasy; pure cholestasis, no inflammation
Miscellaneous acute/subacute	Variable, usually unknown
Chronic liver disease Chronic hepatitis (e.g., isoniazid, methyldopa)	Idiosyncrasy; ? immune, ? metabolic
Chronic cholestasis (e.g., chlorpromazine)	Unknown; rare
Fibrosis/cirrhosis (e.g., methotrexate)	Dose-related, insidious toxic metabolic damage
Tumor: adenomas (oral contraceptives)	Unknown

The prognosis is variable. Acute damage usually resolves when the offending agent is withdrawn, but cases of severe acute necrosis can be fatal or result in postnecrotic scarring. In cases of chronic injury, further hepatocellular damage and inflammation will generally cease when the drug is stopped, but any concomitant fibrosis will be irreversible.

No physician can know the innumerable drugs capable of producing liver injury. Rather, it is best to maintain a constant awareness of the possibility, to understand the general types of damage, and to learn the most common agents responsible for each. Table 14 gives an arbitrary classification and examples of drug-induced hepatic injury. A few of the more important examples are briefly discussed below.

7.1 Acute Hepatocellular Injury
This takes at least two distinct forms, both characterized clinically and biochemically by features of acute liver cell destruction.

7.1.1 *TOXIC NECROSIS*

This involves direct membrane damage by the parent drug or a toxic metabolite. It is therefore dose-related and a predictable occurrence in anyone ingesting a sufficient quantity of the drug. Sometimes the histologic injury is characteristic – e.g., zonal necrosis and fat in carbon tetrachloride toxicity.

Acetaminophen is the most important example. This widely used analgesic is largely excreted as harmless conjugates, but a portion is transformed by hepatic microsomes to toxic intermediate metabolites. Normally these are safely eliminated by conjugation with hepatic glutathione, but a large enough dose of acetaminophen will deplete the available glutathione stores. Once this occurs, cell necrosis results from binding of the toxic intermediates to liver macromolecules. The threshold injurious dose of acetaminophen is usually about 10–15 g acutely; this is far beyond the normal dosage and is generally ingested only in suicide attempts. Alcoholics are susceptible at much lower dosage, however, as a result of heightened microsomal transformation coupled with nutritional depletion of glutathione. Acetaminophen should be suspected in an alcoholic with extremely high AST/ALT levels, as values rarely exceed 300 µmol/L in uncomplicated alcoholic hepatitis. Another clue to acetaminophen toxicity is a disproportionately elevated INR.

Acetaminophen hepatotoxicity typically becomes apparent only 36 to 48 hours after ingestion; by then it is too late to modify the process. Fortunately, injury is successfully aborted by early therapy with N-acetylcysteine, which repletes hepatic glutathione levels. This should be given within 10 to 16 hours of acetaminophen ingestion to be effective, though some benefit may be achieved even at 24 to 36 hours. To guide therapy, nomograms are available relating the probability of liver injury to blood acetaminophen levels and to the amount of time since ingestion.

7.1.2 *ACUTE HEPATITIS*

This pattern of injury closely mimics acute viral hepatitis clinically, biochemically and histologically. Unlike toxic necrosis, it occurs unpredictably, is not dose-related and affects only rare individuals exposed to the drug. Reasons for the idiosyncratic susceptibility are obscure. Numerous agents can produce this injury pattern; methyldopa, isoniazid and halothane are classic examples, the latter usually producing damage only after repeated exposure to the anesthetic. Other relatively common examples include propylthiouracil, phenytoin, sulfonamides and various nonsteroidal anti-inflammatory drugs. Acute hepatitis from isoniazid or diclofenac occasionally develops only after several months of drug therapy. This is an exception to the general rule of a temporal relationship, and the association may therefore be overlooked.

TABLE 15. Hepatobiliary reactions to oral contraceptives

Cholestasis

Tumors
    Adenomas
    Focal nodular hyperplasia?
    Hepatocellular carcinoma (rare)

Vascular
    Budd-Chiari syndrome (↑ clotting tendency)
    Peliosis hepatis (subclinical)

Gallstones (↑ lithogenicity of bile)

"Unmasking" of other cholestatic disorders

7.2 Cholestasis
This type of reaction also takes at least two distinct forms.

7.2.1 *INFLAMMATORY TYPE*
Chlorpromazine and other phenothiazines, carbamazepine, chlorpropamide, erythromycin estolate, amoxicillin–clavulinic acid and many other drugs can produce an acute periportal necro-inflammatory reaction. This is characterized clinically and biochemically by a predominant cholestatic disorder with variable features of concomitant hepatocellular inflammation. Differentiation from extrahepatic biliary obstruction may be required.

7.2.2 *PURE TYPE*
Certain steroid hormonal drugs, most notably oral contraceptives and methyltestosterone, can produce relatively pure impairment of bile flow with little or no associated hepatocellular injury (bland cholestasis). This appears to be due to an idiosyncratic exaggeration of the physiologic effect of sex hormones on bile canalicular transport, and may have a genetic component. The patient typically develops insidiously progressive pruritus, dark urine, and jaundice without associated systemic symptoms. Laboratory tests show high ALP with normal or minimally elevated AST/ALT levels. The liver biopsy is usually unremarkable aside from histologic cholestasis. Women who develop this reaction to oral contraceptives are predisposed to cholestasis of pregnancy, which appears to be similar or identical in pathogenesis (see Section 17).

Oral contraceptives are also associated with other, less common hepatobiliary effects. These are listed in Table 15.

7.3 Miscellaneous Acute and Subacute Reactions

Many hepatic drug reactions involve a variable mixture of hepatocellular and excretory impairments that do not neatly fit any of the above categories. Laboratory and histologic features are variable and nonspecific. Occasionally granulomatous inflammation occurs (e.g., with sulfonamides or quinidine), often with acute systemic features. Differentiation from an infective granulomatous disorder may be challenging. A few drugs can produce an alcoholic hepatitis–like picture, including typical histologic features (e.g., amiodarone). Other unusual patterns of drug injury have also been described. Various herbal remedies are increasingly recognized as a cause of liver damage, with variable manifestations.

7.4 Chronic Liver Disease

Though the large majority of drug-induced hepatic injury is acute or subacute, in a few reactions there is an insidious development of chronic disease. These vary in type.

7.4.1 CHRONIC HEPATITIS

A few agents that induce acute hepatitis are also capable of producing chronic inflammation if drug ingestion continues. Methyldopa and isoniazid are the prime examples. Clinically, biochemically and histologically the reaction may be indistinguishable from idiopathic or immune chronic hepatitis. The disorder typically resolves when the drug intake ceases.

7.4.2 CHRONIC CHOLESTASIS

In rare instances cholestatic injury from chlorpromazine or other agents becomes prolonged and self-perpetuating even though the drug is discontinued. This is termed drug-induced "vanishing duct syndrome" and can simulate primary biliary cirrhosis, though immunologic features of the latter are lacking. Hepatic intra-arterial chemotherapy with floxuridine can produce a sclerosing cholangitis-like picture, probably owing to ischemic injury of the bile ducts.

7.4.3 FIBROSIS/CIRRHOSIS

Insidiously progressive hepatic fibrosis and eventual cirrhosis can occur from methotrexate, some chemotherapeutic agents, and chronic ingestion of arsenicals or vitamin A in megadoses. Scarring typically develops subclinically and with little or no biochemical evidence of hepatic dysfunction. Liver biopsy is therefore the only way to establish the diagnosis. Patients receiving long-term methotrexate therapy for psoriasis or rheumatoid arthritis should generally undergo biopsy after cumulative drug dosage reaches about 1.5 g, and at occasional intervals thereafter.

7.4.4 *TUMORS*

Prolonged intake of oral contraceptives is associated with an increased risk of developing benign hepatic adenomas. These are usually asymptomatic but occasionally produce an acute abdomen due to intraperitoneal rupture and hemorrhage. In rare instances, oral contraceptive–induced adenomas become malignant.

Other unusual drug-related tumors are known to occur as well – e.g., angiosarcoma from chronic exposure to vinyl chloride.

8. INHERITED LIVER DISEASE / P. Adams

8.1 Hemochromatosis

Hemochromatosis is an iron-storage disorder in which there is an inappropriate increase in the absorption of iron from the gut. This leads to iron deposition in various organs with eventual impairment, especially of the liver, pancreas, heart and pituitary gland. The term *hemochromatosis* is preferred for genetic hemochromatosis, with other diseases associated with iron overload such as thalassemia or a sideroblastic anemia referred to as *secondary iron overload*. The term *hemosiderosis* merely describes the appearance histologically of increased stainable tissue iron.

Genetic hemochromatosis is an inherited disease known to be associated with an abnormal gene tightly linked to the A locus of the HLA complex on chromosome 6. A candidate gene has been described (HLA-H) that encodes for a protein with similarities to MHC class-I proteins. It is one of the most common genetic diseases, inherited as an autosomal recessive trait affecting 1 in 300 of the Caucasian population. The heterozygous individual has normal or minor derangements in iron metabolism that have no clinical significance. The homozygote has continued iron accumulation leading to target organ damage. Normally the body iron content of 3–4 g is maintained such that the absorption of iron is equal to iron loss. In hemochromatosis, the absorption of iron is inappropriate to the needs of the body, resulting in the absorption of 4 mg/day or more. In advanced disease, the total body iron accumulation may be 40–60 g.

Most patients are asymptomatic until the fifth or sixth decade, at which time they may present with nonspecific symptoms of arthritis, diabetes, fatigue or hepatomegaly. Other symptoms include pigmentation of the skin, impotence and dyspnea secondary to congestive heart failure. The classic triad of skin pigmentation (melanin deposition), diabetes and liver disease ("bronze diabetes") occurs in a minority of patients and is a late stage of the disease.

A patient with suspected hemochromatosis or unexplained liver disease should be screened for the disease with a serum ferritin and transferrin saturation (serum iron/TIBC). These test abnormalities increase with age and are more marked in males than females because of the regular menstrual blood loss in women. The diagnosis was previously confirmed by liver biopsy demonstrating marked parenchymal iron deposition with iron staining of the tissue. The hepatic iron concentration and the hepatic iron index (hepatic iron concentration/age) are the most helpful in distinguishing genetic hemochromatosis from the increased iron overload that is seen in other chronic liver diseases such as alcoholic liver disease and chronic hepatitis C. MRI scanning can detect moderate to marked iron overload in the liver. Genetic testing has led to a re-evaluation of the role of liver biopsy in hemochromatosis, with liver biopsy moving away from a diagnostic test done in most cases to a pragmatic test done in selected cases with liver dysfunction. C282Y homozygotes detected as young adults with a serum ferritin <1,000 μg/L, a normal AST and without hepatomegaly will not require a liver biopsy. Genetic testing is particularly useful in the evaluation of a patient with other risk factors for iron overload such as alcoholic liver disease or viral hepatitis.

The heterozygous individual may have normal iron metabolism or minor derangements that have no clinical significance. A patient who carries both the major mutation (C282Y) and the minor mutation (H63D) is called a compound heterozygote. These patients may have mild to moderate iron overload but are often normal.

The treatment of hemochromatosis involves the removal of excess body iron. Iron is best removed from the body by weekly or twice-weekly phlebotomy of 500 mL of blood until the body iron stores are within normal limits. The duration of treatment varies with the age and sex of the patient, but older males may require weekly venesections for more than three years. Serum ferritin is measured every three months to assess progress. When the serum ferritin is in the low normal range (50 μg/L) the frequency of venesections is decreased to three or four per year. The goal of therapy is to prevent any further tissue damage. Unfortunately, many of the symptoms do not improve following iron depletion. The most common cause of death is liver failure and/or hepatocellular carcinoma.

Siblings of the patient with hemochromatosis must be screened with serum ferritin, transferrin saturation and genetic testing, as the siblings have a 1 in 4 chance of being affected. Screening of a spouse with genetic testing can be helpful in predicting the risk in children. Screening of the general population

TABLE 16.   Interpretation of C282Y genetic testing for hemochromatosis

	C282Y +/C282Y +	C282Y +/C282Y –	C282Y –/C282Y –
1. Patient found to have elevated transferrin saturation and ferritin without other risk factors	Hemochromatosis homozygote	Hemochromatosis heterozygote	Normal
Action required	Venesection therapy and family investigations	Consider investigations in siblings, consider further genetic testing for H63D	Consider another diagnosis. Likely a small group of C282Y (–/–) hemochromatosis cases. Venesections based on clinical judgment
2. Asymptomatic patient with normal transferrin saturation and ferritin	Non-expressing homozygote (incomplete penetrance)	Typical heterozygote	Normal
Action required	Family investigations and repeat iron studies every 2 years	Testing of siblings and spouse to be considered	No further studies
3. Alcoholic patient HCV + with elevated ferritin	Hemochromatosis homozygote	Hemochromatosis heterozygote with secondary iron overload	Most likely secondary iron overload
Action required	Venesection therapy and family investigations	Consider investigations in siblings, consider further genetic testing for H63D	No venesections or family studies

for hemochromatosis has been predicted to be cost-effective but has not been widely implemented. Genetic screening has the potential to identify cases at birth but raises ethical issues such as genetic discrimination. Chelating agents such as deferoxamine (parenteral) are reserved for the patient with iron overload secondary to an iron-loading anemia such as thalassemia (see Table 16).

8.2 Alpha₁-Antitrypsin Deficiency

Alpha$_1$-antitrypsin, a glycoprotein produced by the liver, constitutes the majority of the α_1 globulin fraction seen on protein electrophoresis. Its deficiency is inherited, resulting in pulmonary emphysema and hepatic disease. Various presentations are possible, including neonatal hepatitis, chronic hepatitis, cirrhosis and hepatocellular carcinoma.

Alpha$_1$-antitrypsin is a protease inhibitor. Its production is controlled by multiple alleles in the Pi system. Normal individuals are PiMM. The inheritance is autosomal codominant. Patients with liver disease most frequently have PiZZ and possess only 20% of the normal amount of serum α_1-antitrypsin.

Diagnosis of α_1-antitrypsin deficiency is suggested by the absence of the α_1 peak on protein electrophoresis and is confirmed by α_1-antitrypsin levels and phenotyping. The characteristic changes seen on liver biopsy include the presence of PAS-positive, diastase-resistant granules in the cytoplasm of the hepatocytes; these granules are α_1-antitrypsin collections within the endoplasmic reticulum. There is an inability to transfer synthesized α_1-antitrypsin from the cytoplasm of the hepatocyte to the serum. Cirrhosis will develop in 10–15% of patients with PiZZ. The risk to heterozygotes of developing liver disease is uncertain. Experimental medical therapies including infusion of recombinant α_1-antitrypsin and gene therapy may become a possibility in the future. Patients with advanced forms of liver disease may be candidates for liver transplantation.

8.3 Wilson's Disease

Wilson's disease is an inherited disorder characterized by the pathological accumulation of copper in the liver, central nervous system and other organs. The disease has a prevalence of 1:30,000. The gene responsible has been localized to the long arm of chromosome 13 (ATP7B). The gene product is a copper-transporting ATPase that is highly expressed in the liver. It is an autosomal recessive disease that may present as pediatric liver disease or may have a neuropsychiatric presentation in adults. The hepatic presentation of the disease is variable, and may include fulminant hepatic failure (often with hemolysis), chronic active hepatitis and cirrhosis. Copper deposition in the central nervous system results in extrapyramidal symptoms of rigidity, choreoathetoid movements and ataxia. Biochemical abnormalities include a low serum ceruloplasmin and high urinary copper concentration. The diagnosis of Wilson's disease is made on the basis of clinical and biochemical features with the addition of genotype analysis in family studies. The diagnostic utility of individual biochemical abnormalities depends on the manner in which a patient presents. In most patients the presence of a serum ceruloplasmin level

TABLE 17.   Major causes of cholestasis

Intrahepatic
Common
  Drugs
  Viral hepatitis
  Alcoholic hepatitis ± cirrhosis

Less common
  Primary biliary cirrhosis
  Chronic hepatitis ± cirrhosis
  Metastatic carcinoma
  Cholestasis of pregnancy
  Sepsis, TPN, etc.

Extrahepatic
Common
  Common bile duct stone(s)
  Pancreatic/periampullary cancer

Less common
  Benign biliary stricture
  Sclerosing cholangitis
  Bile duct carcinoma
  Benign pancreatic disease
  Extrinsic duct compression

< 20mg/dL and the finding of Kayser-Fleischer rings by slit lamp examination is diagnostic. In patients with only one of these abnormalities an elevated liver copper level > 250 μg/gram dry weight on liver biopsy will confirm the diagnosis. Liver histology is often not diagnostic. Copper stains are unreliable, and hepatic copper concentration is required. If liver biopsy is contraindicated, an elevated 24-hour urinary copper excretion > 100 μg/24 hours, an abnormal radiocopper scan or increased non-ceruloplasmin–bound serum copper levels >12 μg/dL may be helpful.

The mainstay of drug treatment for Wilson's disease for the past 40 years has been penicillamine. This drug given at a dose of 1.5–2.0 g/day has proven to be an effective copper chelating agent and will reverse or improve the symptoms and signs of Wilson's disease. It also prevents the onset of symptoms in asymptomatic patients. Side effects occur in 20% of patients within the first month, but most are due to hypersensitivity and respond to drug cessation and reintroduction of penicillamine at small doses (250 mg/day) with gradual increases and short-term prednisolone. Long-term penicillamine treatment needs to be ceased in only 5% of patients. Pyridoxine deficiency may rarely be induced by penicillamine, and 25 mg daily supplements are recommended. Unfortunately, penicillamine causes significant symptomatic deterioration in 20% of patients presenting with neurological symptoms, and alternative drugs may be required in this situation. A small number of alternative agents have been shown to be effective in the treatment of Wilson's disease. Trientine at a dose of 1–2 g/day is an effective copper chelating agent and may be used in patients who suffer severe reactions to penicillamine or develop deteriorating neurological symptoms with this drug. Zinc therapy of 75–150 mg/day has been shown to maintain low copper levels in those patients already on maintenance therapy by increasing gastrointestinal copper excretion. It may be useful in patients unable to tolerate either penicillamine or trientine. Patients with advanced disease can be successfully cured of the disease by liver transplantation.

9. CHOLESTASIS / J. Heathcote

Cholestasis simply means failure of flow of bile. The cause of this failure can arise anywhere in the biliary system, from the liver cell down to the ampulla of Vater. For clinical purposes it is easiest to think of cholestasis as being either intra- or extrahepatic (Table 17).

9.1 Intrahepatic Cholestasis
Drug toxicity is the commonest cause of cholestasis occurring at the cellular level. The injury may be predictable, as with estrogens (for example), or unpredictable, as with most idiopathic drug reactions. (However, as more intracellular mechanisms become understood – e.g., the polymorphic nature of drug-metabolizing enzymes – fewer reactions will be found to be "unpredictable.") Histologically and clinically, cholestatic drug reactions can be considered as "bland" or "inflammatory."

Systemic sepsis is often associated with cholestasis. Endotoxins have been shown to affect both intracellular and canalicular function. If sepsis occurs on a background of cirrhosis, the cholestasis is much more profound.

Most acute and chronic liver diseases exert a cholestatic effect via interruption of intracellular transport mechanisms or damage to the small interlobular bile ducts. Damage to small bile ducts is not at all unusual in acute and chronic hepatitis, particularly with hepatitis C. Cholestasis is also a common feature of relapsing hepatitis A, but does not carry any particular significance.

Several chronic liver diseases specifically target the intrahepatic and sometimes the extrahepatic bile ducts. The diseases of the liver that are associated with paucity of bile ducts are numerous. Primary biliary cirrhosis (PBC) and primary sclerosing cholangitis (PSC) are the best-known examples; other dis-

TABLE 18. Diagnostic features of primary biliary cirrhosis

Elevated serum alkaline phosphatase
Elevated serum cholesterol
Antimitochondrial antibody positive
Typical liver histology
Normal ERCP

eases that destroy bile ducts are chronic drug reactions, chronic rejection, graft-versus-host disease and chronic septic cholangitis, to name but a few.

In children, intrahepatic bile duct paucity may be syndromatic (Alagille's) or nonsyndromatic (e.g., postviral, PSC). PSC is commonly misdiagnosed as autoimmune hepatitis in children, as overt cholestasis may be absent. Cystic fibrosis may give rise to focal biliary cirrhosis as a result of inspissated bile in the ducts.

Many infiltrations may cause a biochemical cholestatic pattern of liver disease, generally anicteric – e.g., sarcoidosis, lymphomas, amyloid and granulomas of any etiology.

There is a very rare condition called "benign recurrent cholestasis" whose mechanism is not understood at all. Several rare congenital conditions, often associated with secretion of abnormal bile acids, result in severe chronic cholestasis in infants. In children, total parenteral nutrition is a well-recognized cause of cholestasis that is thought to be due to the amino acid content interrupting bile acid uptake by the liver.

9.2 Extrahepatic Cholestasis

Diseases of the large bile ducts are generally due to stones, strictures or tumors. The AIDS epidemic has brought its own forms of cholestatic problems: fungal, protozoal and viral cholangitis. Malignant tumors causing biliary obstruction now include Kaposi's sarcoma, lymphoma, and the more common pancreatic and bile duct carcinomas.

9.3 Primary Biliary Cirrhosis (PBC)

9.3.1 DIAGNOSIS

The more accurate term for this disease is chronic nonsuppurative granulomatous cholangitis. It predominantly affects women in middle age and is frequently associated with autoimmune phenomena outside the liver (renal tubular acidosis, vitiligo, thyroiditis, sicca syndrome, CREST syndrome, rheumatoid arthritis and, less often, glomerulonephritis and vasculitis). It is

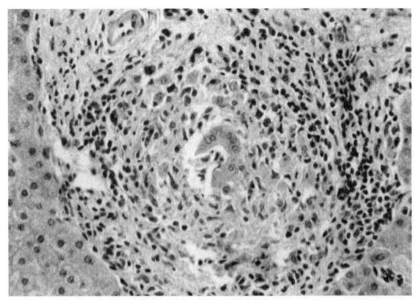

FIGURE 21. Typical bile duct lesion in early primary biliary cirrhosis.

therefore presumed that PBC is also an autoimmune disease, although the inciting antigen has not been identified.

PBC is rarely diagnosed at the first visit, because one-third or more of patients are asymptomatic. The biochemical pattern seen in PBC is typically cholestatic: elevated alkaline phosphatase, GGT and 5′-nucleotidase, with modest elevations of the aminotransferases. An elevated bilirubin is associated with progressive, symptomatic disease, indicating a poor prognosis. The most common symptom of this illness is fatigue, very hard to define yet very distressing to the patient. Other symptoms include pruritus, xanthelasma and, later in the course of the disease, ascites, jaundice and encephalopathy. Portal hypertension occurs early in this disease, as it is presinusoidal in nature; thus, variceal hemorrhage may be a presenting symptom. Many patients with PBC first present with nonhepatic associations. Raynaud's syndrome, osteoporosis with vertebral collapse, sicca syndrome and rheumatoid arthritis are the most common. Some patients with PBC have been misdiagnosed as having the chronic fatigue syndrome.

The diagnostic hallmarks for PBC include a cholestatic serum biochemistry as described above, elevated serum cholesterol, elevated serum IgM and a positive mitochondrial antibody test. If all these features are present, a diagnostic liver biopsy is not essential (Table 18; Figure 21). The biopsy

TABLE 19. Comparison of PBC and PSC

	PBC	PSC
Symptoms	Often none/pruritus	Often none
Biochemistry	Elevated ALP	Elevated ALP
Serum bilirubin	Slow rise	Fluctuates
Non-organ specific Ab	AMA+ve	AMA–ve
Liver histology	Helpful in diagnosis/staging	Helpful in staging
ERCP	Normal	Abnormal

is subject to great sampling error and all four "stages" may be seen in one specimen.

9.3.2 MANAGEMENT

The management of PBC includes symptomatic, preventive and specific measures.

There is little one can do for the fatigue, although a sympathetic and understanding ear helps. Pruritus can generally be controlled by using the anion exchange resin, cholestyramine. There are, however, many who suffer gastrointestinal side effects from this drug, so rifampin 150 mg b.i.d. or t.i.d. can be tried instead. Ultraviolet light also helps, so that pruritus is less in the summer. A trip down south always helps in the winter!

For the most part, the complications of long-term cholestasis can be prevented, except for the osteoporosis. Once the serum bilirubin is elevated, steatorrhea may occur with subsequent malabsorption of fat-soluble vitamins. Vitamin A and D supplements are available in water-soluble form, and vitamin K is best given parenterally. The fat intake should not be reduced. Although this may reduce the steatorrhea, it will also result in massive weight loss and will not affect the serum cholesterol. Despite the hypercholesterolemia, there is no increase in frequency of ischemic heart disease in PBC. A low-cholesterol diet will not affect the high serum cholesterol as the elevation is due to failure of biliary excretion. Calcium supplementation of the diet and vitamin D supplements are recommended but have limited effect on the osteoporosis. Hormone replacement is probably safe via the transdermal route in postmenopausal PCB patients. Bisphosphonates have been used with some success.

Many specific therapies for PBC have been tried, none with resounding success. Some are definitely contraindicated – notably prednisone, because it promotes osteoporosis. Ursodeoxycholic acid (UDCA) has very few side effects, causes a dramatic fall in all the biochemical markers for this disease, and recently has been shown to improve survival in PBC patients. Untreated, the mean survival of symptomatic PBC is 8 years. Treatment with UDCA in a dose

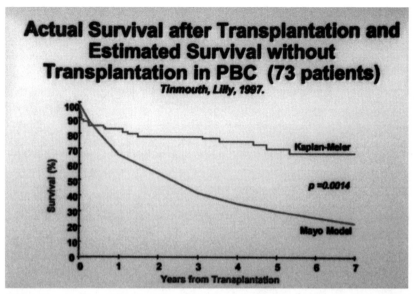

FIGURE 22.   Actual post–liver transplant survival versus predicted survival for primary biliary cirrhosis.

of 13–15 mg/kg/day results in a 31% increase in survival after four years of therapy. The survival of those with asymptomatic disease is much longer. The ultimate treatment is liver transplantation; PBC patients do very well, with a 92% one-year survival rate and a 68% seven-year survival rate (Figure 22).

9.4 Secondary Biliary Cirrhosis

Any disease that permanently and progressively damages bile ducts and is not caused by PBC may lead to secondary biliary cirrhosis, sometimes (although not usually) in the absence of overt jaundice. The most obvious cause is biliary atresia; other pediatric conditions include the various hypoplastic duct syndromes, other biliary tree abnormalities – Caroli's disease, choledochal cysts, sclerosing cholangitis – and cystic fibrosis, which causes focal biliary cirrhosis. In adults the commonest cause of secondary biliary cirrhosis is probably primary sclerosing cholangitis (PSC), although iatrogenic bile duct strictures also feature.

Primary sclerosing cholangitis is the most common cause of secondary biliary cirrhosis in adults. It affects about 10% of patients with ulcerative colitis or Crohn's colitis, although 30% of patients with PSC have no background of inflammatory bowel disease at the time of presentation. Patients are commonly asymptomatic. Just as with PBC, PSC causes presinusoidal portal

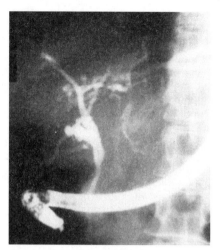

FIGURE 23.   ERCP in primary sclerosing cholangitis (intra- and extrahepatic strictures).

hypertension, so variceal bleeding may present early – i.e., prior to the onset
of jaundice (Table 19). A cholestatic enzyme pattern in any patient with liver
problems should prompt the suspicion of PSC. The diagnosis is made only by
ERCP, never by liver biopsy (Figure 23). As magnetic resonance imaging
(MRI) improves, magnetic resonance cholangiography (MRC) may replace
ERCP, currently the diagnostic test of choice for PSC. Because liver biopsy is
not helpful diagnostically it is performed only to see if the patient is cirrhotic. If PSC is suspected prior to ERCP, then antibiotic coverage should be given
at the time of the procedure. Sepsis is the major complication of this disease
and needs to be avoided if possible, as infection outside the liver precludes
liver transplantation – the treatment of choice for decompensated disease.
Prior to transplantation the only treatment available is symptomatic, as
described for PBC. As yet there have been no therapeutic trials of any reasonable size performed in PSC and hence there is no standard therapeutic
intervention. UDCA therapy leads to a fall in the serum markers of cholestasis and theoretically should improve the bile flow.

9.5 Approach to the Patient with Cholestasis

9.5.1 DIAGNOSIS
The history in any patient is always of utmost importance. A complete drug
history should be taken, including prescribed and over-the-counter drugs. A
past history of cholecystectomy should never be forgotten; common bile duct

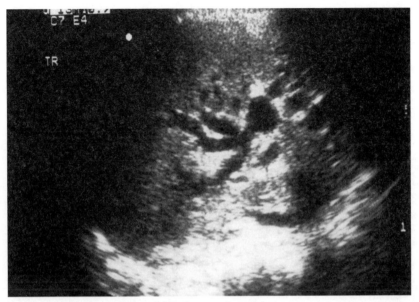

FIGURE 24. Dilation of intrahepatic bile ducts on ultrasound.

stones are not unusual, even in the absence of symptoms and/or dilated bile ducts on ultrasound. Manifestations of other autoimmune disease should be sought. A history of chills and fever would make one suspect extrahepatic (nonmalignant) biliary disease.

Examination should make special note of the patient's temperature. Signs of chronic cholestasis include scratch marks, shiny nails, increased skin pigmentation, xanthelasma, xanthomatous neuropathy, and jaundice, which in its later stages takes on a greenish hue. Hepatosplenomegaly is common in PBC, PSC and biliary atresia, and with infiltrations like lymphoma.

9.5.2 *LABORATORY CONFIRMATION*
The standard biochemical tests are most helpful. Liver function tends to remain normal for long periods in patients with anicteric cholestasis, but the enzyme markers – alkaline phosphatase, GGT, 5′-nucleotidase – are always elevated. In those with prolonged jaundice, coagulation abnormalities (correctable with vitamin K) are common. If the results of these tests confirm the clinical suspicion, then the next step is an ultrasound to look at the bile ducts. Jaundice associated with fever or chills demands prompt ultrasound examination of the abdomen.

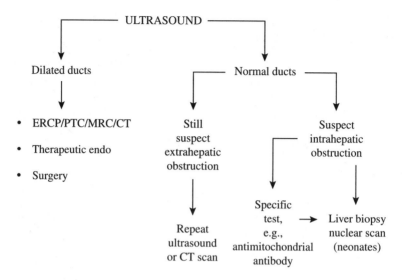

FIGURE 25.   Algorithm for investigation of the cholestatic patient.

9.5.3 FURTHER MANAGEMENT

Further management will depend entirely on whether the bile ducts are dilated (Figure 24). If the ducts are dilated, the management will be interventional. If the ducts are not dilated but there is still a suspicion that the problem lies in the extrahepatic biliary system (common bile duct stones following cholecystectomy, PSC), then an ERCP may still be indicated. In most circumstances, an ERCP is a more helpful and safer method of investigating extrahepatic biliary obstruction, although if the local expertise is not available, a percutaneous cholangiogram (PTC) may be necessary. Magnetic resonance cholangiography (MRC) is a noninvasive means to make a diagnosis as a preliminary screen before contemplating ERCP/PTC therapeutic intervention.

If the history, physical and ultrasound all support a diagnosis of intrahepatic cholestasis, then a liver biopsy may be indicated to make a diagnosis, if this is not already obvious at the bedside (e.g., sepsis, drug reactions). Cholestatic drug reactions may take many months to clear after the drug has been withdrawn. A clinical diagnosis of PBC needs to be confirmed by a positive antimitochondrial antibody test +/– a liver biopsy (Figure 25).

There will always be patients in whom no diagnosis can be made immediately. In the absence of jaundice, the physician has time to observe.

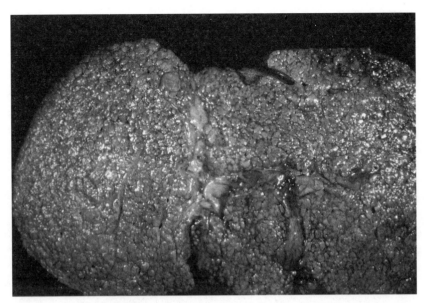

FIGURE 26.   A cirrhotic liver (posterior view).

Granulomas of the liver are the most likely cause of a "missed" diagnosis on biopsy. Electromicroscopy may be helpful when a drug reaction is suspected.

10. CIRRHOSIS OF THE LIVER / J. Heathcote

Cirrhosis is a chronic diffuse liver disease that is characterized by fibrosis and nodule formation (Figure 26). Fibrosis is not synonymous with cirrhosis. Nodule formation with disturbed architecture is essential for the diagnosis of cirrhosis. The condition results from liver cell necrosis and the collapse of hepatic lobules due to many factors such as inflammation or ischemia. Recovery occurs with formation of diffuse fibrous septa and nodular regrowth of hepatocytes. Thus, the ultimate histologic pattern is the same regardless of etiology. Liver cell necrosis is often absent when the liver is ultimately examined either by biopsy or at post mortem.

10.1 Etiology
Known causes of cirrhosis account for about 90–95% of the cases. The most common etiology is chronic viral hepatitis +/– alcoholism (Table 20). Less common causes are hemochromatosis, primary biliary cirrhosis, sclerosing cholangitis, autoimmune hepatitis, drug-induced liver disease and chronic bil-

TABLE 20. Causes of cirrhosis

Alcohol

Viral hepatitis B, C and D ± alcohol

Metabolic
  Hemochromatosis
  Wilson's disease
  α_1-antitrypsin deficiency
  Galactosemia
  Type 4 glycogenosis

Autoimmune
  Primary biliary cirrhosis
  Autoimmune hepatitis
  Primary sclerosing cholangitis

Drug-induced

Congestive

Cystic fibrosis

iary obstruction. Other causes include α_1-antitrypsin deficiency, severe steato-hepatitis in the morbidly obese and Wilson's disease. The remaining 5–10% of patients with cirrhosis of the liver have no known cause, a condition termed *cryptogenic cirrhosis*. Over the last 10 years, the rate of cryptogenic cirrhosis has fallen from 30% to current levels. The most likely cause for this fall has been the availability of testing for hepatitis C.

The etiology of the cirrhosis usually cannot be determined by the pathologic appearance of the liver (with some notable exceptions, including hemochromatosis and α_1-antitrypsin deficiency) (Figure 27).

10.2 Pathology

Micronodular cirrhosis is characterized by thick, regular septa, by regenerating small nodules of uniform size and by involvement of every lobule. Often associated with the persistence of the injurious agent, this may represent the liver's relative impairment for regeneration, as may be seen in alcoholism, old age, ischemia and malnutrition.

Macronodular cirrhosis is characterized by nodules of variable size, some containing large areas of intact or regenerating parenchyma within each large nodule.

Mixed macronodular and micronodular cirrhosis may result from vigorous regrowth in a previous micronodular cirrhosis (Figure 28).

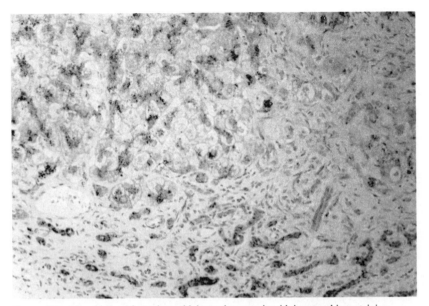

FIGURE 27. Liver biopsy of a patient with hemochromatosis with increased iron staining.

10.3 Clinical Features

The clinical features of cirrhosis relate to the particular cause of the cirrhosis but more importantly to the magnitude of the hepatocellular failure and the presence of portal hypertension, along with the ability of the surviving hepatocytes to compensate for the loss.

Thus, patients are often characterized as having compensated disease or decompensated disease. In the fully compensated state, there may be no symptoms whatsoever, the disease being suspected by the finding of an enlarged liver and/or spleen. With hepatocellular failure, patients may complain of weakness, fatigue, weight loss and a general deterioration of health. Physical examination may reveal the stigmata of chronic liver disease, although these are often missing in those with chronic viral hepatitis (see Section 2 and Figure 29).

The ease of diagnosis of cirrhosis is dependent on the degree of liver decompensation. A high index of suspicion is necessary; the condition may be revealed only by a positive history of excess alcohol ingestion along with the finding of hepatomegaly. Thorough inquiry into all the risk factors for acquisition of viral hepatitis needs to be made, including blood transfusion, injection drug use (ever), snorting cocaine, tattoos, body piercing and multi-

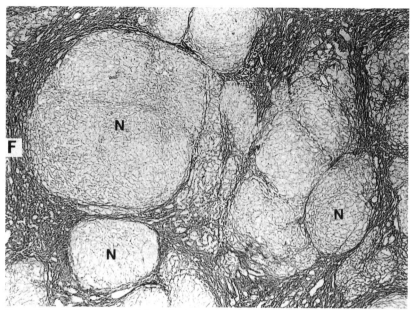

FIGURE 28.   A mixed macronodular and micronodular cirrhosis. The hepatic lobular architecture has been destroyed and replaced by nodular masses of regenerated cells (N). Fibrous tissue surrounds the nodules. (Retic. stain, original magnification × 37)

ple sexual partners. In decompensated disease, the diagnosis is much easier; the clinical features of ascites, asterixis, variceal hemorrhage, jaundice and other signs of hepatocellular failure may be present.

Biochemical tests attempt to identify the specific etiology of the liver disease and to assess the degree of hepatocellular dysfunction. With deteriorating hepatic function, albumin falls, serum bilirubin rises and the INR/prothrombin time becomes increased and not correctable by parenteral vitamin K. Liver enzymes, while helpful in assessing ongoing activity, do not assess the functional severity, as serum aminotransferases may be only mildly elevated despite severe liver disease. Alkaline phosphatase is usually raised, but the level does not reflect the degree of hepatic dysfunction. Commonly a normochromic, normocytic anemia is found, with target cells noted in the blood smear. Occasionally a macrocytic anemia presents. If gastrointestinal bleeding has been occurring, the anemia may be microcytic as a result of iron loss. Depressed leukocyte and platelet counts may be present secondary to hypersplenism. The urine often contains urobilinogen and bilirubin if the patient is jaundiced. Patients with ascites exhibit a marked reduction in urinary sodium excretion. Ultrasound of the abdomen, the most helpful imaging

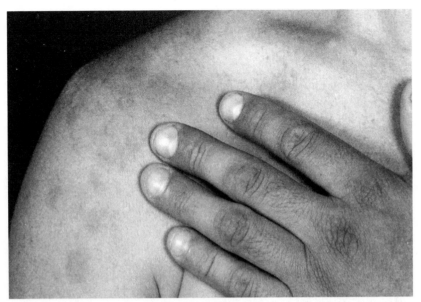

FIGURE 29. Spider nevi, "paper money" skin and clubbing in a patient with cirrhosis.

test, will reveal an inhomogeneous nodular liver with splenomegaly. A CT scan is rarely needed. These tests do not establish the diagnosis of cirrhosis, which can be made only by a liver biopsy with histologic examination. Liver biopsy may also be helpful in establishing an etiology and the degree of activity of the underlying process. When persistent coagulopathy or ascites is present, biopsy via the transjugular route is necessary.

Prognosis depends on the degree of hepatocellular function and the etiology, as well as on whether any causative agents can be removed. Clearly the prognosis is improved if the alcoholic patient can abstain, if the patient with hemochromatosis has iron removed by venesection or if excessive copper is chelated in those with Wilson's disease. In addition, vigorous medical care may prolong life and delay or prevent eventual complications such as ascites and variceal bleeding. All cirrhotics should be advised to avoid aspirin or NSAIDs (which promote GI bleeding and ascites), aminoglycoside antibiotics (which promote renal failure), ACE inhibitors (which promote ascites) and narcotics (which promote encephalopathy). All episodes of infection should be treated promptly, as septicemia leads to rapid deterioration in a cirrhotic. Beta blockers should be considered for prophylaxis against variceal hemorrhage in all cirrhotics with grade 2 or larger varices. Once decompensated

TABLE 21.   Criteria for Child-Pugh classification

Group designation	A	B	C
Serum bilirubin (µmol/L)	Below 34.2	34.2–51.3	Over 51.3
Serum albumin (g/L)	Over 35	30–35	Under 30
Ascites	None	Easily controlled	Poorly controlled
Neurological disorder	None	Minimal	Advanced "coma"
Nutrition	Excellent	Good	Poor, "wasting"

liver disease is present (jaundice, ascites, neurologic impairment, bleeding, coagulopathy, hyponatremia) the prognosis is poor and liver transplant should be considered, if appropriate.

10.4 Treatment

Clearly, where there is a specific treatment for the underlying etiology of the liver disease this should be offered. All patients should consume a healthy, adequate diet and avoid alcohol. Otherwise the management is that of regular surveillance and early detection of hepatocellular failure. Hepatocellular failure or decompensated cirrhosis may be manifested by any of the following: coagulopathy, jaundice (in noncholestatic liver disease), hepatic encephalopathy, variceal bleeding or ascites. The Child-Pugh classification of cirrhosis, which is a very useful guide to calculate the risk of an invasive procedure, takes into account these variables, plus nutritional status (Table 21). Once decompensation occurs, management includes the control of ascites, avoidance of drugs that are poorly metabolized by the liver and the prompt treatment of infection and variceal hemorrhage. Liver transplantation is now becoming the treatment of choice for many with end-stage decompensated liver disease (see Section 15).

11. PORTAL HYPERTENSION / S.S. Lee

Portal hypertension is defined as increased pressure in the portal vein. With the right atrial pressure as a zero reference, normal portal venous pressure is approximately 4–8 mm Hg. The portal vein is formed by the confluence of the splenic and superior mesenteric veins. Its flow rate normally averages about 1–1.2 L/min. The simple phenomenon of increased pressure in this venous circulation unleashes a wide array of hemodynamic and metabolic consequences, including some of the most lethal and distressing complications of chronic liver disease.

TABLE 22. Causes of portal hypertension

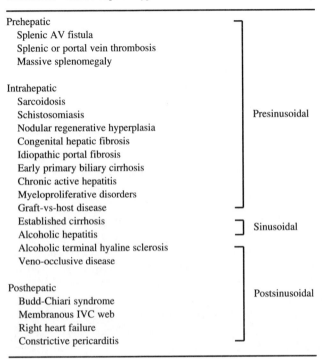

Prehepatic	
Splenic AV fistula	
Splenic or portal vein thrombosis	
Massive splenomegaly	
Intrahepatic	
Sarcoidosis	
Schistosomiasis	Presinusoidal
Nodular regenerative hyperplasia	
Congenital hepatic fibrosis	
Idiopathic portal fibrosis	
Early primary biliary cirrhosis	
Chronic active hepatitis	
Myeloproliferative disorders	
Graft-vs-host disease	
Established cirrhosis	Sinusoidal
Alcoholic hepatitis	
Alcoholic terminal hyaline sclerosis	
Veno-occlusive disease	
Posthepatic	Postsinusoidal
Budd-Chiari syndrome	
Membranous IVC web	
Right heart failure	
Constrictive pericarditis	

11.1 Etiology

The causes of portal hypertension are diverse (Table 22). Since portal pressure is the product of portal blood flow and intrahepatic resistance, any condition causing an increase in flow or resistance will increase portal pressure. An example of a "pure" flow increase is postsurgical or traumatic splenic arterio-venous fistula. The marked increase in splenic and thus portal venous flow leads to the development of portal hypertension. Almost all other causes of portal hypertension are mediated predominantly by increasing resistance, although evidence indicates that most high-resistance syndromes are also accompanied by increases in portal venous flow. In many conditions, the cause of the increased resistance is evident: inflammation and fibrosis lead to vascular distortion, architectural disturbance and impingement of the intravascular spaces. Other less evident factors are predominant in other conditions. For example, in acute alcoholic hepatitis, swelling of hepatocytes and collagen deposition in the space of Disse lead to narrowing and distortion of sinusoidal spaces. The reasons for the increased mesenteric (and thus portal venous) blood flow in high-resistance states remain unclear. One theory postulates that a circulating vasodilatory humoral factor that would normally be inactivated by the liver escapes into the systemic circulation through shunts or hepatocellular insufficiency.

There are two separate and sometimes overlapping classification systems for the causes of portal hypertension, using either the liver or the hepatic sinusoid as the reference point. The former classifies conditions into pre-hepatic, intrahepatic and posthepatic causes, while the latter divides conditions into presinusoidal, sinusoidal and postsinusoidal causes (Table 22). However, the exact site of increased resistance in many intrahepatic causes of portal hypertension has recently been questioned, and it is likely that the predominant resistance sites could change according to the stage of some disease processes. For example, early primary biliary cirrhosis is thought to produce mainly presinusoidal hypertension, but as dense cirrhosis supervenes, sinusoidal hypertension becomes more important. Similarly, an early lesion of alcoholic liver disease, the central or terminal hyaline sclerosis, characterized by zone 3 fibrosis, would cause postsinuoidal hypertension, with sinusoidal hypertension predominating as cirrhosis becomes established. In practical terms, there are reasons for trying to correctly classify resistance sites. One is for predicting responses to surgical shunting procedures: presinusoidal conditions generally have well-preserved hepatocellular function and thus respond well to diversion of portal blood, whereas sinusoidal and postsinusoidal conditions tend to be associated with varying degrees of hepatic insufficiency. Another is that ascites generally occurs only with sinusoidal and postsinusoidal hypertension.

11.2 Pathophysiology

Portal pressure can be measured by several methods. A catheter inserted into a hepatic vein and then wedged provides a good estimate of the upstream portal venous pressure, unless the site of resistance is proximal to the intrahepatic portal vein (as in portal vein thrombosis wherein the wedged hepatic vein pressure will be normal in the presence of significant portal hypertension). The spleen, liver or portal vein can be directly percutaneously punctured by small-gauge (19–22 gauge) needles to obtain reliable estimates of portal pressure. Measurement of portal pressure is mostly used for research purposes, as its invasiveness precludes wide clinical use.

Portal hypertension leads to many clinical complications. Ascites is directly related to the development of sinusoidal or postsinusoidal hypertension. Portosystemic collateral vessels form in an attempt to decompress the portal hypertension (Table 23). The most troublesome site of collateral formation is around the proximal stomach and distal esophagus (gastroesophageal

TABLE 23. Common sites of portosystemic collateral formation

Location	Portal circulation	Systemic circulation	Clinical consequence
Proximal stomach and distal esophagus	Coronary vein of stomach	Azygos vein	Submucosal gastroesophageal varices
Anterior abdominal wall	Umbilical vein in falciform ligament	Epigastric abdominal wall veins	Caput medusae
Retroperitoneal	Splenic vein branch Sappey's veins (around liver and diaphragm)	Left renal vein Retzius's vein	Usually none Usually none
Anorectal	Middle and superior hemorrhoidal veins	Inferior hemorrhoidal vein	May be mistaken for hemorrhoids

varices). Bleeding from such varices (or the gastric mucosa) and hepatocellular failure are the two commonest causes of death in cirrhosis. Indeed the mortality rates for variceal bleeding range from 15–50% depending on the degree of hepatic function: Child-Pugh class A, B and C patients have, respectively, 15%, 20–30% and 40–50% mortality rates when their varices bleed.

The risk of bleeding from gastroesophageal varices is related to several factors. First, a threshold minimum level of portal pressure of approximately 12 mm Hg appears necessary for varices to form. However, above this level it is unclear whether absolute height of portal pressure affects the bleeding risk. Factors such as intrathoracic pressure gradients induced by coughing, straining or sneezing, and damage to the variceal wall by acid reflux into the esophagus appear not to play a role. The two factors most important in determining bleeding risk are variceal size and local variceal wall characteristics. Several studies have shown that small varices almost never bleed, while the bleeding risk of medium-sized varices is approximately 10–15% over two years, and that of large varices, approximately 20–30% over the same period. During the past decade, it has become clear that certain endoscopic characteristics of the varices are also predictive of high bleeding risk. These endoscopic features are the red and blue color signs. Small localized wall defects such as thin-walled blebs or sacs in the wall look like red spots or streaks and have variously been termed "red wale markings," "cherry-red spots" or "red streaks," while a diffuse pronounced blue color indicates a large varix (vein) with a stretched mucosa covering it.

TABLE 24. Comparison of portal hypertensive gastropathy and inflammatory gastritis

	Portal hypertensive gastropathy	Inflammatory gastritis
Endoscopic appearance	Mosaic pattern, speckled red spots	Discrete red erosive lesions
Site	Predominantly fundus	Predominantly antrum
Histology	Scant inflammatory cell infiltrate, prominent vascular dilatation, mucosal and submucosal lesions	Heavy inflammatory cell infiltrate, mucosal lesions
Treatment	Surgery, ? beta blockers, ? cytoprotective agents	Acid suppression, cytoprotective agents

Approximately 30–50% of upper GI bleeding episodes in patients with portal hypertension originate from nonvariceal sources. Cirrhotic patients have an increased incidence of acid-peptic disease, mostly erosive gastritis. This is probably due to the alcohol abuse that is common in this population. It has recently become clear that the majority of nonvariceal upper GI bleeding in cirrhosis is due to a peculiar form of gastropathy seen in the stomach in portal hypertension. Several features distinguish this portal hypertensive gastropathy from the erosive or inflammatory gastritis seen in nonhypertensive patients (Table 24). The major symptom of portal hypertensive gastropathy is bleeding. Pain or dyspepsia is uncommon as a presenting feature of this type of gastropathy. The appropriate treatment for this condition is still unclear, but it probably responds to measures to decrease portal pressure, although a possible role for cytoprotective agents has also been suggested.

11.3 Diagnosis

Diagnosing portal hypertension is usually easy. The patient often has concomitant ascites and splenomegaly, along with the stigmata of chronic liver disease. In contrast, all the prehepatic and many of the presinusoidal conditions have well-preserved liver function and no ascites. Abdominal wall collaterals radiate outward from the umbilicus. When they are very prominent, it is easy to see why this condition is termed "caput medusae," after the fearsome creature in Greek mythology with the serpentine hairdo. Dilated abdominal wall veins, especially in the upper abdomen, are common, but caput medusae is rare. Another diagnostic clue may be the presence of anorectal varices masquerading as hemorrhoids. Gastroesophageal variceal bleeding produces large-volume, brisk bleeding with hematemesis and, later, melena or hematochezia. Portal hypertensive gastropathy may also produce brisk bleeding, but can occasionally cause low-volume oozing manifested only by melena.

11.4 Management

Managing the acute bleeding episode consists of the general resuscitative measures such as volume and blood replacement, and specific measures to stop the bleeding. Various pharmacological, mechanical and surgical modes of arresting hemorrhage are used, usually in that order. Vasoconstrictive drugs to stop bleeding include vasopressin and somatostatin or their longer-acting analogues such as glypressin and octreotide, respectively. Vasopressin infusions induce generalized arteriolar and venous constriction, with resultant decreased portal venous flow and thus pressure, and at least temporary cessation of bleeding in 50–80% of cases. However, the generalized vasoconstriction also may result in peripheral vascular ischemia, myocardial ischemia or infarction and renal tubular damage. Concurrent nitrate administration has been suggested to attenuate some of these side effects, but whether it actually does so is still unproven. A safer alternative may be somatostatin or octreotide. Their mechanism of action is still unclear but probably relates to a suppressive effect on the release of vasodilatory hormones such as glucagon, leading to a net vasoconstrictive effect. Side effects are minimal. Whatever drug is used, it is generally inadvisable to continue drug therapy for more than one to two days.

Mechanical modes of therapy include inflatable balloons for direct tamponade. The Sengstaken-Blakemore tube has both an esophageal and a small gastric balloon; the Linton-Nachlas tube, with only a large gastric balloon, is attached to a small weight to stanch the cephalad flow of blood in the varices. Both tubes carry significant complication rates (15%), especially in inexperienced hands. The most common complications of esophageal balloon therapy for varices include aspiration, esophageal perforation and ischemic (pressure) necrosis of the mucosa.

The most common and probably the most effective nonsurgical therapies are endoscopic variceal sclerotherapy and ligation. Highly irritant solutions such as ethanolamine, polidocanol or even absolute ethanol are injected through endoscopic direct vision into and around the bleeding varix. The subsequent inflammation leads to eventual thrombosis and fibrosis of the varix lumen. Possible complications include chest pain, dysphagia, and esophageal ulceration and stricturing. The injection of irritant solutions that eventually lodge in the pulmonary circulation can result in lung function abnormalities, although these tend to be subclinical. A newer and probably safer method of endoscopic therapy is ligation or banding, similar to the rubber band ligations used to fibrose anorectal hemorrhoids. Initial studies suggest that its efficacy is similar to sclerotherapy, with fewer esophageal complications. The combination of endoscopic therapy and either balloon tamponade or drug therapy to control actively bleeding varices is successful in 80–95% of cases.

When all the above measures fail, emergency surgery may be tried. Emergency portacaval shunt surgery has been abandoned because of a 30–50% operative mortality rate. The simplest and probably best choice in the emergency situation is esophageal transection, in which a mechanical device transects and removes a ring of esophageal tissue, and then staples the ends together. Another type of "surgery" is the transjugular intrahepatic portosystemic shunt (TIPS). In this procedure, an intrahepatic shunt between branches of the hepatic and portal veins is made by balloon dilation of liver tissue, and then an expandable metal stent of approximately 1 cm diameter is lodged into the fistula. The procedure can be done by a radiologist using fluoroscopy-guided catheterization, and requires only light sedation and local anesthesia.

Once the acute bleeding episode has been treated, how do we reduce the risk of future rebleeding? Before considering any other therapy, some obvious common-sense measures should be taken. For example, patients with cirrhosis caused by alcohol (the cause of approximately 50–60% of cirrhosis in Canada) absolutely must stop drinking; the rebleeding and mortality rates in patients who continue their alcohol use are much higher than in those who remain abstinent.

Prophylactic therapy to prevent bleeding may be divided into primary (to prevent the first bleed in a patient with varices who has never bled) and secondary prophylaxis (to prevent rebleeds). There is still much conflicting literature on these two topics, but for now, the following preliminary recommendations can be made. First, patients with large varices that have never bled should be started on beta blocker therapy at doses sufficient to reduce the resting heart rate by 20–25%. Beta-adrenergic antagonists are thought to produce arteriolar and venous constriction and significantly reduce blood flow through portosystemic collaterals while modestly reducing portal pressure. Endoscopic sclerotherapy/banding, TIPS and surgery carry risks and are unproven for primary prophylaxis.

The appropriate secondary prophylaxis regimes remain controversial. There is probably a minority subgroup who respond favorably to beta blocker therapy, but they cannot be easily identified. One approach is to perform enough endoscopic sclerotherapy/banding sessions (usually 3–6) to obliterate varices or reduce them to small size. Treatment failures on this regime (e.g., those with recurrent bleeding) could be considered either for TIPS or surgery (portacaval shunt). Decompression of the portal venous system should not be done in patients with a history of, or active, encephalopathy; it would only change the mode of death (encephalopathy vs variceal blood), not the outcome.

Prehepatic causes of portal hypertension such as portal vein thrombosis generally respond well to some type of portal-mesenteric diversion procedure such as mesocaval or portacaval shunting. In these cases, normal liver function protects against the development of encephalopathy or hepatic insufficiency when portal blood is diverted from the liver.

The definitive treatment for most of the complications of end-stage liver disease, including recurrent GI bleeding due to severe portal hypertension, is orthotopic liver transplantation. The presence of a surgical portacaval or mesocaval shunt greatly complicates the transplantation procedure, limiting the use of shunting operations in patients with cirrhosis.

12. ASCITES / N. Girgrah and F. Wong

Ascites is a detectable collection of free fluid in the peritoneal cavity. The risk of developing ascites after the diagnosis of cirrhosis is approximately 50% over 10 years. The two-year survival after the onset of ascites is 50%. This is reduced to six months with the development of refractory, or diuretic-resistant, ascites. This contrasts with a two-year survival rate of 80% following liver transplantation. Therefore, the development of ascites is now recognized as an indication for referral for assessment for liver transplantation.

The pathogenesis of ascites in cirrhosis is controversial. The peripheral arterial vasodilation hypothesis proposes that, in cirrhosis, arterial vasodilation leads to a decrease in splanchnic and systemic vascular resistance with pooling of blood in the splanchnic circulation, resulting in a reduction of the effective arterial blood volume. This in turn activates various neurohumoral pressor systems to promote renal sodium and water retention in an attempt to restore the effective arterial blood volume and maintain blood pressure. When the increased renal sodium and water retention cannot keep pace with the arterial vasodilation, the cascade of further activation of neurohumoral pressor systems follows, leading to further sodium and water retention. In the presence of sinusoidal portal hypertension, some of the excess fluid is preferentially localized to the peritoneal cavity as ascites (Figure 30).

However, recent evidence suggests that peripheral arterial vasodilation is not the only factor responsible for renal sodium retention in cirrhosis. For example, pre-ascitic cirrhotic patients usually have low-normal neurohormones despite retaining sodium when challenged with a sodium load. Also, one-third of early ascitic patients have normal levels of neurohormones despite avid sodium retention. That is, in both instances, there is no evidence of effective arterial underfilling despite the presence of renal sodium retention. A hepatorenal interaction has been suggested as the initiating mechanism, with sinusoidal portal hypertension and/or hepatic dysfunction as the

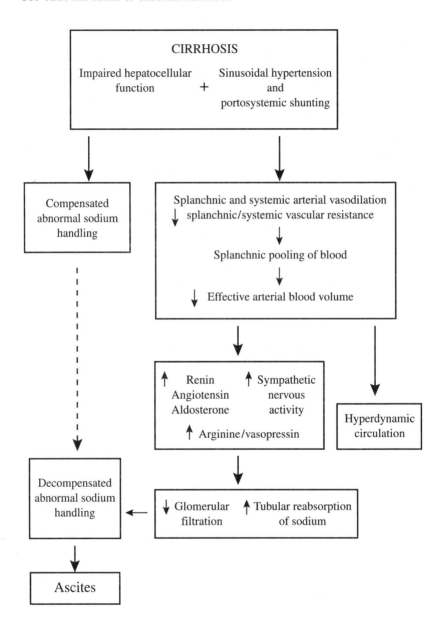

FIGURE 30.   Pathogenesis of ascites.

TABLE 25. Indications for diagnostic paracentesis

New-onset ascites
Hospital admission of the cirrhotic patient
Development of:
– peritoneal signs/symptoms – e.g., fever, abdominal pain
– alterations in GI motility
– encephalopathy
– renal insufficiency
Ascitic patient with GI hemorrhage

TABLE 26. Variants of spontaneous bacterial peritonitis

	Ascitic fluid analysis	
	PMN count	Organisms
Spontaneous infection		
Spontaneous bacterial peritonitis	>250 cell/μL	single
Monomicrobial non-neutrocytic bacterascites (MNNB)	<250 cell/μL	single
Culture-negative neutrocytic ascites (CNNA)	>250 cell/μL	negative culture
Secondary infections	>250 cell/μL	multiple

stimulus and the renin-angiotensin-aldosterone system and sympathetic nervous system as the messengers to the kidneys to retain sodium.

Clinically, the first evidence of ascites is weight gain. Peritoneal fluid of less than 2 L is difficult to detect clinically, and ultrasound is useful in defining small amounts of ascites. The abdomen is distended. Bulging flanks and the presence of flank dullness are the most sensitive physical signs for ascites, whereas eliciting a fluid wave or confirming shifting dullness are the most specific. Other findings may include umbilical hernia and scrotal and leg edema. A pleural effusion, usually right-sided, can accompany ascites. This is due to the presence of a diaphragmatic defect allowing ascitic fluid to pass into the pleural cavity. Patients also demonstrate signs and symptoms of a hyperdynamic circulation, such as systemic hypotension, resting tachycardia and a warm periphery, as well as evidence of portal hypertension such as distended abdominal wall veins radiating from the umbilicus.

Diagnostic paracentesis to examine ascitic fluid should be performed at first presentation, or when there is alteration of the patient's clinical state, such as a sudden increase in the amount of ascitic fluid, worsening of encephalopathy, abdominal pain or presence of fever, in order to rule out other complications such as spontaneous bacterial peritonitis (SBP), hepatocellular carcinoma or other noncirrhotic causes of ascites (Table 25). Ascitic fluid analysis should include a total polymorphonuclear (PMN) count, protein and albumin concentrations and cultures. At least 10 mL of ascitic fluid should be directly inoculated into blood culture bottles at the bedside. This increases the diagnostic yield from 50% to >80% when the PMN count is >250 cells/μL, which is diagnostic of SBP. Variants of SBP are shown in Table 26. A serum-ascitic fluid albumin gradient of >11 g/L has a >97% accuracy in predicting cirrhotic ascites. A serum-ascitic albumin gradient of <11 g/L effectively excludes portal hypertension as a cause of the ascites. A high protein content may be associated with congestive heart failure or Budd-Chiari syndrome and may be seen in pancreatic ascites. A low ascitic protein count (<10 g/L) puts the cirrhotic patient at increased risk for developing SBP. Either abdominal ultrasound or CAT scan of the abdomen may be used for detection of ascites. In particular, abdominal ultrasound can detect even a few milliliters of ascitic fluid and is highly sensitive (>95%) and specific (>90%). It can also direct the site of paracentesis.

The management of cirrhotic ascites begins with treatment of the etiologic factors, if possible, such as abstinence from alcohol. Although bed rest will result in redistribution of body fluid, salt and fluid restriction is required to mobilize the ascites. The patient is usually prescribed a low-salt diet containing 44–66 mmol sodium per day, which is lower than that contained in a no-added-salt diet. Professional dietary advice is necessary. Patients require specific instructions regarding where to purchase low-salt food. Salt substitutes are contraindicated, as they often contain potassium chloride and therefore can predispose patients who are taking potassium-sparing diuretics to hyperkalemia. Patients should be carefully monitored with daily weights and frequent 24-hour urinary sodium excretion. Urinary creatinine is measured simultaneously to assess completeness of the collection. Random urine sodium assessments are unreliable, as urine sodium excretion varies over the course of the day. However, a urine Na/K ration of >1 predicts a urinary sodium excretion of >78 mmol/day with >95% accuracy. Measurement of abdominal girth is unreliable, as gaseous distention is common. The rate at which ascitic patients gain or lose weight can be used to assess compliance with the low-salt diet and efficacy of treatment (Figure 31).

Diuretic therapy, in addition to salt and fluid retention, will be required in 90% of patients to manage ascites. Combination diuretic therapy, with both a potassium-sparing and a loop diuretic, is now the standard of care. The potassium-sparing diuretic spironolactone is usually started at a dose of 100 mg/day. Spironolactone has a slow onset and offset of action because its half-

Scenario I	Urinary sodium excretion	= 100 mmol/day
	Na intake	= 44 mmol/day
	Na output	= 100 mmol/day
	Na balance	= (44–100) mmol/day
		= –56 mmol
	Ascitic [Na]	= 130 mmol/L
	Therefore, fluid loss	= –56 mmol / 130 mmol/L
		= –0.41 L
	Weight loss/day	= 0.41 kg
Scenario II	Urinary sodium excretion	= 0 mmol/day
	Na intake	= 44 mmol/day
	Na output	= 0 mmol/day
	Na balance	= (44–0) mmol/day
		= +44 mmol
	Ascitic [Na]	= 130 mmol/L
	Therefore, fluid loss	= +44 mmol / 130 mmol/L
		= 0.34 L
	Weight gain/day	= 0.34 kg

FIGURE 31. Predicting weight change in patients compliant with low-salt (44 mmol Na/day) diet.

life in cirrhotic patients can be as long as 35 hours. Therefore, frequent dose adjustments are unnecessary and patients should still be monitored even after spironolactone is discontinued. One of its unacceptable side effects is painful gynecomastia. Amiloride, another potassium-sparing diuretic, is a less potent but certainly acceptable alternative. The starting dose is 5 mg/day. Either potassium-sparing diuretic is usually combined with furosemide, starting at 40 mg/day. The combination can be increased in a stepwise fashion (Table 27). Electrolyte abnormalities and renal dysfunction are common, and patients should be monitored regularly. Initial outpatient management may be attempted if the volume of ascites is small and in the absence of concomitant gastrointestinal hemorrhage, encephalopathy, infection or renal failure. Hypokalemia and hypochloremic alkalosis can precipitate encephalopathy. Too rapid mobilization of fluid will result in worsening of renal function, and one should aim at a weight loss of 0.5 L (0.5 kg) per day. Patients with peripheral edema can have their fluid mobilized more rapidly, as the edema fluid can easily be absorbed to replenish the intravascular volume. Symptoms of encephalopathy, a serum sodium of <125 mmol/L or a serum creatinine of >130 mmol/L should be dose-limiting. Daily weights and at least twice-weekly electrolytes and renal function should be monitored initially.

Refractory ascites is defined as ascites unresponsive to 400 mg of spirono-lactone or 30 mg of amiloride plus up to 160 mg of furosemide daily for two

TABLE 27.   Stepwise approach to the use of diuretic therapy for the management of ascites

	I	II	III	IV
Spironolactone/	100 mg	200 mg	300 mg	400 mg
Amiloride	5 mg	10 mg	15 mg	20 mg
Furosemide	40 mg	80 mg	120 mg	160 mg

Increase diuretics if	1. weight loss < 1.5 kg in 1 week, and
	2. patient is compliant with low-Na diet, and
	3. renal function is normal, and
	4. no electrolyte abnormalities or encephalopathy
Monitor	1. daily weights
	2. weekly postural symptoms/signs
	3. twice-weekly electrolytes, renal function
	4. symptoms/signs of encephalopathy

weeks in a patient who has been compliant with sodium restriction. Noncompliance with sodium restriction is a major and often overlooked cause of refractory ascites. Other causes of refractory ascites include the development of SBP, hepatocellular carcinoma and intrinsic renal pathology. Refractory ascites without any underlying cause usually indicates a grave prognosis, with only 50% survival at six months. Large-volume paracentesis is now recognized as a safe and effective therapy for the treatment of refractory ascites. Removal of ascitic fluid volume of up to 5 L without the simultaneous infusion of plasma expanders is safe in non-edematous patients. Larger volumes can be removed in edematous patients. Albumin infusion of 6–8 g per liter of ascitic fluid removed should be considered for repeated large-volume paracenteses. Other plasma expanders, such as Hemaccel®, dextran 70 and Pentaspan®, are limited by availability. In one large randomized controlled trial, large-volume paracentesis was safer and more effective than diuretic therapy for management of ascites with reduced length of hospitalization. There was, however, no difference in survival outcome between the two groups.

A peritoneovenous shunt may be considered in selected patients with good liver reserve. It can be dramatically effective in resolving the ascites, decreasing frequency of hospitalizations and decreasing diuretic requirement. But in patients with severe liver dysfunction, there is higher morbidity and mortality with the procedure. Previous abdominal surgery, SBP and large varices are relative contraindications to the procedure. Early complications include pulmonary edema and disseminated intravascular coagulopathy. Late complica-

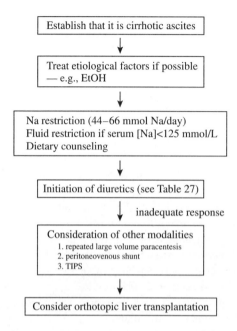

Establish that it is cirrhotic ascites

↓

Treat etiological factors if possible
— e.g., EtOH

↓

Na restriction (44–66 mmol Na/day)
Fluid restriction if serum [Na]<125 mmol/L
Dietary counseling

↓

Initiation of diuretics (see Table 27)

↓ inadequate response

Consideration of other modalities
1. repeated large volume paracentesis
2. peritoneovenous shunt
3. TIPS

↓

Consider orthotopic liver transplantation

FIGURE 32.   Management of ascites.

tions include thrombosis of the superior vena cava, infection and blockage or dislodgement of the shunt, all of which require its immediate removal. Successful peritoneovenous shunt placement can significantly improve patient well-being and nutritional status. Peritoneovenous shunts are not inserted often these days, as there are better treatment modalities for ascites and fewer surgeons are technically skilled in the procedure.

A transjugular intrahepatic portosystemic stent shunt (TIPS) has recently been shown to be an effective means of managing refractory ascites. When recent studies including up to 400 patients with TIPS inserted for refractory ascites were analyzed, complete resolution of ascites was seen in approximately two-thirds of patients and a partial response in the other third. Liver transplantation should always remain as a treatment option in these patients. An algorithm for the management of ascites appears in Figure 32.

12.1 Spontaneous Bacterial Peritonitis

Spontaneous bacterial peritonitis (SBP) is a common and often fatal complication of cirrhosis. In this clinical syndrome, ascites becomes infected in the absence of a recognizable cause of peritonitis. Its increased inci-

TABLE 28. Micro-organisms that can cause spontaneous bacterial peritonitis

Gram-negative bacilli	Gram-positive bacilli	Anaerobes
E. coli	Streptococcus	Bacteroides
Klebsiella	Group D streptococcus	Clostridia
C. freundii	S. pneumoniae	Lactobacillus
Proteus	S. aureus	
Enterobacter		

dence over the past decade may be due to greater recognition. The yearly risk of developing SBP after the onset of ascites is approximately 20–30%. Risk factors include prior episodes of SBP, recent variceal hemorrhage, an ascites fluid protein of less than 10 g/L and bilirubin >43 mmol/L. In most cases, the infection occurs after admission into hospital. About one-third of cases of SBP are asymptomatic; therefore, the clinician should not hesitate in performing a diagnostic paracentesis (Table 25).

Typically, SBP presents with fever and/or abdominal pain. It more commonly presents atypically, with worsening encephalopathy or renal dysfunction. The "gold standard" for diagnosis of SBP is a polymorphonuclear (PMN) count of >250 cells/μL. A variant of SBP known as *culture-negative neutrocytic ascites* occurs as culture-negative cases of suspected SBP with an ascitic fluid PMN count of >250 cells/μL. The patients with culture-negative neutrocytic ascites have the same clinical presentation and carry the same unfavorable prognosis as those with SBP. Positive culture results may take 48 hours and Gram's stains of ascitic fluid are positive in only 10–50% of infected patients (Table 26). Therefore, treatment for suspected SBP should start immediately after the diagnostic PMN count rather than waiting for positive culture results. Another variant of SBP is *monomicrobial non-neutrocytic bacterascites*. In this scenario, the ascitic PMN count is <250 cell/μL, but the subsequent ascitic culture is positive. It is not known whether this represents an early stage of SBP. It is recommended that the patient undergo repeat paracentesis. If the ascitic culture is again positive or if the PMN count is >250 cells/μL, then the patient should be treated as presumed SBP. Gram-negative bacilli account for 70% of cases of SBP. E. coli is the most common pathogen isolated (Table 28). Anaerobic organisms are uncommon causes of SBP, as the oxygen tension in the ascitic fluid is too high for their survival. Among these, Bacteroides species appear to be more common than other anaerobes. A management algorithm for SBP is shown in Figure 33. Cefotaxime, a broad-spectrum, third-generation cephalosporin, is now recognized as the treatment of choice for SBP. Its spectrum includes most organisms responsi-

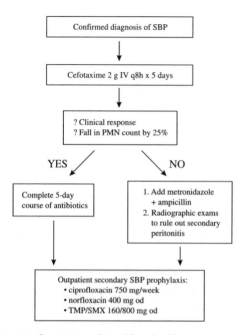

FIGURE 33. Management of spontaneous bacterial peritonitis.

ble for SBP and it is not nephrotoxic in the therapeutic range. A 5-day course of cefotaxime 2 g IV every 8 hours has been shown to be as effective as a 10-day course. Aminoglycosides should not be used since cirrhotic patients are particularly sensitive to their nephrotoxic effects, and monitoring serum levels of aminoglycosides is no guarantee against aminoglycoside-induced nephrotoxicity.

It is recommended to assess the response to treatment by both periodically evaluating the symptoms and signs of infection and performing at least one follow-up paracentesis after 48 hours of antibiotic therapy. Clinical improvement should parallel a fall in the ascitic PMN count. Although no specific PMN decrease cut-off has been established, a reduction of less than 25% in relation to the pretreatment value is often considered to represent failure of antibiotic treatment. Secondary bacterial peritonitis should be considered if the following features are present: (1) poor clinical response to antibiotic therapy; (2) multiple organisms are grown from the ascitic fluid; (3) ascitic fluid protein concentration >10 g/L or ascitic glucose <3 mmol/L; (4) PMN count remains high despite antibiotic therapy. Antibiotic coverage should then be broadened with the addition of metronidazole and ampicillin. Radiographic

TABLE 29.   Grading of hepatic encephalopathy

Grade	Level of consciousness	Intellectual function	Neurological findings	EEG
1	Lack of awareness Personality change Day/night reversal	Short attention	Incoordination Mild asterixis	Slowing (5–6 cps) Triphasic
2	Lethargic Inappropriate behavior	Disoriented	Asterixis Abnormal reflexes	Slowing Triphasic
3	Asleep Rousable	Loss of meaningful communication	Asterixis Abnormal reflex	Slowing Triphasic
4	Unrousable	Absent	Decerebrate	Very slow (2–3 cps), delta

examinations are required to exclude perforation of the gastrointestinal tract, and emergency surgery performed only if gut perforation is confirmed.

Despite successful treatment of SBP, the prognosis of these patients remains poor. The one-year probability of recurrence is 40–70%. Selective intestinal decontamination with oral nonabsorbable antibiotics has proved effective in reducing the recurrence of SBP. Norfloxacin 400 mg daily has the advantages of rarely causing bacterial resistance and having a low incidence of side effects when administered chronically. Trimethoprim/sulfamethoxazole 160/800 mg daily is an alternative and may confer greater gram-positive coverage. Cirrhotic patients with upper gastrointestinal bleeding are at a high risk for developing severe bacterial infections, including SBP, within the first days of the hemorrhagic episode. One randomized controlled trial using norfloxacin 400 mg twice daily for 7 days showed a significant reduction in both bacteremia and SBP. A meta-analysis also reported that antibiotic prophylaxis was effective in improving survival in cirrhotic patients with gastrointestinal hemorrhage. Short-term inpatient prophylaxis therefore is recommended. It may also be prudent to consider primary SBP prophylaxis in ascitic patients with significant jaundice or low protein ascites. Despite decreased SBP recurrence rates with prophylactic antibiotics, no change in mortality has yet been demonstrated. All patients who have experienced one episode of SBP should be considered for liver transplantation.

13. HEPATIC ENCEPHALOPATHY / L.J. Worobetz

Hepatic encephalopathy (HE) is a complex, potentially reversible neuropsychiatric condition that occurs as a consequence of acute or chronic liver failure. The clinical manifestations of this syndrome range from subtle abnormalities detectable only by psychometric testing to coma. Hepatic encephalopathy is characterized by changes of personality, consciousness, behavior and neuromuscular function and has been the subject of a number of grading systems (Table 29). HE may be present in as many as 50–75% of all patients with cirrhosis. Early features include reversal of sleep pattern, apathy, hypersomnia, irritability and personal neglect. In later stages, delirium and coma may occur. Neurologic signs may include hyperreflexia, rigidity, myoclonus and asterixis. Asterixis is not diagnostic of hepatic encephalopathy, however, as it may occur in other causes of metabolic encephalopathy. Clinically, a number of encephalopathic patterns can be observed. Hepatic encephalopathy associated with acute liver failure is rapid in onset and progression and is almost always complicated by cerebral edema, which can lead to seizures and lateralizing signs. Encephalopathy associated with chronic liver disease may present acutely or in a chronic recurring fashion. Finally, a minority of patients may exhibit chronic refractory encephalopathy with progression to debilitating syndromes such as dementia, spastic paraparesis, cerebellar degeneration and extrapyramidal movement disorders.

Factors of importance in the pathogensis of encephalopathy are the shunting of portal venous blood around the liver into the systemic circulation and the presence of hepatocellular dysfunction. Encephalopathy probably results from one or more toxic products of gut origin that are usually metabolized by the liver entering the systemic circulation and reaching the brain. Abnormalities of ammonia metabolism are most frequently implicated in the pathophysiology of HE. The normal gut flora produces a urease that enzymatically cleaves NH_3 from protein in the lumen. Ammonia derived from colonic bacteria and from deamination of glutamine in the small bowel is absorbed into the portal circulation and reaches the systemic circulation because of shunts and the inability of the liver to metabolize the ammonia. Increased blood–brain barrier permeability likely facilitates the entrance of ammonia and other toxic metabolites into the brain. Alternative proposals of gut-derived toxins include benzodiazepine-like substances, neurotoxic short-chain fatty acids, phenols and mercaptans. Other hypotheses propose that increased levels of short-chain fatty acids and aromatic amino acids associated with decreased levels of branched-chain amino acids cause production of false neurotransmitters. As well, the principal neuro-inhibitory neurotransmitter γ-aminobutyric acid (GABA) is increased in encephalopathy. Different concepts include other false neurotransmitters, including an endogenous modulator of GABA receptors, suggesting involvement of the GABA-diazepam receptor complex in the pathogenesis of HE.

There is no specific diagnostic test for hepatic encephalopathy. The history and the results of the clinical examination, including a complete mental status and neurologic examination, are the most important tools for diagnosing HE and distinguishing it from other causes of neurologic disease and encephalopathy. The presence of asterixis is helpful but is not pathognomonic for HE. Blood tests help verify the presence and severity of liver disease and rule out other causes of encephalopathy such as renal failure, hypoxia, CO_2 retention and drug overdose. Blood tests are also helpful in identifying precipitating factors of HE such as hypoglycemia, azotemia, electrolyte imbalance and infection. An elevated serum ammonia is often observed but correlates poorly with the degree of encephalopathy and may be normal in 10% of cases with HE. Lumbar puncture and brain imaging studies such as CT scan may be necessary to rule out other CNS pathology. The cerebrospinal fluid is usually normal or may show increased protein with increased GABA levels. The EEG shows slow, triphasic wave activity mainly over frontal areas, but although this is characteristic of HE, it is not specific for this condition. In patients with clinical symptoms of HE, neuropsychological testing is not necessary but may be helpful in establishing the diagnosis in the so-called subclinical HE.

Hepatic encephalopathy occurring in acute liver failure is usually accompanied by cerebral edema and carries with it a poor prognosis. Unless the liver shows signs of spontaneous recovery, these patients should be considered for orthotopic liver transplantation. Patients with grade 3 to 4 encephalopathy are usually managed in intensive care, as there is often associated multi-organ failure. Management may include elective ventilation, mannitol infusion and intracranial pressure monitoring.

Most HE occurs in patients with chronic liver disease and is due to a clinically apparent precipitating event or the development of spontaneous or surgically created portosystemic shunt (Table 30). The most important aspect of management is the prompt recognition and treatment of these precipitating factors. Exogenous factors include increased dietary protein, administration of certain drugs (such as sedatives), gastrointestinal bleeding, azotemia, electrolyte imbalance (often from diuretic therapy), hypoxia and infection (urinary, respiratory, spontaneous bacterial peritonitis). Provision of meticulous care to these confused and often comatose patients is important. The next goal of therapy is to lower the level of neurotoxic substances by reducing or excluding protein from the diet and by emptying nitrogenous materials from the gut. Dietary protein may be restricted to 20 g/day and gradually increased until the patient's protein tolerance has been established. Vegetable protein is much better tolerated, and increasing the calorie:nitrogen ratio may improve protein tolerance. Constipation is avoided by the use of laxatives and, in more urgent cases, cleaning of the gut with enemas or colonic lavage. A commonly used laxative is lactulose, a synthetic disaccharide that is degraded by intestinal bacteria into lactate and acetate to produce stool acidification and an

TABLE 30.   Common precipitants of hepatic encephalopathy

Increased nitrogen load
Gastrointestinal bleeding
Excess dietary protein
Azotemia
Constipation

Electrolyte imbalance
Hyponatremia
Hypokalemia
Metabolic alkalosis/acidosis
Hypoxia
Hypovolemia

Drugs
Narcotics, tranquilizers, sedatives

Miscellaneous
Infection
Surgery
Superimposed acute liver disease
Progressive liver disease
Transjugular intrahepatic portosystemic shunt (TIPS)

osmotic diarrhea. The acidification of colonic contents reduces ammonia absorption in part by trapping nitrogenous compounds in the lumen. The daily dose of lactulose should be titrated to produce 2–4 soft, acidic (pH <6) stools a day. For most patients, this will be between 45 and 90 g. Patients in coma or with small bowel ileus can receive lactulose by enema. An excessively sweet taste, flatulence, diarrhea and cramping are the most common side effects. Too much diarrhea can result in fluid and electrolyte depletion with renal failure and can worsen HE. Lactulose can be used chronically to reduce the frequency of episodes of encephalopathy. Alternatively, antibiotics such as neomycin and metronidazole may be used. These inhibit urea-splitting and -deaminating bacteria, reducing the production of ammonia and other potential toxins. Neomycin has the potential for ototoxic and nephrotoxic side effects. Because of their potential toxicity, antibiotics are not recommended for prolonged periods. Limited data support the combined use of lactulose and antibiotic therapy in selected cases.

Other potential therapeutic approaches exist, particularly when HE becomes refractory. On the basis of increased aromatic amino acids and decreased branched-chain amino acids (BCAA) found in HE (and the resulting effect on neurotransmitter synthesis), nutritional support with formulas rich in BCAA but low in aromatic amino acids has been suggested. Most studies with oral BCAA have shown clinical improvement of low-grade HE and increased protein tolerance, whereas studies with IV BCAA have produced inconclusive and conflicting results. Intravenous ornithine aspartate has been proven helpful, and the efficacy of the oral form is being tested in controlled trials. Two of the five enzymes involved in the metabolism of ammonia to urea are zinc-dependent. On the basis of this, the significant incidence of zinc deficiency in cirrhosis and some studies showing improvement of HE with zinc replacement, this deficiency should always be looked for and corrected if present.

Decreased dopaminergic neurotransmission activity has also been suggested to play a role in HE. However, controlled trials failed to demonstrate any beneficial effect of levodopa or bromocriptine treatment. In controlled trials, benzodiazepine receptor antagonists such as flumazenil showed only modest success, which argues against a major role of endogenous benzodiazepines in the pathogensis of HE.

HE as a complication of spontaneous or surgically created portosystemic anastomoses or transjugular intrahepatic portosystemic shunts (TIPS) is usually managed successfully with conventional therapy. Transhepatic embolization or surgical ligation of shunts may benefit refractory cases. Refractory HE complicating TIPS can be helped by implanting a reducing stent to reduce blood flow through the TIPS.

Orthotopic liver transplantation has the potential to entirely reverse HE. Thus, this procedure should be considered in all patients with HE whose liver disease makes them suitable for liver transplantation.

14. HEPATORENAL SYNDROME / L.J. Worobetz

The hepatorenal syndrome (HRS) represents advancing renal failure occurring in patients with severe liver failure. Although usually seen in patients with advanced cirrhosis, it can also be seen in acute or chronic liver disease such as alcoholic hepatitis and acute liver failure. It is characterized by impaired renal function and abnormalities in the arterial circulation and the endogenous vasoactive systems. As a result, the kidney demonstrates marked renal vasoconstriction with resulting low glomerular filtration rate (GFR). However, the external circulation demonstrates a reduction in total vascular resistance, resulting in arterial hypotension.

The main pathophysiologic hallmark of HRS is vasoconstriction of the circulation to the kidney. The histology of the kidneys is virtually normal; some kidneys have been used for transplantation and have functioned normally.

TABLE 31. Diagnostic criteria for the hepatorenal syndrome

Major criteria
Low GFR, with serum creatinine > 134 mmol/L or creatinine clearance < 40 mL/min
Absence of shock, presence of bacterial infection, fluid loss and no current treatment with nephrotoxic drugs
No sustained improvement in renal function after diuretic withdrawal and expansion of plasma volume with 1.5 L of a plasma expander
Proteinuria < 500 mg/day and no ultrasound evidence of obstructive uropathy or parenchymal renal disease
Additional criteria
Urine volume < 500 mL/day
Urine sodium < 10 meq/L
Urine osmolality > plasma osmolality
Urine RBC < 50 per high-power field
Serum sodium concentration < 130 meq/L

Conversely, if hepatic function is restored by liver transplantation, kidney function may return to normal. The mechanism of the renal vasoconstriction is not completely understood, but likely reflects an imbalance between systemic vasodilators and renal vasoconstricting mechanisms. Currently, two theories are proposed to explain HRS. The arterial vasodilation hypothesis proposes that because of general systemic arterial vasodilation, there is progressive baroreceptor-mediated activation of the vasoconstrictor systems that cause the renal vasoconstriction. An alternative theory suggests that HRS is a consequence of a direct relationship between the liver and the kidney. This link may be a vasodilator factor whose hepatic synthesis is reduced in liver failure. Alternatively, the link may be a hepatorenal reflex that causes renal vasoconstriction.

Patients usually do not have HRS at the time of admission to hospital, but rather develop HRS subsequently. The incidence of HRS in patients hospitalized with cirrhosis and ascites is 10%. There are two different clinical patterns of HRS. Type 1 HRS is characterized by rapid, progressive renal dysfunction with a doubling of serum creatinine > 220 mmol/L or a 50% reduction in the initial 24-hour creatinine clearance to < 20 mL/min in less than two weeks. Clinical features include progressive oliguria, marked sodium retention with a reduction in the urinary sodium to < 10 meq/L and progressive hyponatremia. Ascites is usually present. Half of the patients with HRS appear to develop these symptoms spontaneously, whereas they occur in others in association with a complication or therapeutic intervention (infection, including spontaneous bacterial peritonitis; paracentesis; GI bleeding). Type 2 HRS is characterized by a moderate, stable reduction in glomerular filtration rate. It occurs in patients with relatively well preserved liver function, resulting usually in diuretic-resistant ascites.

Although criteria for the diagnosis of HRS have been established, no specific test is diagnostic of HRS (Table 31). The diagnosis is based on the exclusion of other causes of renal failure that may be seen in severe liver disease. These include prerenal azotemia, acute tubular necrosis, glomerulonephritis and drug-induced renal failure (aminoglycosides, NSAIDs). Although prerenal azotemia may show similar tubular function, this is ruled out by the clinical setting in which the hepatorenal syndrome occurs and the lack of sustained benefit by expansion of intravascular volume with colloid replacement.

Prognosis of patients with HRS is very poor. The median survival for type 1 HRS is < 2 weeks, whereas the survival for type 2 HRS is several months. Treatment of established HRS is difficult. Thus, emphasis is on prevention by avoiding intravascular volume depletion from excessive diuretic use and treating ascites slowly. Complications of electrolyte imbalance and GI bleeding should be recognized early. Volume expansion with colloid infusion results only in transient improvement. Isotonic saline is usually avidly retained, worsening ascites and possibly precipitating pulmonary edema. Dialysis does not improve survival. Recent reports suggest that (1) the administration of systemic vasoconstrictors combined with volume expansion with albumin or (2) the insertion of TIPS may be useful. The only effective treatment for HRS is liver transplantation, but a significant number die before transplantation because of their extremely short survival rate. Thus, liver transplantation should be considered in those with end-stage liver disease before the development of HRS.

15. LIVER TRANSPLANTATION / G. Malkan, L.B. Lilly and G.A. Levy

Starzl performed the first human liver transplant in 1963 in a 3-year-old boy with biliary atresia. The first successful liver transplant was not performed until 1967 when a 1½-year-old girl with hepatocellular carcinoma was transplanted; she died of recurrent tumor after 17 months. One-year survival in the early years was 25–35% using methylprednisolone and azathioprine as immunosuppressives. The introduction of cyclosporine in the early 1980s allowed liver transplantation to become a clinical reality, with one- and five-year survivals in excess of 85% and 70% respectively.

Liver transplantation is now the recognized management for end-stage liver disease. The number of liver transplant centers in North America was more than 170 in 1998, and more than 3,000 liver transplants are performed yearly

TABLE 32. Liver transplantation: indications

Cirrhosis related to viral hepatitis
- B ± D (HBV-DNA negative)
- C
- Non A–E

Cholestatic liver disease
- Primary biliary cirrhosis
- Primary sclerosing cholangitis
- Biliary atresia
- Cholestatic sarcoidosis
- Graft-vs-host disease
- Chronic ductopenic rejection
- Secondary sclerosing cholangitis
- Drug-induced cholestasis and biliary cirrhosis

Alcoholic cirrhosis
Fulminant hepatic failure (viral hepatitis A–E, herpes, adenovirus, Wilson's disease, drugs, Reye's syndrome)
Neoplasms (hepatoma, hepatoblastoma, fibrolamellar CA, cholangiocarcinoma, hemangiosarcoma)
Metabolic liver disease (α_1-antitrypsin deficiency, Wilson's disease, hemochromatosis, glycogenosis type 4, tyrosinemia, Gaucher's disease, cystic fibrosis)
Vascular disease (Budd-Chiari syndrome, veno-occlusive disease)
Congenital (Caroli's disease, choledochal cyst, polycystic disease, hemangioma)

---

in the United States, while over 300 liver transplants are performed yearly in Canada. One-year survival rates of 80–90% are now expected. The rate-limiting step in the application of transplantation to liver disease has become donor availability.

15.1 Assessment for Transplantation

A patient should be considered for liver transplantation when the diagnosis of irreversible, acute or chronic liver failure is made for which no alternative medial or surgical therapy exists. The most common indications for liver transplantation in adults and children and the expected results are shown in Tables 32 and 33. Given the scarcity of donor organs, the selection of the patient and the timing of the transplantation require individual assessment. The patient with decompensated cirrhosis should not be moribund, which would increase the risk of the procedure to an unacceptable degree, nor should the patient be in such a stable condition that she or he may be able to live an independent life without liver transplantation. At the time of listing for transplantation the expected one-year survival should be < 90% – i.e., a survival

TABLE 33.   Results of liver transplantation by cause of liver failure

Result	Cause of liver failure	Comments
Excellent	Cholestatic liver disease	Low recurrence rates
	Autoimmune hepatitis	
	Alcoholic cirrhosis	
	Metabolic disease	
	Congenital disease	
Good	HCV	Moderate recurrence rates
	HBV	
	HCC (small tumors)	
Fair	Fulminant hepatic failure	Results affected by the pretransplant status of
	Retransplantation	the patient
	Biliary atresia	
Poor	Large tumors	High recurrence rates
	Cholangiocarcinoma	

less than that expected with orthotopic liver transplantation (OLT). The indications for referral for transplantation in patients with chronic liver disease are outlined in Table 34.

Transplantation for hepatitis B remains somewhat controversial, with high recurrence rates in the absence of effective antiviral therapy. The use of HBIG (not uniformly available in Canada) and/or the antiviral agent lamivudine (Heptovir®) have significantly reduced disease recurrence, resulting in patient and graft survival rates similar to those for other transplantation indications. The results of transplantation for primary hepatic malignancies have been disappointing, the best results being achieved in patients with unifocal tumor that is less than 5 cm in diameter and with no evidence of vascular or lymphatic invasion. However, transplant may be curative for patients with compensated cirrhosis and incidental tumors discovered on screening protocols. Physicians should be aware of their transplant center's policy when considering patients for referral. The exclusion of patients with contraindications to liver transplantation (outlined in Table 35) allows the best use of scarce donor resources while maximizing benefit.

15.2 Preoperative Workup

The principles behind the liver transplant workup are to definitively establish the etiology of the liver disease and to identify contraindications to surgery. Assessment by a multidisciplinary team that includes medical, surgical, anes-

TABLE 34.   Criteria for referral of patients for liver transplantation

Chronic liver disease in general Portal hypertensive bleeding Intractable ascites Spontaneous bacterial peritonitis Portosystemic encephalopathy Child-Pugh Score $\geq$ 7
Primary biliary cirrhosis and primary sclerosing cholangitis* Progressive jaundice Intractable pruritus Progressive hepatic osteodystrophy Ascending cholangitis (in PSC)

*In addition to those criteria listed above.

thetic, social and psychiatric specialists is performed in patients to ensure the success of the transplantation process.

Once the patient is declared a candidate for liver transplantation, he or she goes on a waiting list until a suitable organ becomes available. In the allocation of an available organ, consideration is given to ABO blood group compatibility, medical urgency and waiting time. As a rule, the sickest patient on the waiting list for the longest time is given priority. Patients may deteriorate in the course of their disease and become too sick to tolerate transplantation. Many programs expect 15–20% of listed patients to die or be delisted before an organ becomes available.

15.3 Timing of Transplantation
With improving results of liver transplantation, quality of life criteria may merit consideration in referral for transplantation; however, at present the scarcity of organs permits only the sickest to benefit from transplantation (Tables 32–35). It is clear that transplantation is best considered prior to the development of catastrophic complications and the need for life support, although waiting times can be expected to increase as patients are referred and listed earlier.

15.4 Operative Procedure
Technical details of the procedure are beyond the scope of this discussion; however, there are several salient points to be reviewed. During the procedure the liver is mobilized and both inflow to the liver and inferior vena caval return to the heart are interrupted. This may cause hemodynamic instability, which, if not correctable, may require the use of venovenous bypass (in which

TABLE 35.   Liver transplantation: contraindications

---

1. Absolute
Sepsis outside the biliary tree
Extrahepatic malignancy
Advanced cariopulmonary disease
Severe pulmonary hypertension (PA pressure 60 mm of Hg)
AIDS
Active alcohol and/or substance abuse
Inability to accept the procedure, understand its nature, or cooperate in the medical care
required following liver transplantation

2. Relative
Chronic renal insufficiency
Age
Vascular problems (portal and superior mesenteric vein thrombosis or prior shunt surgery)
Noncompliance
Inadequate psychosocial support
Other significant extrahepatic disease(s)

IVC and portal blood are diverted through a bypass circuit to the axillary vein) or an alternative surgical approach. The liver is subsequently removed and the new graft sewn in place. Although the liver is flushed of the high potassium preservation solution prior to reperfusion, there can be significant cardiac abnormalities upon removing the clamps and reperfusing the liver. These intraoperative events demand a thorough preoperative assessment of cardiac status.

15.5 Postoperative Management

Issues that must be addressed in the postoperative period include management of fluid and electrolytes, respiratory function, monitoring of neurologic status, immunosuppression and graft function.

In most cases patients are quickly extubated within 24 hours of surgery. However, ventilatory support may be needed for an extended period, particularly when there is delayed graft function, presence of large pleural effusions, pulmonary infiltrate and diaphragmatic dysfunction or paralysis. Patients who were deeply encephalopathic before transplantation typically require an extended period of ventilatory support and ICU care.

Most patients are in a state of fluid overload after transplantation. These patients usually have a low serum albumin and respond well to colloid supplementation and diuretics. Renal insufficiency, occasionally requiring dialysis, is not uncommon postoperatively. Renal failure may be due to a combination of factors including pre-existing renal disease, hepatorenal syndrome, intraoperative blood loss and hypotension leading to tubular necrosis, drug-induced nephrotoxicity (especially cyclosporine or FK-506), poor liver function and sepsis.

Graft function resumes almost immediately following transplantation; abnormalities of coagulation are sensitive markers of hepatic dysfunction and coagulation parameters should return to normal levels within 48 hours in most patients. Delayed graft function and primary nonfunction are rare events and may present with coagulopathy, encephalopathy, hypoglycemia, hyper-kalemia or renal failure. The failure of coagulation parameters to normalize is therefore an ominous sign of graft failure and suggests the need for retrans-plantation.

The causes of significant hepatic dysfunction within first 48 hours include accelerated cellular rejection, primary nonfunction and hepatic artery throm-bosis. These can be difficult to differentiate on clinical grounds, and radio-logical investigations such as ultrasound Doppler or angiography may be required for diagnosis.

Most patients wake up within several hours of liver transplantation, where-as patients with fulminant hepatic failure may require one to three days to return to normal neurological status after liver transplantation. Monitoring intracranial pressure in fulminant liver failure may help both with patient selection for transplantation and in perioperative management. Immediately following transplantation, narcotics and sedatives are kept to a minimum. Confusion and seizures can occur, and are usually related to metabolic distur-bances (e.g., low serum magnesium levels), but are a recognized complication of both cyclosporine and FK-506. Some centers place all patients on a con-tinuous infusion of magnesium sulfate for the first 72–96 hours postopera-tively, followed by oral supplementation for three months.

15.6 Immunosuppression

15.6.1 IMMUNOSUPPRESSIVE AGENTS CURRENTLY IN USE

15.6.1.1 Cyclosporine
The introduction of cyclosporine is one of the most important factors that has improved the results of liver transplantation. Cyclosporine binds to a specific cell protein, cyclophillin, and through a series of intracellular events prevents activation of T cells and the production of interleukin-2 (IL-2). The drug is given preferentially by the oral route or by slow intravenous infusion. The dosage of cyclosporine is adjusted to maintain a trough cyclosporine level of 300–400 ng/mL (monoclonal radioimmunoassay) in the early postoperative

period, although there is some evidence that peak (C2) cyclosporine level monitoring may be a better guide to therapeutic efficacy. Neoral®, which is less bile acid–dependent in its absorption than the original formulation (Sandimmune®), has all but eliminated the need for the intravenous formulation. Daily monitoring of cyclosporine levels in the immediate postoperative period is mandatory, as the compound has a narrow therapeutic index (efficacy vs toxicity). Cyclosporine interacts with many drugs, such as antibiotics and calcium channel blockers. Caution must therefore be exercised in giving any drug to patients who are taking cyclosporine.

Common side effects of cyclosporine include renal dysfunction, hypertension, increased susceptibility to infections, malignancy (especially post-transplant lymphoproliferative disease), hypertrichosis, tremor, headaches and gum hyperplasia. Other less common side effects include confusion, seizures, agitation, hearing loss, anorexia, diarrhea, nausea and vomiting, abdominal discomfort and gynecomastia.

15.6.1.2 FK-506 (Tacrolimus®; Prograf®)

FK-506, a calcineurin inhibitor, binds to FK-binding protein before inhibiting T-cell activation by blocking IL-2 production in a similar fashion to cyclosporine. Toxicity and efficacy are similar to those of cyclosporine, although recent multicenter trials suggest there may be a slightly decreased incidence of rejection using Tacrolimus®, and that it may play a role in the management of chronic rejection, which to date has not translated into improved graft survival.

15.6.1.3 Corticosteroids

All activated mononuclear cells express high levels of steroid receptors. The major action of steroids is to reduce or eliminate the production of inflammatory mediators (IL-1 and TNF) and reduce activated lymphocytes by inducing apoptosis. All patients receive methylprednisolone preoperatively. There are probably as many steroid protocols as transplant programs. One uses a preoperative dose of 500 mg Solu-Medrol®, which subsequently is reduced rapidly to a dose of 20 mg/day. Steroids are discontinued within the first six months to a year in the majority of patients. Short-term side effects include an increased incidence of infections (bacterial and fungal), hyperglycemia and impaired wound healing.

15.6.1.4 Antilymphocyte products

Antilymphocyte products can be monoclonal (OKT3) or polyclonal (ALG, RATS, ATG). In either case the aim of therapy is to prevent or treat rejection by lymphocyte depletion. The use of these products has been associated with higher rates of viral infections, in particular cytomegalovirus (CMV) as well as an increased risk of lymphoproliferative disorders. OKT3 has been associated with side effects secondary to the release of tumor necrosis factor and IL-1 that can range from mild flu-like symptoms to life-threatening pulmonary edema and circulatory collapse. In liver transplantation the use of these drugs is generally limited to induction of immunosuppression in the presence of renal failure to spare the use of calcineurin inhibitors, and treatment of steroid-resistant rejection.

15.6.2 NEW IMMUNOSUPPRESSIVE AGENTS

15.6.2.1 Mycophenolate mofetil (CellCept®)
Mycophenolate mofetil (MMF) is a potent reversible noncompetitive inhibitor of inosine monophosphate dehydrogenase. It acts as a selective inhibitor of T- and B-cell proliferation by blocking the production of guanosine nucleotides and interfering with glycosylation of adhesion molecules. The main side effect of MMF is bone marrow suppression. It has no nephrotoxicity and is an important agent in triple drug regimens, allowing a decrease in the cyclosporine dosage (and in its nephrotoxicity) while at the same time decreasing the incidence of rejection.

15.6.2.2 Rapamycin
Rapamycin is a secondary macrolide metabolite that has a distinctly different mechanism of action than calcineurin inhibitors. It binds to the FK-binding protein and inhibits the growth factor–dependent proliferation of hematopoietic and nonhematopoietic cells at G1 to S phase through calcium-independent signals. It has been shown to effectively prevent allograft rejection as well as reverse ongoing rejection in animal models. No major side effects on other organ systems have been observed. A number of formulations are undergoing Phase II clinical trials in Canada.

15.6.2.3 IL-2 receptor antagonists
Baxiliximab (Simulec®) and diaclizumab (Zenapax®) are IL-2 receptor–specific monoclonal antibodies which inhibit proliferation of T cells by binding to the alpha chain of the IL-2 receptor complex on activated T cells. They have been shown to reduce the incidence of acute allograft rejection in kidney transplantation and improve the one-year graft and patient survival. Phase II clinical trials in liver transplantation are ongoing.

15.7 Postoperative Complications
Complications common to any surgical procedure can occur with liver trans-

plantation. However, there are several adverse events peculiar to liver transplantation. The most concerning of postoperative complications is *primary nonfunction* (PNF) of the new graft. The incidence of PNF ranges from 2 to 10% and becomes evident by coagulation parameters that worsen and cannot be corrected, increasing acidosis and deterioration in the patient's mental status. The etiology of PNF is unclear, and the treatment is urgent retransplantation. Primary graft dysfunction of a less significant degree has been managed with some success with prostaglandin E_1 and/or N-acetylcysteine.

Vascular thromboses that occur in the early postoperative period are generally technical in nature. Although thrombectomy of both portal vein and hepatic artery has been reported with some success, retransplantation is usually required should these vessels thrombose.

The *bile duct* has been termed the Achilles heel of liver transplantation. Problems occur in 10–30% of cases. Early leaks are secondary to ischemia, sepsis or severe rejection. The bile duct can be irreversibly damaged in hepatic artery thrombosis immediately post-transplant.

Acute allograft rejection occurs in 40–60% of transplant patients, usually in the first three months after transplantation. Rejection is suspected in patients with rising liver enzymes. Patterns of enzyme elevation can be either hepatocellular (high AST) or cholestatic (high bilirubin and alkaline phosphatase). Fever, malaise and right upper quadrant discomfort are late signs and should not be required for diagnosis of rejection. Diagnosis is confirmed by liver biopsy. Histologic findings include periportal inflammation with mononuclear cells and eosinophils, bile duct injury and endophlebitis. Episodes of cellular rejection usually respond to high-dose steroid therapy. Those patients whose rejection fails to respond to steroids are usually treated with a 7–14 day course of antithymocyte globulin (monoclonal or polyclonal). Recently, FK-506 has shown some success in treating rejection refractory to either steroids or OKT3. Failure to respond to immunosuppressive therapy may result in ductopenic rejection (chronic rejection) leading to biliary cirrhosis, which may result in the need for retransplantation in 5–10% of all transplanted patients.

The major cause of death following liver transplantation is related to *infections*. The three main determinants of risk of infection in transplant patients are those related to surgical problems; the net state of immunosuppression; and environmental exposure. There are similar patterns of infection in all forms of organ transplantation and a consistent timetable for when different infections occur. Immunosuppressed patients are at risk for bacterial, viral and fungal infections. Bacterial infections with non-opportunistic organisms are usually seen in the early postoperative period. Opportunistic bacterial infections are seen one to two months or more after transplantation. Wound infections and intra-abdominal sepsis account for the majority of bacterial infections seen in transplanted patients. Viral infections are seen frequently in immunosuppressed patients and usually occur at six weeks or later. The most important pathogen affecting transplant patients is cytomegalovirus (CMV), which causes both direct effects including tissue injury and clinical disease, and a variety of indirect effects. Seronegative recipients of organs from seropositive donors have > 50% risk of symptomatic disease. Diagnosis of disease due to CMV is accomplished by demonstrating viremia or tissue invasion. The prevention of CMV infection is of great importance. The intensity of prophylaxis (e.g., use of ganciclovir during ALG therapy) must be proportional to the intensity of immunosuppression and to the risk of viral reactivation. Prophylaxis is initiated before reactivation of the virus – i.e., in seronegative recipients of seropositive donors. The therapy for CMV infection includes the reduction of immunosuppression and the use of anti-viral agents such as ganciclovir. Other viral infections seen in transplanted patients include herpes simplex, Epstein-Barr virus, varicella zoster and adenovirus. Fungal infections have been noted in up to 20% of patients and carry with them a 20–100% mortality rate. Infections in general are usually proportional to the degree of immunosuppression.

15.8 Results of Liver Transplantation
A one-year survival of ≥80% after liver transplantation is now not uncommon. Most mortality occurs within the first 90 days. After one year, few patients or grafts are lost. Furthermore, 60% of patients return to gainful employment, demonstrating that this procedure is not only of benefit to the patient, but also to society as a whole. Though there are few reports of cost effectiveness, investigators in Pittsburgh have demonstrated that liver transplantation is less expensive than costs of caring for similar patients treated for complications of cirrhosis. Patients with diseases such as cholestatic liver disease that tend not to recur after liver transplantation have an excellent long-term prognosis (greater than 80% five-year survival). In contrast, patients transplanted for viral hepatitis B and C have a poorer long-term outlook because of the problem of recurrent disease. At least 95% of hepatitis C patients develop virological recurrence. At least 20% progress to cirrhosis within five years. Pretransplant high HCV-RNA titres and the occurrence of rejection requiring steroid therapy are probably the most important determinants of post-transplant recurrence and survival. The use of high-dose HBIG and the advent of new antiviral agents such as lamivudine are markedly reducing the recurrence rate of hepatitis B. Long-term results on the impact of lamivudine resistance are awaited. Studies of combination therapy with HBIG and lamivudine are underway.

15.9 Recent Advances and Future Directions

Liver transplantation in the pediatric age group is limited by the shortage of pediatric donors. As a result, reduced-size liver transplantation, where an adult liver is cut down to pediatric size, has been developed. Split liver transplantation, whereby a donor liver is given to two recipients, has been performed with success and is being applied with increasing frequency now that many of the technical hurdles have been overcome. Living-related liver transplantation is performed routinely in some centers with greater than 80% one-year survival.

Isolated hepatocyte transplantation may offer treatment of metabolic liver diseases and has been successful in the laboratory setting. Artificial support systems have shown initial promise in fulminant hepatic failure and may reduce the need for transplantation.

The elusive goal of tolerance has been produced in animal models and if induced in humans would obviate the need for immunosuppression and its associated complications. Xenotransplantation sits on the horizon; the use of transgenic animals may eventually offer a solution to the shortage of donor organs and permit a wider application of liver transplantation to liver disease.

16. NEOPLASMS OF THE LIVER / L.J. Worobetz

Neoplasms of the liver can be divided into benign and malignant, with malignant tumors being either primary or secondary from a cancer that has metastasized from elsewhere. The sites from which metastases occur frequently include lung, colon, pancreas, breast, stomach and ovary. In North America, primary hepatic neoplasms are uncommon, with metastatic tumor being the most common malignant tumor of the liver. Worldwide, especially in areas such as the Far East, hepatocellular carcinoma (HCC) is much more prevalent than metastatic disease.

16.1 Benign Tumors of the Liver

Benign tumors of the liver are detected more frequently than in the past, in part as a result of the increased use of diagnostic imaging tests, including ultrasound and CT scanning, for reasons unrelated to the tumors. Benign tumors are divided into three categories: hepatocellular, cholangiocellular and non-epithelial.

16.1.1 *HEPATOCELLULAR ADENOMA*

Hepatocellular adenomas are benign tumors seen primarily in females in their third and fourth decades. The increasing prevalence has paralleled the introduction of the oral contraceptive, suggesting a hormonal influence in their pathogenesis. The estimated risk for women on oral contraceptives for seven years is 5 times the normal rate and increases to 25 times with use longer than nine years. The tumors may be multiple, usually involving the right lobe, and may be > 10 cm in diameter. Clinical features include an asymptomatic presentation, pain in the right hypochondrium or palpable mass. The most alarming presentation is an acute hemoperitoneum following rupture of the adenoma, which carries an appreciable mortality. Diagnosis is usually established with imaging techniques including ultrasound, CT scanning, angiography and radionuclear scanning. Hepatic arteriography is useful for diagnosis. About 50% of adenomas are avascular with hepatic arteries surrounding the lesion; the remainder are hypervascular. Because adenomas mimic normal hepatic tissue, liver biopsy is of limited diagnostic use. The risk of malignancy is up to 10% with an increased risk in the larger, multiple tumors. Management includes stopping oral contraceptives and resection of larger, symptomatic tumors.

16.1.2 FOCAL NODULAR HYPERPLASIA
Focal nodular hyperplasia differs from the adenoma in that this usually solitary solid tumor is composed of nodules of benign hyperplastic hepatocytes surrounding a central stellate fibrous scar and includes other cell types such as atypical hepatocytes, Kupffer's cells and inflammatory cells. The lesion is vascular and because of the presence of Kupffer's cells will appear as an area of increased uptake on radionuclear scanning. Although also more common in women, it does not appear related to the oral contraceptive. No treatment is needed if the patient is asymptomatic, which is usually the case. These lesions rarely rupture.

16.1.3 CAVERNOUS HEMANGIOMA
Hemangiomas are the most common benign tumor of the liver and are seen in about 0.5–7% of the general population. These are usually detected by imaging techniques done for other reasons. These vascular lesions are usually asymptomatic and are more common in women. Hemangiomas present at all ages but are most common in the third to fifth decades. Lesions larger than 4 cm are called *giant cavernous hemangiomas.* If hemangiomas are symptomatic, pain is the most common complaint. The only physical sign may be an enlarged liver with an arterial bruit heard over the lesion. Ultrasound findings include an echogenic lesion with diagnosis being confirmed by RBC-labeled nuclear scan, bolus-enhanced CT scan or, if necessary, angiography. The lesion does not require any treatment as there is no malignant potential and hemorrhage is rare.

16.2 Malignant Tumors of the Liver

16.2.1 *PRIMARY HEPATOCELLULAR CARCINOMA*

Hepatocellular carcinoma (HCC) is an extremely common tumor in Africa and Southeast Asia. In Africa, it makes up 50% of all malignant tumors in men and is usually found in young adults. In North America, it represents only 1–2% of malignant tumors and is generally a disease of older people.

Although many factors potentially contribute to HCC, the disease is usually limited to individuals with pre-existing liver disease. Approximately 60–80% of patients in North America with HCC have a cirrhotic liver, and more than 10% of individuals with cirrhosis will develop HCC. The risk is greatest in patients with hemochromatosis or hepatitis B or C infection. Other causes that can lead to HCC include alcohol abuse, schistosomal infection and homozygous α_1-antitrypsin deficiency.

Hepatitis B virus has a clear association with the development of HCC, with the tumor occurring 22 times more frequently among carriers of hepatitis B surface antigen than among the general population. Integrated DNA sequences of hepatitis B virus have been identified in the genome of both tumor cells and normal hepatocytes of patients with HCC, suggesting that viral integration occurs before the development of the tumor. Hepatitis C also appears to be a causative agent for the development of HCC. Antibodies to hepatitis C have been found in more than 50% of cases of HCC who had no evidence for hepatitis B infection. The hepatitis C virus does not appear to integrate into the host genome, and thus the mechanism for the hepatocarcinogenesis is unclear.

Noncirrhotic causes of HCC include the ingestion of aflatoxins (metabolites of the mold Aspergillus flavus) and ingestion of hormone supplements, including oral contraceptives and exogenous androgens.

The clinical recognition of HCC may be difficult, as the tumor often occurs in patients with underlying cirrhosis and the signs and symptoms may simply suggest progression of the underlying liver disease. The most frequent feature is the development of a painful mass in the right upper quadrant accompanied by weight loss. In the patient with cirrhosis, the presentation may include the development of ascites, portal hypertension or abrupt clinical deterioration. A hepatic friction rub or bruit may be heard over the lesion. Patients may present with one of the many paraneoplastic syndromes, including erythrocytosis, hypercalcemia, dysproteinemia or hypoglycemia. Abnormal liver enzymes are common, but normal enzymes do not rule out the diagnosis. The oncofetal antigen, α_1-fetoprotein (AFP), is usually elevated in the serum, with levels > 500 µg/L in 70–80% of cases. However, the antigen lacks specificity, with elevations occurring in metastatic disease from germ cell tumors of the testis or ovary, or carcinoma of the pancreas or stomach. The level of AFP does correlate with extent of the HCC. Ultrasound and CT scan are useful in diagnosis and localization for percutaneous sampling of the tumor mass. Angiography and MRI are more useful imaging studies in distinguishing HCC from metastatic disease and determining whether the lesion can be resected.

The prognosis for patients with HCC is very poor, with the median survival of North American patients only four to six months. Radical resection represents the only opportunity for cure, but resection is often complicated by the presence of underlying cirrhosis, the occasional multicentric nature of the tumor and the presence of micrometastases. Up to 70% have metastatic disease at the time of diagnosis. Liver transplantation may be considered, but recurrence of tumor and presence of metastases after transplantation have limited its usefulness. The induction of tumor necrosis by ligation of the hepatic artery or by nonoperative arterial embolization with gel-foam fragments along with chemotherapy (chemoembolization) may provide palliation of pain. Other approaches include percutaneous injections of alcohol, cryotherapy, external-beam irradiation or systemic chemotherapy with doxorubicin or 5-fluorouracil (5-FU). Newer therapies include monoclonal antibodies with chemotherapy and gene therapy with cytotoxic agents.

Screening strategies for HCC have included ultrasound and/or AFP determinations every 6 to 12 months in high-risk patients. This approach identifies tumors at an earlier stage but has not yet been shown to improve morbidity or mortality rates.

16.2.2 HEPATOBLASTOMA
Hepatoblastoma is a malignant tumor that develops in children under the age of five years, with over 50% of the cases occurring before the age of two years. About one-third of patients with hepatoblastoma have birth defects in other organs. Patients may present with failure to thrive, weight loss or a rapidly enlarging liver mass. The tumors are composed of immature hepatocytes occasionally accompanied by a mesenchymal component such as bone, and have the potential for growth to a large size. Treatment consists of surgical resection followed by radiotherapy and chemotherapy. The five-year survival rate is 15–35%.

16.2.3 METASTATIC TUMORS
In North America, the most common malignant tumor to affect the liver is metastasis from primary carcinoma elsewhere. Common sources include colorectal, breast, lung or urogenital cancer as well as neuroendocrine tumors. It is sometimes difficult to distinguish primary from metastatic carcinoma in the

liver. Metastases are often multiple with smaller lesions, whereas HCC have a dominant larger mass. In most cases, metastases are readily imaged by ultrasound, CT or MRI. The diagnosis is usually confirmed by needle biopsy. Occasionally, metastases have histologic or immunohistochemical features that suggest a primary site.

For most cases, metastatic disease implies advanced disease with poor prognosis and few therapeutic options. Exceptions include metastatic colorectal carcinoma and neuroendocrine tumors. Surgical resection for metastatic colorectal carcinoma confined to the liver may increase five-year survival rates up to 40%. Cryotherapy and chemotherapy for unresectable colorectal disease may prolong survival. Resection for localized neuroendocrine tumors and drug therapy (interferon, octreotide) for more advanced disease may help prolong survival and reduce symptoms from hormone release (carcinoid syndrome, Zollinger-Ellison syndrome).

17. LIVER DISEASE IN PREGNANCY / R.J. Hilsden and E.A. Shaffer

17.1 Normal Pregnancy

The pregnant state normally is mildly cholestatic from the increase in endogenous estrogens. This changes several biochemical tests, but primary liver disease is an uncommon complication. When features of liver disease do occur during pregnancy, prompt evaluation is essential as some conditions, such as acute fatty liver of pregnancy, rapidly progress to become fatal to both mother and fetus.

The anatomic and physiologic changes that accompany pregnancy alter physical findings and liver biochemistries. Yet normal pregnancy does not significantly affect liver metabolism or function.

Pregnancy does not change liver size. In the third trimester, the enlarging uterus displaces the liver superiorly and posteriorly. Therefore, a palpable liver suggests significant hepatomegaly and underlying liver disease. A small amount of peripheral edema is also common during pregnancy, as are some findings that usually connote chronic liver disease, such as spider angiomas and palmar erythema. These findings are signs of high circulating estrogen levels.

Pregnancy does not alter the expected values for serum bilirubin, aminotransferases, γ-glutamyl transpeptidase or 5′-nucleotidase, or the INR/prothrombin time. Dilution from the expanded plasma volume causes a 10 g/L fall in serum albumin and in total protein. Alkaline phosphatase, primarily of placental and skeletal origin, increases 1.5 times normal after the fifth week. Alkaline phosphatase may remain elevated for up to six weeks after delivery. There is an increase in serum globulin, total cholesterol and triglyceride.

TABLE 36. Differential diagnosis in major liver diseases during pregnancy

	Intrahepatic cholestasis of pregnancy	Acute fatty liver of pregnancy	Toxemia of pregnancy	Hyperemesis gravidarum	Viral hepatitis
Clinical features					
Onset (trimester)	3	3	3	1	1, 2, 3
Family history	+	–	–	–	–
Pruritus	+	–	–	–	–
Jaundice	+/–	+	–	–/+	+
Abdominal pain	–	+	+	–	–
Nausea and vomiting	–	+	+	+	+
Tender hepatomegaly	–	–	+	–	+
Biochemical features					
Cholestasis	++	–	–	+	–
Aminotransferases	Normal or <250 units	<300 units	100–300 units to >500 units	<200 units	>1,000 units
Hepatitis serology	–	–	–	–	+
Thrombocytopenia +/–DIC	–	+	+	–	–
Hypoglycemia	–	+	+	–	–
Pre-eclampsia/eclampsia	–	+	++	–	–

Liver diseases occurring during pregnancy can be divided into three categories: (1) acute liver disease coincident with pregnancy; (2) pregnancy occurring in a patient with established chronic liver disease; and (3) liver diseases unique to pregnancy. When assessing a pregnant woman presenting with liver disease, the nature of her symptoms, stage of gestation and liver biochemistry provide important clues to the underlying etiology. Liver diseases unique to pregnancy usually occur only during certain trimesters, whereas liver disease coincident with pregnancy may occur at any time (Table 36).

17.2 Acute Liver Disease Coincident with Pregnancy

Any liver disease that can afflict young women may arise during pregnancy. Of these, viral hepatitis is the most common cause of jaundice in pregnancy. Pregnancy does not affect the course of viral hepatitis, except for hepatitis E, which occurs in epidemics in underdeveloped countries. In such settings, the combination of pregnancy and hepatitis plus any indigenous malnutrition results in a significant mortality rate (up to 20%). In developed areas, hepatitis B poses a high risk of neonatal infection (vertical transmission). Neonates born to mothers who are hepatitis B surface antigen (HB_sAg) positive must receive immunoprophylaxis with hyperimmune globulin and hepatitis B vaccine to prevent the long-term sequelae of chronic hepatitis B: cirrhosis and hepatocellular carcinoma. Perinatal transmission of hepatitis C occurs in up to 18% of pregnancies in HCV-positive, HIV-negative women. Breastfeeding has not been associated with transmission of HCV. Current information does not support routine immunoprophylaxis of infants born to HCV-positive women.

Gallstones and their complications, and the rupture of a hepatic adenoma, have an increased frequency during pregnancy.

17.3 Pregnancy Occurring in Chronic Liver Disease

Pregnancy is unusual in patients with chronic liver disease. Fertility becomes nearly normal when cirrhosis is well compensated or the active liver disease improves with appropriate therapy (e.g., autoimmune hepatitis on steroids). The degree of hepatic impairment determines the risk for the mother during the pregnancy. Hemorrhage from esophageal varices is the most significant complication of cirrhosis in pregnancy. The increased blood volume and flow through the azygous system that are a part of any normal pregnancy raise the pressure in the esophageal veins; in established cirrhosis this increases variceal size and the likelihood of bleeding. Women who have undergone liver transplantation can have successful pregnancies. There is an increased risk of prematurity and low birth weight, but no increase in congenital anomalies. Immunosuppressive agents must be continued throughout pregnancy, but adjustments to the immunosuppressive regime may be required.

17.4 Liver Diseases Unique to Pregnancy

17.4.1 *ACUTE FATTY LIVER OF PREGNANCY*

Acute fatty liver of pregnancy is characterized by fatty infiltration of the liver. It may rapidly progress to hepatic failure and death. Acute fatty liver may be uncommon (1 in 13,000 deliveries), but is important, having a maternal mortality of 18% and fetal mortality of 23%. The etiology is unknown, but the microvesicular fat that accumulates in hepatocytes probably represents mitochondrial injury causing disordered intermediary fat metabolism.

Acute fatty liver of pregnancy almost invariably presents in the third trimester, with a peak frequency around 36–37 weeks gestation. Occasionally, it will become apparent only after delivery. There is an association with nulliparity, twin gestations, male fetus and pre-eclampsia or eclampsia. Presentation can vary from nonspecific symptoms to fulminant hepatic failure. Nausea and vomiting with or without abdominal pain are common. Examination may reveal a tender liver. Pruritus is uncommon and would suggest the possibility of a different liver problem such as intrahepatic cholestasis of pregnancy. Progressive hepatic failure then rapidly supervenes, with the development of jaundice, generalized bleeding from coagulopathy, hypoglycemia, hepatic encephalopathy and renal failure. Such severe cases have an inexorable downhill course unless the fetus is delivered; even then, deterioration may continue for a further 48 to 72 hours.

Laboratory features include a moderately elevated aminotransferase, which is usually around 300 IU/L but may range from normal to 1,000 IU/L. Alkaline phosphatase and serum bilirubin are elevated. Liver biopsy reveals tiny droplets of fat (microvesicular fat) inside hepatocytes.

Diagnosis requires a high degree of suspicion, as the presentation is often nonspecific. Acute fatty liver of pregnancy should be considered whenever marked nausea and vomiting develop in the third trimester of pregnancy. Suspicion increases with a twin pregnancy, nulliparity or signs of toxemia. Ultrasound or CT scans may detect the increased fat in the liver and help exclude complications such as a subcapsular hematoma or another entity such as choledocholithiasis. Liver biopsy is diagnostic. Biopsy even via the transvenous route (necessary when a coagulopathy makes percutaneous liver biopsy hazardous) should be done if the results will alter management. For example, differentiation of acute viral hepatitis from acute fatty liver is important to determine whether rapid delivery is indicated. Delivery can be life-saving in acute fatty liver.

Management involves aggressive supportive care. The only definitive treatment for the condition is prompt delivery. Liver transplantation has been used when women have failed to improve with delivery and supportive care. The risk of acute fatty liver of pregnancy is not increased in subsequent pregnancies.

17.4.2 INTRAHEPATIC CHOLESTASIS OF PREGNANCY

Intrahepatic cholestasis of pregnancy accounts for 20–25% of cases of jaundice during pregnancy. The etiology is unknown. There is a clear genetic predisposition, likely autosomal dominant, with an increased frequency in women of Scandinavian or Chilean descent. The cholestasis (failure of bile formation) represents an exaggerated response of the liver to the normal increase in endogenous estrogens during pregnancy.

Presentation typically is in the third trimester with the insidious onset of pruritus. In half of these patients, jaundice follows within one to four weeks. Other cholestatic features include dark urine and, occasionally, pale stool. Otherwise women generally feel well, without nausea, vomiting or abdominal pain. Serum alkaline phosphatase and cholesterol rise, but aminotransferases are only modestly elevated. Ultrasound and cholangiography, if performed, are normal. The appropriate laboratory and ultrasound evaluation of the pregnant woman with cholestasis involves excluding other causes of jaundice and pruritus including viral hepatitis, primary biliary cirrhosis, biliary tract disease and medications. Liver biopsy, which shows only cholestasis without inflammation, may be necessary in some atypical cases.

Although a benign condition for the mother (other than the inexorable pruritus), intrahepatic cholestasis decreases fetal survival and increases the risk of prematurity. Treatment is supportive with bile salt–binding agents such as cholestyramine. Ursodeoxycholic acid therapy improves bile formation, perhaps washing out "toxic" bile acids and pruritogenic agents. It can alleviate maternal pruritus, although whether it improves fetal outcome is unclear at present. S-adenosylmethionine, which alters membrane fluidity, and rifampin, which increases the excretion of pruritogenic agents, also work. Treatment for cholestasis and pruritus, however, frequently is unsatisfactory. Delivery should occur as soon as fetal lung maturity is documented, to prevent the increased risk of stillbirth. Parenteral vitamin K may be needed to correct a prothrombin deficiency.

Symptoms usually abate within two weeks of delivery. There is a significant risk of recurrence with subsequent pregnancies and with the use of oral contraceptives or other estrogens.

17.4.3 PREGNANCY TOXEMIAS AND THE HELLP SYNDROME

Pre-eclampsia (hypertension, proteinuria and edema) and eclampsia (signs of pre-eclampsia plus seizures and/or coma) begin in the late second or in the third trimester. In severe pre-eclampsia or eclampsia, liver involvement is evident by abdominal tenderness and abnormal liver biochemistry. Hepatocellular necrosis can occur from endothelial damage and platelet and fibrin deposition in the sinusoids. Subcapsular hematoma and hepatic rupture rarely develop.

The HELLP syndrome (hemolysis, elevated liver enzymes, low platelets) is usually associated with pre-eclampsia; occasionally, it may arise in the absence of either hypertension or proteinuria. Liver complications are similar to those in pre-eclampsia. Differentiation of acute fatty liver of pregnancy from the HELLP syndrome may be clinically difficult, but the treatment – prompt delivery and supportive care – is identical for both.

17.4.4 HYPEREMESIS GRAVIDARUM

Abnormalities in serum liver enzymes may be found in up to 50% of women hospitalized for hyperemesis gravidarum. Aminotransferases may be increased up to 200 IU/L. Mild hyperbilirubinemia may also be seen, returning to normal after the resumption of adequate nutrition. Some of these cases may be Gilbert's syndrome.

18. VASCULAR DISORDERS OF THE LIVER / L.J. Worobetz

The most frequent abnormality of the circulation to affect the liver is congestive heart failure, which leads to reduced outflow of blood from the liver.
Other causes of hepatic congestion include constrictive pericarditis, obstruction of the inferior vena cava and hepatic veins (Budd-Chiari syndrome) and
occlusion of the small hepatic veins (veno-occlusive disease). Increased resistance to hepatic venous outflow results in congestive hepatomegaly, dilation
of hepatic venules and sinusoids, and hypoxia. The hypoxia in turn leads to
hepatocyte damage with possible fibrosis and cirrhosis, the latter termed *cardiac cirrhosis*.

18.1 Congestive Heart Failure

The clinical features of congestive heart failure can include tender
hepatomegaly and abdominal discomfort. In tricuspid insufficiency, the liver
may be pulsatile. Ascites, which may be present, often has a high protein content. Characteristic biochemical abnormalities are mild hyperbilirubinemia
with a moderate elevation of aminotransferases (<300) and a mild elevation of
alkaline phosphatase, especially in acute congestion. In acute ischemic liver
insult, aminotransferase values can be quite high, simulating hepatitis – hence
the term *ischemic hepatitis*. The prognosis is directly related to the severity of
the heart failure and the response to therapy.

18.2 Hepatic Vein Thrombosis (Budd-Chiari Syndrome)

Hepatic vein thrombosis is a rare disorder that may occur alone or in association with inferior vena cava thrombosis. It may be associated with polycythemia vera, paroxysmal nocturnal hemoglobinuria, hypercoagulability, use
of oral contraceptives or neoplasia, or it may be secondary to obstruction by
a membranous web. The presentation may be acute, with rapidly developing
hepatomegaly, ascites, and abdominal pain leading to liver failure and coma.
The chronic presentation is usually that of progressive ascites. The degree of
aminotransferase elevation is variable, depending on the rapidity of the onset.
The liver biopsy shows large hemorrhagic areas with congestion, atrophy and
necrosis around the center of the lobule. Diagnosis was traditionally by liver-
spleen colloid scan showing decreased uptake in areas that are otherwise normally drained by the hepatic vein. The caudate lobe of the liver demonstrates
a normal uptake in that it has a different drainage, that being directly into the
vena cava. Doppler ultrasound is now the diagnostic procedure of choice. The
typical ultrasound features include inability to visualize normal hepatic
venous connections to the vena cava and absence of any wave form in the
hepatic vein. MRI and CT scan usually do not add much more information. In

difficult diagnostic cases, IVC hepatic venography may reveal blocked hepatic veins. The decision regarding treatment depends on etiology, anatomy and acuteness of the illness. Those with a fulminant form with liver failure should be considered for liver transplantation. Causes may be local (tumor, web) or transient (pregnancy). Treatment with anticoagulants and streptokinase is rarely successful. Patients with chronic hepatic vein thrombosis and adequate hepatic reserve may benefit from a portacaval shunt.

18.3 Veno-occlusive Disease

Veno-occlusive disease refers to the obstruction of small and medium-sized intrahepatic veins. Causal factors include pyrrolizidine alkaloids, hepatic irradiation, azathioprine and graft-versus-host disease related to bone marrow transplantation. The presentation mimics the Budd-Chiari syndrome. In the acute form, presentation may include hepatomegaly, ascites and liver failure. The chronic form leads to cirrhosis and portal hypertension with esophageal varices. The liver biopsy characteristically shows intense congestion around the hepatic venule with thickened obstructed hepatic veins. There is no effective therapy available. Control of the ascites may be required. Some patients have a spontaneous recovery, while others develop cirrhosis with sequelae of portal hypertension, varices and ascites. Liver transplantation may be the only hope for many.

18.4 Portal Vein Thrombosis

Thrombosis of the portal venous system may result from trauma, pancreatitis, neoplasia (e.g., hepatoma), neonatal umbilical sepsis, pylephlebitis or a complication of cirrhosis, or may be idiopathic. Patients usually present with massive hematemesis that is recurrent. Splenomegaly is present. Biochemical tests of the liver are normal or only mildly elevated. Because liver function is usually preserved, ascites and encephalopathy are uncommon and bleeding episodes are better tolerated. Diagnosis may be confirmed by special Doppler ultrasound studies of the portal vein or a venous phase of hepatic angiography. If treatment is required for recurrent hematemesis from esophageal varices, sclerotherapy or banding may be necessary. Because of normal liver parenchyma, surgical approaches such as mesocaval shunt may be considered and are generally better tolerated than by patients with chronic liver disease.

SUGGESTED READING LIST

General
Schiff L, Schiff ER (eds.). Diseases of the liver. 8th ed. Philadelphia: JB Lippincott, 1999.

Sherlock S, Dooley J (eds.). Diseases of the liver and biliary system. 10th ed. Oxford: Blackwell Scientific Publications, 1997.

Section 2 Approach to the Patient with Liver Disease
Aranda-Michel J, Sherman KE. Tests of the liver: use and misuse. Gastroenterologist 1998; 6:34–43.
Davern TJ II, Scharschmidt BF. Biochemical liver tests. In: Feldman M, Scharschmidt BF, Sleisenger MH (eds.), Sleisenger & Fordtran's Gastrointestinal and liver disease. 6th ed. Toronto: WB Saunders, 1998:1112–1122.
Saini S. Imaging of the hepatobiliary tract. N Engl J Med 1997; 336:1889–1894.
Van Leeuwen DJ, Wilson L, Crowe DR. Liver biopsy in the mid-1990s: questions and answers. Semin Liver Dis 1995; 15:340–359.
Zoli M, Magalotti D, Grimaldi M, et al. Physical examination of the liver: is it still worth it? Am J Gastroenterol 1995; 90:1428–1432.

Section 3 Congenital Hyperbilirubinemia
Okolicsanyi L, Cavestro GM, Guatti-Zuliani C. Hyperbilirubinemia: does it matter? Can J Gastroenterol 1999; 13:663–670.

Section 4 Acute Viral Hepatitis
Fattovich G, Giustina G, Degos F, et al. Morbidity and mortality in compensated cirrhosis type C: a retrospective follow-up study of 384 patients. Gastroenterology 1997; 112:463–472.
Margolis HS, Alter MJ, Hadler SC. Hepatitis B: evolving epidemiology and implications for control. Semin Liver Dis 1991; 11:84–92.
Poynard T, Leroy V, Cohard M, et al. Meta-analysis of interferon randomized trials in the treatment of viral hepatitis C: effects of dose and duration. Hepatology 1996; 24:778.
Proceedings of the National Institutes of Health Consensus Development Conference on the Management of Hepatitis C. Hepatology 1997; 26(Suppl 1).

Section 5 Chronic Hepatitis
Krawitt EL. Autoimmune hepatitis. N Engl J Med 1996; 334:897–903.
Sheth SG, Gordon FD, Chopra S. Nonalcoholic steatohepatitis. Ann Intern Med 1997; 126:137–145.

Section 6 Alcoholic Liver Disease
Lieber C. Medical disorders of alcoholism. N Engl J Med 1995; 333:1058–1065.
Sherlock S. Alcoholic liver disease. Lancet 1995; 345:227–229.
Wong F. Alcoholic liver syndromes. Medicine North Am 1997; 20:27–34.

Section 7 Drug-Induced Liver Disease
Beaune PH, Lecoeur S. Immunotoxicity of the liver: adverse reactions to drugs. J Hepatol 1997; 26(Suppl 2):37–42.
Erlinger S. Drug-induced cholestasis. J Hepatol 1997; 26(Suppl 1):1–4.
Farrell GC. Liver disease caused by drugs, anesthetics, and toxins. In: Feldman M, Scharschmidt BF, Sleisenger MH (eds.), Sleisenger & Fordtran's Gastrointestinal and liver disease. 6th ed. Toronto: WB Saunders, 1998:1221–1253.

Huet P-M, Villeneuve J-P, Fenyves D. Drug elimination in chronic liver diseases. J Hepatol 1997; 26(Suppl 2):63–72.

Lee WM. Drug-induced hepatotoxicity. N Engl J Med 1995; 333:1118–1127.

Section 8   Inherited Liver Disease

Adams PC. Population screening for hemochromatosis. Hepatology 1999; 29:1324–1327.

Bacon BR, Olynyk JK, Brunt EM, et al. HFE genotype in patients with hemochromatosis and other liver diseases. Ann Intern Med 1999; 130:953–962.

Bacon BR, Powell L, Adams PC, et al. Molecular medicine and hemochromatosis: at the crossroads. Gastroenterology 1999; 116:193–207.

Eriksson S. Alpha-1-antitrypsin deficiency. J Hepatol 1999; (Suppl 1):34–39.

Forbes JR, His G, Cox DW. Role of the copper-binding domain in the copper transport function of ATP7B, the P-type ATPase defective in Wilson disease. J Biol Chem 1999; 274:12408–1.

McDonnell S, Preston B, Jewell S, et al. A survey of 2,851 patients with hemochromatosis: symptoms and response to treatment. Am J Med 1999; 106:619–625.

Olynyk J, Cullen D, Aquilla S, et al. A population-based study of the clinical expression of the hemochromatosis gene. N Eng J Med 1999; 341:718–724.

Steindl P, Ferenci P, Dienes H, et al. Wilson's disease in patients presenting with liver disease: a diagnostic challenge. Gastroenterology 1997; 113:212–218.

Section 9   Cholestasis

Boberg KM, Lundin KEA, Schrumph E. Etiology and pathogenesis of primary sclerosing cholangitis. Scand J Gastroenterol 1994; 204:47–58.

Heathcote J. Review: treatment of primary biliary cirrhosis. J Gastroenterol Hepatol 1996; 11:605–960.

Kaplan MM. Primary biliary cirrhosis. N Engl J Med 1996; 335:1570–1580.

Section 10   Cirrhosis

MacSween RNM, Anthony PP, Scheuer PJ, et al. Pathology of the liver. 3d ed. Edinburgh: Churchill Livingstone, 1994.

Section 11   Portal Hypertension

De Franchis R, Primignani M. Why do varices bleed? Gastroenterol Clin North Am 1992; 21:85–96.

Hilsden RJ, Lee SS. Suspecting variceal bleeding in portal hypertensive patients. Can J Diag 1993; 10:91–103.

Sections 12 and 14   Ascites/Hepatorenal Syndrome

Andreu M, Sola R, Sitges-Serra A, et al. Risk factors for spontaneous bacterial peritonitis in cirrhotic patients with ascites. Gastroenterology 1993; 104:1133–1138.

Arroyo V, Gines P, Gerbes A, et al. Definition and diagnostic criteria of refractory ascites and hepatorenal syndrome in cirrhosis. Hepatology 1996; 23:164–176.

Bataller R, Gines P, Guevara M, et al. Hepatorenal syndrome. Semin Liver Dis 1997; 17:233–247.

Gines P, Arroyo V, Vargas V, et al. Paracentesis with intravenous infusion of albumin as compared with peritoneovenous shunting in cirrhosis with refractory ascites. N Engl J Med 1991; 325:829–835.

Runyon BA. Management of adult patients with ascites caused by cirrhosis. Hepatology 1998; 27:264–272.

Wong F, Sniderman K, Liu P, et al. The effects of transjugular intrahepatic portosystemic shunt on systemic and renal hemodynamics and sodium homeostasis in cirrhotic patients with refractory ascites. Ann Intern Med 1995; 122:816–822.

Section 13   Hepatic Encephalopathy
Haussinger D. Pathogenesis and treatment of chronic hepatic encephalopathy. Digestion 1998; 59(Suppl 2):25–27.
Mizock BA. Nutritional support in hepatic encephalopathy. Nutrition 1999; 15:220–228.
Seery JP, Aspinall RJ, Taylor-Robinson SD. Diagnosis and treatment of chronic hepatic encephalopathy. Hosp Med 1998; 59:200–204.

Section 15   Liver Transplantation
Chung SW, Greig PD, Cattral M, et al. Evaluation of liver transplantation for high-risk indications. Br J Surg. 1997; 84:189–195.
Lilly LB, Ding JW, Levy GA. The immunology of hepatic allograft rejection. In: Sorrell MF (ed.), Transplantation of the liver. 3d ed. Lippincott Williams and Wilkins, in press.
Maddrey WC, Van Thiel DH. Liver transplantation: an overview. Hepatology 1988; 8:948–959.
Munoz SJ. Long-term management of the liver transplant recipient. Med Clin North Am 1996; 90:1103–1120.
Penko ME, Tirbaso D. Overview of liver transplantation. AACN Clinical Issues 1999; 10:176–184.
Wiesner RH. U.S. FK506 Study Group. A long-term comparison of tacrolimus (FK506) versus cyclosporine in liver transplantation. Transplantation 1998; 66:493–499.

Section 16   Neoplasms Of The Liver
Bennet W, Bova J. Review of hepatic imaging and a problem-oriented approach to liver masses. Hepatology 1990; 12:761–775.
Bruix J. Treatment of hepatocellular carcinoma. Hepatology 1997; 25:259–262.
Okuda K, Wands J. Hepatocellular carcinoma. Semin Liver Dis 1999; 19:233–338.
Reddy K, Schiff E. Approach to a liver mass. Semin Liver Dis 1993; 43:423–435.
Rubin R, Mitchell D. Evaluation of the solid hepatic mass. Med Clin North Am 1996; 80:907–928.

Section 17   Liver Disease in Pregnancy
Fallon HJ, Riely CA. Liver diseases. In: Burrow GN, Ferris TF (eds.), Medical complications during pregnancy. 4th ed. Philadelphia: WB Saunders, 1995.

Section 18   Vascular Disorders of the Liver
Dunn GD, Hayes P, Breen KJ, et al. The liver in congestive heart failure: a review. Am J Med Sci 1973; 265:174–189.
Gitlin N, Serio KM. Ischemic hepatitis: widening horizons. Am J Gastroenterol 1992; 87:831–836.
Langnas AN, Sorrell MF. The Budd-Chiari syndrome: a therapeutic Gordian knot? Semin Liver Dis 1993; 13:352–359.
Wang ZG, Jones RS. Budd-Chiari syndrome. Curr Probl Surg 1996; 33:83–211.

OBJECTIVES

Jaundice/Ascites/Hepatic Encephalopathy/Liver Failure

1. Describe normal bilirubin metabolism.
2. Describe pathophysiologic mechanisms of jaundice.
3. Outline the diagnostic tests used in approaching patients with jaundice and discuss the utilization of liver function tests and liver enzymes.
4. Define jaundice.
5. Describe mechanisms of ascites formation.
6. Discuss the causes of ascites.
7. Describe the techniques and diagnostic tests used to detect ascites.
8. Discuss the indications for abdominal paracentesis and interpret the findings.
9. Distinguish between primary and secondary bacterial peritonitis.
10. Outline the management of ascites.
11. Interpret serum and urinary electrolytes in patients with ascites.
12. Discuss the mechanisms of action and side effects of drugs used in the treatment of ascites.
13. Demonstrate clinical skills in approaching patients with hepatic encephalopathy and hepatic failure.
14. List the stigmata of chronic liver disease.
15. List neurotransmitters that have possible pathophysiologic roles in hepatic encephalopathy.
16. List precipitating factors of hepatic encephalopathy.
17. Discuss the use of ammonia blood level in hepatic encephalopathy.
18. Outline the management of hepatic encephalopathy.
19. Discuss the mechanisms of action of lactulose and antibiotics in the treatment of hepatic encephalopathy.
20. Discuss the role of liver transplantation.
21. Differentiate between hepatorenal failure and prerenal azotemia.
22. Discuss the management of hepatorenal failure.

Cirrhosis

1. List underlying causes of cirrhosis.
2. List complications of cirrhosis.
3. List major mechanisms contributing to portal hypertension.
4. Discuss diagnostic methods used in patients with cirrhosis.
5. Describe indications for and complications of liver biopsy.
6. Classify portal hypertension.
7. List the consequences of portal hypertension.
8. Describe the management of patients with bleeding esophageal varices.
9. Discuss the efficacy, mechanisms of action and side effects of vasopressin and somatostatin used in treating bleeding esophageal varices.

10. Discuss the role of sclerotherapy and banding in patients with bleeding esophageal varices.
11. List major complications of sclerotherapy and banding.
12. Discuss the surgical management of portal hypertension, including the placement of a TIPS.

Hepatitis

1. List causative agents for acute hepatitis.
2. Discuss serologic tests used in hepatitis.
3. Discuss the significance of delta agent.
4. Give indications for hepatitis A and B vaccination.
5. Discuss the clinical manifestations of hepatitis A and hepatitis B infections.
6. Discuss the natural history of hepatitis C.
7. List causes of chronic liver disease.
8. Describe histologic features of mild, moderate and severe chronic hepatitis.
9. Discuss the role of corticosteroids and/or azathioprine in the treatment of autoimmune hepatitis.
10. List possible complications of corticosteroids.
11. Describe major drug-metabolizing pathways of the liver.
12. List five drugs that cause chronic liver disease.
13. Describe alcohol metabolism.
14. Give the spectrum of alcohol-related liver diseases.
15. Discuss clinical manifestations of alcoholic hepatitis.
16. Discuss the management of alcoholic hepatitis.

Cholestasis/PBC/Hemochromatosis/Wilson's Disease

1. Define cholestasis.
2. List conditions associated with cholestasis.
3. Discuss the approach to neonatal jaundice.
4. Discuss diagnostic tests used in patients with cholestasis.
5. Define primary biliary cirrhosis.
6. Discuss the clinical manifestations of and diagnostic tests for primary biliary cirrhosis (PBC).
7. Give histologic staging of PBC.
8. Discuss the treatment of PBC.
9. List the complications of PBC.
10. Discuss normal iron metabolism.
11. Describe the clinical features of hemochromatosis.
12. Discuss diagnostic tests used in hemochromatosis.
13. Discuss genetic testing for hemochromatosis and its use in patient management.

14. Discuss the management of hemochromatosis.
15. Define Wilson's disease.
16. Describe clinical manifestations of Wilson's disease.
17. Discuss the diagnostic tests for Wilson's disease.
18. Discuss the use and side effects of penicillamine in treating Wilson's disease.
19. List the diagnostic methods that differentiate liver abscesses, neoplasms and cysts.

Jaundice and Liver Disease in Children

1. Understand bilirubin metabolism in the neonate. Understand the significance of bilirubin metabolism in the fetus, and the changes that occur during the first 72 hours after birth.
2. Understand "physiologic jaundice of the newborn."
   a. Why does it occur?
   b. What brings it to an end?
   c. Under what circumstances will it be "unphysiologic"?
   d. What treatment modalities are available to modify and treat this disorder?
3. Understand the importance of careful choice of drugs in the newborn and in the nursing mother.
4. Understand the significance of unconjugated versus conjugated bilirubin in the plasma.
5. Be aware of kernicterus and its various manifestations.
6. Be aware of "hydrops fetalis," "RhoGAM®," Rh and ABO immunization.
7. Be aware of "neonatal hepatitis syndrome," and understand that it is a spectrum of specific and nonspecific disorders of the liver.
8. Be aware of "giant cell hepatitis," including its histologic abnormality.
9 Be aware of "biliary atresia," including its pathology.
10. Be aware that a number of metabolic disorders may present as "neonatal hepatitis syndrome," including galactosemia, α_1-antitrypsin deficiency, tyrosinemia, cystic fibrosis.
11. Be aware that a number of perinatal infections may present as "neonatal hepatitis syndrome," including first-degree cytomegalovirus infection and rubella.
12. Understand the significance in investigation of:
   a. HIDA scan
   b. Liver biopsy
   c. Mini lap and operative cholangiogram
   d. Alpha-fetoprotein
13. Know the prognosis of giant cell hepatitis and biliary atresia.

15

Manifestations of Gastrointestinal Disease in the Child

R.B. Scott, G. Withers, D.J. Morrison, S.A. Zamora,
H.G. Parsons, J.D. Butzner, R.A. Schreiber,
H. Machida and S.R. Martin

1. RECURRENT ABDOMINAL PAIN / R.B. Scott

1.1 Definition

Recurrent abdominal pain (RAP) is defined as at least three episodes of pain occurring over a period of at least three months in children 3 years of age or older, and which are of sufficient severity that the discomfort interferes with their activities. The overall incidence of recurrent abdominal pain is 10.8%, with 12.3% of girls and 9.5% of boys being affected. The prevalence of RAP at any given age is quite constant in school-age boys, but in girls prevalence reaches a peak between the ages of 8 and 10.

1.2 History

The discomfort of RAP is typically localized in the periumbilical region and is nonradiating. In almost all other respects it is variable in character from patient to patient – often vague and ill-defined, a dull ache or a crampy feeling, but occasionally a sharp and colicky pain. It is generally mild to moderate in intensity; the child will stop playing, sit or lie down, but in a minority of affected children the pain will be sufficiently severe to cause crying. The temporal occurrence, frequency and duration of pain are also highly variable. Pain may occur at any time of the day, be reported upon awaking, or be present until the child falls asleep. However, the discomfort will only rarely awaken the child from sleep at night. The occurrence of pain generally bears no consistent relation to the ingestion of specific foods or to meals, physical activity, defecation, urination or (in girls) menstruation. Episodes may occur infrequently or several times a day, and last from a few minutes to several hours at a time. Although aggravating factors are frequently absent, a relationship between recurrent attacks of abdominal pain and stressful situations is reported in approximately one-third of affected children. A brief rest is often cited as a relieving factor. Characteristically, treatment with antacids, anticholinergics, H_2 antagonists, barbiturates and analgesics provides no consistent relief. Episodes of RAP are commonly associated with nonspecific symptoms: pallor, nausea, headaches, limb or "growing" pains and drowsiness after attacks. Sporadic vomiting may occur, but repetitive or bilious emesis should suggest the possibility of an organic disorder. Diarrhea and documented elevation of temperature are occasionally reported but are atypical, and should also suggest an alternative etiology. Characteristically, the children are otherwise well and active between episodes.

There is nothing specific or diagnostic with respect to the past or family history of the child who presents with RAP. However, as a group, the parents and siblings of children with RAP are much more likely than those of unaffected children or those with organic disease to experience somatization of stress and to provide a history of recurrent abdominal pain/irritable bowel syndrome, peptic ulcer, severe headaches and disorders that were in the past very loosely labeled as "nervous breakdown."

1.3 Physical Signs
Except for subjective abdominal tenderness, the physical examination of children with RAP is striking in its normality. Plots of the previous and currently measured heights and weights demonstrate a normal growth velocity, and objective physical signs of disease are absent.

1.4 Psychosocial Factors
The intellectual abilities of children with RAP are identical to those of unaffected children, but certain personality traits are more commonly recognized in children with RAP than in those without. These children have been described as overachievers, overconscientious, high-strung, fussy or particular, anxious, and timid or apprehensive – generalizations that do not always apply in the individual case, however.

There is a close association between emotional status and function of the gastrointestinal tract, and the literature contains numerous anecdotal reports of children presenting with recurrent abdominal pain in whom there is (1) no organic cause, (2) a temporal relationship between discomfort and a specific stress, and (3) resolution of the pain in response to measures that relieve the stress. However, objective evidence of psychological difficulties – and not just the absence of an organic etiology – is necessary before a "psychogenic" label is applied. Using these criteria, psychological or emotional disturbance will be a primary diagnosis in only a very small number of children presenting with RAP.

1.5 Differential Diagnosis and Approach to Investigation

Although the differential diagnosis of abdominal pain is extensive, a complete history and physical examination with limited laboratory investigations should enable the physician to make a positive diagnosis of recurrent abdominal pain. In 90–95% of affected children, RAP is functional; organic disease is identified in only 5–10%. The approach to diagnosis should not be one of extensive investigation to exclude organic disease. In the majority of cases of recurrent abdominal pain, the extent of appropriate investigation should be limited to a complete blood count, urinalysis, and perhaps a stool occult blood test. Comprehensive lists of organic causes of chronic abdominal pain are available but need be referred to only when features of the history and physical examination, or the CBC and urinalysis, strongly suggest an organic problem that is not readily apparent. Specific aspects of the history that should signal concern on the part of the physician include significant recurrent pain in a child under the age of 3; consistent localization of pain away from the umbilicus; frequently being woken from sleep by pain; repetitive or bilious emesis; and any constellation of symptoms and signs that are typical of a specific organic etiology.

Urogenital and alimentary disorders are the most common organic causes of RAP. Genitourinary diseases such as recurrent infection and hydronephrosis or obstructive uropathy can present with abdominal pain. In patients with these disorders who present without urinary tract symptoms, an abnormal urinalysis and pyuria will frequently bring attention to the underlying problem.

Constipation is a common disorder and patients may experience crampy abdominal discomfort in association with the urge to defecate. A suggestive history and the demonstration on physical examination of bulky stool retained in the rectum should initiate a trial of appropriate treatment.

A history of abdominal pain, bloating, flatus and watery diarrhea that occurs with heavy ingestion of "sugarless" gums or confections suggests the possibility of malabsorption of nonabsorbable carbohydrates. The same history occurring with milk intake in individuals whose ethnic background might predispose to lactase deficiency (oriental, black or peri-Mediterranean) suggests lactose malabsorption.

Pernicious vomiting or bilious emesis in the presence of abdominal pain should always alert the clinician to the possibility of an intestinal obstruction. Malrotation or incomplete rotation of the mid-gut is a disorder that may present as a bowel obstruction and also predisposes to intestinal volvulus. Whenever malrotation is suspected an upper gastrointestinal series should be performed to determine the position of the duodenojejunal flexure, and a barium enema may be required to ensure proper location of the cecum in the lower right quadrant.

Primary peptic ulcer disease is much less common in children than in adults and frequently lacks the typical meal-related characteristics that are common with the adult presentation. A family history of peptic ulcer disease, vomiting, nighttime awakening with pain, hematemesis or melena, or unexplained anemia should suggest the diagnosis.

1.6 Pathophysiology and Treatment

A thorough history, careful physical examination and a minimum of laboratory examinations are essential to provide the data that allow a physician to reach a positive diagnosis of RAP. This care and thoroughness are crucial to the success of subsequent management because they demonstrate that the complaint has been seriously evaluated by the physician and lend credibility to the diagnosis that is subsequently rendered. Having made a positive diagnosis, it is then important to cease investigation and to educate and reassure the patient and parents. If this is not done the parents' perception that there is a significant probability of an underlying organic problem may be reinforced. On the other hand, reassurance in the absence of explanation (i.e., simply saying "Don't worry") is of little value.

It must be made clear that the discomfort of RAP is genuine, not imagined or manufactured for gain or manipulation. It is important to point out that this is a common complaint. Identify for the parent those criteria upon which you based the diagnosis of RAP: the periumbilical location of the discomfort, the absence of any constellation of historical or objective physical findings that suggest underlying organic disease, continued normal growth and development (show the parents the growth chart), continued general well-being between episodes, and a family history of similar functional complaints, if that exists. In those cases where they can be identified note the positive association of RAP with stressful situations or events and any characteristics of the child's personality that might serve to exaggerate the stress. Try to elicit and allay any specific concerns on the part of the child or parents (e.g., "Does my child have appendicitis?").

Encourage the parents to discuss potential stressful contributing events with the child, and recommend a positive approach to coping that includes a return to all normal activities. Insist on attendance at school. Discuss the prognosis of this condition with the parents and provide reassurance by offering to reassess the child should there be any change in the symptoms.

Patient education is generally very effective in relieving the parents' anxiety. Drugs, and specifically analgesics or sedatives, are not considered effective or appropriate. However, a recent prospective, double-blind, randomized control trial demonstrated a significant decrease in RAP in children given additional dietary fiber as compared to placebo.

1.7 Prognosis

Many children and their parents experience considerable immediate relief at having organic disease excluded. In the long term one-third of patients managed in this fashion are completely free of pain as adults, one-third experience continuing abdominal pain, and one-third develop alternative symptomatology such as headaches. Almost all lead unrestricted lives. The goal of management should be to develop, through education, the increased understanding and constructive coping mechanisms that will prevent symptoms from generating dysfunctional behavior.

2. VOMITING AND REGURGITATION / G. Withers and R.B. Scott

2.1 Definitions
Gastroesophageal reflux is the apparently effortless passage of gastric contents into the esophagus due to impairment of the antireflux mechanism at the gastroesophageal junction. Reflux is facilitated by the presence of a gradient in pressure between the positive pressure within the abdominal cavity and the negative pressure within the intrathoracic cavity. Vomiting, however, is a complex coordinated reflex mechanism that may occur in response to a variety of stimuli and results in forceful expulsion of gastric contents through the mouth. The vomiting reflex is controlled by the nervous system, specifically via the vomiting center in the brainstem.

2.2 The Vomiting Child

2.2.1 INTRODUCTION
The approach to the vomiting child is one of the most difficult problems in pediatrics, as the differential diagnosis is not limited to the gastrointestinal tract and includes conditions that are pediatric emergencies. In addition, persistent vomiting can lead to complications such as dehydration, electrolyte abnormalities, Mallory-Weiss tears and aspiration of gastric contents. The following comments on history, examination, diagnosis and management provide guidance as to the approach to the vomiting child, but cannot substitute for a broad knowledge of pediatrics and clinical experience that allows differentiation of the sick child from the child that is less unwell.

2.2.2 HISTORY
A number of features of the history are particuarly helpful in reaching a diagnosis:

2.2.2.1 Age
Vomiting in the neonatal and early infant period may frequently be due to structural abnormalities of the bowel, inborn errors of metabolism and withdrawal secondary to maternal drug addictions (Table 1). A complete history of the pregnancy (including drug history, past pregnancies and abortions), deliv-

TABLE 1.   Causes of vomiting according to age of presentation

---

Neonate/infancy

Gastrointestinal disorders	*Nongastrointestinal disorders*
Common	Common
Gastroenteritis	Upper respiratory tract infection
Gastroesophageal reflux	Septicemia/meningitis
Pyloric stenosis	Pneumonia
Intussusception	Urinary tract infection
Anatomic obstruction	
Atresia – esophagus, small intestine	
Malrotation and volvulus	
Hirschsprung's disease	
Rare	Rare
Meconium ileus	Inborn error of metabolism
	Raised intracranial pressure –
	tumor/hydrocephalus
	Endocrine deficiency – adrenal, thyroid
	Renal tubular acidosis
	Genetic syndromes (trisomy 21, 13, 18)

Child/adolescent

Gastrointestinal disorders	*Nongastrointestinal disorders*
Common	Common
Gastroenteritis	Infection – URTI, OM, UTI
Appendicitis	Toxin/drug ingestion
Intussusception	Bulemia
Pancreatitis	Pregnancy
Celiac disease	
Inflammatory bowel disease	
Rare	Rare
Hepatitis	Cyclic vomiting syndrome/migraine
Intestinal obstruction	Brain tumor
Peptic ulcer	Testicular torsion
Achalasia	Ovarian cyst/salpingitis
Reye's syndrome	

---

ery and postpartum period is vital. Some conditions will occur in specific age ranges: pyloric stenosis at 2 to 8 weeks of age; intussusception at 3 to 18 months. Appendicitis is rare before the age of 12 months. In older children, other conditions, especially gastroenteritis, otitis media and respiratory tract infections are more common.

2.2.2.2 *Diet*
Food allergy, the most common cause being cow's milk protein intolerance,

occurs primarily in formula-fed infants. Infant celiac disease presents only after prolonged exposure to gluten in the diet. Enzyme-deficiency diseases such as galactosemia and fructosemia manifest only after the introduction of the offending sugar into the diet.

2.2.2.3 Nature of the vomitus
Bile-stained vomitus suggests intestinal obstruction distal to the second part of the duodenum, while hematemesis suggests esophageal, gastric or duodenal mucosal disease.

2.2.2.4 Onset and duration of vomiting
Acute onset and short duration suggest a transient illness, while a longer history of vomiting suggests chronic disease, especially if associated with growth failure.

2.2.2.5 Associated symptoms
Diarrhea is a common feature accompanying gastrointestinal infection, but some looseness of stools can be found in association with other conditions such as urinary tract infections. A bloody stool resembling red currant jelly is seen classically in intussusception. If abdominal pain is present, the nature, severity and location are important. Obstruction of the GI tract often presents with central, colicky, intermittent pain, as do the cramps of gastroenteritis. Colicky pain may be accompanied by pallor, especially in intussusception. Other conditions are associated with a more constant pain, or pain in specific locations – eg., in the right iliac fossa with appendicitis, epigastric/central pain radiating to the back with pancreatitis. Fever suggests an infectious origin, and foci outside the GI tract as in meningitis should be considered. Neurological symptoms such as headache, confusion and loss of developmental skills may indicate a primary CNS pathology.

2.2.3 EXAMINATION
A complete physical assessment is required, for it is important to determine whether the child is well or sick. An initial assessment is often possible by careful observation from the end of the bed. The height, weight and head circumference should be plotted (with past recordings if possible) on a growth chart to determine whether there has been a fall-off in recent months. A rapidly expanding head circumference suggests intracranial pathology. An assessment of dehydration (including tissue turgor, mucous membranes, capillary return, pulse and blood pressure) as well as a thorough examination of each system is essential. When examining the abdomen, it is particularly important to detect any distention, masses, tenderness and especially rigidity or guarding that suggests the need for urgent surgical review.

2.2.4 INVESTIGATION

Investigation of the vomiting child is dependent on the history and the results of physical examination. An acutely ill febrile neonate requires different investigation than an older child. Investigation may include:

2.2.4.1 Blood tests

A complete blood count may show an elevated white cell count with infection or inflammation, but is relatively nonspecific. Anemia may be present and be secondary to an acute bleed, or be of a long-term nature in the presence of chronic disease (normochromic) or ongoing blood loss (hypochromic, micro-cytic). Electrolytes, urea, creatinine and anion gap provide information regarding fluid balance and metabolic status. Generally, frequent vomiting results in hypochloremic, hypokalemic alkalosis; however, acidosis may occur if dehydration is severe or secondary to an underlying metabolic disor-der. Abnormalities of urea are found in dehydration (high) and in urea cycle disorders (low). Hypo- or hypernatremia may occur if inappropriate fluid replacement is given.

2.2.4.2 Radiology

Any child with symptoms that suggest a surgical problem such as intestinal obstruction requires an urgent radiograph of the abdomen with both supine and erect films. Intestinal obstruction is suggested by dilated loops of bowel with air-fluid levels, although a similar appearance can occur with an ileus accompanying gastroenteritis. The history and examination usually allow dif-ferentiation. Other conditions have more specific appearances, such as the right upper quadrant mass in intussusception, the double-bubble appearance of duodenal atresia and a distended loop of bowel with volvulus. An abdomi-nal ultrasound may be of help in the diagnosis of pyloric stenosis (hyper-trophic mass at outlet of stomach), liver disease (gallstones and thickened gallbladder wall in cholecystitis, liver enlargement in hepatitis), pancreatitis (swollen, edematous pancreas), renal disease (hydronephrosis or small kid-neys). A child who presents with persistent bile-stained emesis requires an upper GI contrast study to exclude anatomical causes of obstruction including intestinal malrotation, webs, rings and strictures. The contrast study may include a follow-through of the small intestine to identify more distal prob-lems such as terminal Crohn's disease.

2.2.4.3 Microbiology

Urinalysis is important to exclude urinary pathology such as infection. Stool examinations for bacterial culture, ova and parasites, and viruses are indicat-ed if diarrhea is present, and for Clostridium difficile toxin if there is a recent history of antibiotic use. In the severely ill and/or febrile child with emesis and suspected sepsis or meningitis, cultures of the blood and cerebrospinal fluid are required.

2.2.4.4 *Endoscopy*

Upper gastrointestinal endoscopy may be employed to exclude mucosal disease in the esophagus (esophagitis), stomach (H. pylori gastritis, ulceration) or duodenum (ulceration, Crohn's disease, celiac disease).

2.2.5 *MANAGEMENT*

Management of the vomiting child centers on establishing an accurate diagnosis and stabilizing the patient's condition with regard to fluid and electrolyte abnormalities. Specific conditions require specific treatment, such as surgery for appendicitis and antibiotics for meningitis. Acute management of dehydration requires an accurate assessment as mild (<5%), moderate (5–10%) or severe (>10%). Fluid requirements are then calculated to replace the deficit (usually over 8, 12 or 24 hours), provide maintenance fluids (age-dependent), and replace continuing GI losses. Mild to moderate dehydration can usually be managed via the oral route unless contraindicated (e.g., preoperative conditions such as appendicitis or intestinal obstruction), while severe dehydration usually requires intravenous replacement, often with colloid as well as crystalloid solutions.

2.3 Gastroesophageal Reflux Disease (GERD)

2.3.1 *INTRODUCTION*

Effortless reflux of stomach contents is noted in approximately 50% of healthy newborn infants. In the majority of affected children it resolves over the first year of life, especially in the second six months when the dietary intake of solids increases and sitting and standing are achieved. In all children, occasional reflux after a meal is a normal event. Pathological reflux is defined as being secondary to an underlying disorder or when the reflux is complicated by failure to thrive, esophagitis or respiratory conditions such as asthma or aspiration pneumonia.

2.3.2 *PATHOGENESIS*

Reflux of gastric contents into the esophagus is prevented by the antireflux mechanism at the gastroesophageal junction, which consists primarily of the diaphragmatic crura and the lower esophageal sphincter (LES). The LES is a physiologically defined region of the lower esophagus that is maintained in a partial contractile condition to create a high-pressure zone, but relaxes as part of the swallowing reflex to allow food passage into the stomach. The primary cause of reflux is transient relaxation of the LES unrelated to swallowing, rather than a consistently low pressure of the sphincter. Although gastric volume and composition of gastric contents are important influences, the mechanism of this transient relaxation is not understood. Other factors important in the prevention of complications of reflux include esophageal peristalsis, which clears refluxed contents from the esophagus; salivary secretions, which assist in neutralizing refluxed gastric acid; esophageal mucosal resistance; and the protective pulmonary reflexes that prevent reflux into the respiratory tree.

2.3.3 CLINICAL FEATURES

A thorough history and physical examination are required to establish if possible whether the child is refluxing or vomiting. Gastroesophageal reflux is often effortless and vomiting forceful, but some overlap occurs. The onset of gastroesophageal reflux in infants is usually soon after birth. A sudden onset of reflux in a child with no past history or bilious emesis requires a search for a secondary cause. Feeding history is important. Feeds of inappropriately large volume are more likely to be refluxed. The physician should always determine whether the child is otherwise well and if not, identify symptoms or signs that suggest an underlying disorder or predispose to reflux or vomiting (Table 1). The frequency and volume of the reflux episodes should be established and any symptoms or signs of complications of gastroesophageal reflux sought.

2.3.4 COMPLICATIONS OF GASTROESOPHAGEAL REFLUX (Table 2)

2.3.4.1 *Failure to thrive*

Failure to thrive occurs in association with gastroesophageal reflux when caloric intake is insufficient as a result of the loss of milk through reflux, or when children with esophagitis limit intake due to pain or dysphagia associated with feeding.

2.3.4.2 *Esophagitis*

Esophagitis may be indicated by dysphagia, hematemesis, anemia, hypoalbuminemia and thrombocytosis. While dysphagia may occur secondary to esophageal ulceration or strictures, it may also be secondary to the impaired motility that is associated with esophagitis and often presents as food sticking.

2.3.4.3 *Respiratory complications*

Aspiration of gastric contents causing pneumonia is relatively common in the neurologically impaired child, but aspiration of food during its ingestion may also occur as a result of incoordinate swallowing. Some children with asthma, especially nocturnal asthma, may have symptoms secondary to reflux. Gas-

TABLE 2. Complications of GER

Systemic
Failure to thrive

Esophageal
Pain
Esophagitis
Hematemesis
Anemia
Hypoproteinemia
Dysphagia secondary to stricture or dysmotility
Sandifer's syndrome – an unusual posturing of head and
  upper body in infants with reflux esophagitis

Respiratory
Apnea
Bronchospasm
Laryngospasm
Aspiration pneumonia

troesophageal reflux is a less common cause of apnea in premature infants, most apnea in this age group being of central origin. Gastroesophageal reflux is not responsible for SIDS.

2.3.5 INVESTIGATION

The vast majority of infants with gastroesophageal reflux do not require additional investigation. Infants whose reflux is persistent, severe or associated with symptoms or signs of an underlying disorder require further investigation. Initial investigations should include a complete blood count, electrolytes, urea, anion gap, urinalysis and, in older infants, liver function tests and a lipase or amylase. An upper gastrointestinal contrast study (upper GI) should be performed to exclude predisposing anatomic abnormalities such as malrotation or strictures. Reflux seen during this test is a poor indicator of pathologic reflux. If the infant or child is suspected of having a complication of gastroesophageal reflux, then more extensive investigation may be required. These tests are usually available only at a tertiary center and include 24-hour pH probe monitoring of the distal esophagus to quantify the frequency, duration and pattern (postprandial, nocturnal) of reflux episodes and their association with other events. A pH probe is best performed in conjunction with respiratory monitoring to determine whether respiratory symptoms such as apnea or wheezing coincide with reflux.

Esophageal manometry may be performed to exclude motor disorders of the esophagus such as achalasia, and nuclear medicine gastric emptying studies can document those children in whom delayed gastric emptying contributes to reflux. To determine if esophagitis is present, esophageal mucosal tissue may be obtained either by endoscopic or suction biopsy. Features of esophagitis on biopsy include esophageal inflammatory infiltrate (especially an increased number of eosinophils), increased thickness of the basal layer, increased papillary height and ulceration with a neutrophil infiltrate. Bronchoscopy and bronchial-alveolar lavage to look for lipid-laden macrophages may be of help in the diagnosis of reflux-related respiratory infection.

2.3.6 MANAGEMENT

Management of most children with gastroesophageal reflux often requires no more than an explanation to parents that reflux is a normal phenomenon in infants. Conservative measures may be helpful. These include positioning the infant and smaller, more frequent thickened feedings; rarely, continuous drip feedings may be necessary. Positioning the child in a head-elevated prone position after feeds can be useful, but the use of infant seats has been shown to make reflux worse. Thickening of feeds (usually with rice formula) decreases the number of emeses and time crying, but has not been shown to decrease the time spent refluxing, as shown by esophageal pH monitoring.

For those children with complicated or severe reflux unresponsive to conservative management, drug therapy may be necessary. This usually entails the use of a prokinetic agent and/or an acid suppressant. Cisapride is the prokinetic agent of choice as it lacks the neurological and respiratory side effects of other prokinetic agents such as metoclopramide and bethanechol. Cisapride acts peripherally to increase the release of acetylcholine from the intestinal myenteric plexus and has been shown to be effective in the treatment of gastroesophageal reflux in children. It is given orally approximately 30 minutes prior to feedings at a dose of 0.2mg/kg/dose q.i.d. up to a maximal dose of 0.3 mg/kg/dose. It is well tolerated and side effects are generally limited to an increased stool frequency. However, recent reports have shown that cisapride can induce life-threatening ventricular arrhythmias in individuals with conduction abnormalities such as a prolonged Q–T interval; it should be used with extreme caution in such patients. Acid suppression is helpful in those patients with evidence of esophagitis or reflux-associated pain. An H_2 antagonist such as ranitidine or cimetidine is often sufficient for pain relief, but patients with esophagitis may require more powerful acid suppression with a proton pump inhibitor such as omeprazole to achieve healing.

Surgery may be necessary in patients with gastroesophageal reflux who fail medical therapy or who have life-threatening reflux-associated apnea. Nissen fundoplication, where the fundus of the stomach is wrapped 360° around the lower esophagus to produce an esophageal high-pressure zone, is the operation of choice. Fundoplication is effective, and a successful clinical outcome is seen in almost 90% of patients at five years, but major complications such as postoperative adhesions, wound infection and pneumonia occur in approximately 10–20% of patients. Fundoplication is less successful in controlling reflux in neurologically impaired children, where clinical success rates are of the order of 50–60% and complication rates are higher. Recently, newer surgical techniques such as partial wraps (<360°) and laparoscopic fundoplication have become available, but it is not yet known whether the long-term success rates or complications of these procedures differ from the open Nissen technique.

3. COLIC / D.J. Morrison

The term *colic* is used to describe intense or excessive crying or fussiness in an otherwise healthy infant. This typically starts in the second or third week of life and resolves by three to four months (although it can persist longer). A variety of definitions of excessive crying have been used. Perhaps the most useful is Wessel's "rule of threes": more than three hours per day for more than three days per week for more than three weeks. The most common time of day seems to be early evening. In extreme cases the crying may occur throughout the day and night. Prospective studies have shown that colic is common. Dr. T.B. Brazleton, using crying diaries kept by parents, found that 35% of 6-week-old infants cried for more than three hours per day. Typically these infants cry longer, though not more frequently, than other infants and are more difficult to console.

The etiology of colic is unknown. The fact that it occurs in healthy babies, follows the crying pattern of normal infants and resolves without later sequelae has prompted its description as a disorder of development.

Colic occurs with equal frequency in breastfed and formula-fed infants. The question of milk intolerance as a possible cause of colic is frequently raised, and formula changes are a commonly tried intervention. Cow's milk protein sensitivity probably does cause colic in a small subgroup of infants. These infants may also experience weight loss, vomiting and diarrhea. With such a history, a trial of casein-hydrolyzed formula would be appropriate. The incidence of lactose or carbohydrate malabsorption does not appear to be different in patients with colic compared to those without.

Intestinal immaturity with delayed development of normal patterns of intestinal motor activity and resulting poor propulsion has been proposed as an etiology. Many infants with colic appear uncomfortable, draw their legs up and pass wind. This may be secondary to air swallowing with crying. Antispasmodics and antiflatulents have generally not been shown to help. There is evidence that one antispasmodic, dicylomine hydrochloride, may be effective; however, concern regarding respiratory distress and apnea preclude its use.

Intestinal hormones may play a role in colic; this role is incompletely understood at this time, however.

At one time, colic was blamed on "overanxious mothers," but there is no scientific confirmation of this etiology. Certainly, prolonged crying in an infant can itself give rise to anxiety in parents.

In the evaluation of a patient with colic it is first essential to take a thorough history to rule out pathological causes of crying, inquire about feeding practices (including formula preparation and burping procedure) and soothing techniques. For an accurate description of duration of crying it is useful to have the mother keep a diary over a few days. A thorough physical examination must be performed to assess growth and development as well as rule out illness (particularly infection) or intestinal obstruction.

If no apparent cause is found for the crying it is first essential to relieve parental guilt and reassure parents that they do not cause the colic. Explaining the natural history of colic (frequency and duration) can be very helpful. Trials of soothing techniques (carrying the baby in a body carrier, car rides or automatic rockers) may be useful. Advising parents on obtaining relief – babysitting or even a weekend away – is often the best intervention. Finally, a trial of casein-hydrolyzed formula for the infant or a milk-free diet for the breastfeeding mother may be useful, particularly if additional symptoms suggesting food allergy are present.

4. CHRONIC CONSTIPATION, ENCOPRESIS AND SOILING /
R.B. Scott

4.1 Definition
Constipation is a symptom indicative of an abnormality in stool or its elimination: the stool is too large or too hard; passage is too infrequent, painful or incomplete. There is an extremely wide range in what constitutes normal bowel habit, and this changes markedly between birth and adolescence. As a generalization, stool frequency is less in the formula-fed than in the breastfed infant. The formula-fed infant tends to pass 3 to 5 bowel motions per day; breastfed infants, however, can be very well and pass soft stool without difficulty with a frequency that may range from 10 stools per day to 1 stool every 10 days. At 2 to 3 years of age the modal frequency of defecation is 2 bowel motions per day. From age 3 to adulthood bowel motions are passed between 3 times per day and 3 times per week in 96% of individuals. One-quarter of all cases of chronic constipation begin during the first year of life, but the majority of children affected develop problems in the preschool years. Chronic constipation is a very common cause of referral to pediatric gastroenterology practices and tends to affect males slightly more often than females (by a ratio of 1.5:1).

Encopresis is a term that has become synonymous with a voluntary or involuntary passage of stool in an inappropriate place (usually the underclothing). *Soiling* refers to the constant involuntary seepage of stool associated with fecal impaction. Chronic constipation complicated by encopresis or soiling is reported to make up 3% of referrals to large teaching hospital clinics. It occurs in 1–2% of 7-year-old primary school children, and is more prevalent in males than females (by a ratio of 5:1).

4.2 Pathophysiology

The colon absorbs water and electrolytes, and collects and packages indigestible residue as a formed stool for later evacuation. Colonic motor function is specialized to perform these functions. Repeated ring contractions or haustral contractions cause to-and-fro shuttling of luminal contents, delaying their transit and enhancing absorption. One to three times a day mass movements transport colonic contents distally. Normal defecation is a combination of autonomic and voluntary functions. Distention of the rectum is the stimulus that initiates reflex defecation. When the fecal bolus distends the rectum, sensory receptors in the rectal wall are stimulated, leading to conscious perception of rectal distention and involuntary relaxation of the internal anal sphincter. In the absence of voluntary contraction of the puborectalis muscle and the external anal sphincter, the fecal bolus is expelled.

Intestinal transit time is closely related to defecation frequency. The reduction of frequency of defecation with age is associated with an increase in intestinal transit time. In the first month of life transit time is 8 hours, at age 2 it is 16 hours, between 3 and 13 years it is 26 hours and in an adult it is 48 hours or more. Transit time is largely influenced by the amount of fiber in the diet. Fiber-rich diets favor the retention of water and result in increased stool weight and volume, shorter transit time and more frequent defecation. Normal stools have a water content of 60–85% of mass. An increase or decrease in volume of stool water of as little as 100 mL in the adult can represent diarrhea or constipation, respectively. In constipation the increased desiccation of colonic contents is due to increased duration of mucosal contact rather than an alteration of mucosal absorptive function.

4.3 Differential Diagnosis

In the child who presents as having a difficulty with elimination, the physician must determine whether the problem is functional, organic or a parental misinterpretation of symptoms. Examples of the latter include the healthy, breastfed infant who passes a soft stool without difficulty once every 10 days and the normal infant who passes soft stools on a regular basis but frequently becomes fussy, cries or turns red and grunts while defecating. Similarly, 1- to 2-year-old children will interrupt their other activities, become flushed, stand in a rigid posture, and appear to be concentrating on the passage of a bowel motion that is difficult to pass. Often there is no difficulty and these children are in fact attempting to utilize a newly acquired skill and withhold passage of a bowel movement.

Organic constipation may be the result of mechanical obstruction, perianal difficulties causing painful defecation, metabolic or medical disorders, neuromuscular disorders or medications that favor the development of constipation. Mechanical obstruction may occur as a result of congenital, post-surgical or inflammatory stenosis at the level of the anal canal; obstruction by an intrinsic mass such as adenocarcinoma in the adult; or obstruction by an extrinsic mass such as neoplasia or pregnancy. Painful defecation may result from trauma or surgery to the anorectal region, anal fissures, thrombosed hemorrhoids or a perianal abscess/infection. Metabolic and medical disorders that have been associated with organic constipation include hypercalcemia, hypokalemia, hypothyroidism, porphyria and conditions leading to polyurea and dehydration, including diabetes insipidus, diabetes mellitus and chronic renal failure. Organic constipation can result from dysfunction at all levels of the neuromuscular axis: central nervous disorders such as cerebral palsy or stroke; abnormalities of the peripheral nervous system, including myelomeningocele, trauma, polio or diabetic nephropathy; conditions affecting the enteric nervous system such as Hirschsprung's disease; and skeletal or smooth-muscle myopathies. Medications known to predispose to constipation include the opiates, anticholinergics, tricyclic antidepressants and phenothiazines, aluminum-containing antacids, diuretics, iron and vincristine.

Precipitants of functional constipation include decreased fluid intake or increased fluid losses; decreased physical activity; a diet that is low in fiber, contains excessive milk or is nutritionally insufficient; and anything that leads to chronic involuntary inhibition of defecation. Imposed schedules and some children's reluctance to use different facilities are examples of the latter; children may also be simply too busy to attend to the urge to defecate.

In the child who presents with encopresis, the physician must consider whether the incontinence of stool is due to a congenital or acquired neuromuscular disorder, or a behavioral disturbance. However, most of these children have soiling secondary to chronic fecal impaction and overflow. In such cases children may have secondary behavioral disturbance but their primary problem is one of gross rectal distention with loss of the rectal–anorectal angle and the continence function of the puborectalis sling. Whenever there is a mass movement the only residual continence mechanism in these children is the external voluntary anal sphincter, which rapidly fatigues, leading to involuntary soiling. It is not unusual for younger children to deny any knowledge that this is occurring, because if they admit to awareness their parents often expect

TABLE 3. Differentiating features of functional constipation and aganglionic megacolon (Hirschsprung's disease)

	Functional constipation	Hirschsprung's disease
Age of onset	Acquired sometime after birth	Present from birth
Growth	Normal	Poor
History	Coercive bowel training Colicky abdominal pain Rarely abdominal distention Periodic voluminous stools Soiling	Lack of coercive bowel training Rarely abdominal pain Abdomen distended Pellet-like or ribbon-like stools No soiling
Past history	No episodes of intestinal obstruction	Frequent episodes of intestinal obstruction
Physical exam	Well child Feces-packed, capacious rectum	Nutritional status poor Empty rectum
Barium enema	Absence of transition zone and a distended distal colon	Presence of transition zone
Manometry	Rectoanal inhibitory reflex intact	Absent rectoanal inhibitory reflex
Biopsy	Normal	Absence of ganglia in myenteric plexus and hypertrophy of nerve trunks
Course	Negligible mortality Variable morbidity	High mortality, depending on promptness of diagnosis, and variable morbidity, depending on type and outcome of surgical management

them to be able to prevent soiling. Such children will regain continence only if their gross rectal distention is relieved.

4.3.1 DIFFERENTIATION OF CHRONIC FECAL RETENTION FROM HIRSCHSPRUNG'S DISEASE

The most frequently considered organic problem in the differential diagnosis of patients presenting with functional constipation is Hirschsprung's disease. These two conditions can frequently be distinguished by significant differences in the history and physical examination. These are detailed in Table 3.

4.4 Treatment

If an organic cause of constipation is suspected, it should be investigated and treated; however, most patients with constipation have no underlying organic abnormality. In patients with mild constipation, dietary modification with an increase in fluid or fiber intake, establishment of a regular bowel habit with a prompt response to the urge to defecate, and appropriate physical activity may be a sufficient remedy. Many individuals will require a laxative in addition. Patients whose constipation is complicated by fecal impaction and soiling require very aggressive management, including education, clearing of the impaction, establishment of a regular bowel habit, laxative therapy titrated to achieve the passage of a soft bowel motion daily, appropriate diet and exercise, and (in younger children) positive reinforcement for appropriate behavior. Therapy must be aggressive and persist for three to six months until the distended and dysfunctional colon has an opportunity to return to normal caliber, tone and sensitivity.

The fecal impaction can generally be cleared by administration of Fleet® enemas at intervals of 12 hours (generally 2–4 are sufficient). There is a variety of laxatives on the market whose mechanism of action includes hydrophilic (dietary fiber), lubricant (mineral oil), osmotic (glycerin suppositories, lactulose, magnesium citrate/sulfate and sodium phosphate/biphosphate), secretory (ricinoleic acid, free hydroxy fatty acids, dihydroxy bile acids, and dioctyl sodium sulfosuccinate) and motor stimulants (anthraquinones and diphenylmethene derivatives). Natural bran, methylcellulose, polycarbophil and psyllium are all forms of fiber that by virtue of their ability to bind water within their structure lead to an increase in stool bulk and weight, and are associated with more rapid transit and more frequent bowel motions. These are safe and effective in children if sufficient amounts are taken, but children's compliance is often poor. Mineral oil is the lubricant laxative of choice in the pediatric age group because of better compliance. It is an indigestible, tasteless oil that adds bulk, softens and lubricates the stool and exerts an additional osmotic effect. Its aspiration can lead to lipoid pneumonia; therefore this form of treatment should be avoided in patients known to aspirate or with a history of reflux. Taken with meals mineral oil will result in a degree of fat-soluble vitamin malabsorption. This problem can be addressed by giving it as a single dose several hours after the evening meal. Properly used, mineral oil is an inexpensive, well-tolerated, effective and safe children's laxative. In those children who refuse mineral oil the osmotic agent lactulose is a more expensive but effective alternative.

Constipation in the very young infant can often be managed by adding prune juice to the diet or brown sugar to the formula, or by feeding the infant purées with a natural laxative action (containing prunes, for example). Mineral oil is frequently not a good choice in this age group because of the frequency of gastroesophageal reflux.

5. GROWTH FAILURE AND MALNUTRITION / S.A. Zamora and H.G. Parsons

5.1 Definitions

Failure to thrive (FTT), a widely used term in industrialized countries, is not distinct from protein-energy malnutrition encountered in children in developing countries [1]. Both terms describe a spectrum of pathologic states resulting from childhood undernutrition. FTT accounts for 1–5% of tertiary hospital admissions for infants and is reported in about 10% of low-income preschool children seen in community-based settings.

FTT is used to describe infants and young children whose growth is substantially less than that of their peers. Although no consensus exists on anthropometric indicators of FTT [2], most commonly used systems for selection of samples of FTT in hospital or clinic studies include children with a weight less than the 5th percentile on reference growth charts [1]. The key to the identification of FTT is ascertainment of longitudinal progression of growth with serial measurements over time. A weight decrement of more than two major channels of growth (centiles) from a previously established growth channel or the loss of 10% of an infant's weight is evidence of FTT [1, 3]. A reduction in growth velocity is a particularly helpful indicator of abnormality in the 5% of otherwise normal children who plot out below the 5th percentile, but follow a growth channel parallel to the normal growth curves.

Acute malnutrition typically results in "wasting," where weight is depressed out of proportion to height. Chronic malnutrition will also affect height and may lead to "stunting," in which weight and height are proportionally decreased. Head circumference is the last parameter to be affected by malnutrition.

Extreme conditions of protein-energy malnutrition are rarely encountered in industrialized countries. Marasmus occurs after severe deprivation, primarily of calories, and is characterized by growth retardation and wasting of muscle and subcutaneous fat. Kwashiorkor results from a protein deficiency exceeding the calorie deficiency and is manifested by edema (secondary to hypoalbuminemia) and muscle wasting.

5.2 Diagnostic Categories

FTT can be categorized as organic, nonorganic, or of mixed etiology. Organic FTT involves children who have a specific diagnosable disorder implicated in the failure to grow and accounts for a minority of cases: about 20–30% of children hospitalized for FTT [5, 6] and a lower proportion of children seen in outpatient clinics. Organic causes of FTT can be attributed to prenatal influences (congenital anomalies, in utero insults such as infections or toxins, prematurity) or to ongoing or recurring illnesses after the neonatal period. Nonorganic FTT suggests that the cause is primarily external to the infant; it accounts for the majority of cases. It may result from the individual temperament of the child (sickly, difficult child), difficult interactions between the child and the caregiver, nonfeeding, family poverty, stress or loss.

For both organic and nonorganic FTT, the main pathophysiologic denominator resulting in growth delay is an imbalance between nutrient availability and requirements. This imbalance results from a suboptimal intake (psychosocial factors, organic disease interfering with feeding); increased losses (gastroesophageal reflux, vomiting, diarrhea) or malabsorption of nutrients; and more rarely, increased needs (hyperkinetic states, hyperthyroidism). Inborn errors of metabolism may result in FTT despite an adequate balance between nutrient availability and requirements.

A useful diagnostic approach recognizes three types of FTT according to the deviance of head circumference, height and weight on growth charts [8] (Table 4).

5.2.1 TYPE I

Head circumference is normal and weight is reduced out of proportion to height (Figure 1). This pattern results from an imbalance between calorie availability and requirements. The majority of patients with FTT fall into this category; adverse psychosocial factors are the most frequent contributors.

5.2.2 TYPE II

Head circumference is normal or enlarged and weight is reduced in proportion to (or slightly more than) the reduction in height (Figure 2). This pattern is mainly represented by children with constitutional growth delay, familial short stature or endocrinopathies. Chronic malnutrition resulting in stunting may also fall into this group (celiac disease). Comparison of the children's height age and bone age with chronologic age (see Section 5.4.2) further identifies three subgroups:

Type IIa – Most frequently bone age and height age are proportionally delayed beyond chronologic age (e.g., constitutional growth delay).

Type IIb – Bone age is in accordance with chronologic age but height age is retarded (e.g., familial short stature).

Type IIc – Bone age is significantly more delayed than chronologic age (e.g., malnutrition).

5.2.3 TYPE III

Head circumference is subnormal and weight and height are proportionally reduced (Figure 3). These children are frequently described as dysmorphic and may present with associated developmental delay or seizures. Patients in

TABLE 4.   Differential diagnosis of failure to thrive based on anthropometric criteria

Type I – HC normal	*W reduction >>> H reduction*
Inadequate caloric intake	
Nonorganic FTT (psychosocial factors)*	Genitourinary diseases (e.g., UTI)
Neurologic and neuromuscular diseases	Malignancy
Chronic infection	Cardiovascular disorders
Increased losses	
Gastroesophageal reflux or vomiting	
Diarrhea	
Malabsorption	
Cystic fibrosis	Parasitic infestation
Milk protein enteropathy	Immunodeficiency
Celiac disease	Inflammatory bowel disease
Shwachman syndrome	Hepatobiliary disorders
Short gut	Intermittent midgut volvulus
Impaired caloric utilization	
Glycogen storage disease	Chronic infection
Galactosemia	Renal disease
Fructose intolerance	Malignancy
Phenylketonuria	Anemia
Increased metabolic requirements	
Hyperthyroidism	Hyperkinesia (attention deficit disor-
Diencephalic syndrome	ders, athetoid cerebral palsy)

Type II – HC normal or enlarged	*W reduction = or > H reduction*
a. Bone age delay = height age delay	
Constitutional growth delay	Metabolic disease
Celiac disease	Chronic diseases
b. Bone age not delayed; height age delayed	
Familial short stature	
c. Bone age delay >>> height age delay	
Endocrine disorder (growth hormone deficiency,	Maternal deprivation syndrome
hypothyroidism, hypopituitarism)	(deprivation dwarfism)

Type III – HC subnormal	*W reduction = H reduction*
Dysmorphic	
Chromosomal abnormalities	Birth asphyxia
Congenital infections	CNS abnormalities
Toxic intrauterine exposure (alcohol, drugs,	Familial
anticonvulsants)	

FTT = failure to thrive; HC = head circumference; W = weight; H = height or length
*Environmental causes are the most common source of problems.
SOURCE: Adapted from Roy CC, Silverman A, Alagille D (eds.). Pediatric clinical gastroenterol-
ogy. 4th ed. St. Louis: Mosby-Year Book, 1995:3–10.

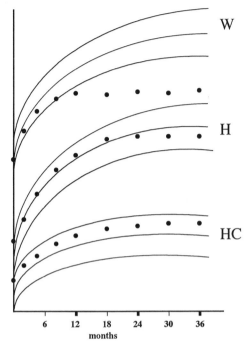

FIGURE 1.   Type I failure to thrive. *W* refers to weight, *H* to height or length, *HC* to head circumference.

this category may have chromosomal abnormalities, intrauterine or perinatal insults (congenital infections, alcohol, drug or anticonvulsant exposure during pregnancy, severe prematurity, birth asphyxia), CNS abnormalities and more rarely a familial phenotype.

5.3 Pitfalls in Diagnosis

The size of an infant at birth is more related to maternal size and intrauterine influences than to genetic factors. Consequently, growth across percentiles (increased or decreased growth velocity) between birth and 2 years of age is to be expected in some children owing to genetic adjustment. Patterns of normal growth in the first two years of life can then present as factitious FTT [2]: familial short stature and constitutional growth delay. Term infants born small for gestational age and premature infants can also present diagnostic problems.

5.3.1 *FAMILIAL (GENETIC) SHORT STATURE*

Familial short stature is genetically determined, and these children are short

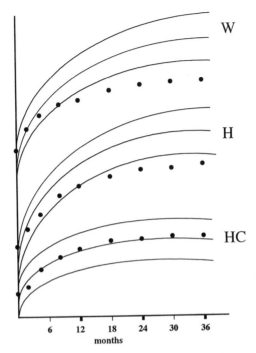

Figure 2. Type II failure to thrive. W refers to weight, H to height or length, HC to head circumference.

throughout life. The final height is determined by mid-parental height, and a readjustment with drop in percentiles may take place in the first two years of age. After this deceleration phase, these children grow normally at constant rates and enter puberty at an appropriate age. Weight in these children is usually proportional to length, and they have no bone age delay. The diagnosis of familial short stature is confirmed on the basis of a normal history and physical examination and if, during follow-up, the child maintains the new growth channel appropriate to his or her genetic potential.

5.3.2 CONSTITUTIONAL GROWTH DELAY

Children with constitutional growth delays are "slow growers" and "late bloomers." They present with marked deceleration of growth in the first three years of life and then follow a lower growth channel into adolescence, when a late pubertal growth spurt occurs and they catch up to their original growth channel [4]. The deceleration begins usually between 3 and 6 months, will be greatest in the first two years of life and frequently results in these children

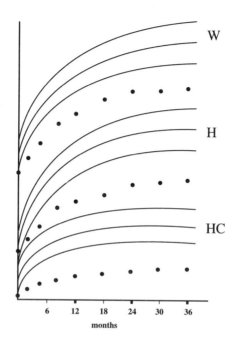

FIGURE 3.   Type III failure to thrive. W refers to weight, H to height or length, HC to head circumference.

falling well below the 5th percentile both for weight and height. These children have a two- to four-year delay in skeletal maturation and will enter puberty late. There is frequently a family history of this type of delayed growth and pubertal development.

5.3.3 *SMALL FOR GESTATIONAL AGE AND PREMATURE INFANTS*
Small for gestational age infants are a heterogeneous group who fail to grow in utero (intrauterine growth retardation, or IUGR) as a result of environmental, maternal, placental or fetal factors. Asymmetric IUGR (birth weight disproportionally more depressed than length or head circumference) frequently results from placental insufficiency. These newborns have a good prognosis for catch-up growth if they are provided with enhanced postnatal nutrition. Symmetric IUGR may result from intrauterine infections, chromosomal abnormalities or prenatal exposure to toxins such as alcohol, drugs or anticonvulsants. Infants who are symmetrically growth retarded at birth have a poor prognosis for later growth. Because of the initial small size, the weight gain and growth progression of these patients may give the false impression

of FTT; however, if the patient doubles the birth weight by 4 months of age and triples it by 1 year of age, FTT must be excluded.

In premature infants corrected age should be used in growth monitoring or they will be inappropriately labeled as FTT. The age at measurement should be corrected for the number of weeks the child was premature (the difference between 40 weeks and gestational age). Corrected age should be used to 18 months for head circumference, 24 months for weight and 40 months for height [5]. Premature infants without serious medical problems may show catch-up growth in the first year of life, whereas more severely affected premature infants may not show catch-up growth but should at least parallel reference curves [1].

5.4 Assessment of FTT

Assessment of infants with FTT always demands a very careful history and physical examination in order to minimize the need for investigations. Particularly important are a thorough dietary assessment, documentation of adverse psychosocial factors and an anthropometric evaluation.

5.4.1 *DIETARY HISTORY AND PSYCHOSOCIAL FACTORS*

The dietary history should document the child's feeding history (breastfeeding and/or method of formula preparation, concentration and volume of formula consumed, age at introduction and acceptance of solids, ability to feed independently), food allergies and difficulties in chewing or swallowing. A three- to seven-day dietary record should ideally be evaluated by a nutritionist or dietitian for adequacy of calories, protein intake and micronutrients. Parents' misconceptions about nutrition may be detrimental. Families concerned with cardiovascular diseases or obesity may restrict and limit the nutritional intake of the infants (through use of skim milk or restriction of sweet food). "Therapeutic fasting" for treatment of diarrhea and elimination diets employed in suspected cases of "food allergy" may also result in caloric insufficiency. Excessive fruit juice intake may result in an unbalanced diet with decreased consumption of milk and snacks.

Considering that the majority of cases of FTT have no organic basis, contributing psychosocial factors should be evaluated in detail: poverty, familial dysfunction, disordered parent–child interaction, chronic illness, depression or intellectual impairment of the caregiver. A feeding disorder is best appreciated by direct observation of a meal. Is the child correctly positioned? Are there inappropriate distractions? Is the interaction between child and caregiver appropriate?

5.4.2 *ANTHROPOMETRIC EVALUATION*

Repeated, rather than cross-sectional, accurate anthropometric measurements are essential in establishing FTT. Head circumference should always be recorded in children of less than 36 months. Length should be measured recumbent before 2 years of age. Extrapolation of weight and length horizontally to the 50th percentile on growth charts will define the child's weight age and height age, which can be compared to chronologic age and bone age (skeletal maturation). Parental heights and weights will give an idea of the child's genetic growth potential. Mid-parental height is obtained by averaging the parents' height and then adding 6.5 cm for boys or subtracting 6.5 cm for girls.

The most accurate technique for classifying growth deficiency uses Z scores, where the deviance from the median reference value is expressed in units of standard deviations for that population:

$$\text{Z score} = \frac{\text{actual measured value} - \text{median reference value}}{\text{standard deviation for age of reference population}}$$

A Z score of 0.00 is equivalent to the 50th percentile. A Z score of -2.00 SD corresponds to a percentile of 2.3 and is currently recommended by the WHO as a cut-off value for growth deficiencies [1]. Z scores are very sensitive to growth deviances but their calculation necessitates the use of computer software [6].

Other systems commonly used to categorize malnutrition express the child's weight as a percent of the median weight-for-age (Table 5) or as a percent of the median weight-for-height (Table 6). Percent of the median weight- (or height-) for-age is obtained by dividing the actual measurement by the median value for that age. Median weight-for-height (ideal weight for height) is obtained by extrapolating height horizontally to the 50th percentile and taking the median weight for that age. Comparing the child's height to the median height-for-age gives an idea of the severity of stunting or chronic malnutrition. It must be noticed that these methods applied to the same population may classify children in different grades of malnutrition [7]. Therefore, appreciation of the severity of malnutrition should not rely exclusively on these ratios.

On physical examination a clinical appreciation of nutritional status is readily available by inspecting the child's buttocks (flat in malnutrition) and subscapular and limb muscles. Evaluation of the triceps skin fold (index of fat tissue) and mid-arm muscle circumference requires the use of published nomograms and reference tables [8, 9]. Among other physical signs that may be associated with malnutrition are a distended abdomen (malabsorptive states), edema (hypoalbuminemia) and clubbing (chronic disease). More severe cases may show pallor (anemia), glossitis-stomatitis, pellagroid dermatitis, ecchymosis (vitamin K deficiency) and bone deformities (vitamin D deficiency).

TABLE 5. Classification of severity of underweight

Grade of malnutrition	Percent of median weight-for-age
Normal	90–110
I. Mild	75–89
II. Moderate	60–74
III. Severe	<60

SOURCE: Data from Gomez F et al. Malnutrition in infancy and childhood, with special reference to kwashiorkor. Advance Pediat 1955; 7:131–169.

TABLE 6. Classification of severity of wasting and stunting

Grade of malnutrition	Percent of median weight-for-height (wasting)	Percent of median height-for-age (stunting)
Normal	90–110	95
I. Mild	80–89	90–94
II. Moderate	70–79	85–89
III. Severe	<70	<85

SOURCE: Data from Waterlow JC. Classification and definition of protein-calorie malnutrition. BMJ 1972; 3:566–569.

5.5 Investigations

Because poor nutrition and psychosocial factors are the major contributors to FTT, investigations are of very limited diagnostic help. Large series of hospitalized children have documented that only about 1% of laboratory studies performed helped identify an organic etiology to FTT. Furthermore, no test was useful in the absence of a specific indication from the history and physical exam. If the clinical evaluation is normal, children with decreased growth should be followed at regular intervals without extensive investigations; frequently, one of the physiologic variations of growth (Table 4) will be identified. Basic tests may be indicated: urine analysis, CBC and differential, albumin, calcium, phosphorus and alkaline phosphatase. Particularly useful is a stool smear for fat. In cases of moderate and severe malnutrition, nutrient deficiencies should be documented (especially iron, zinc, vitamin D).

5.6 Management

Management of FTT generally necessitates a multidisciplinary approach to address both psychosocial and medical factors (nutritionist and/or dietitian, physician and/or nurse, social worker and/or psychologist). Parental education regarding the infant's nutritional needs is essential. Financial difficulties and family dysfunction should be addressed in order to obtain compliance with treatment. The goal of nutritional treatment is to promote compensatory catch-up growth, which is achieved only if the child receives nutrients in excess of the normal requirements for age. Daily caloric needs may be estimated in calories per kilogram as follows:

$$\text{kcal/kg} = \frac{120 \text{ kcal/kg} \times \text{median weight for current height}}{\text{current weight (kg)}}$$

Protein intake should be 1.5–2 times the RDNI[1] for age. As it is not generally possible for a child to eat twice the normal volume, the usual diet must be fortified to increase nutrient density. This is achieved in infants by increasing the caloric density of the formula (normal dilution = 20 kcal/oz or 0.67 kcal/mL) to 24 kcal/oz (by increasing the formula concentration) or 28–30 kcal/oz (by adding polycose or oil). In toddlers, food preferred by the child should be enriched by adding cheese, peanut butter, butter, vegetable oil or carbohydrate additives. Small frequent feedings should be offered. In cases of moderate and severe malnutrition a multivitamin supplement containing iron and zinc should be prescribed routinely during nutritional rehabilitation.

Management of severe malnutrition should be done in hospital with close monitoring of electrolytes and fluid imbalances, which can be lethal if not managed prospectively. Potassium and phosphorus depletion are particularly worrisome. Levels should be monitored daily. Phosphorus supplementation should be routinely instituted with refeeding. Initial caloric intakes should be low, 25 kcal/kg in infants and 50 kcal/kg in children, and advanced daily in 25 kcal/kg increments if tolerated [1].

5.7 Prognosis

Provided that intervention is early and effective, and depending on the primary underlying psychosocial or organic factors, there is a potential for catch-up growth in children with FTT. Long-term follow-up studies on children hospitalized for FTT demonstrate impairment of both physical and mental development in a substantial number. Malnutrition produces functional alterations of behavior at any age, but the brain is particularly vulnerable during the critical period of brain growth that extends from mid-gestation to 3 years of life. In the absence of any organic disease, the duration of malnutrition in the first year of life and the disturbed environment in which the child remains seem to determine the adverse long-term sequelae.

---

[1] Recommended daily nutritional intake (RDNI) identifies the adequate intake of essential nutrients judged to meet the needs of all healthy people in Canada. Except for energy, the RDNI is established at two standard deviations above the estimated mean requirements.

6. ACUTE DIARRHEA IN CHILDREN / J.D. Butzner

6.1 Introduction

A North American child will develop between 6 and 12 episodes of acute diarrhea before the age of 5. This contributes to approximately 12% of childhood hospitalizations and approximately 300 deaths per year. Worldwide, acute diarrheal disease is the leading cause of childhood morbidity and mortality, accounting for three million deaths each year. Most deaths are caused by failure to treat acute dehydration properly and to correct electrolyte imbalances. Studies from both the developing and developed world demonstrate that hospitalization can be avoided and morbidity and mortality can be drastically reduced by the prompt introduction of two simple treatments: oral rehydration therapy and early refeeding. In spite of recommendations to use oral rehydration therapy and to continue or resume feeding early in mild to moderate diarrheal illnesses, the use of unsuitable treatments persists. These include unnecessary intravenous therapy, inappropriate oral fluids (unbalanced sugar-electrolyte solutions), prolonged starvation with a slow introduction of limited feeds, and the inappropriate use of antibiotics as well as antimotility and antidiarrheal agents.

6.2 Pathophysiology of Acute Diarrheal Disease

An understanding of the physiology of intestinal fluid, electrolyte and nutrient transport provides a basis for understanding the mechanisms of acute diarrheal disease and successful oral rehydration therapy. Water absorption occurs primarily in the small intestine, driven by osmotic gradients that depend on the transport of the electrolytes sodium and chloride, as well as nutrients such as glucose and amino acids. Sodium, glucose and several amino acids are transported through the apical membranes of intestinal epithelial cells by sodium-dependent nutrient cotransporters. Sodium is then transported from the cell across the basolateral membrane to the extracellular space by the enzyme Na^+/K^+-ATPase. This enzyme utilizes energy to reduce the intracellular sodium concentration, which produces a negative extracellular electrical charge. The resultant electrochemical gradient facilitates sodium absorption by the epithelial cell, which drives the sodium-dependent nutrient cotransporters. The anion chloride is absorbed to maintain electrical neutrality across the epithelium, and water is passively absorbed in response to the transport of these electrolytes and nutrients. Successful oral rehydration therapy with balanced sugar-salt solutions depends upon these simple physiologic principles.

Diarrhea associated with small intestinal injury in infants and children is caused by four major mechanisms. These include (1) increased osmotic fluid losses, (2) inappropriate secretion, (3) inflammation associated with exudative fluid and protein losses and finally, (4) altered intestinal motility. The most frequent cause of osmotic diarrhea and acute infectious diarrhea worldwide is viral enteritis due to the rotavirus. This virus stimulates the shedding of mature absorptive epithelial cells from the small intestinal villi. These cells are replaced by immature cells with inadequately developed transporters, including the sodium-dependent glucose cotransporter and Na^+/K^+-ATPase. When unbalanced sugar-electrolyte solutions such as fruit juice, soda pop and broth are provided as treatments, the intestine's immature transport capacity is overwhelmed. The osmotic forces created by nonabsorbed nutrients that remain in the lumen stimulate watery diarrheal fluid losses. Children with intestinal injury caused by an acute enteritis may also develop secondary disaccharidase deficiencies, which contribute to osmotic diarrhea by the malabsorption of the disaccharides lactose and sucrose. Interestingly, the frequency of this complication has been markedly decreased in children with mild to moderate dehydration by the prompt implementation of treatment protocols that stress oral rehydration and early refeeding. Osmotic diarrhea is also caused by infections due to Giardia lamblia, Cryptosporidium, Salmonella and enteroadherent E. coli. Medications that contain nonabsorbable sugars such as sorbitol, lactulose and mannitol and poorly absorbable ions such as magnesium, sulfate, phosphate and citrate may also provoke osmotic diarrhea. Healthy children who ingest excessive quantities of fruit juice, soda pop or sugar-free products such as sorbitol-containing gum or mints may develop osmotic diarrhea due to the malabsorption of the fructose and sorbitol found in these products. This is a major cause of chronic nonspecific diarrhea of childhood.

The second major mechanism of diarrheal disease results from the active secretion of the anions chloride and bicarbonate, followed by passive water secretion. Luminal secretagogues include bacterial enterotoxins produced by V. cholerae, heat-labile and heat-stable E. coli, staphylococcal enterotoxins, Clostridium perfringens and Bacillus cereus, as well as hydroxy fatty acids from malabsorbed dietary lipids and nonabsorbed bile acids. Recently, investigators described rotavirus-induced intestinal secretion. Endogenous secretagogues include hormones secreted by intestinal tumors and inflammatory mediators released in response to food allergy, inflammatory bowel disease and systemic infections. These mediators include histamine, eicosanoids, platelet-activating factor, serotonin and IL-1. They are released after direct activation of inflammatory cells or through stimulation of these cells by the enteric nervous system. Cholera toxin was the first described and remains the classic cause of secretory diarrhea. The B subunit of this toxin binds to the luminal surface of the microvillus membrane of the enterocyte. The A subunit is then internalized and irreversibly activates adenylate cyclase, which stimulates the formation of cyclic adenosine monophosphate (cAMP). This activates protein phosphorylation, which triggers chloride secretion and impairs Na^+Cl^- absorption. In secretory diarrhea no morphologic epithelial injury is present and the sodium-dependent glucose transporter and the enzyme Na^+/K^+-ATPase function normally. This permits successful oral rehydration therapy in the face of ongoing intestinal secretion.

The third mechanism causing diarrhea results from exudation of fluid and protein secondary to inflammation and ulceration of intestinal or colonic mucosa. This results in bloody diarrhea or dysentery caused by the bacteria Shigella, Campylobacter jejuni, Salmonella, Yersinia enterocolitica, enteroinvasive and enterohemorrhagic E. coli, as well as the protozoa Entamoeba histolytica. This type of diarrhea is also seen in inflammatory bowel disease, particularly ulcerative colitis. The diarrheal stools contain mucus, exudate and blood. As mentioned above, the release of inflammatory mediators also stimulates fluid secretion.

Finally, both hyper- and hypomotility result in diarrheal fluid losses. Hypermotility occurs in intestinal infections, hyperthyroidism, functioning tumors and irritative-type laxative abuse. Hypomotility is observed in the intestinal pseudo-obstructive syndromes and with partial anatomic obstruction that results in the intestinal blind loop syndrome. With decreased motility, bacterial contamination develops with resultant malabsorption of nutrients and stimulation of secretory diarrheal fluid losses.

6.3 Clinical Assessment

The infant or child with an acute watery diarrheal illness has most likely contacted a viral enteritis. However, these symptoms can be presenting features of other gastrointestinal and nongastrointestinal illnesses, including otitis media, urinary tract infection, bacterial sepsis, meningitis, pneumonia, allergy and toxic ingestion. Children who develop loose, watery stools in conjunction with infections such as those involving the middle ear or urinary tract usually do not become dehydrated. This is known as "parental diarrhea" and is likely due to the release of inflammatory mediators. A careful history and physical examination play a crucial role in differentiating an acute gastroenteritis from the other causes of acute diarrhea. In addition, accurate assessment of the degree of dehydration, ongoing fluid losses and the ability to drink are required to ensure adequate fluid replacement and maintenance of intake.

6.3.1 HISTORY

Specific questions about the frequency, volume and duration of vomiting and diarrhea are required to determine the severity of fluid deficit and electrolyte imbalance. Significant dehydration can also be manifested by a decreased activity level, reduced urine volume and weight loss. A summary of the assessment of dehydration appears in Table 7. Information about the consistency of stool as well as the presence and quantity of blood aids in establishing a diagnosis and in determining appropriate investigation. In infants sus-

TABLE 7. Dehydration assessment and management

Degree of dehydration; % deficit	General	Thirst	Eyes; tears	Mouth	Skin	Urine	Rehydration therapy within 4 hrs.	Replacement of fluid losses
None; <2%	Well, alert	Drinks normally	Normal; tears present	Moist	Normal	Normal	Not required; proceed with maintenance and replacement of ongoing losses	10 mL/hr or $^{1}/_{2}$–1 cup of ORS for each diarrheal stool; 2–5 mL/kg for each emesis
Mild; 3–5%	Well	Drinks eagerly	Normal; decreased tears	Decreased moisture	Normal	Decreased	ORS 50 mL/kg	As above
Moderate; 6–9%	Restless, irritable	Drinks eagerly	Sunken; absent	Dry	Pallor; delayed capillary refill; tenting < 2 sec.	Absent	ORS 100 mL/kg	As above
Severe; ≥ 10%	Lethargy, floppy, decreased consciousness, rapid weak pulse, rapid breathing	Drinks poorly or not able to drink	Very sunken and dry; absent	Very dry	Pallor; delayed capillary refill; tenting > 2 sec.	Absent	IV fluids (normal saline, Ringer's lactate) 20 mL/kg/hr until pulse and mental status return to normal; then ORS 50–100 mL/kg	As above

SOURCE: Modified from Butzner JD. Acute vomiting and diarrhea. In: Walker-Smith JA, Walker WA, Hamilton JR (eds.), Practical pediatric gastroenterology. 2d ed. Toronto: BC Decker, 1996:51–69.

pected of having a gastrointestinal infection, a history of illness among contacts, including playmates, siblings and day-care attendees, as well as exposure to visiting travelers may provide clues to the source of infection. Mild upper respiratory infections in parents or older children may result in acute vomiting and diarrhea in the infant or toddler. In addition to person-to-person contact, exposure to animals and contaminated drinking water and food may lead to enteric infections. Foods cause acute vomiting and diarrhea by multiple mechanisms. These include immunologic reactions resulting in food allergies as well as metabolic, pharmacologic and toxin-induced reactions to food and its contaminants. Lactose intolerance due to adult-onset lactase deficiency; "Chinese restaurant syndrome" due to monosodium glutamate ingestion; and staphylococcal food poisoning occurring one to six hours after the ingestion of preformed toxins are examples of the nonimmunologic causes of food poisoning. Infants who suffer an acute diarrheal illness in the first few weeks of life are more likely to have a congenital anatomic abnormality of the GI tract or an inherited metabolic disease such as abetalipoproteinemia, cystic fibrosis or one of the rare intestinal transporter deficiencies.

6.3.2 PHYSICAL EXAMINATION

The inaccurate assessment of fluid deficits and ongoing fluid losses is the most important cause of the morbidity and mortality associated with acute vomiting and diarrhea in children. Infants are particularly susceptible to the development of dehydration for they sustain greater fluid losses because of an increased intestinal surface area per kilogram of body weight compared to adults. An immature renal concentrating ability, increased metabolic rate and dependence on others to provide fluids also contribute to the rapid development of severe fluid deficits in the pediatric patient. An immediate pre-illness weight provides the most sensitive mechanism of determining severity of dehydration. Unfortunately, this is rarely available. A weight should be obtained at the time of initiation of treatment in order to judge ongoing losses and gauge successful therapy. As outlined in Table 7, the severity of dehydration used to gauge the level of rehydration therapy can be assessed rapidly with history and physical examination. Watery diarrhea sometimes is mistaken for urine in the diaper. This may result in an underestimation of fluid losses. Evidence of particulant matter or a positive dipstick for sugar or protein suggests watery stool. Rapid, deep breathing may suggest an uncomplicated metabolic acidosis. In the child with a distended abdomen, auscultation of bowel sounds should be performed to rule out a paralytic ileus, and a rectal exam should be performed to determine if fluid is being third-spaced in the gut lumen. Examination of the stool for blood, white blood cells, reducing substances, pH, fat and fatty acid crystals may provide valuable clues about the etiology of a diarrheal illness.

6.3.3 INVESTIGATIONS

The majority of episodes of acute watery diarrhea in previously healthy children are self-limited and associated with only mild dehydration. In this situation, the performance of biochemical or microbiologic examination is rarely required. When an advanced stage of dehydration is suspected, assessment of serum electrolytes, urea nitrogen, and acid/base chemistry will aid in tailoring ongoing rehydration therapy. Virologic and microbiologic examination should be performed only when results will be utilized to alter patient management or treat patient contacts, or for the protection of other hospitalized patients. Examples that require further investigation include an outbreak of diarrheal disease in a day-care center or hospital, diarrhea in a patient with a recent history of travel to an area of endemic diarrheal disease, and evaluation of the immunocompromised patient or of the patient where initial therapeutic measures are unsuccessful. In the infant or child with bloody diarrhea, stool cultures and antibiotic sensitivities should be performed to guide appropriate antibiotic therapy, if treatment is indicated. In areas where enterohemorrhagic E. coli causes bloody diarrhea, additional laboratory investigations including a CBC with a platelet count, blood smear for evidence of intravascular hemolysis, serum electrolytes, serum creatinine and serial urinalyses are warranted to aid in the diagnosis and management of hemolytic-uremic syndrome, the leading cause of acute renal failure in children under the age of 6.

6.4 Management – Oral Rehydration Therapy

6.4.1 ORAL REHYDRATION

In children with acute diarrhea associated with mild to moderate dehydration, the administration of a balanced oral rehydration solution (ORS) should be immediately instituted as described in Table 7. Parents should be instructed in the proper administration of oral rehydration therapy as part of preventive health care. An oral rehydration solution with a carbohydrate-to-sodium ratio of less than 2:1 and an osmolality that is similar to or slightly less than plasma is recommended. In North America, most oral rehydration solutions have a sodium content of 45–75 mmol/L because stool sodium losses (approximately 35–45 mmol/L) in viral enteritis are much less than those in secretory diarrheas such as cholera (90–140 mmol/L). For children with continued high purging rates (>10 mL/kg/hr), solutions with a higher sodium content may be required. When solutions with a sodium content of >60 mmol/L are used for maintenance, low-sodium fluids such as breast milk, infant formula, diluted juice or water must be provided simultaneously to prevent the development of hypernatremia. In North America, intravenous electrolyte solutions are used to manage children with severe dehydration because of their wide availability and high degree of success. In the developing world, children suffering from severe dehydration can usually be successfully rehydrated with oral solutions. More than 90% of vomiting infants can be successfully rehydrated and maintained with oral hydration providing 5–10 mL every 2 to 3 minutes and gradually increasing the amount administered.

About 5–10% of children fail initial oral rehydration therapy as a result of either persistent vomiting or a persistently high stooling rate of > 10 mL/kg/hr. Parents should be instructed to seek further care if the child develops (1) irritability or lethargy that inhibits drinking, (2) intractable vomiting, (3) worsening fluid deficits associated with persistent diarrhea, (4) bloody diarrhea, or (5) decreased urinary output. These children require re-evaluation and intravenous rehydration similar to that provided for the severely dehydrated child. Their hydration status should be monitored, and when rehydration is complete, maintenance therapy to replace ongoing losses can be commenced. If dehydration persists, the fluid deficit should be recalculated and rehydration therapy continued for an additional 2 to 4 hours with ongoing assessment of fluid losses.

There are only a few contraindications to the use of oral rehydration therapy for the initial management of acute diarrheal disease. These include (1) severe (>10%) dehydration associated with hemodynamic instability, (2) refusal to drink due to extreme irritability, lethargy, stupor or coma, and (3) intestinal ileus. These children should be managed initially with intravenous fluids and switched to oral rehydration therapy when they can safely drink. Homemade oral rehydration solutions are not recommended because electrolyte abnormalities caused by inappropriate mixing are a well-recognized complication.

6.4.2 EARLY REFEEDING

Recommendations for the dietary management of acute diarrheal disease stress the importance of continued breastfeeding throughout the illness and early refeeding of the formula-fed infant and older child. Continued feeding throughout a diarrheal illness improves nutritional status, stimulates intestinal repair, and diminishes the severity as well as the duration of illness. Breastfed infants should be allowed to nurse as often and as long as they want throughout a diarrheal illness. The refeeding of the non-breastfed infant remains somewhat controversial. Recent evidence suggests that the infant with mild to moderate dehydration should receive the full-strength infant formula that was fed prior to illness. There is no need to routinely switch to a lactose-free milk or to refeed with dilute formula. Treatment failure rates of 10–15% when refeeding is carried out in this manner are no higher than with more cautious approaches. Infants with severe dehydration, pre-existing intestinal injury and severe malnutrition, and those who have failed initial refeeding, should receive a lactose-free formula; they occasionally require a more predigested formula during refeeding.

The older child, who is established on a wider variety of foods, should receive a well-balanced, energy-rich, and easily digestible diet. Complex carbohydrates including rice, noodles, potatoes, toast, crackers and bananas should be offered initially, with the rapid addition of vegetables and cooked meats. Foods to avoid include those high in simple sugars such as soft drinks, undiluted fruit juice, caffeinated beverages, presweetened gelatins and sugar-coated cereals. Foods high in fat may be poorly tolerated because of delayed gastric emptying that results in increased vomiting. In some children watery stools will persist for longer than 10 days, but not to the extent where they cause recurrent dehydration. In these cases infection should be excluded and stools examined for reducing substances to rule ongoing carbohydrate malabsorption.

6.4.3 *USE OF MEDICATIONS*
The prescription of antiemetic, antimotility and antidiarrheal agents for the treatment of acute diarrhea seldom benefits the child and may be associated with serious complications. In children with acute diarrheal disease, these agents do not reduce stool volume or duration of illness. They often have anorexic or sedating effects, which prevent successful oral rehydration therapy. Their use results in a third spacing of fluid, which leads to an underestimation of ongoing losses. This results in inadequate fluid replacement therapy.

Antibiotics should be used in the treatment of diarrheal disease only when specifically indicated. Antibiotics are not effective for the treatment of viral enteritis. Giardiasis should be treated when the diarrheal illness persists and when cysts or trophozoites are identified in the stool. There is no benefit to treating asymptomatic carriers of Giardia lamblia. Antibiotic therapy for the bacterial diarrheas remains controversial because most infections are self-limiting and antibiotic therapy does not shorten the duration of illness. Antibiotic therapy is indicated (1) when a treatable pathogen has been identified, (2) in the immunocompromised host, (3) as an adjunctive therapy in the treatment of cholera and (4) in infants less than 3 months of age with positive stool cultures. Infants at this age are at increased risk to develop septicemia. Infants and children with diarrhea who display signs of septicemia should be treated with parenteral antibiotics.

7. MALABSORPTION / R.A. Schreiber

7.1 **Introduction**
Growth and development are fundamental to the general health and well-being of any infant, child or adolescent. In order to achieve a normal growth velocity, the pediatric patient requires a sufficient intake of appropriate dietary

Dietary
Components   Intraluminal Phase   Intestinal Phase   Delivery
Phase

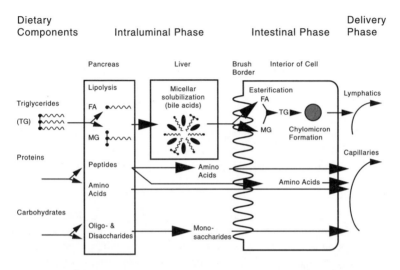

FIGURE 4.   Digestion and absorption of triglycerides, proteins and carbohydrates.
SOURCE: Adapted from Silverman A, Roy CC. Pediatric clinical gastroenterology. 3d ed. St.
Louis: CV Mosby, 1983:250.

nutrients as well as an intact and functional digestive system. In North America, failure to thrive occurs most often because of an inadequate intake of calories. Malabsorption, however, is another important cause of failure to thrive in the pediatric population.

Malabsorption may be defined as a clinical syndrome characterized by defective digestion and absorption of any dietary constituent. A large number of diseases can cause malabsorption. Moreover, the clinical manifestations of this syndrome may be quite diverse, depending upon the dietary constituents that are malabsorbed. The following section reviews the mechanisms for normal digestion and absorption and presents a practical approach to the evaluation of the pediatric patient with malabsorption.

7.2 Physiology and Pathophysiology of Digestion and Absorption

The normal process of intestinal digestion can be divided into three phases (Figure 4). During the intraluminal phase, ingested carbohydrates, proteins and lipids are hydrolyzed within the intestinal lumen by enzymes released by the salivary glands, the stomach and the pancreas. In the intestinal phase, further digestion of peptides and disaccharides continues at the level of the intestinal brush border and the resulting amino acids, small peptides, monosaccharides, monoglycerides and fatty acids are subsequently absorbed into the enterocyte. The movement of nutrients from the intestinal epithelial cell into the vascular or lymphatic circulation defines the delivery phase. The overall absorptive capacity of the intestinal tract depends upon its length and available surface epithelium. In addition, some dietary substances have specific intestinal sites of uptake. Bile acids, for example, are absorbed in the ileum. Vitamin B_{12} first binds to intrinsic factor secreted by the gastric parietal cell and is then absorbed by a specific receptor-mediated process on ileal enterocytes.

An understanding of the determinants of the digestion and absorption of dietary products can provide a basic framework for the clinical approach to the pediatric patient with malabsorption.

7.2.1 CARBOHYDRATES
Dietary carbohydrates are comprised of polysaccharides (starch), disaccharides (sucrose and lactose) and traces of monosaccharides. Polysaccharides first undergo intraluminal digestion by salivary and pancreatic amylases. The hydrolysis of disaccharides occurs at the intestinal brush border by the disaccharidases sucrase-isomaltase, maltase and lactase. The monosaccharides glucose, galactose and fructose are then absorbed into the enterocyte by simple or facilitated diffusion or by a sodium carrier–mediated active transport. From the enterocyte, monosaccharides diffuse into the vascular circulation.

Symptoms of carbohydrate malabsorption are characterized by gaseous distention, borborygmi, cramps and watery nonbloody diarrhea having an acidic pH (4.0–5.5) and containing unabsorbed reducing sugars. The most common cause of carbohydrate malabsorption in infancy is lactase deficiency secondary to viral gastroenteritis. However, lactase deficiency may also complicate any disease that disrupts the small intestinal brush border, including celiac disease, Crohn's disease and HIV enteropathy. Congenital lactase deficiency, sucrase-isomaltase deficiency and other inherited deficiencies of brush-border enzymes are extremely rare. In each case simply excluding the malabsorbed carbohydrate from the diet will promptly resolve the symptoms.

7.2.2 PROTEIN
Protein digestion begins in the stomach, where gastric acid causes protein denaturation and activates pepsin. In the small intestine brush border, enterokinase converts pancreatic trypsinogen into trypsin which, in turn, activates the pancreatic enzymes chymotrypsin and elastase. Digested protein in the form of free amino acids, di- and tripeptides is rapidly absorbed into the enterocyte and then into the circulation. In contrast to carbohydrate malabsorption, diseases that significantly disrupt the intestinal mucosa do not result in protein malabsorption. Rather, in cases of severe gastroenteropathy, intestinal protein loss develops because of a "back-leak" of protein from the sys-

Dietary   Delivery

Components   Intraluminal Phase   Intestinal Phase   Phase

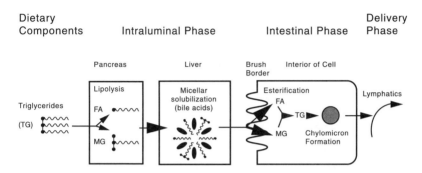

FIGURE 5.   Phases in the digestion of lipids.
SOURCE: Adapted from Silverman A, Roy CC. Pediatric clinical gastroenterology. 3d ed. St. Louis: CV Mosby, 1983:250.

temic circulation across the damaged bowel wall into the intestinal lumen – aptly termed a protein-losing enteropathy.

7.2.3 FAT

The digestion of fat begins in the stomach, where fundal lipase hydrolyzes medium- and long-chain fats. This phase of fat digestion is particularly important in neonates whose pancreatic lipase activity is relatively low compared with the mature adult. In the duodenum, hydrophobic long-chain triglycerides are first emulsified by bile salts and then hydrolyzed by pancreatic lipase. Free fatty acids and monoglycerides solubilize into micelles and approach the luminal surface, where they then diffuse across the enterocyte cell membrane. In the enterocyte the free fatty acids and monoglycerides are re-esterified and packaged along with apoprotein B-48 into chylomicrons. Chylomicrons are excreted via the intercellular spaces into the lymphatic circulation, and then through the thoracic duct into the systemic circulation. In contrast to long-chain fats, medium-chain triglycerides are water-soluble and are absorbed by the enterocyte directly into the bloodstream. Medium-chain triglycerides therefore do not require bile salts for digestion or an intact lymphatic system for circulation.

With fat malabsorption the stools are greasy, soft but not liquid, foul smelling and bulky. Growth failure is a dominant feature, because the intestinal loss of high-energy fat nutrients (9 kcal/g of fat) leads to a profound deficiency in the total calories absorbed daily. In addition to the steatorrhea and failure to thrive, the clinical manifestations of fat-soluble vitamin deficiency (vitamins A, D, E, K) may also be present.

Fat digestion is a complex process involving many organ systems (Figure 5). It is not surprising that a variety of disease states can present with signs and symptoms of fat malabsorption. Impaired bile salt excretion associated with any cholestatic liver disease or disorders of bile salt metabolism including bacterial overgrowth, ileal Crohn's disease or the short gut syndrome can lead to fat malabsorption. Pancreatic insufficiency associated with cystic fibrosis or with the Shwachman syndrome, intestinal mucosal abnormalities such as celiac disease and cow's milk protein intolerance, and rare conditions like abetalipoproteinemia and lymphangiectasia are other important causes of fat malabsorption.

7.3 Diagnosis

A complete history and thorough physical examination are the necessary first steps for establishing a diagnosis of malabsorption and sorting out the potential etiologies. Diarrhea is often a principal clinical symptom, and it is important to determine by the history whether steatorrhea is present. The duration, fluidity, frequency, size, consistency and color of the stools should be documented. Another cardinal presenting symptom for malabsorption is weight loss. However, since failure to thrive in infancy is most often secondary to poor dietary intake, it is critical to obtain a complete dietary history. The physician should ask about the quantity and type of formula the infant is receiving or whether the child is breastfed. The age at which new foods were introduced should be established and the physician should try to ascertain whether there is any correlation between the onset of symptoms and the dietary modifications. The average daily caloric intake should be estimated. Consultation with a pediatric dietitian can be very helpful with this assessment. The physician should inquire about the child's growth and review the record of the child's weight and height. These should be plotted on standard infant growth curves.

A complete birth history should also be obtained. All neonatal complications or prior abdominal surgery should be documented. For a patient who presents with a family history of similar gastrointestinal complaints or with gastrointestinal complaints and a background of consanguinity, an underlying genetic disorder should be considered. Information about travel or recent contacts may help to exclude infectious etiologies. A history of frequent infections may point to an underlying immunodeficiency disorder. Recurrent pulmonary disease might suggest a diagnosis of cystic fibrosis.

On physical examination, accurate measurements of the child's current weight, height and head circumference should be obtained and plotted on a standard pediatric growth curve graph along with all previous measurements. The physician should examine the head, eyes, mouth and tongue, looking for features of fat-soluble or water-soluble vitamin or trace mineral deficiencies. For example, pallor and cheilosis might implicate an iron deficiency anemia.

Alopecia may be a feature of zinc deficiency. The cardiovascular and pulmonary examination should be thorough. Abdominal distention may be a manifestation of organomegaly or intestinal gas. Buttock wasting and excess skin folds, particularly in the groin, are features of subcutaneous fat loss. Edema of the lower extremities may develop with hypoalbuminemia. Clubbing may occur in celiac disease or inflammatory bowel disease.

7.4 Laboratory Tests

7.4.1 *BASELINE STUDIES*
The stools should be analyzed for leukocytes and blood which, if present, suggest a colitis. Determination of the stool pH and a search for reducing substances will support or exclude a diagnosis of carbohydrate malabsorption. A stool smear staining positively for fat globules or fat crystals suggests the presence of fat malabsorption. It is useful to obtain a complete blood count. Iron deficiency anemia may be associated with celiac disease, inflammatory bowel disease or cow's milk protein intolerance. Megaloblastic anemia is a feature of folate or B_{12} deficiency. Acanthocytes are the hallmark of abetalipoproteinemia. The presence of eosinophilia may support a diagnosis of milk protein intolerance. Low serum protein and albumin are features of a protein-losing enteropathy. A urinalysis and urine culture should be obtained to exclude an occult urinary tract infection. Infants and children who present with failure to thrive despite a sufficient caloric intake should have a sweat test to screen for cystic fibrosis.

7.4.2 *72-HOUR STOOL FAT COLLECTION*
If fat malabsorption is suspected, the gold standard test is a 72-hour stool collection for fat. In this instance a complete and accurate 72-hour dietary history must be obtained concomitantly with the three-day stool collection so that the coefficient of fat absorption can be calculated. Infants less than 6 months of age should absorb >85% of fat intake. By one year of age the fat absorption should be at an adult level of >95%.

7.4.3 *D-XYLOSE*
D-xylose is a sugar that is absorbed by the intestinal enterocyte independent of brush-border enzymes or pancreatic function. The D-xylose test is used to assess the integrity of the intestinal mucosa. A standard dose of D-xylose is given by mouth, and a serum level is drawn one hour later. A level greater than 25 mg/dL is normal. A low one-hour serum level suggests mucosal damage. The usefulness of this test in the evaluation of malabsorption is controversial.

7.4.4 *BREATH HYDROGEN TEST*

The breath hydrogen test is most often used to diagnose lactose malabsorption. In this instance a standard dose of lactose is given by mouth and serial breath samples are obtained. If lactose is malabsorbed, colonic bacteria ferment the sugar, producing hydrogen ion, which is subsequently absorbed by the colon into the blood, circulated to the lungs and then exhaled. A significant rise in breath hydrogen 60–90 minutes after lactose ingestion is consistent with incomplete lactose absorption. Hydrogen breath tests may also be used for the diagnosis of sucrase deficiency or small intestinal bacterial overgrowth.

7.4.5 *IMAGING STUDIES*

Contrast radiographic studies are useful to exclude congenital anatomical abnormalities of the gastrointestinal tract as a cause for the malabsorption. Ulceration and strictures are features of Crohn's disease. Intestinal dilation and hypomotility support a diagnosis of bacterial overgrowth.

7.4.6 *ENDOSCOPY*

Upper endoscopy with multiple biopsies permits both gross and microscopic assessment of the intestinal mucosa. The histologic features of a small intestinal biopsy may be highly indicative or even diagnostic for the etiology of the malabsorption. The diagnosis of celiac disease is established only by an intestinal biopsy. The presence of fat-laden vacuoles in intestinal villus cells suggests a disorder in the delivery phase of fat digestion, such as abetalipoproteinemia or hypobetalipoproteinemia. The histological presence of dilated lacteals is a feature of lymphangiectasia.

7.5 **Management**

There are a few basic principles to the management of the pediatric patient who presents with a malabsorption syndrome. First, it is important to determine the cause of the disorder and direct treatment accordingly. For example, patients with celiac disease recover on a gluten-free diet. Infants with cow's milk protein allergy respond to a modification of the protein in the diet. The manifestations of secondary lactase deficiency will resolve with a lactose-free formula or with the use of enzyme supplements (Lactaid®). The fat malabsorption in cystic fibrosis is corrected with pancreatic enzyme replacement. Second, it is usually necessary to provide ample supplemental calories in order to achieve catch-up growth. A good supply of extra calories is especially important for the young infant with marked failure to thrive. High-calorie formulas are frequently introduced early, often before a specific diagnosis has been established. Third, any vitamin, mineral and trace element deficiencies should be corrected. Anemias are treated with the appropriate supplements.

Fat-soluble vitamins are required for infants with ongoing steatorrhea, especially those with cholestatic liver disease. Vitamin B_{12} supplementation may be necessary for patients with ileal resection.

7.6 Summary

The malabsorption syndrome is characterized by a constellation of signs and symptoms associated with a wide variety of disorders, each having a distinct etiopathogenesis. Two common manifestations of this syndrome in the pediatric population are diarrhea and failure to thrive. A careful evaluation of the infant with malabsorption based on a thorough knowledge of the normal physiology of digestion will help the physician to secure a diagnosis and institute an appropriate management plan. The judicious treatment of an infant with malabsorption should lead to a rapid resolution of the symptoms. The reestablishment of a normal growth velocity is ultimately required in order to ensure the healthy development of any infant, child or adolescent.

8. CYSTIC FIBROSIS / H. Machida

Cystic fibrosis (CF) is an autosomal recessive disease that causes chronic morbidity and decreases the life-span of most affected individuals. Because of a defect at a single gene locus that encodes a protein, the cystic fibrosis transmembrane regulator (CFTR), individuals with cystic fibrosis have defective cyclic adenosine monophosphate–regulated chloride transport in epithelial cells of exocrine organs. Although the exact pathophysiology remains to be clarified for each involved organ, there is an accumulation of viscous secretions associated with progressive obstruction and subsequent destruction of excretory ducts.

Chronic pulmonary disease is the major cause of morbidity in the majority of patients. These individuals have progressive bronchiectasis and associated bacterial endobronchial infections, most often secondary to Pseudomonas species.

Although the pulmonary disease is most prominent, the GI manifestations of cystic fibrosis are extensive and contribute to significant morbidity and even mortality. This section will review the clinical problems related to the gastrointestinal tract, particularly the pancreatic insufficiency and hepatic disease in cystic fibrosis.

8.1 Pancreatic Insufficiency

Approximately 80% of patients with cystic fibrosis are born with pancreatic insufficiency, and another 5–10% develop pancreatic insufficiency in subsequent years. These patients have marked impairment of pancreatic exocrine function, including decreased secretion of water, bicarbonate, lipase, amylase and proteinases from the pancreas into the duodenum. In the very young, the endocrine function of the pancreas is usually normal, but many gradually develop evidence of glucose intolerance; a small number develop clinical diabetes requiring insulin therapy. Patients with pancreatic insufficiency may present with any of the following clinical entities with or without pulmonary disease.

8.1.1 MECONIUM ILEUS
Meconium ileus is partial or complete obstruction of the intestine, commonly the ileum, with thick inspissated meconium. This occurs in approximately 15% of infants with cystic fibrosis. Any infant with meconium ileus must have cystic fibrosis excluded. These infants may present with delayed passage of meconium, abdominal distention, vomiting or other signs of obstruction. Meconium ileus may be complicated by antenatal or postnatal volvulus, atresia, perforation of the bowel and meconium peritonitis. In cases with complications, infants may require surgery shortly after birth. Extensive bowel resection may leave them with the short bowel syndrome.

These infants are investigated initially with a plain abdominal x-ray for evidence of obstruction or perforation. If the bowel perforates in utero the perforation often seals, and the x-ray may show calcifications from the meconium in the peritoneum. If meconium ileus is a possibility, surgery should be considered immediately. As long as the x-ray shows no evidence of free air (implying a perforation), most infants are given a gentle water-soluble contrast enema to attempt to relieve the obstruction or at least outline the obstruction for the surgeon. These enemas can cause significant fluid shifts in small neonates, so an IV must be running during the procedure. If the procedure is unsuccessful, surgery is required. The majority of infants with meconium ileus also have pancreatic insufficiency, but this condition can occur in pancreatic-sufficient patients as well.

8.1.2 CHRONIC DIARRHEA
After the neonatal period, chronic diarrhea with or without failure to thrive is common. These infants have loose stools essentially from birth, and one may obtain a history of delay in the passage of meconium. The parents may describe the diarrheal stools as being pale, foul smelling, fatty and/or soupy. The diarrhea is primarily secondary to fat malabsorption because of the pancreatic insufficiency. However, infants who have had small bowel resection, such as for bowel atresia secondary to meconium ileus, may have mucosal disease secondary to bacterial overgrowth. This will contribute significantly to the diarrhea and may cause it to become more watery. Initially, if they do not have respiratory problems, infants with cystic fibrosis tend to have a relatively good appetite and can in some cases compensate for the extreme loss of

nutrients by increasing their intake. As they develop pulmonary symptoms or become gradually malnourished, however, their appetite will decrease.

8.1.3 FAILURE TO THRIVE

In cystic fibrosis, failure to thrive is usually a result of a combination of decreased intake, loss of fat in the stools and increased metabolic requirements. The requirements of the average cystic fibrosis patient have been reported to be 120% of normal. Nevertheless, some patients have essentially normal caloric requirements, and others may have requirements in excess of 150% of normal. Many in the early childhood years are able to maintain their nutritional status well with pancreatic enzyme supplementation and good nutrition. Unfortunately, the increased caloric requirements of puberty coupled with deteriorating lung function often make it impossible for the most severely affected patients to maintain their nutrition and normal growth. In addition, CF patients may have anorexia of chronic disease and difficulty eating due to chronic cough. They present with a gradual decrease in growth percentiles, first of the weight and subsequently of the height. Puberty may be delayed or arrested in the early stages. At this time, nutritional supplementation becomes extremely important. Pancreatic enzyme supplementation must be maximized, and nutritional supplementation given either orally or by enteral tube feeding. Total parenteral nutrition is rarely required. If enteral feeds are needed, we use nasogastric tubes in all our patients except those who have nasal polyps. These patients are taught to put their nasogastric tubes down five to six nights a week to obtain 10 hours of nocturnal supplementary feedings. We have had patients as young as 4 years of age who are able to put their own tubes down. The optimal supplement to use is still being debated. We have been most successful with regular high-calorie formula such as Ensure® with fiber, particularly in patients who have evidence of glucose intolerance. Some centers do not give pancreatic enzyme supplements with the tube feeding; others give enteric-coated enzymes at the initiation of tube feeds; still others add pancreatic enzyme powder to the feeds. We have had the most success with the last approach. With infants, we use the enteral tube feeds in those who present with significant failure to thrive and are unable to take enough calories for catch-up growth, and also in those who have had small bowel resections. Generally, these infants will require the tube feeding only for several weeks to months. We have had only two children between the ages of 2 and 9 who have needed enteral tube feeding. In the adolescent group who require enteral feeding supplementation, we find that about 50% require the supplementation for only a transient period of six months to two years while they are experiencing the significant growth of puberty. A small number of our patients have had to remain on the enteral tube feeding program for years in order to maintain their weight and nutritional status.

8.1.4 *FAT-SOLUBLE VITAMIN DEFICIENCY*

As a result of significant malabsorption prior to treatment, patients may present with overt evidence of bruising or bleeding due to vitamin K deficiency. We have seen one infant female who presented with this condition as well as evidence of xerophthalmia, apparently due to vitamin A deficiency. The clinical effects of vitamin E deficiencies in cystic fibrosis are not well documented, but this vitamin must be given to patients in a supplement and in adequate doses. We also supplement with vitamin D, although vitamin D deficiency, particularly evidence of rickets, is very uncommon in patients with cystic fibrosis.

8.1.5 *HYPOALBUMINEMIA AND EDEMA*

In spite of their pancreatic insufficiency, most patients with cystic fibrosis do not have difficulty with hypoalbuminemia secondary to protein malabsorption. Protein malabsorption, however, is a problem in infants who are fed a soy protein formula, and sometimes in those who are breastfed. These infants will present with significant hypoalbuminemia, edema and usually a history of diarrhea. We have had at least one infant who presented with heart failure secondary to severe hypoalbuminemia. Feeding with soy formula must be discontinued, but often those who are receiving breast milk may have their albumin corrected with pancreatic enzyme supplementation. Older patients with severe malnutrition or cor pulmonale may also develop hypoalbuminemia.

8.1.6 *RECTAL PROLAPSE*

An infant with untreated pancreatic insufficiency becomes increasingly malnourished and continues to pass numerous stools, and thus may begin to have regular rectal prolapse. This is not infrequently the complaint that brings the infant to medical attention. In these cases, a diagnosis of cystic fibrosis must be made quickly and the child renourished. The prolapse will resolve with appropriate nutrition and pancreatic enzyme supplementation to decrease the stooling. In most of these infants the rectal prolapse reduces spontaneously. If it does not, it must be gently reduced manually.

8.1.7 *DISTAL INTESTINAL OBSTRUCTION SYNDROME*

The distal intestinal obstruction syndrome (DIOS), also known as meconium ileus equivalent, is partial or complete obstruction of the bowel resulting from fecal masses, usually in the cecum. This can occur in any age of child with cystic fibrosis, but we find it most often in the older child. Younger children with DIOS present with decreased appetite, decreased stooling, distention and often vomiting. Older patients complain of grumbling or crampy abdominal pain and a gradual decrease in stooling. In most patients, the fecal masses are easily palpated and an x-ray is not always required. If the diagnosis is made early, most can be treated with N-acetylcysteine given orally. We give a loading dose in a cola drink and 3 subsequent doses (1 dose every 6 hours over 24 hours). Fluids must be encouraged during this time. If there is evidence of marked obstruction, we admit the patients to hospital and give them polyethylene glycol–salt solution (GoLYTELY™) orally or by nasogastric tube. This completely clears the obstructive fecal masses. It is essential to ensure that patients with DIOS get adequate enzymes, as the syndrome seems to occur most often in patients who are not getting enough enzymes or in whom the duodenal pH is too low for optimal efficacy of the enzymes.

8.1.8 PANCREATITIS
Five to 10% of patients with cystic fibrosis will remain pancreatic-sufficient throughout their life. Unfortunately, some pancreatic-sufficient patients develop pancreatitis, which may present with vomiting and acute pain that radiates to the back or with recurrent low-grade abdominal pain and perhaps a change in appetite. Those who present with acute pancreatitis should be treated as any other patient with pancreatitis. The bowel is rested until the enzymes return essentially to normal and the patient is asymptomatic. In patients who are found to have mild abdominal pain and only slight increase in enzymes, management is less definitive. We have treated these patients with pancreatic enzymes to try to decrease the amount of stimulation of the pancreas. Unfortunately, the pancreatitis tends to be a recurrent problem in some individuals.

8.2 Hepatobiliary Disease
Hepatobiliary disease in cystic fibrosis is well documented. Fortunately, although a significant number of patients have subtle manifestation of hepatobiliary abnormalities, only a small number have severe liver disease. Given the increasing life expectancy of patients with cystic fibrosis there may be an increasing need to manage patients with severe liver problems. The following briefly outlines the clinical features of some of the hepatobiliary problems associated with cystic fibrosis.

8.2.1 NEONATAL JAUNDICE
Prolonged conjugated hyperbilirubinemia is reported to occur in neonates with cystic fibrosis. In some cases, the hyperbilirubinemia may be secondary to a problem unrelated to the cystic fibrosis; nevertheless, any infant with conjugated hyperbilirubinemia of unknown origin should be investigated for cystic fibrosis.

8.2.2 ELEVATED LIVER ENZYMES
A significant portion of patients with cystic fibrosis have mildly elevated liver enzymes, including alkaline phosphatase, γ-glutamyl transferase (GGT),

aspartate aminotransferase (AST) and alanine aminotransferase (ALT). This is not uncommon in patients who had a meconium ileus as a neonate and are pancreatic-insufficient. In most of these patients, the enzymes either normalize or remain slightly elevated throughout their life. A small proportion develop serious liver disease.

8.2.3 HEPATOSPLENOMEGALY

Many patients with cystic fibrosis have a slightly large liver secondary to fatty infiltration, probably because of poor nutrition. In these patients, the liver is smooth and soft. In those who develop progressive liver disease, the liver is initially large; it gradually begins to feel hard and often nodular. Splenomegaly is usually not detected until the patient is aged 6 or older. On histologic examination, these patients have multinodular or biliary cirrhosis. The liver disease tends to progress slowly and the prominent clinical problems are secondary to hypersplenism. It can be years before there are changes in the albumin, INR/PT or PTT, or an elevation of the bilirubin. With the significant portal hypertension, the patients are at risk for bleeding from esophageal or small bowel varices. As the life-span of patients with cystic fibrosis increases, one would expect to see increasing morbidity and mortality from liver failure.

In very recent years, ursodeoxycholic acid has been used to try to improve the liver disease in cystic fibrosis. Short-term studies report that patients treated with ursodeoxycholic acid show improvement in their liver enzymes and, in some cases, in liver function studies. It has yet to be determined whether long-term treatment will actually prevent progression of the liver disease and perhaps protect some children from developing cirrhosis.

8.3 Management of Pancreatic Insufficiency

As there are numerous gastrointestinal problems in cystic fibrosis and their interrelationship can be quite complex, it is beyond the scope of this section to discuss the management in detail. In the majority of cases, the problem must be identified, assessed and managed as in patients without cystic fibrosis. Nevertheless, because the pancreatic insufficiency causes most of the gastrointestinal problems, an approach to its management will be outlined.

There are several indirect methods that assess pancreatic insufficiency, but the only direct measurement of pancreatic function is a pancreatic stimulation test. Unfortunately, this test requires intubation of the duodenum, it is invasive and uncomfortable for the patient, and generally it will not contribute significantly to the patient's management. Therefore, this test is usually reserved for complicated cases. We usually assess the pancreatic insufficiency by a 72-hour fecal fat collection, which measures the percentage of fat lost in the stools daily. If possible, this test is done before the patient is placed on pancreatic enzyme supplementation and post-enzyme supplementation.

Once the pancreatic insufficiency is diagnosed, it is treated with supplementary pancreatic enzymes. The aim of treatment is to control the fat malabsorption so that the patient has normal growth and good nutrition. (In the majority of cases it is impossible to reduce fecal fat loss to less than 12%, even on optimal enzyme supplementation.) Commonly, the enzymes given are in capsule form and contain enteric-coated spheres of lipase, amylase and proteinases. These enteric-coated spheres are released in the alkaline environment of the duodenum. The strength of these preparations varies; usually the dosage is expressed in lipase units. We find that the appropriate dosage of lipase is best determined empirically.

We begin giving infants under 6 months of age at diagnosis 1 enteric-coated capsule with 4,000 units of lipase per feed. By 1 year of age, the majority will be on 8,000 to 10,000 lipase units per feed and 4,000 per small snack. Subsequently, the enzymes are evaluated and increased as the patient grows and whenever there is evidence of increasing malabsorption. By age 8 the majority of patients with pancreatic insufficiency will require 80,000 to 100,000 lipase units per meal. In most cases an increase in lipase above this level does not improve their fat absorption. In older children, we generally use capsules containing 20,000 lipase units each, so that the child can take fewer capsules per meal. The disadvantage with this is that the child may be taking more enzymes than required for small meals or snacks.

With the lack of bicarbonate secretion from the pancreas, the duodenal pH may be too low for optimal activity of the pancreatic enzyme supplements. In patients in whom the number of enzymes seems maximal for age and weight, ranitidine is started at 2 mg/kg b.i.d. to enhance the efficacy of the enzymes.

8.4 Summary

The gastrointestinal effects of cystic fibrosis are extensive. Most of the prominent problems are secondary to the pancreatic disease. Once this is treated adequately with enzymes, vitamin replacement and adequate nutrition, many problems will resolve. Severe liver disease is less common; it can be devastating in the patients in whom it occurs and may be of more concern as the lifespan of the patients increases. Research into the pathophysiology of the liver disease and into pharmacologic agents such as ursodeoxycholic acid is ongoing. Because failure to thrive and liver disease can present insidiously, it is essential to monitor these patients on a regular basis, including documentation of height and weight, a complete physical examination and a regular biochemical evaluation.

9. APPROACH TO THE JAUNDICED NEONATE / S.R. Martin

Jaundice is caused by the deposition of bile pigment in the skin and other tissues as a result of an elevated serum bilirubin concentration. Bilirubin is formed from the degradation of hemoglobin as well as other heme-containing

TABLE 8.   Factors contributing to physiological jaundice in the neonate

Absence of placental bilirubin metabolism
Reduced hepatic blood flow via ductus venosus shunting
Decreased red blood cell survival
Increased red blood cell mass
Reduced enteric bacterial flora
Presence of intestinal β-glucuronidase
Immature liver function
Delayed oral feeding

proteins, mainly within cells of the reticuloendothelial system. Bilirubin is carried in the circulation bound to albumin and taken up in the liver by the hepatocytes, where it is conjugated with glucuronic acid before being secreted into bile. Conjugated bilirubin is then converted to urobilirubins by intestinal bacteria, preventing its reabsorption and permitting its excretion in the feces. Jaundice in the neonatal period (<1 month) is present in up to 60% of full-term and 80% of premature infants; usually it is a physiological phenomenon related to the developmental nature of bilirubin metabolism. Infants of certain racial background (oriental, Greek, North American native) may be particularly susceptible.

9.1 Physiological Jaundice

Physiological jaundice generally appears around the third to fifth day, rises by no more than 85 μmol/L/day and resolves by the end of the second week of life. Hyperbilirubinemia is always of the unconjugated fraction. Peak levels rarely exceed 150 μmol/L in full-term infants, although in premature infants levels of 200 μmol/L are not uncommon and the resolution may be slower. Several mechanisms that contribute to the development of physiological jaundice, including increased bilirubin load and decreased capacity to process bilirubin, are shown in Table 8.

After birth the placenta is no longer available for bilirubin metabolism and the immature liver has a limited capacity for uptake of bilirubin from plasma and for its binding, conjugation and secretion into bile. Blood flow may not immediately favor hepatic perfusion (shunting via the ductus venosus). An increased bilirubin load derives from the neonate's elevated hematocrit combined with a reduced red blood cell life-span. Delayed feedings result in retention of meconium containing significant amounts of bilirubin within the intestine, which initially has reduced bacterial flora. This limits the conversion of conjugated bilirubin into urobilinogens. Also present is β-glucuronidase, which converts conjugated bilirubin into a reabsorbable form.

9.2 Pathological Jaundice

Jaundice is quantified by measuring the serum bilirubin composed, in general, of unconjugated and conjugated fractions. Because it is impossible to differentiate visually between jaundice caused by unconjugated hyperbilirubinemia and that caused by conjugated hyperbilirubinemia, each of which has different etiologies, therapies and prognosis, the first step in evaluating a jaundiced baby is to determine the total and conjugated bilirubin concentrations. Potentially life-threatening illnesses may present with neonatal jaundice, so it is important that the initial evaluation distinguish between physiological and pathological causes of jaundice in order to start any therapy without delay. Pathological jaundice is suggested and requires investigation when any of the following conditions arises:

1. jaundice appearing within the first 24 hours;
2. a rate of rise of more than 85 µmol/L/24 hours;
3. total bilirubin >250 µmol/L in breastfed infants, or >200 µmol/L in formula-fed infants;
4. persistence of jaundice beyond 2 weeks of age; or
5. a conjugated fraction >34 µmol/L, or >15% of the total bilirubin concentration.

9.2.1 UNCONJUGATED HYPERBILIRUBINEMIA

In practice, jaundice is caused either by increased production or decreased clearance of bilirubin by the liver. The pathological causes of unconjugated hyperbilirubinemia are shown in Table 9.

9.2.1.1 Increased bilirubin production

Any process that presents a greater bilirubin load to the liver than can be processed will result in hyperbilirubinemia. Thus, red blood cell hemolysis from a variety of causes, including maternal–infant blood group incompatibility (Rh, ABO, minor groups), membrane defects, red cell enzyme deficiencies and toxic effects of drugs, increases the load of unconjugated bilirubin presented to the liver. Hemoglobinopathies rarely present in the neonatal period because of the presence of a large proportion of the relatively stable fetal hemoglobin (Hgb F). Massive hemolysis may occasionally also raise *conjugated* bilirubin levels to 25–30% of the total, possibly resulting from the toxic effects of bilirubin secretion into bile. Conditions resulting in increased red cell breakdown, especially hematomas, elevate the serum bilirubin; these are relatively more important in smaller premature infants. Finally, some conditions accentuate the normally high neonatal hemoglobin, resulting in polycythemia. Examples are maternal–infant transfusion, delayed umbilical

TABLE 9.   Causes of unconjugated hyperbilirubinemia in the neonate

---

Increased bilirubin production
Hemolytic disease
   Blood group incompatibility (Rh, ABO, minor groups)
   Membrane defects (spherocytosis, elliptocytosis, infantile pyknocytosis)
   Enzyme deficits (G6-PD, hexokinase, pyruvate kinase)
   Drugs (oxytocin, vitamin K)
Increased breakdown
   Infection
   Hematoma, swallowed maternal blood
Increased RBC mass
   Polycythemia (maternal diabetes, delayed cord clamp, small for gestational age, altitude)

Decreased bilirubin metabolism
Reduced uptake
   Portacaval shunt, hypoxia, sepsis, acidosis, congenital heart disease
Decreased conjugation
   Crigler-Najjar type I, II
   Gilbert's syndrome
   Lucey-Driscoll syndrome
   hypothyroidism
   panhypopituitarism

Altered enterohepatic circulation
Breastfeeding
   Free fatty acids, steroids, breast milk β-glucuronidase
Intestinal hypomotility
   Retained meconium
Reduced intestinal flora
   Newborn, antibiotic use

---

cord clamping at birth, and conditions that result in relative intrauterine hypoxia (maternal diabetes mellitus, high altitude, newborn small for gestational age).

9.2.1.2 *Altered bilirubin metabolism*

At any stage in the processing of bilirubin – uptake, transport, conjugation, excretion – abnormalities may affect the unconjugated bilirubin concentration. The Crigler-Najjar syndrome is an inherited disorder characterized by absent or low hepatic glucuronyl transferase activity. Type I is associated with very high levels of bilirubin and with kernicterus, whereas type II has lower bilirubin levels and is responsive to enzyme induction with phenobarbital to lower the serum bilirubin. Gilbert's syndrome, an autosomal dominant condition, is a mild form of elevated bilirubin with reduced glucuronyl transferase activity, in which jaundice (which is rarely observed in the newborn) is often provoked by stress or fasting. It requires no treatment. The Lucey-Driscoll syndrome is a transient form of acquired reduction in glucuronyl transferase activity in the newborn, caused by a factor in maternal serum. Endocrine disorders such as panhypopituitarism and hypothyroidism affect bile conjugation by unclear mechanisms.

9.2.1.3 *Altered enterohepatic circulation*

Jaundice induced by breast milk occurs in approximately 1 in 200 infants. Jaundice may present in the first week in the early form or after the first week in the late form, which is associated with higher bilirubin levels. The degree of hyperbilirubinemia is quite variable (171–462 μmol/L) and may last from 3 to 10 weeks. Despite the occasional presence of very elevated unconjugated bilirubin levels, kernicterus has not been reported in normal term newborns with breast milk–induced jaundice. Several breast milk components have been implicated, including free fatty acids, an isomer of naturally occurring steroids and β-glucuronidase. Hyperbilirubinemia may also be caused by antibiotic-induced reductions in intestinal flora that increase the level of intestinal conjugated bilirubin, the preferred substrate for β-glucuronidase, whose action produces unconjugated bilirubin that is readily absorbed.

9.2.1.4 *Kernicterus*

The importance of determining an etiology for unconjugated hyperbilirubinemia lies in directing appropriate treatment to prevent kernicterus. Severe unconjugated hyperbilirubinemia is associated with brain toxicity possibly secondary to cellular hypoxia induced by bilirubin. Early symptoms are nonspecific – e.g., lethargy, vomiting, poor feeding and loss of the Moro reflex. Progressive injury leads to respiratory difficulties, bulging fontanelles, a high-pitched cry, loss of deep tendon reflexes and opisthotonos, finally resulting in gaze paresis, convulsions and death. In survivors long-term sequelae include choreoathetosis, spasticity, seizures and sensorineural hearing loss.

Although the lowest level of bilirubin predictive of kernicterus is not known, it is almost universal at levels >500 μmol/L, present in one-third of full-term infants >342 μmol/L, and rare below this latter level. However, numerous factors play a role in increasing bilirubin toxicity at lower levels. Some concern exists that more subtle long-term effects may occur in any infant with raised unconjugated bilirubin concentration; motor development may be affected by levels greater than 255 μmol/L. Bilirubin toxicity may be increased by factors that reduce binding to albumin, such as hypoproteinemia, acidosis, hypothermia, hypoglycemia-induced elevations of plasma free fatty acids and drugs (sulfa, salicylates, heparin, hematin, ceftriaxone, sodium benzoate), or by factors affecting the permeability of the blood–brain barrier, such as prematurity, asphyxia, hyperosmolarity, infection, respiratory distress syndrome, acidosis and intraventricular hemorrhage. Such factors are frequent in very low birth weight infants, in whom kernicterus may occur at unconjugated bilirubin levels as low as 255 μmol/L.

9.2.1.5 *Management*

In contrast to cholestatic infants, those with unconjugated hyperbilirubinemia have normal colored stools, the urine is not dark and the liver is only rarely enlarged and is not firm or nodular. When unconjugated hyperbilirubinemia is confirmed, initial management should identify maternal and infant risk factors according to the causes shown in Table 9. Correction of underlying illnesses (sepsis, hypothermia, acidosis, hypoxia) should be initiated. Specific investigations should include maternal and infant blood group, Coombs' test, hemoglobin or hematocrit, red cell indices and morphology to identify polycythemia, hemolysis or red blood cell disorders. Early feedings should be instituted where possible. For high-risk infants with early jaundice (appearing within the first 24 hours), rapidly rising levels of bilirubin (>85 μmol/L/24 hours) or elevated levels of bilirubin (>250 μmol/L in breastfed or >200 μmol/L in formula-fed infants), specific therapy usually includes phototherapy, exchange transfusion or occasionally oral administration of bilirubin binding agents such as charcoal or agar. Phenobarbital may be given to stimulate the enzymes responsible for bilirubin conjugation. Inhibition of bilirubin formation from its heme precursors may in the future be achieved with agents like tin-protoporphyrin, an inhibitor of heme oxygenase. Breast milk jaundice usually does not require treatment other than maintaining good hydration of the infant with more frequent feedings and occasionally supplemental water or formula, as well as periodic serum bilirubin determinations. Cessation of breast milk feedings for 36 to 48 hours will significantly reduce bilirubin levels that are of concern.

9.2.2 *CONJUGATED HYPERBILIRUBINEMIA IN THE NEONATE*

Conjugated hyperbilirubinemia in the newborn is a sign of cholestasis and always requires further investigation. Because cholestasis implies impairment of bile flow at any point from its formation in the hepatocyte to its excretion from the common bile duct, the causes of neonatal cholestasis are many. However, therapeutic interventions that will significantly affect the outcome are relatively few. For certain conditions, notably infections, some metabolic and endocrine disorders and biliary atresia, early intervention is associated with better outcome. The goal, therefore, is to identify treatable causes as early as possible.

The more common causes of cholestatic jaundice in the neonate are out-

TABLE 10.   Causes of conjugated hyperbilirubinemia in the neonate

Infection
Bacterial urinary tract infection/sepsis
Cytomegalovirus
Rubella
Herpes viruses: simplex; type 6
Toxoplasmosis
Syphilis
Other viruses: adenovirus, Coxsackie virus, echovirus, parvovirus B19

Metabolic
Galactosemia
Fructosemia
Tyrosinemia
Peroxisomal disorders
Bile acid synthesis disorders
α_1-antitrypsin deficiency
Cystic fibrosis
Niemann-Pick disease
Endocrine disorders: hypopituitarism, hypothyroidism
Neonatal hemochromatosis

Bile duct disorders
Extrahepatic
   Biliary atresia
   Bile duct perforation, stenosis
   Neonatal sclerosing cholangitis
   Choledochal cyst
   Cholelithiasis
   Intra/extrahepatic masses
   Inspissated bile/bile plug

Intrahepatic
   Alagille's syndrome
   Byler's disease (familial progressive cholestasis)
   Nonsyndromic bile duct paucity

Miscellaneous
Parenteral nutrition
Intestinal obstruction
Shock
Trisomy 21

lined in Table 10. Although several groups of illnesses are recognized (infectious, metabolic/endocrine, disorders of the bile ducts, cholestatic syndromes), in practice the diagnostic approach consists initially of differentiating biliary obstruction (which requires surgical intervention) from intrahepatic causes of cholestasis. Idiopathic neonatal cholestasis is commonly, but less precisely (because true hepatitis is not often present), referred to as neonatal hepatitis. Neonatal hepatitis is used as a general name for a wide variety of different disorders that present similarly and together with biliary atresia account for 70–80% of all neonatal cholestasis. As specific diseases are elucidated the proportion accounted for by true idiopathic neonatal hepatitis appears to be diminishing. A possible diagnostic approach is shown in Figure 6.

A maternal history of unexplained illness, rash, exposure to cats or uncooked meat may provide clues to infectious causes. A history of blood transfusion or intravenous drug abuse should be sought, although cholestasis is unusual in the neonate with vertically transmitted hepatitis B or C, or human immunodeficiency virus. The family history is especially important for metabolic disorders such as galactosemia, fructosemia, tyrosinemia, Niemann-Pick, α_1-antitrypsin deficiency, peroxisomal disorders or cystic fibrosis as well as familial disorders such as Alagille's syndrome or familial progressive intrahepatic cholestasis (Byler's disease). A history of previous infant deaths in the family due to unexplained liver disease may be important now that previously lethal familial diseases (such as bile acid synthesis defects) can be successfully treated.

The infant's presentation may also suggest a particular etiology. Lethargy, poor feeding or vomiting may signify sepsis or hypoglycemia associated with pituitary dysfunction. Forceful vomiting may indicate intestinal obstruction, but may also occur with galactosemia and fructosemia. While the normal neonate usually does not have fructose in the diet, several medications have a sucrose-based vehicle that is metabolized to fructose. Jaundice with acholic stools in the first 24 hours of life may suggest a bile duct lesion (stone, stricture, perforation). A well appearing infant of full-term gestation and normal birth weight with gradual onset of persistently acholic stools is likely to have extrahepatic biliary atresia.

The physical examination frequently may guide subsequent investigations. The particular facies and high-pitched cry associated with the murmur of peripheral pulmonic stenosis may suggest Alagille's syndrome. A small for gestational age infant with petechiae, rash, retinal lesions, hepatosplenomegaly and adenopathy portrays the clinical appearance of congenital viral infection. An enlarged, firm and/or nodular liver suggests fibrosis, most commonly due to biliary atresia. Biliary atresia also may be associated with situs inversus and a murmur of congenital heart disease. A palpable right upper quadrant mass may signify a choledochal cyst. A micropenis in the male, optic disk atrophy or midline facial defects such as cleft lip may be a clue to hypopituitarism. Severe hypotonia is associated with peroxisomal disorders. Finally the rectal examination may provide stool to determine the presence or absence of bile.

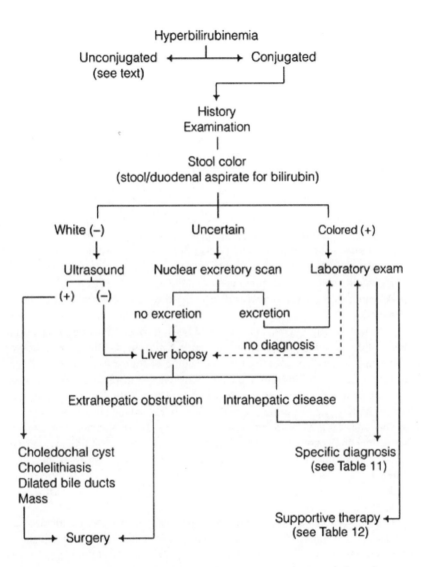

FIGURE 6.   Algorithm for diagnostic evaluation of neonatal cholestasis.

9.2.2.1 Management

If the stool is persistently white, investigations should be directed toward possible extrahepatic biliary obstruction. Although acholic stools may occasionally occur with severe intrahepatic disease, Alagille's syndrome and cystic fibrosis, additional clinical features and laboratory investigations usually are diagnostic. An abdominal ultrasound will detect a choledochal cyst, cholelithiasis, dilated bile ducts from obstruction or stenosis, and intrahepatic or extrahepatic masses. Elements of the polysplenia syndrome (preduodenal portal vein, situs inversus, abnormal inferior vena cava), associated with biliary atresia, may also be detected. At this stage it would be appropriate to refer to a pediatric surgeon for surgery and intraoperative cholangiogram. Sometimes the color of the stool is uncertain and tests for bilirubin in the stool (Ictotest®) are equivocal. (Confusion may arise because yellow secretions or urine will color otherwise acholic stools. This often can be avoided by obtaining stool by rectal examination or by breaking open the stool to reveal its true color.) In such cases hepatobiliary scintigraphy using a ^{99m}Tc-labeled iminodiacetic acid derivative, following five days of treatment with phenobarbital to enhance excretion, may demonstrate patency of the biliary tree. If excretion into the intestine is demonstrated, further diagnostic laboratory investigations are indicated. The absence of excretion is less specific and may arise with intrahepatic cholestasis, as previously mentioned.

A percutaneous liver biopsy will usually differentiate extrahepatic biliary obstruction, particularly biliary atresia, from intrahepatic causes of cholestasis. Typically, biliary atresia is associated with fibrous expansion of the portal tracts, bile ductular proliferation and portal bile plugs. Idiopathic neonatal cholestasis is characterized by disorganization of the structure of the lobule, mononuclear cell infiltration, focal hepatocyte necrosis and more diffuse presence of giant cells than found with other disorders. Bile duct paucity is suggested by absence of intralobular bile ducts, but an adequate number of portal spaces must be present to confirm the diagnosis. Early biopsies may suggest idiopathic cholestasis, requiring clinical suspicion and repeat biopsy to arrive at the correct diagnosis. The less common nonsyndromic forms of bile duct paucity may ultimately be shown to be secondary forms because the list of diseases associated with this histological picture appears to be increasing with time.

Laboratory investigations useful in the evaluation of the cholestatic neonate are outlined in Table 11. Serum bilirubin measures the degree of cholestasis. Alkaline phosphatase and γ-glutamyl transpeptidase (GGT) are greatly elevated with biliary obstruction. However, with prolonged cholestasis alkaline phosphatase may be elevated on the basis of the effects of vitamin D malabsorption on bone; γ-glutamyl transpeptidase is normally elevated in the neonatal period. A measure of hepatic synthetic function is provided by INR/prothrombin time, serum albumin and, where available, factor V levels. The most urgent investigations search for possible bacterial infection and certain metabolic/endocrine disorders for which prompt therapy will reverse the cholestasis as well as treat the underlying disease state. Thus, bacterial cultures of the

TABLE 11. Laboratory evaluation of conjugated hyperbilirubinemia

---

Total and direct serum bilirubin
Alkaline phosphatase, aminotransferases, γ-glutamyl transpeptidase
Prothrombin time or INR, serum albumin (factor V levels, if available)
Complete blood cell count, differential
Urine culture (blood/cerebrospinal fluid, if indicated)
Serology for cytomegalovirus, rubella, herpes simplex, herpes type 6, toxoplasmosis, syphilis
  (adenovirus, Coxsackie virus, reovirus III, parvovirus B19, if available)
Urine for reducing substances, serum galactose-1-phosphate uridyltransferase, serum/urine
  amino acids and organic acids
Sweat chloride
α_1-antitrypsin level and Pi phenotype
Urine for bile acid metabolites
Ophthalmologic examination
Radiograph of vertebral column, long bones, skull
Serum ferritin

---

urine and/or blood; urine for reducing substances (while the infant is ingesting lactose in the form of breast milk or lactose-based formula) or serum galactose-1-phosphate uridyltransferase to diagnose galactosemia; and tests of pituitary function (thyroxin, thyroid stimulating hormone, cortisol and growth hormone levels), in the appropriate clinical setting, are indicated. Serum for very long chain fatty acids may aid in the diagnosis of peroxisomal disorders. Recently, bile acid synthesis defects have been described that respond to specific bile acid replacement therapy if begun early in the course. The presentation and liver biopsy resemble idiopathic neonatal cholestasis (neonatal hepatitis), although the GGT is normal. The diagnosis requires bile acid metabolite analysis of the urine, a technique available in only a few tertiary pediatric centers. The only other cause of neonatal cholestasis with normal or low GGT is progressive familial intrahepatic cholestasis (Byler's disease). The diagnosis of many infections is made serologically, particularly with specific IgM antibody titers. Maternal titers may be required to interpret elevated IgG titers in the face of possible placental transfer. The sweat chloride test is specific for cystic fibrosis but requires a sufficient collection of sweat to be interpretable. Ophthalmologic evaluation may detect the chorioretinitis common in congenital infections, cataracts that develop with galactosemia or the posterior embryotoxon of Alagille's syndrome. Vertebral radiographs may demonstrate the butterfly vertebrae of Alagille's syndrome and long bone radiographs may be abnormal in some congenital infections. Intracranial calcifications that accompany congenital infections may be detected with skull films, ultrasound or CT scan.

TABLE 12. Management of chronic cholestasis

Malnutrition
Increase caloric intake, if necessary by enteral feedings
Supplement with medium-chain triglycerides
Supplement with water-soluble vitamins and minerals

Fat-soluble vitamin deficiency
Vitamin A 5,000–25,000 IU po qd as Aquasol® A, or 50,000 IU IM/month where available
Vitamin E 50–100 IU po qd (polyethylene glycol–based form)
Vitamin K_1 2.5–5.0 mg po qd, or 10 mg IM twice monthly
Vitamin D_2 5,000–8,000 IU po qd, or preferably 5 mg IM/3 months where available, or 3,000 IU IV/1–4 weeks with crystalline cholecalciferol IV

Pruritus
Hydroxyzine
Ursodeoxycholic acid
Rifampin
Cholestyramine
Ultraviolet B light therapy
Biliary diversion

9.2.3 *TREATMENT*

Treatment for many of these disorders is supportive. Ensuring optimal caloric intake for growth may at times require nasogastric tube feeding to supplement a poor intake. Fat malabsorption is common as a result of lack of intestinal luminal bile acids; it may be treated with supplemental medium-chain triglycerides, which can be absorbed in the absence of luminal bile acids. Supplemental fat-soluble vitamins are required to prevent rickets (vitamin D), coagulopathy (vitamin K), peripheral neuropathy (vitamin E) or xerophthalmia (vitamin A). Only vitamin E is available in a well-absorbed oral form (d-alpha-tocopheryl polyethylene glycol succinate); intramuscular administration of other fat-soluble vitamins is frequently necessary. Pruritus is treated with variable success with the agents and procedures listed in Table 12. Progression of cholestasis requires monitoring the child for the development of cirrhosis and treating its complications of ascites, portal hypertension and liver failure.

REFERENCES

Section 5 Growth Failure and Malnutrition
1. Peterson KE. Failure to thrive. In: Queen PM, Lang CE (eds.), Handbook of pediatric nutrition. Gaithersburg, MD: Aspen, 1993:366–383.

2. Wilcox WD, Nieburg P, Miller DS. Failure to thrive: a continuing problem of definition. Clin Pediatr 1989; 28:391–394.
3. Maggioni A, Lifshitz F. Nutritional management of failure to thrive. Ped Clin North Am 1995; 42:791–810.
4. Horner JM, Thorsson AV, Hintz RL. Growth deceleration patterns in children with constitutional short stature: an aid to diagnosis. Pediatrics 1978; 62:529–534.
5. Altagiani M, Murphy JF, Newcombe RG, Gray OP. Catch-up growth in preterm infants. Acta Paediatr Scand 1989; 357(Suppl):3–19.
6. Dean AG, Dean JA, Burton AH, Dicker RC. Epi Info, V.5: a word processing, database, and statistics program for epidemiology on microcomputers. Stone Mountain, GA: USD, 1990.
7. Wright JA, Ashenburg CA, Whitaker RC. Comparison of methods to categorize undernutrition in children. J Pediatr 1994; 124:944–946.
8. Gurney JM, Jelliffe DB. Arm anthropometry in nutritional assessment: nomogram for rapid calculation of muscle circumference and cross-sectional muscle and fat areas. Am J Clin Nutr 1973; 26:912–915.
9. Frisancho AR. New norms of upper limb fat and muscle areas for assessment of nutritional status. Am J Clin Nutr 1981; 34:2540–2545.

SUGGESTED READING LIST

Section 1 Recurrent Abdominal Pain
Boyle JT. Chronic abdominal pain. In: Walker WA, Durie PR, Hamilton JR, Walker-Smith JA, Watkins JB (eds.), Pediatric gastrointestinal disease: pathophysiology, diagnosis and management. Toronto: BC Decker, 1991:45–54.

Section 2 Vomiting and Regurgitation
Sondheimer JM. Vomiting. In: Walker WA, Durie PR, Hamilton JR, Walker-Smith JA, Watkins JB (eds.), Pediatric gastrointestinal disease: pathophysiology, diagnosis and management. 2d ed. St. Louis: Mosby-Year Book, 1996:195–205.
Orenstein SR. Gastroesophageal reflux. In: Hyman PE (ed.), Pediatric motility disorders. New York: Academy Professional Services, 1994.

Section 3 Colic
Barr RG. Colic. In: Walker WA, Durie PR, Hamilton JR, Walker-Smith JA, Watkins JB (eds.), Pediatric gastrointestinal disease: pathophysiology, diagnosis and management, vol. 1. 2d ed. St. Louis: Mosby-Year Book, 1996:241–250.
Symptoms. In: Roy CC, Silverman A, Alagille D (eds.), Pediatric clinical gastroenterology. 4th ed. St. Louis: Mosby-Year Book, 1995:39–43.

Section 4 Chronic Constipation, Encopresis and Soiling
Read NW, Timms JM. Defecation and the pathophysiology of constipation. Clin Gastroenterol 1986; 15:937–965.
Leoning-Baucke V. Chronic constipation in children. Gastroenterology 1993; 105:1557–1564.

Section 6 Acute Diarrhea in Children
Jin S, Kilgore PE, Holman RC, Clarke MJ, Gangarosa EJ, Glass RI. Trends in hospitalizations for diarrhea in United States children from 1979 through 1992: estimates of the morbidity associated with rotavirus. Pediatr Infect Dis J 1996; 15:397–404.
Centers for Disease Control. The management of acute diarrhea in children: oral rehydration, maintenance, and nutritional therapy. MMWR 1992; 41(RR-16):1–20.
Canadian Pediatric Society. Oral rehydration therapy and early refeeding in the management of childhood enteritis. Can J Pediatr 1994; 1:160–164.
Nazarian LF, Berman JH, Brown G, et al. Practice parameter: the management of acute gastroenteritis in young children. Pediatrics 1996; 97:424–435.
Butzner JD. Acute vomiting and diarrhea. In: Walker-Smith JA, Walker WA, Hamilton JR (eds.), Practical pediatric gastroenterology. 2d ed. Toronto: BC Decker, 1996:51–69.
Field M, Semrad CE. Toxigenic diarrheas, congenital diarrheas, and cystic fibrosis: disorders of intestinal ion transport. Ann Rev Physiol 1993; 55:631–655.
Cohen M. Etiology and mechanisms of acute infectious diarrhea in infants in the United States. J Pediatr 1991; 118:S34–S39.
Mackenzie A, Barnes G, Shann F. Clinical signs of dehydration in children. Lancet 1989; 2:605–607.
Brown KH, Peerson JM, Fontaine O. Use of nonhuman milks in the dietary management of young children with acute diarrhea: a meta-analysis of clinical trials. Pediatrics 1994; 93:17–27.
Wolf DC, Giannella RA. Antibiotic therapy for bacterial enterocolitis: a comprehensive review. Am J Gastroenterol 1993; 88:1667–1683.

Section 7 Malabsorption
Malabsorption. In: Roy CC, Silverman A, Alagille D (eds.), Pediatric clinical gastroenterology. 4th ed. Toronto: CV Mosby, 1995:299–362.

Section 9 Approach to the Jaundiced Neonate
Keating JP. Jaundice. In: Walker WA, Durie PR, Hamilton JR, Walker-Smith JA, Watkins JB (eds.), Pediatric gastrointestinal disease: pathophysiology, diagnosis and management. 2d ed. Toronto: CV Mosby, 1996:395–401.
Dellert SF, Balistreri WF. Neonatal cholestasis. In: Walker WA, Durie PR, Hamilton JR, Walker-Smith JA, Watkins JB (eds.), Pediatric gastrointestinal disease: pathophysiology, diagnosis and management. 2d ed. Toronto: CV Mosby, 1996:999–1015.

OBJECTIVES

Recurrent Abdominal Pain

1. Recognize the characteristic clinical presentations (history, physical exam, psychosocial factors) of benign recurrent functional abdominal pain in the child.
2. Be aware of the common organic causes of abdominal pain in children.
3. Be able to identify features of the history or physical exam that are not consistent with functional pain and suggest an organic basis.

4. Understand the approach to the investigation and management of recurrent abdominal pain in children.

Vomiting and Regurgitation

1. Understand the definitions of, and distinction between, vomiting and regurgitation.
2. Be aware of the range of gastrointestinal and nongastrointestinal causes of vomiting characteristic of neonates, infants, children and adolescents.
3. Be aware of an age- and presentation-appropriate approach to the investigation and management of vomiting in neonates, infants, children and adolescents.
4. Be aware of the pathophysiology and natural history of gastroesophageal reflux in infancy, the potential complications of gastroesophageal reflux, the features of history and physical exam that suggest GER-induced disease, available investigations and appropriate treatment of GERD.

Colic

1. Understand that colic describes a pattern of crying or fussiness the etiology of which is not yet clear.
2. Know the possible etiologies for colic that have been proposed.
3. Develop an approach to history taking, physical exam and management of the infant presenting with colic.

Chronic Constipation, Encopresis and Soiling

1. Understand the definitions of constipation, encopresis and soiling.
2. Understand the role of age, colonic motility, dietary fiber and transit time in determining defecation frequency, fecal water and electrolyte content.
3. Recognize normal variations in patterns of elimination in infants (e.g., breastfed vs formula-fed babies).
4. Be aware of the functional and organic causes of constipation.
5. Be able to differentiate chronic fecal retention from Hirschsprung's disease.
6. Understand the mechanism(s) and management of functional constipation and soiling.

Growth Failure and Malnutrition

1. Define the terms *failure to thrive* and *malnutrition*.
2. Learn to categorize failure to thrive in order to facilitate diagnoses.
3. Review appropriate methods for the assessment and management of failure to thrive.

Acute Diarrhea in Children

1. Understand the pathophysiology of acute diarrheal disease in the pediatric patient.
2. Be able to assess severity of dehydration in infants and children.
3. Understand the use of oral rehydration therapy for the management of acute diarrheal disease.

Malabsorption

1. Understand the physiology of digestion and absorption in order to develop an approach to the clinical evaluation of a pediatric patient with the malabsorption syndrome.
2. Be aware of the role of history and physical examination in the assessment of children with the malabsorption syndrome, and in particular, the importance of the dietary record, growth parameters and the need to plot growth curves.
3. Be aware of the various laboratory tests used for the evaluation of children with malabsorption.
4. Understand basic concepts regarding the management of the infant with failure to thrive.

Approach to the Jaundiced Neonate

1. Be aware of the factors contributing to physiological jaundice in the newborn.
2. Be aware of the various causes of unconjugated hyperbilirubinemia in infancy. Know the symptoms and sequelae of unconjugated hyperbilirubinemia. Be aware of options for management.
3. Be aware of the various causes of neonatal conjugated hyperbilirubinemia.
4. Be aware of an approach (algorithm) for the investigation and management of neonatal hyperbilirubinemia.

16
The Applications of Recombinant DNA Technology in Gastrointestinal Medicine and Hepatology: The Basic Paradigms of Molecular Cell Biology

G.E. Wild, P. Papalia, M.J. Ropeleski, J. Faria
and A.B.R. Thomson

1. INTRODUCTION [1–8]

For most gastroenterologists, the principles of cell and molecular biology have not played a major role in day-to-day clinical practice.[1] However, tremendous advances in the discipline of molecular medicine have provided new insights into the cellular and molecular pathologic basis of disease. This ever-increasing expansion of our knowledge base has transformed our understanding and management of an array of diseases. The cumulative research efforts in cell and molecular biology have translated into clinically relevant information in every medical subspecialty. For example, hematologists have defined the molecular basis of the hemoglobinopathies. Endocrinologists have defined the cellular and molecular networks that mediate the action of hormones. Neurologists have identified a host of gene mutations that lead to neurodegenerative disorders. Finally, the identification of the cystic fibrosis transmembrane regulator has facilitated the molecular diagnosis of the disease and as a result, gene therapy protocols are being conducted at several centers.

Many of the recent advances in molecular medicine have been driven by the Human Genome Project. It is apparent that molecular biology has accounted for a dramatic paradigm shift in both the teaching and the practice of medicine. This chapter constitutes a framework for integrating new information into the core knowledge base of concepts related to the pathogenesis of gastrointestinal disorders and liver disease. We hope to provide the reader with a set of tools for understanding some basic concepts of recombinant DNA technology and its role in unraveling the intricate molecular pathophysiology of

[1] A list of selected terms and their abbreviations is found at the end of this chapter.

disease. As well, we wish to give the reader a sense of the impact of molecular medicine in the areas of gastroenterology and hepatology. The goal of this chapter is to review the basic principles of eukaryotic gene expression. In contrast to prokaryotes (where all genes are transcribed by a single RNA polymerase that binds directly to gene promoter sequences), transcription in eukaryotic cells involves several different RNA polymerases that interact with a variety of transcription factors to initiate transcription. This increased complexity characteristic of eukaryotic transcription facilitates the sophisticated and orderly regulation of gene expression that ultimately determines the activities of the diverse cell types seen in multicellular organisms.

Three distinct nuclear RNA polymerases are found in eukaryotic cells. Genes that encode proteins are transcribed into messenger RNA (mRNA) by RNA polymerase II. Ribosomal RNAs (rRNAs) and transfer RNAs (tRNAs) are transcribed by RNA polymerase I and III, respectively. Some small nuclear and cytoplasmic RNAs are transcribed by RNA polymerase II and III. Finally, mitochondrial genes are transcribed by a separate group of RNA polymerases. RNA polymerases are composed of 8 to 14 different subunits. Although they recognize distinct promoters and transcribe different classes of genes, these RNA polymerases share many common features, including a clear dependence on other proteins to initiate transcription.

The transcription of DNA into RNA is the primary level at which gene expression is controlled in eukaryotic cells. Only a fraction of the transcribed RNA is translated into polypeptides. This is explained on the basis of the following:

1. Some transcription units code for RNA molecules only, as in the case of rRNAs, tRNAs and a host of small nuclear and cytoplasmic RNA molecules.
2. The initial transcription product of those transcription units that do not encode polypeptides is subject to events known as RNA processing. With RNA processing, much of the initial RNA sequence is trimmed to yield smaller mRNA molecules.
3. Only the central region of mRNA is translated; variable portions of the 5' and 3' ends of mRNA remain untranslated.

Transcription is mediated by the enzyme RNA polymerase, using DNA as a template and ATP, CTP, GTP and UTP as RNA nucleoside precursors. RNA is synthesized in the 5'-to-3' direction as a single-strand molecule. Only one of the two DNA strands serves as a template for transcription. Since the growing RNA molecule is complementary to this template strand, the transcript has the same 5'-to-3' orientation and base sequence (except that U replaces T) as the opposite, nontemplate strand of the DNA double helix. Thus, the nontemplate strand is called the *sense strand*, and the template strand is called the *antisense strand*. Gene sequences listed in various databases show only the sequence of the sense strand. Orientation of sequences relative to a gene sequence is dictated by the sense strand and by the direction of transcription (e.g., the 5' end of the gene refers to the sequences of the 5' end of the sense strand, and "upstream" or "downstream" of the gene refers to sequences that clamp the gene at the 5' or 3' ends of the sense strands, respectively).

The processes of DNA replication and transcription occur inside the nucleus. By contrast, protein synthesis takes place in the cytoplasm. Protein synthesis is termed *translation* and is directed by mRNA templates. The translation of mRNA is only the first step in the formation of a functional protein. Importantly, the polypeptide chain must subsequently fold into the appropriate three-dimensional configuration and undergo various processing steps prior to being converted into its active form. In eukaryotic cells, these processing steps are closely related to the sorting and transport of different proteins to their appropriate destinations within the cell.

While the regulation of gene expression occurs primarily at the level of transcription, the expression of many genes can also be controlled at the level of translation. Most proteins can be regulated in response to extracellular signals and, in addition, intracellular protein levels can be controlled by differential rates of protein degradation. Thus, the regulation of both the amounts and activities of intracellular proteins ultimately determines all aspects of cell behavior.

Proteins are synthesized on mRNA templates by a process that is remarkably similar in both prokaryotes and eukaryotes. The mRNAs are translated in the 5'-to-3' direction, and polypeptide chains are synthesized from the amino to the carboxy terminus. The amino acids incorporated into the polypeptide chains are specified by three bases (A, U, and C or G – i.e., a *codon*) in the mRNA, determined by the genetic code. Translation occurs on ribosomes with tRNAs serving as adapters between the amino acids being incorporated into the nascent protein strand and the mRNA template. Thus, protein synthesis involves interactions between three species of RNA molecules: mRNA templates, rRNAs, tRNAs.

At the 5' end of the mRNA is the Cap sequence, followed by the 5' untranslated region (UTR), and then by the AUG codon that signals the initiation of translation. Toward the 3' end of the mRNA there is a signal for the termination of translation (UAA, UAG or UGA) followed by the 3'-UTR. At the extreme 3' end of the mRNA is the poly A tail. Protein synthesis starts at the AUG codon and proceeds in the 5'-to-3' direction until a termination codon is reached, which heralds the end of protein synthesis.

The genetic code comprises 64 codons, each containing three bases (A, U, and either C or G). This accounts for the permutations of the four bases in

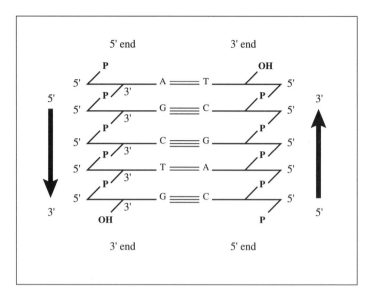

Figure 1.   Base pairing and the antiparallel orientation of DNA. The two DNA strands in the helix have opposite polarity, with one strand running in a 5'-to-3' direction and the other running in the 3'-to-5' direction. Four bases (A, T, C and G) reside on the inside of the helix to allow hydrogen bonding between purine and pyrimidine residues.

groups of three. The 64 codons code for 61 amino acids and termination signals. The genetic code, with some minor exceptions, is ubiquitous: the same codons always code for the same amino acid. Minor variations do occur in the mitochondria. More than one codon can code for the same amino acid in a species-specific fashion. This is known as "redundancy of the genetic code."

2. EUKARYOTIC GENE STRUCTURE AND DNA REPLICATION

2.1 Nucleic Acids and Information Transfer in Cells [1–8]

DNA (deoxyribonucleic acid) is the storage form of genetic information in cells. The structure of DNA was determined by Watson and Crick in 1953, a discovery that has revolutionized the thinking in modern cell biology. All DNA molecules consist of four types of nucleotides joined together by phosphodiester bonds to form polynucleotides. The nitrogenous bases found in DNA consist of purines (i.e., adenine [A] and guanine [G]) and pyrimidines (i.e., cytosine [C] and thymine [T]) (Figure 1). The nucleotides are linked together by covalent phosphodiester bonds that join the 5' carbon of one deoxyribose to the 3' carbon of the adjacent deoxyribose to form polynucleotide genes. The double-stranded DNA helix with its two polynucleotide strands of DNA run in an antiparallel orientation, and the DNA strands are held together by hydrogen bonding between A and T residues and G and C residues. The antiparallel orientation in base pairing is an important concept in nucleic acid biochemistry. One strand runs in a 5'-to-3' direction, and the complementary strand runs in the 3'-to-5' direction (Figure 1). Thus, the two strands of the double helix are complementary. For example, the sequence CTGAAGCGCTTA on one strand of DNA will have the complementary sequence GACTTCGCGAAT on the opposite strand of DNA in an antiparallel orientation. The variation of the sequence of nucleotides along the DNA strand determines the function of each section of the DNA molecule, as well as its ability to transmit information to RNA and protein.

RNA (ribonucleic acid) molecules consist of nucleotides linked together by phosphodiester bonds. RNA generally occurs as single-stranded polynucleotides and contains ribose in place of the deoxyribose found in DNA. RNA is made up of the bases A, G and C, but contains uracil (U) in place of T as the fourth base. Since U has the ability to bind with A in the same way that T binds with A, the four bases found in RNA—A, U, G and C—can form complementary pairs with other RNA bases as well as with the bases found in DNA. These biochemical properties highlight the major function of the RNA molecule in the transfer of information from DNA to protein in eukaryotic cells. RNA often contains intramolecular hydrogen bonding that gives rise to secondary structures. Intrastrand base pairing creates structures known as *stem loop structures*, with the base pairing sections forming the stem and noncomplementary bases forming the loop.

Eukaryotic cells contain five classes of RNA: (1) messenger RNA (mRNA), (2) transfer RNA (tRNA), (3) ribosomal RNA (rRNA), (4) heterogenous nuclear RNA (hnRNA) and (5) small nuclear RNA (snRNA). mRNA makes up a small percentage of the total RNA (1–5%) in eukaryotic cells, has a short half-life and demonstrates a large variation in base sequence from one mRNA molecule to another. mRNA is the chemical messenger that carries information from the DNA helix to the protein-synthesizing machinery in the cytoplasm.

tRNA molecules are polynucleotides ranging from 75 to 95 nucleotides in length that carry specific amino acids to the ribosomes during protein synthesis. There is a unique tRNA that specifically recognizes each of the 20 amino acids. In some instances, there is more than one tRNA species for a single amino acid.

rRNA is the most abundant of the RNA species in eukaryotic cells, and it is found associated with proteins in structures called *ribosomes*. These specific rRNAs of eukaryotic cells are designated by their sedimentation coefficients (S values). Human ribosomes contain 28S, 18S, 5.8S and 5S rRNA species.

Heterogenous nuclear RNA and small nuclear RNA species are located in the nucleus of eukaryotic cells. hnRNA is the immediate product of transcription, and is complementary to one strand of the DNA helix. hnRNA is the precursor to mRNA before it undergoes further processing. snRNA is associated with specific proteins that are involved in the processing of the hnRNA to mRNA prior to departure of the mRNA from the nucleus to the cytoplasm. The role of these RNA molecules in transcription and translation will be discussed in detail in subsequent sections.

2.2 Molecular Anatomy of Eukaryotic Genes [4, 8]

Eukaryotic genomes are larger and more complex than those of primitive prokaryotes (bacteria). For example, the human genome contains approximately 100,000 genes, and much of its complexity arises from the abundance of several different types of noncoding DNA sequences.

A gene can be defined as a segment of DNA that is expressed to yield a functional product that may be either an RNA or a peptide. The structural features common to all eukaryotic genes are illustrated in Figure 2. The sequence of base pairs confers gene specificity and determines the specificity of the product that it encodes. However, not all of the nucleotides present in the gene are expressed in the final product. Eukaryotic genes are often split into (1) *exons* – sequences that remain in the final mature mRNA, and (2) *introns* – sequences that are removed from the primary mRNA transcript early during processing, most which have no known function. In addition to encoding sequence information that ultimately defines the protein product, exons contain other sequences that are essential to the organized functioning of mRNA. Thus, an exon is defined as a sequence in the primary RNA transcript that is conserved during the processing of the transcript into a mature mRNA molecule.

Unique sequences that signal the start of transcription are present in each gene. These sequences represent promoter sequences and they determine the site at which the initiation of transcription begins on the DNA molecule. Transcription is initiated when RNA polymerase and transcription factors bind to the promoter site and catalyze the synthesis of RNA. RNA polymerase transcribes RNA using the sequence of bases from one strand of the DNA double helix, which serves as a template. RNA is synthesized as a single-stranded molecule in the 5′-to-3′ direction.

Further processing of mRNA transcripts to yield a mature RNA product involves a series of steps that include the addition of a Cap structure at the 5′ end of the mRNA and the addition of a poly A tail at the 3′ end. Untranslated

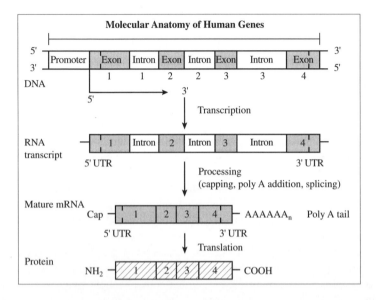

Figure 2. A typical human gene contains exon and intron sequences that are transcribed by RNA ploymerase into the primary transcript. This primary transcript is subsequently processed by the addition of a Cap structure at the 5′ end and the addition of a poly A tail at the 3′ end. The intron sequences are removed and the exonic RNA sequences are spliced together. The mature mRNA contains only exonic RNA sequences that have information for protein sequences as well as signals for the initiation and termination of protein synthesis. UTR = untranslated regions.

regions called UTRs are situated at both the 3′ and 5′ ends of the mRNA and represent sequences in the exons that remain in the mRNA but are not translated into proteins. These regions contain signals required for processing of mRNA and its subsequent translation into protein.

2.3 Organization of Eukaryotic Genomes [4, 8]

The average polypeptide is approximately 400 amino acids long. Thus, the average size of the coding sequence of a gene is 1,200 base pairs. Each amino acid is determined by a set of three nucleotides (a codon). In contrast to E. coli and yeasts, the human genome contains large amounts of noncoding DNA. Thus, only a small proportion of the total 3×10^9 base pairs of the human genome is expected to correspond to protein-coding sequences. The average gene spans 10,000 to 20,000 base pairs (including introns) such that the human genome consists of approximately 100,000 genes, representing 3% of the total human DNA.

Several types of highly repeated sequences exist in eukaryotic genomes. One class, called *simple-sequence DNA*, contains tandem arrays of thousands of copies of short sequences ranging from 5 to 200 nucleotides. Such repeat-sequence DNA accounts for approximately 10–20% of the DNA in higher eukaryotes and is referred to as *satellite DNA*. Other repetitive DNA sequences are scattered throughout the genome rather than being clustered as tandem repeats. These sequences are classified as either *short (SINEs)* or *long (LINEs) interspersed elements*. The major SINEs in the mammalian genome are *Alu sequences,* which contain a signal site for the restriction endonuclease *AluI*. These Alu sequences (300 base pairs long) are dispersed throughout the genome and account for nearly 10% of the total cellular DNA. The major human LINEs are about 6,000 base pairs in length and repeat approximately 50,000 times in the human genome. In contrast to Alu sequences, LINE sequences are transcribed, and some encode proteins of unknown function.

Eukaryotic DNA is tightly associated with small, basic proteins (i.e., rich in arginine and lysine) called *histones*. The complexes between eukaryotic DNA and proteins consist of *chromatin*, which contains about twice as much protein as DNA. The basic amino acids contained in histones have been identified: H1, H2A, H2B, H3 and H4. In addition, chromatin contains a variety of nonhistone chromosomal proteins that are involved in DNA replication and gene expression. The association of DNA and protein to form chromatin is illustrated in Figure 3.

The basic structural unit of chromatin is called the *nucleosome*, which is composed of repeating 200 base pair units. Nucleosomes contain a core particle that contains 146 base pairs of DNA wrapped 1.75 times around a histone core consisting of two molecules each of H2A, H2B, H3 and H4. The other structural feature of the nucleosome is the *chromatosome,* which contains two full turns of DNA (166 base pairs) held in place by one molecule of H1. The structure (i.e., degree of condensation) of chromatin is closely linked to the control of gene expression in eukaryotes. The extent of chromatin condensation varies during the life cycle of the cell. In nondividing cells, most of the chromatin, called *euchromatin*, is decondensed and distributed throughout the nucleus. Genes are transcribed during this period of the cell cycle and the DNA is replicated in preparation for mitosis. By contrast, about 10% of interphase chromatin is in a very highly condensed state called *heterochromatin*. Heterochromatin is transcriptionally inactive and contains highly repeated DNA sequences.

The human genome is distributed among 24 chromosomes (22 autosomes and the two sex chromosomes), each containing between 5×10^4 and 26×10^4 kilobases of DNA. The chromosomes have three well-defined structures that

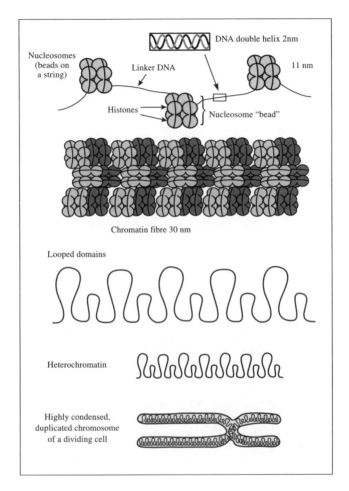

Figure 3. The packaging of DNA in the nucleus. A model is depicted for the progressive stages of DNA coiling and folding in the nucleus. The hierarchy of structural features arising from the DNA double helix includes nucleosomes, chromatin fibers and their looped domains, and heterochromatin, which makes up the arms of chromosomes.

are essential for their replication: (1) DNA replication origins, (2) centromeres and (3) telomeres. The DNA replication origins will be considered in detail in Section 2.6. *Centromeres* consist of highly repetitive DNA sequences and are the site where the two sister chromatids (daughter strands of a duplicated chromosome) are attached. The function of the centromere is to ensure the equal distribution of each chromosome to the daughter cells at cell division.

The *telomere* is an important structure associated with the ends of all human chromosomes. Telomeric DNA consists of multiple tandem repeats of the sequence TTAGGG, located at both ends of each chromatid. Telomeres perform a variety of functions in human cells, including the following:

1. Telomeres maintain chromosomal stability and prevent the formation of end-to-end fusions. The presence of telomeric sequences protects chromosomal ends from nuclease degradation.
2. They ensure the proper replication of the ends of chromosomes. DNA ends are not completely replicated during DNA replication and require the presence of the enzyme *telomerase* to add nucleotides to the extreme ends of the DNA molecule. The presence of noncoding telomeric sequences at the chromosomal ends protects the coding sequences of the DNA located near the terminal ends of a chromosome from being lost during each cycle of replication.
3. They serve as markers of chromosomal integrity. In the event that a chromosome is damaged, the cell cycle stops temporarily so that DNA repair mechanisms can repair the damage.

2.4 The Flow of Genetic Information in Eukaryotic Cells [1–8]

The expression of genetic information in all eukaryotic cells is largely a one-way system. DNA directs the synthesis of RNA, and RNA specifies the synthesis of polypeptides that subsequently form proteins. Because of its universality, the *DNA → RNA → protein* flow of genetic information is called the "central dogma of molecular biology." The synthesis of RNA by RNA polymerase using DNA as a template is called *transcription.* Transcription occurs in the nucleus of eukaryotic cells, and to a limited extent in mitochondria. The second step involves polypeptide synthesis and is called *translation.* Translation occurs on ribosomes, which are large RNA protein complexes found in the cytoplasm. The RNA molecules that specify polypeptides are known as messenger RNAs (mRNAs).

Gene expression has been held to follow a *colinearity principle* where the linear sequence of the nucleotides in DNA is decoded to give a linear sequence of nucleotides in RNA. This linear sequence can be decoded in turn to give rise to a linear sequence of amino acids in the polypeptide product. This concept has been challenged by recent findings that eukaryotic cells, including mammalian cells, contain nonviral chromosomal DNA sequences that encode cellular *reverse transcriptases.* Many different classes of viruses have a genome that consists of RNA. Retroviruses such as HIV are a subclass of RNA viruses in which the RNA replicates via a DNA intermediate, using reverse transcriptase, which is an RNA-dependent DNA polymerase. Because

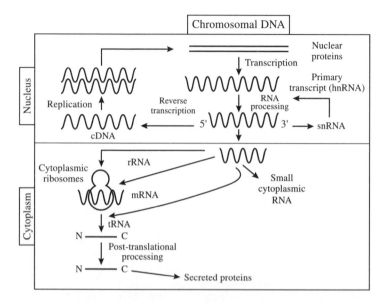

Figure 4. Gene expression in the eukaryotic cell. The expression of genetic information in eukaryotic cells is very largely a one-way system. DNA specifies the synthesis of RNA, and RNA specifies the synthesis of polypeptides, which subsequently form proteins. A small proportion of nuclear RNA molecules can be converted to cDNA by reverse transcriptases and subsequently integrate into chromosomal DNA.

some nonviral RNA sequences in eukaryotic cells are known to act as templates for cellular DNA synthesis, the principle of unidirectional flow of genetic information is no longer strictly valid. The overall flow of genetic information and gene expression in eukaryotic cells is illustrated in Figure 4.

2.5 The Cell Cycle [9–13]

The cellular processes that determine DNA replication and mitosis are the keys to normal cell growth and development. These processes occur in a well-regulated and orderly progression through the mammalian cell cycle (Figure 5). The regulation of the cell cycle ultimately determines how a cell progresses between growth, differentiation and division phases. Cell cycle control is a key determinant of either cell differentiation or the decision to halt the cycle. The loss of control of the cell cycle leads to abnormal cell growth, which results in tumorigenesis, developmental defects or premature programmed cell death (i.e., apoptosis).

The mammalian cell cycle comprises four distinct phases: G1 (G = gap), S

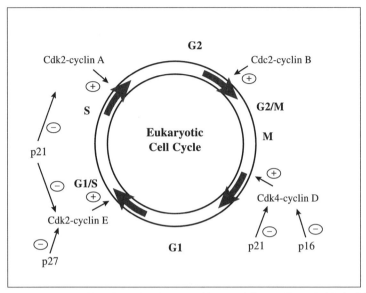

Figure 5.   Eukaryotic cell cycle. Cyclin-dependent kinases (Cdks), cyclins and Cdk inhibitors (CKIs) interact during the cell cycle. Progression during the cell cycle is regulated by interaction of positive and negative regulatory factors. The positive progression is directed by multiple cyclin-Cdk complexes, which act by phosphorylating various proteins at the different stages of the cycle. Negative regulatory factors include CKIs such as p16, p21 and p27, which inhibit phosphorylation of proteins by kinase and stop the cell cycle.

(synthesis), G2 and M (mitosis). The period between one M phase and the next – consisting of the three remaining phases G1, S and G2 – is called *interphase*. The G1 phase is the interval between the completion of M phase and the onset of S phase. The G2 phase is the interval between the end of S phase and the beginning of M phase. DNA is replicated during the S phase and is distributed equally to two daughter cells during the M phase. The cells prepare for the S phase during G1, and for the M phase during G2, the interval when proteins are synthesized in preparation for mitosis. Cells that do not undergo division, such as neurons, exit the cell cycle and enter a phase called G0. If cells in G0 are stimulated to grow, they move from G0 into the G1 phase. Progression through the cell cycle is mediated by multiple cyclin-dependent kinases (Cdks) that are sequentially activated by the binding of cyclins. The activated Cdk-cyclin protein complex phosphorylates specific proteins that are required for the reactions unique to each distinct phase of the cell cycle. Cyclins vary dramatically during the cell cycle. For example, cyclin B levels increase during interphase and subsequently decline during M phase.

TABLE 1. Cyclin-dependent kinases (Cdks), cyclins and cyclin-dependent kinase inhibitors
(CKIs) at different stages of the cell cycle

Cell cycle phase	Cdk	Cyclin	CKI	
			KIPᵃ	INKᵇ
G1	Cdk4	Cyclin D	p21, p27	P15, P16
G1/S	Cdk2	Cyclin E	p21, p27	
S	Cdk2	Cyclin A	p21	
G2/M	Cdc2	Cyclin B	p21	
M	Cdc2	Cyclin B, cyclin A		

ᵃKIP proteins (p21, p27) bind multiple cyclin-Cdk complexes that prevent activation or inhibit
kinase activity.
ᵇINK proteins (p15, p16) are specific for Cdk4/6 and cyclin D. They bind Cdk and inhibit the
binding of cyclin D.

The changes in the level of cyclin B are correlated with the activity of a specific Cdk called Cdc2, which is active when cyclin B levels peak and becomes
inactive as cyclin B levels decline. Thus, the phosphorylating activity of Cdc2
is modulated during the cell cycle by the availability of cyclin B. The activation of Cdc2 also depends on phosphorylation of a specific threonine residue,
thus adding a second layer to the control of the kinase activity. A variety of
cell-cycle "checkpoints" monitor progression through the cell cycle. Deviation from the normal cell cycle impedes progression beyond the checkpoint
and the cell cycle is halted until the defect is corrected. Thus, the orderly progression through the cell cycle depends on both positive factors that drive the
cell cycle forward and negative factors that halt the cycle at a particular stage.
Cdks and specific cyclins are the main positive factors that function at each
stage of the cell cycle. Negative factors that block the activity of the specific
Cdks are called cyclin-dependent kinase inhibitors (CKIs) (Table 1).

Several mechanisms may be responsible for the inactivation of an active
Cdk-cyclin complex:

1. The cyclin molecule can be degraded through the ubiquitin protein-degrading system.
2. The critical phosphate required for activation of the kinase activity can be
   removed from the protein by a specific phosphatase.
3. CKI molecules interact with Cdks or Cdk-cyclin complexes and inhibit the
   kinase activity. Two classes of CKIs have been described, the INK (inhibitor
   of Cdk) class and the KIP (kinase inhibitory protein) class (Table 1).

Thus the interplay between the activation and deactivation of the Cdk activities at various stages of the cell cycle is the key determinant of the normal progression and regulation of the cell cycle.

2.5.1 THE G1 PHASE

The G1 phase heralds the onset of the cell cycle. Resting cells (G0 phase) that are stimulated to divide enter the G1 phase. Once the cell passes this point it is committed to entering the S phase and subsequently divides. The key positive regulators of the G1 phase are Cdk4 and cyclins of the D family, which form a complex capable of phosphorylating a host of proteins required for cell function in the G1 phase. The retinoblastoma protein (pRb) is a key protein phosphorylated by the Cdk4–cyclin D in G1. pRb exists in a nonphosphorylated form during the first two-thirds of the G1 phase and becomes phosphorylated just prior to the transition from G1 to S phase. Nonphosphorylated pRb restricts cell growth, whereas phosphorylated pRb is associated with a loss of growth inhibitory function and allows the cell to proceed through the cell cycle. Thus, pRb functions as a regulator that represses or activates specific promoters through interaction with and modification of the activities of transcription factors that bind to DNA and regulate the expression of cell-cycle genes. The phosphorylation of pRb by the Cdk4–cyclin D complex allows previously repressed genes to be transcribed and allows the cell to progress from G1 to S phase.

The Cdk inhibitor p27 is a second important control that regulates the progression of a cell from G1 to S phase. This protein binds to the Cdk2–cyclin E complex and inactivates it. The cells are unable to proceed to the S phase and remain arrested in G1. Growth-promoting factors result in the degradation of p27, activation of the Cdk2–cyclin E complex and transition to the S phase. The ubiquitin protein-degrading system is responsible for the degradation of p27.

2.5.2 THE S PHASE

Entry into the S phase is determined by a putative cytoplasmic signal that is most likely an active Cdk-cyclin complex. The entrance into S phase from G1 and progression through S phase to G2 depends on the function of specific Cdk-cyclin complexes. Cdk2 initially binds cyclin E as the cells proceed into the S phase. Cyclin A activates Cdk2 and phosphorylation of proteins required for DNA replication.

2.5.3 THE G2/M PHASE

The G2/M phase represents a critical checkpoint where cells decide whether to enter mitosis. The critical proteins involved in the G2/M checkpoint include Cdc2 and cyclin B, which form a complex. The Cdc2–cyclin B complex is essential for the entry into and exit from the M phase, which involves the activation and deactivation of the Cdc2-cyclin B complex through a series of phosphorylation and dephosphorylation steps.

2.5.4 THE M PHASE

The sudden activation of the Cdc2–cyclin B complex by dephosphorylation, which occurs at the G2/M border, results in the phosphorylation of a variety of proteins required for mitosis. Three checkpoints are key to the orderly entry into and exit from mitosis, with each daughter cell receiving an exact copy of the parental genome. These three checkpoints are (1) the transition from G2 to M concurrent with the activation of the Cdc2–cyclin B complex; (2) the M phase checkpoint that occurs during metaphase (the point that regulates the timing of the separation of the chromatids and the initiation of anaphase); and (3) the immediate proteolytic destruction of cyclin B at the onset of anaphase with the concomitant inactivation of Cdc2 (which allows the cell to exit the M phase and enter a new G1 phase). These checkpoints are regulated by the ubiquitin pathway.

2.5.5 THE ROLE OF p53 AND p21 IN THE CONTROL OF
   CELL DAMAGE

The orderly progression within the cell cycle and the cell's ability to sense any perturbation in its normal state are crucial to normal cell growth and development. Cells have evolved negative regulatory mechanisms that sense physiological disturbances, DNA damage, hypoxia, nutrient depletion and viral infection. Either the cell can arrest the cycle at a particular stage or, in some instances, the cell will undergo programmed cell death, which is called apoptosis.

The DNA-binding protein, p53, orchestrates the negative regulatory mechanisms take effect when the cell is damaged. The p53 protein is a tumor-supressor protein and activates transcription of the gene encoding the Cdk inhibitor, p21. The p21 protein binds to multiple cyclin-Cdk complexes and blocks kinase activity. This inhibits the phosphorylation of proteins required for the various stages of the cell cycle. The binding of p21 to the G1 cyclin-Cdk complexes is central to the cessation of the G1 phase that follows DNA damage by radiation. This gives the DNA repair mechanisms time to correct the damage. Another function of p21 is to bind *proliferating cell nuclear antigen (PCNA)*. PCNA is a cofactor required for full expression of DNA polymerase δ (see Section 2.6). DNA replication is inhibited when p21 is bound to PCNA. The roles that p53 and p21 play in damage control in cells are illustrated in Figure 6.

Mutations that lead to the loss or alteration of p53 activity result in cancer

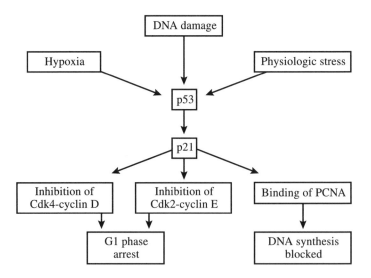

Figure 6.   The control of damage by p53 and p21. Cellular damage results in increased p53 activity. p53 functions as a transcription factor and induces the transcription of p21, a cyclin-dependent kinase inhibitor (CKI). The p21 interacts with multiple cyclin-dependent kinase (Cdk)-cyclin complexes, inhibits the kinase activity, and halts the cells in G1 phase. p21 also binds pro-liferating cell nuclear antigen (PCNA), inhibiting DNA synthesis.

development. Abnormal p53 levels are associated with the loss of the cell's ability to halt the progression of the cell cycle under the aforementioned adverse conditions. Therefore, the cell continues to proliferate, and this results in a defective phenotype.

2.6 DNA Replication [14–19]

As described earlier, the replication of DNA occurs during the S phase of the cell cycle. The S phase occupies approximately 30% of the cell-cycle time. The replication of DNA is a semi-conservative process, wherein each parental strand of the DNA helix serves as a template for the synthesis of a new and complementary daughter strand. In human diploid cells, this involves the replication of 6 billion base pairs of DNA.

Many enzymes and proteins are involved in DNA replication. The key enzyme is *DNA polymerase*, which catalyzes the ligation of the deoxyribonu-cleoside 5′-triphosphates (dNTPs) to generate the growing DNA chain. Eukaryotic cells contain 5 types of DNA polymerases: α, β, γ, δ, ϵ. The prop-

TABLE 2.   The structural and functional properties of human DNA polymerases

DNA polymerase	Size (catalytic subunit) [kilodaltons]	Location	Function in the cell
α	160–185	Nucleus	Lagging strand replication
β	40	Nucleus	DNA repair
γ	125	Mitochondria	Replication of mitochondrial DNA
δ	125	Nucleus	Leading and lagging strand replication
ε	210–230	Nucleus	DNA repair (?)

erties of the various human DNA polymerases are described in Table 2. The DNA polymerase γ is restricted to the mitochondria, where it is responsible for mitochondrial DNA replication. The other four DNA polymerases are localized in the nucleus. DNA polymerase δ is the major replicating enzyme in human cells.

The process of DNA replication on each chromosome is initiated at designated positions, referred to as *origins of replication (ori)*. Each human chromosome has multiple ori placed at every 150–200 kilobase pairs. There are approximately 30,000 initiation sites found over the entire human genome. Thus, multiple sections of the genome are replicated simultaneously. Each small replicating unit is termed a *replicon,* and has its own ori site where DNA synthesis is initiated. The process of DNA replication proceeds bi-directionally on the chromosome until each replicon comes into contact with the next one. Thus, an entire chromosome can be replicated completely during the S phase of the cell cycle.

As the two parent DNA strands unwind and separate, DNA replication begins at ori and proceeds down the two DNA strands (Figure 7). Because of the inherent properties of DNA polymerase, daughter strand synthesis can proceed from the ori only in the 5'-to-3' direction. Thus, one strand is synthesized in a 5'-to-3' direction and the opposite strand is also synthesized in the 5'-to-3' direction. As there is no DNA polymerase that can synthesize DNA in a 3'-to-5' direction, a DNA strand cannot be used as a template in the 3'-to-5' direction. Thus, replication of the 3'-to-5' strand above the ori is accomplished by synthesis of short fragments of DNA, called *Okazaki fragments.* The Okazaki fragments are approximately 200 nucleotides in length, and are synthesized in a 5'-to-3' direction. The resulting fragments are then joined by an enzyme called *DNA ligase* to give one continuous DNA strand. The DNA strand that is synthesized continuously in the 5'-to-3' direction is called the *leading strand of DNA synthesis*, since it starts at a fixed point and dictates DNA synthesis. The strand of DNA that is synthesized in the 5'-to-3' direc-

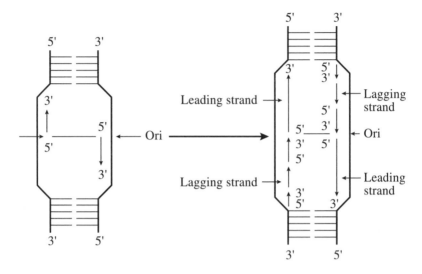

Figure 7. Replicon. DNA polymerase can synthesize DNA only in a 5'-to-3' direction. For both strands of the DNA helix to serve as templates, one strand (i.e., the leading strand) is synthesized continuously in a 5'-to-3' direction while the other strand (i.e., the lagging strand) is synthesized discontinuously in short fragments but still in a 5'-to-3' direction. The short DNA fragments (Okazaki fragments) are subsequently joined together by DNA ligase.

tion in short pieces (i.e., discontinuously) is called the *lagging strand of DNA synthesis.*

The *replication fork* refers to that part of the DNA molecule that is being replicated at a given time, and represents the region between the unreplicated segment of the DNA molecule and a newly replicated portion of DNA. Since DNA is synthesized bi-directionally, each replicon contains two replication forks. A specific initiator protein has the ability to recognize the origin sequence and signals the initiation of DNA synthesis. It has been hypothesized that this initiator protein binds the ori sequence, and attracts the DNA-replicating complex to this particular site on the DNA molecule.

All DNA polymerases must have a *primer* (i.e., a free 3'-OH end of a polynucleotide). The primer in DNA replication is not DNA, but rather is a small segment of RNA measuring 5 to 10 nucleotides in length, which is synthesized by the enzyme *DNA primase.* DNA primase initiates the synthesis of an RNA molecule at the ori, and DNA polymerase uses this RNA primer to add deoxyribonucleotides to the 3'-OH group of the RNA and synthesizes a new DNA strand that is complementary to the template strand. After comple-

TABLE 3. Proteins involved in DNA replication

Protein	Function
DNA helicase	Unwinds DNA and breaks hydrogen bonds
Single-stranded DNA-binding protein (RPA)	Binds single-stranded DNA to prevent hydrogen bonding
Proliferating cell nuclear antigen (PCNA)	Stimulates DNA polymerase δ activity
DNA polymerase δ	Leading and lagging strand DNA replication and 3′–5′ exonuclease proofreading
DNA polymerase α/DNA primase complex	Synthesis of RNA primers and lagging strand synthesis
DNA ligase	Seals 3′ terminal hydroxyl and 5′ terminal phosphate groups of adjacent nucleotides in DNA
Ribonuclease H1 (Rnase H1)	Removes RNA from RNA-DNA hybrid
DNA topoisomerase	Relaxes DNA by breaking and resealing phophodiester bonds

tion of DNA synthesis, the RNA molecule is removed from the DNA helix and the resulting gap in the DNA is filled by a DNA polymerase.

The various proteins that play an important role on the process of DNA replication are listed in Table 3. The separation of the two strands of DNA is catalyzed by an enzyme called *DNA helicase*, which breaks the hydrogen bonds holding the DNA strands together. The DNA helix is subsequently unwound, and the strands remain separated through the action of a protein called *replication protein A (RPA)*. RPA is a single-stranded DNA-binding protein (Figure 8). The DNA helicase acts at the edge of the replication fork, opening and unwinding the DNA as replication proceeds along the DNA molecule. As the helicase unwinds the DNA at the replication fork, the DNA helix downstream becomes tightly wound and supercoiled. The tension on the DNA molecule is released by the action of *DNA topoisomerase,* which breaks phosphodiester bonds, unwinds the downstream DNA helix, and then reseals it by forming new phosphodiester bonds. Both DNA helicases and DNA topoisomerases play a pivotal role in the process of DNA replication and transcription.

The DNA polymerases catalyze the formation of phosphodiester bonds between the adjacent deoxyribonucleotides in the DNA molecule. All DNA polymerases catalyze the synthesis of DNA only in the 5′-to-3′ direction. DNA polymerase δ is the major replicating protein in human cells, and is involved in both leading and lagging strand replication. DNA polymerase α is complexed with another protein, the DNA primase. Together, these proteins are involved in the replication of the lagging strand. DNA primase

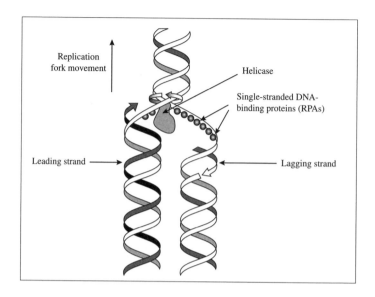

Figure 8. The replication of a DNA molecule, illustrating the interaction of the helicase and DNA-binding proteins at the replication fork.

makes the small RNA primers with DNA polymerase α. Deoxyribonu-cleotides are added to the 3' terminal of the primer for a short distance of about 30 nucleotides. The DNA polymerase α/DNA primase complex sub-sequently falls off the DNA molecule, and is replaced by DNA polymerase δ, which continues the synthesis of the growing DNA chain. The RNA primers used by DNA polymerases must be removed from the DNA mole-cule. This is accomplished by the action of the enzyme *RNase H1*, which specifically degrades RNA present in a DNA/RNA hybrid. DNA polymerase later completes the DNA synthesis of the lagging strand by filling in the gap. Then the ligation of the 3'-OH terminus of the DNA of one Okazaki frag-ment with the 5' terminal phosphate of DNA of the adjacent fragment occurs through the formation of a phosphodiester bond. This reaction is catalyzed by DNA ligase.

DNA polymerase β and ϵ serve in the process of DNA repair, and are not directly involved in replicating the entire genome. Finally, DNA polymerase γ is responsible for replicating the circular double-stranded DNA found in mitochondria.

An additional protein involved in the replication of DNA in human cells is termed *proliferating cell nuclear antigen (PCNA)*. PCNA forms part of the DNA polymerase δ complex and stimulates the activity in the DNA poly-

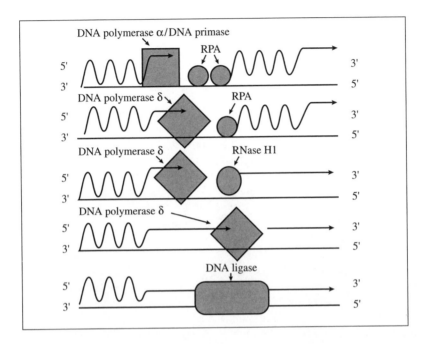

Figure 9. Model for DNA replication in human cells. Replication protein A (RPA), a single-stranded DNA-binding protein, separates the DNA strands to allow the DNA polymerase α/DNA primase complex to bind to the DNA and initiate synthesis of an RNA primer (indicated by the wavy line). DNA polymerase α adds approximately 30 deoxyribonucleotides to the 3' end of the RNA primer. The DNA polymerase δ displaces the RNA polymerase α/DNA primase complex and extends the DNA strand by adding deoxyribonucleotides to the 3' end of the newly synthesized DNA strand. Upon completion of DNA synthesis, RNase H1 removes the RNA primer. The DNA polymerase δ fills in the gap using the opposite DNA strand as a template. Finally, the two Okazaki fragments are joined together. This reaction is catalyzed by DNA ligase.

merase. The interactions of various proteins involved in DNA synthesis in the lagging strand are depicted in the model shown in Figure 9.

Some DNA polymerases (e.g., DNA polymerase δ) have intrinsic 3'-5' *exonuclease* activity, which removes bases sequentially from the end of the DNA molecule (i.e., the 3' end). This nuclease activity plays a critical role in preventing mistakes in base pairing during DNA replication. For example, if a C on the new DNA strand binds to an A on the template strand, subsequent replications of this mistake result in a CG base pair molecule instead of an AT base pair. The substitution of one base pair by another leads to a mutation in the DNA molecule which may have an impact upon cellular function.

The 3'-5' exonuclease recognizes these mispairs as soon as they occur and removes the newly inserted incorrect base. The DNA polymerase then inserts the proper base into the growing DNA chain. This exonuclease activity of DNA polymerase is termed the *proofreading function*.

As mentioned in Section 2.3, the ends (telomeres) of all chromosomes maintain the overall integrity of the chromosomes. Telomeres consist of the base sequence TTAGGG, whose elements are randomly repeated 100 to 1,000 times. Because DNA polymerases function only in the 5'-to-3' direction, they are unable to copy the extreme 5' ends of linear DNA molecules. These sequences (i.e., telomeres) are replicated by the action of the enzyme telomerase, which is a reverse transcriptase. Reverse transcriptases synthesize DNA from an RNA template. Telomerases carry their own template RNA complementary to the telomere repeat sequences. The RNA template allows telomerase to generate multiple copies of the telomeric repeat sequences, thus maintaining telomeres in the absence of a conventional DNA template to direct their synthesis.

Despite the accuracy of DNA replication, cellular genomes are far from static. Gene rearrangements and mutations are required to maintain genetic diversity among individuals. To this end, recombination between homologous chromosomes occurs during meiosis and allows parental genes to be rearranged in new combinations in the next generation of cells. The rearrangements of DNA sequences within the genome create novel combinations of genetic information. In some instances DNA rearrangements are programmed to regulate gene expression during the cellular processes of differentiation and development. A striking example of this is the rearrangement of antibody genes during the development of the immune system. A key feature of both immunoglobulins and T-cell receptors is their enormous diversity, which allows different antibody or T-cell receptor molecules to recognize a variable array of antigens. These diverse antibodies and T-cell receptors are encoded by unique lymphocyte genes that are formed during the development of the immune system as a result of site-specific recombination between distinct segments of immunoglobulin and T-cell receptor genes.

2.7 Mutations and DNA Repair Mechanisms [20–26]

Mutations are the result of permanent changes in the base sequence of the DNA molecule, and are central to the pathogenesis of all human genetic diseases. The various classes of mutations that occur in DNA molecules are listed in Table 4. Many of the concepts concerning the different types of mutations that occur in DNA, and the potential mechanisms associated with the production of these mutations, were originally developed in bacterial cell model systems. Recently, our knowledge base has expanded in the area of the

TABLE 4. The classes of mutations found in human DNA

Single-base pair substitutions (point mutations)	
Altered structure of gene product	
Missense mutation	Single amino acid replacement in the protein
Nonsense mutation	A termination codon in the middle of the gene results in premature termination of protein synthesis
RNA-splicing mutation	The protein may be missing part or all of an exon sequence
Altered quantity of gene product	
Mutations in regulatory sequences	Transcription of the gene is altered, which can reduce or eliminate the gene product
Mutations in RNA processing and translation	The stability of messenger RNA is altered, which may reduce the amount of gene product
Insertions or deletions	
One or two base pairs (frameshift mutations)	The addition or deletion of one or two base pairs can affect the reading frame of the gene, resulting in a grossly altered or absent gene product
Large number of base pairs	Large pieces of the DNA may be lost, or large segments of DNA may insert into the middle of a gene, resulting in loss of function
Expansion of trinucleotide repeat sequences	
	Unstable trinucleotide repeats can suddenly expand in number, resulting in the alteration of production or structure of a particular gene product
Chromosomal alterations	Inversions, translocations, duplications or gene amplification may result

molecular basis of mutations in eukaryotic cells. Studies of diseased human cells have established common mechanisms by which DNA undergoes mutation. More importantly, DNA repair mechanisms have been defined.

Many of the mutations that occur in DNA are the result of *single-base-pair substitutions* in which one base pair (e.g., an adenine–thymine pair) is replaced by a second base pair (e.g., a guanine–cytosine pair). The substitution of one base pair by a second base pair elicits a change of codon that can lead either to a *missense mutation* (where one amino acid replaces another amino acid in a protein) or to a *nonsense mutation* (where one of the terminator codons appears in the middle of a gene). With a nonsense mutation, there is no transfer of an RNA molecule to recognize these codons, and protein synthesis terminates at the site of the nonsense codon. This leads to the production of a truncated polypeptide.

A mutation that alters the splice acceptor or splice donor sequences can result in apparent splicing of an RNA transcript. This leads to the production of an mRNA that may be missing a substantial part of a particular exon, and thus codes for a mutant protein. Other base pair substitutions can occur in regulatory sequences required for the binding of transcription factors or RNA polymerase. In this instance, the quantity of the product produced by the gene that is controlled by these sequences is dramatically altered. In the extreme case, base pair substitutions can lead to a complete absence of the gene product, or to a dramatic increase in the amount of a particular gene product.

Frameshift mutations are caused by the addition or deletion of one or two base pairs within the coding sequence of a gene. This alters the reading frame of the mRNA. Thus, the mRNA is translated out of the frame from the site of the insertion or deletion of the base pair. This results in the production of a protein that is altered in its amino acid sequence, starting from the point of the insertion or deletion of the base pair and continuing to the end of the protein. Often, the altered reading frame also leads to the production of a termination codon in the middle of the gene. This results in premature cessation of protein synthesis.

The insertion and deletion of many base pairs can also occur with DNA molecules. Deletion mutations can occur in a chromosome with the loss of hundreds to thousands of base pairs from the DNA, with the result that the deleted genetic material is permanently lost. Large insertions of DNA sequences have been described. These are caused by transposon-like elements, often repetitive DNA sequences such as long interspersed nuclear element (LINE) repeats.

In summary, the possible changes in DNA that give rise to mutations may be illustrated by considering the following literary masterpiece:

Wild type	The cat sat on the mat.
Substitution	The **r**at sat on the mat.
Insertion (single)	The cat **s**hat on the mat.
Insertion (multiple)	The cat**tle** sat on the mat.
Deletion (single)	The c.t sat on the mat.
Deletion (multiple)	The cat ... .. the mat.
Inversion (small)	The **tac** sat on the mat.
Inversion (large)	**Tam eht no tas tac eht.**

DNA polymerases catalyze the proper pairing of A to T and G to C with very high accuracy. However, mispairing occurs at a frequency of approximately 10^{-5} bases. For example, if an AC pair forms instead of an AT pair, and if such a mispair remains in the DNA molecule, the initial AT pair that has become an AC pair now gives rise to a GC pair during the next replication cycle. In order to keep the mutation rate at a low level, eukaryotic cells have devised mechanisms for correcting base mispairs before they become a permanent feature of the DNA.

Bases that are present in DNA molecules can undergo spontaneous damage or modification. One frequent form of modification occurs with the purine bases A and G. Purine residues may be lost from the DNA molecules by a process called *depurination*. The glycosidic bond between the deoxyribose and the base is hydrolyzed, which leads to a gap in one of the DNA strands. This damage must be corrected before the DNA is replicated, otherwise a mutation ensues. The bases C, A and G are capable of undergoing spontaneous *deamination*, wherein the base loses an amino group and its structure is changed. For example, when cytosine is deaminated it becomes uracil. This leads to the presence of uracil in DNA instead of cytosine. Uracil now appears with an adenine residue during the next replication cycle. The original GC pair, which after deamination is now a GU pair, subsequently becomes an AT pair. Ultraviolet rays from sunlight are a common mutagenic agent that causes bond formation between adjacent pyrimidines on the same DNA strand. The most frequent type of pyrimidine dimer is the TT dimer. The presence of a TT dimer in the DNA molecule blocks DNA replication and leads to the death of the cell if it is not removed. The 3'-5' exonuclease activity associated with DNA polymerase δ and ϵ is responsible for cleaving mispaired nucleotides from the 3' end of newly replicated DNA strands. This allows the polymerase a second opportunity to add the correct base. The entire process is known as the proofreading function.

If base mispairing remains in the DNA, it leads to a mutation at the next DNA replication cycle. However, eukaryotic cells have evolved a mechanism to deal specifically with persistent base mispairing immediately after replication. Human cells have a *methyl-directed mismatch repair system,* which appears to be similar to that of bacterial strains. The methyl-directed mismatch repair system scans the DNA molecule, and when base mispairs as well as insertions and deletions are detected, correction of the error occurs on the nonmethylated, newly synthesized DNA strand. This allows the repair system to correct the nascent strand that has a normal base in the wrong location, and prevents the mispaired bases from giving rise to a permanent mutation.

DNA molecules are methylated at specific sites, either on an A or a C residue. In human cells, C residues located in CpG islands are methylated. Methylation is a postreplication event. During the initial period of DNA replication, one strand (i.e., the template strand) is methylated, while the newly synthesized DNA strand is not methylated.

Mutator (mut) proteins are involved in methyl-directed mismatch repair. Human homologues have been identified for MutS (hMSH2 and GTBP) and MutL (hMLH1 and hPMS2), but at this time, there are no known homologues for MutH. Methyl-directed mismatch repair appears to be similar in bacteria and humans. In human cells, mismatches are recognized by the protein hMSH2 or a dimer composed of hMSH2 and GTBP. Base mispairing creates a bulge in the DNA, which is recognized and bound by the MutS protein. The MutS protein that is bound to the mismatch recruits the MutL homologue to the site. MutH cleaves the nonmethylated DNA strand. This is followed by the stepwise removal of nucleotides by an exonuclease, and the resulting gap in the DNA molecule is repaired by DNA polymerase using the base sequence in the template strand. The final phosphodiester bond is sealed by DNA ligase.

One of the most common hereditary cancers, HNPCC (hereditary nonpolyposis colon cancer), arises from mutations in the methyl-directed mismatch repair system. HNPCC affects 1 in 200 people in North America and accounts for approximately 15% of all colon cancers. There are at least five genetic loci involved in the human mismatch repair process. These include hMSH2, hMLH1, hPMS1, and hPMS2 and the GTBP gene. Cells with HNPCC are characterized by *microsatellite instability*. Microsatellites are repetitive nucleotide sequences (di-, tri- or tetranucleotides) located throughout the human genome. The presence of these repeats in the DNA is a "road block" to the DNA polymerase molecule during DNA replication. When DNA polymerase is confronted with a long, repetitive sequence of DNA, it produces a strand of DNA with extra bases that are not base-paired with the template and that loop away from the DNA helix. The mismatch repair system recognizes these loops as defective and removes them. The loops remain if the repair system is defective. Microsatellite instability signals that the cell has developed a *mut* phenotype and has an increased rate of overall mutation. These cells also develop mutations in such genes as the p53 gene or other tumor supressor genes at a much higher rate than do normal cells.

Another type of DNA mutation is incurred through damage to bases of a DNA molecule that is not undergoing replication. Cells have evolved two major repair systems to deal with this type of DNA damage. The first system is called *base excision repair*. When a uracil residue occurs in a DNA molecule, it is recognized by uracil-DNA glycosylase and is removed from the DNA, leaving behind a gap. The lack of a base in the DNA helix is recognized by specific endonucleases known as *AP endonucleases* (which recognize *a*purinic and *a*pyrimidinic sites in DNA). The AP endonuclease cleaves the DNA at the site of the missing base. The resulting gap is repaired by DNA polymerase, using the base present in the complementary strand as a template.

This is followed by ligation via DNA ligase. If the uracil residue is not removed, it eventually results in a GU mismatch, and the original GC pair becomes an AT pair or a mutation. A more general repair mechanism, known as *nucleotide excision repair,* repairs bulky distortions in the DNA molecule. The overall scheme for nucleotide excision repair resembles that of base excision repair and methyl-directed mismatch repair. All systems have specific proteins that recognize the damaged area of DNA, as well as specific proteins involved in the removal of the damage from the DNA. Following removal of the damage, the gap is filled by repair synthesis. This is catalyzed by DNA polymerase, and sealing is accomplished by DNA ligase.

Xeroderma pigmentosum (XP) is a rare autosomal recessive disorder characterized by skin neoplasms. Skin cells from XP patients are unable to repair DNA damage caused by exposure to ultraviolet (UV) light. UV light damages DNA, resulting in the formation of dimers between adjacent pyrimidines on the same DNA strand (e.g., TT dimer). These TT dimers distort the DNA helix and result in the cessation of replication and transcription at that point until the dimer is removed. The nucleotide excision repair system removes these TT dimers. The initial step is the recognition of the damage by the XPA protein, which binds along with XPF-ERCC1 protein and the single-stranded DNA-binding protein RPA. Helicase activity unwinds the helix and stimulates the excision activity of two endonucleases, XPF and XPG, which cut the DNA. This creates a large gap in the DNA molecule, and the 3′ hydroxyl terminus is recognized by DNA polymerase δ or ε, which carries out repair synthesis using the undamaged DNA strand as a template. The final nick is sealed by DNA ligase.

A new type of mutation has been recently described which results in a number of human genetic diseases. These mutations are the result of the expansion of trinucleotide repeats (CAG, CTG, CGG or GAA) found throughout the human genome. Long runs of these repeat triplets are found in exons at the 5′ or 3′ end of genes. Individuals affected with one of the expansion disorder diseases have an increase in the number of copies of the trinucleotide repeats. The expansion of the repeat sequences can alter either the structure or function of a particular protein. One of the best characterized examples of this is the trinucleotide CAG, which codes for the amino acid glutamine. In *Huntington's disease* the CAG repeat is located in the coding region of the first exon at the 5′ end of the gene. These repeats are translated, and appear as a long stretch of glutamines within the structure of the protein such that the mutant protein has a range of 40 to 100 glutamines at that particular site. All of the CAG repeat diseases are autosomal dominant disorders characterized by late-onset neuronal loss.

3. EUKARYOTIC GENE TRANSCRIPTION AND POST-TRANSCRIPTIONAL RNA PROCESSING

3.1 Chromatin Structure and Transcription [27–31]

The DNA present in all eukaryotic cells is tightly associated to histones, forming *chromatin*. Moreover, the packaging of eukaryotic DNA into chromatin has important ramifications in terms of its availability to serve as a template for transcription. Thus, chromatin structure is a critical aspect of eukaryotic gene expression. Actively transcribed genes are situated in regions of decondensed chromatin. The tight coiling of DNA around the *nucleosome* poses a major obstacle to transcription: the tight coiling impedes the ability of transcription factors to bind to DNA, as well as impeding the ability of RNA polymerase to gain access to the DNA template. This inhibitory effect of nucleosomes is overcome by the action of *nucleosome remodeling factors*. These remodeling factors disrupt chromatin structure, thus allowing transcription factors to gain purchase to nucleosome DNA and coordinate the assembly of the transcription complex with the promoter. A multiprotein complex, initially identified in yeast as the SWI/SNF (switch/sucrose nonfermenting) complex, has been localized in mammalian cells. SWI/SNF disrupts the nucleosome array and facilitates the transcription of DNA that was previously unavailable to the transcription complex.

Eukaryotic transcriptional activators play a dual role in modulating gene expression. In addition to promoting transcription by interacting with basal transcription factors, they stimulate changes in chromatin structure that alleviate repression by histones. The ability of RNA polymerase to transcribe chromatin templates is facilitated through the acetylation of histones, and by the association of the nonhistone chromosomal proteins HMG-14 and HMG-17 with the nucleosomes of actively transcribed genes. The signals that target HMG-14 and HMG-17 to actively transcribe genes remain an enigma.

3.2 Cis-Acting Elements [27, 30–32]

This discussion of the transcriptional control of gene expression is focused on the role of RNA polymerase II, the enzyme responsible for transcribing protein-encoding genes into mRNAs. The production of each mRNA in human cells involves complex interactions of proteins (*trans-acting factors*) with specific sequences on the DNA (*cis-acting elements*). Cis-acting elements are short base sequences adjacent to, or within, a particular gene. Alternatively, they can be sequences that occur several thousand base pairs away from a particular gene. Cis-acting elements are sequences required for the recognition of a gene by RNA polymerase II. These sequences also serve as binding sites for

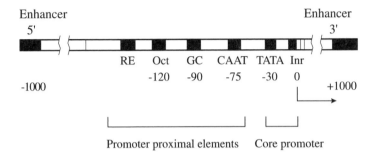

Figure 10. The localization of cis-acting sequences in a typical human gene. The core promoter is composed of TATA and initiator (Inr) sequences. The TATA sequence, located 30 base pairs upstream of the Inr sequence, is the binding site for the TATA-binding protein (TBP). The Inr sequence is where RNA polymerase II binds and initiates transcription. The promoter proximal elements are located 50 to several hundred base pairs upstream of the Inr site and include the common sequences CAAT, GC and Oct. These sequences are the binding sites for upstream transcription factors. Sequences in the promoter proximal regions are the response elements (RE), which are the binding sites for inducible transcription factors. Situated thousands of pairs away, either 5' or 3' to the gene of interest, are enhancer elements that bind activators.

the proteins that regulate the rate and specificity of transcription. The initiation of transcription is dictated by sequences that are present in each gene. The major cis-acting sequences of a gene are illustrated in Figure 10, and include the following:

1. The *core promoter element* is situated 5' to the gene and consists of the sequences where the transcription complex containing the RNA polymerase II assembles on the DNA molecule. There are two fixed sequence elements: the *initiator element (Inr)*, which determines the transcription start site, and the *TATA element*, which is located 25–30 base pairs upstream from the Inr. The promoter initiation site defines the location and the direction of transcription.

2. The *promoter proximal elements* are composed of two types of cis-acting sequences located 50 to a few hundred base pairs upstream from the start site. The first type of promoter proximal element comprises a class of base sequences (e.g., CAAT or GC) found in many genes, and these sequences function as binding sites for proteins called *upstream transcription factors*. The second type of promoter proximal element is the *response element (RE)*. The RE contains sequences that are found in promoters controlled by a particular stimulus, e.g., genes that respond to particular glucocorticoid

stimulation or iron response elements (IRE) implicated in intestinal iron absorption.

3. The *promoter distal elements* are cis-acting sequences found thousands of base pairs away from the start site of transcription. These distal sites are known as *enhancers* or *silencers* and are situated either upstream or downstream from the gene that they regulate. Enhancers, like promoters, act by binding transcription factors that subsequently regulate RNA polymerase. Because of the looping of the DNA helix, this allows a transcription factor bound to a distant enhancer to lie in relative proximity to the upstream promoter and interact with RNA polymerase or basal transcription factors at the promoter. The binding of specific transcriptional regulatory proteins to enhancers is a mechanism responsible for controlling gene expression during development and cell differentiation. In addition, this mechanism also serves to mediate the response of cells to hormones and growth factors.

Transcription is initiated by the binding of a variety of transcription factors and the enzyme RNA polymerase to the promoter site. A large number of transcription factors serve to recruit the RNA polymerase to the promoter site. Transcription factors bind to sequences in the promoter site on the DNA molecule or they can bind to one another in several different areas to determine whether RNA polymerase will or will not transcribe a particular gene. The structural features of typical transcription factors are illustrated in Figure 11. Transcription factors are characterized by the following shared features: (1) binding to specific DNA sequences; (2) interaction with other transcription factors to regulate transcription; (3) a DNA-binding domain made up of the amino acid sequences that recognize and bind specific DNA sequences; and (4) a transactivation domain comprising the amino acid sequences required for the activation of transcription.

Transcription factors may have similar DNA-binding domains but different transactivating domains. Thus, they bind the same sequence of DNA but activate transcription in a different manner. Alternatively, transcription factors have similar transactivating domains but different DNA-binding domains. In this case, the transcription factors bind to different sequences of DNA, although the process of activation is similar. RNA polymerase catalyzes the formation of a phosphodiester bond by attaching the 5'-phosphate of the incoming ribonucleotide to the 3'-hydroxyl of the growing RNA chain. Multiple RNA transcripts may be synthesized from a single DNA molecule through the sequential binding of additional RNA polymerase to the promoter sequence.

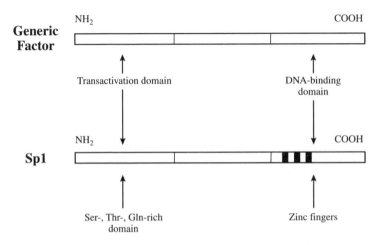

Figure 11. Common functional domains in transcription factors. Many transcription factors contain two common functional domains. The transactivation domain represents the amino acid sequence of the protein that interacts with other protein factors and is responsible for activating the transcription of genes. The DNA-binding domain comprises amino acid sequences that are responsible for interacting with and binding to specific DNA sequences. The upstream transcription factor (Sp1) binds to GC sequences through its DNA-binding domain, which includes three zinc finger motifs. The transactivation domain of Sp1 is rich in the amino acids serine, threonine and glutamine, and interacts with the TAFIID 110 subunit of TFIID.

3.3 Trans-Acting Transcription Factors [27, 30–36]

Trans-acting transcription factors bind to cis-acting elements on the DNA and interact with other transcription factors. These proteins control the initiation of transcription and comprise the following:

1. *General transcription factors* are polypeptides that assemble at the core of the promoter site and recruit RNA polymerase II to that site to form the pre-initiation complex.
2. *Upstream transcription factors* are proteins that bind the common cis-acting sequences proximal to many promoters, such as the sequences CAAT and GC.
3. *Inducible transcription factors* are proteins that respond to external stimuli that activate them and in turn promote their binding to the response element (RE) sequences. This results in increased transcription of genes containing the particular response element sequence.
4. *Activator proteins* are transcription factors that bind enhancers and increase transcriptional initiation of a particular gene.

5. *Repressor proteins* are transcription factors that silence and inhibit transcriptional initiation of a particular gene.

The ability of proteins to bind DNA is a reflection of their amino acid sequences and the formation of specific motifs. A well-characterized DNA-binding domain is the *zinc finger domain*. This contains repeats of cysteine and histidine residues that bind zinc ions within the DNA-binding domain. Zinc finger domains are common among transcription factors that regulate RNA polymerase II promoters, including the common transcription factor Sp1, the general transcription factor TFIIA and the glucocorticoid receptors. The *helix-turn-helix* motif is found in the *homeodomain* proteins, among other eukaryotic cell proteins. These play a central role in the regulation of gene expression during embryonic development. The molecular cloning and analysis of these genes have shown that they contain conserved sequences of 180 base pairs (homeoboxes) that encode the DNA-binding domains (homeodomains of transcription factors). Homeobox genes are highly conserved across a variety of species. Finally, leucine zipper and helix-loop-helix proteins are two other families of DNA-binding proteins that contain DNA-binding domains formed by dimerization of two polypeptide chains. They appear to play important roles in regulating tissue specific and inducible gene expression.

3.4 Initiation of Transcription by RNA Polymerase II [37–40]

A set of *basal transcription factors* interact with the cis-acting core promoter sequences to form a *basal transcription complex* (Figure 12) during the process of the initiation of transcription by RNA polymerase II. These transcription factors are named TFII for transcription factors associated with RNA polymerase II, followed by a letter (A, B, D, E, F or H). Other transcription factors bind to DNA sequences that control the expression of distinct genes and are thus responsible for regulating gene expression.

TFIID is the first TF to bind to the core promoter sequence, and is made up of a variety of proteins. These include a *TATA-binding protein* (TBP) that recognizes the TATA sequence at all promoter sites. The remaining proteins in TFIID are called TBP-associated factors (TAFs). Once TFIID is bound at the TATA sequence, a pre-initiation complex is formed with the recruitment of TFIIA, TFIIB, TFIIF/RNA polymerase II, TFIIE and TFIIH (Figure 12). The synthesis of mRNA then proceeds with the movement of RNA polymerase II away from the promoter region, and elongation of the mRNA transcript.

3.4.1 *ACTIVATION OF TRANSCRIPTION* [30, 31]

A variety of short cis-acting sequences (Figure 10) that are located upstream of the TATA sequence facilitate the efficient and specific recognition of the core

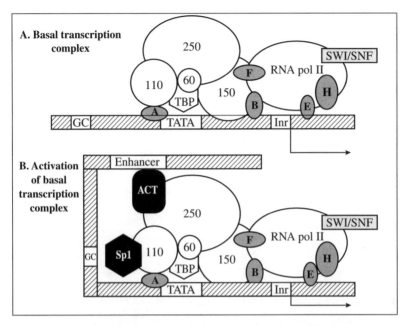

Figure 12. Model of the initiation of transcription by RNA polymerase II. The binding of the general transcription factors (GTFs) is illustrated in panel A, which depicts the formation of the basal transcription complex. RNA polymerase II (RNA pol II) binds to the core promoter. The TATA-binding protein (TBP), a subunit of TFIID, binds to the TATA sequence and facilitates the binding of the TBP-associated factors (TAFs). TBP and some of the TAFs are indicated as 250, 110, 150 and 60. Once TFIID is bound to the TATA sequence, the other GTFs (A, B, F, E and H) and RNA polymerase II bind to the core promoter, thus forming the basal transcription complex. Also indicated is the SWI/SNF multiprotein complex, associated with RNA polymerase II. This multiprotein complex is necessary for the disruption of chromatin structure. The activation of the basal transcription complex is illustrated in panel B: the activation of transcriptional initiation by Sp1 bound to the GC sequence and interacting with TAFIID 110. Further activation results from the binding of an activator protein (ACT) to an enhancer sequence located 1,000 base pairs from the core promoter. The ACT is brought into close proximity with the basal transcription complex by looping away from the DNA between the enhancer sequence and the core promoter to allow the activator to interact with TAFIID 250.

promoter by the basal transcription complex. The sequences include the common sequences found in RNA polymerase II promoters, including CAAT, Oct and GC. Specific upstream TFs recognize these sequences and bind to the DNA through a set of interactions among the DNA-binding domain of the TF, the DNA sequence, and the amino acid sequence of the transcription factor. For example, the upstream transcription factor Sp1 binds to GC sequences and subsequently interacts with the TFIID bound at the TATA box to activate transcription.

The activation mechanism for transcription of some classes/families of genes is shared in common under specific conditions. For example, exposure of cells to glucocorticoids or phorbol esters elicits a specific induction of the transcription of all the genes induced by these molecules. These inducible responses are attributed to upstream RE sequences in special promoters that function as binding sites for specific inducible transcription factors. An example of inducible control is the binding of the factor AP1 (made up of subunits encoded by *fos* and *jun*) to the TRE sequence (TGACTCA) in genes that are activated by phorbol esters, growth factors or cytokines. In the absence of phorbol ester, AP1 is phosphorylated, and then cannot bind to DNA (i.e., it is inactive). The activation of AP1 involves its dephosphorylation, such that it may bind to promoters containing TRE sequences. The binding of AP1 increases the rate of initiation of transcription.

Another example is steroid hormones, which bind to specific receptors to form an activated complex that is capable of binding to RE sequences found in specific genes. Steroid-receptor proteins comprise a DNA-binding domain that contains zinc finger motifs, and a hormone-binding domain. Activated steroid-receptor proteins are essentially TFs that, when bound to RE sites in the DNA, activate transcription of a specific class of genes through activation of the initiation of transcription by RNA polymerase II. All genes that contain the common RE sequence are simultaneously activated. This allows the cell to coordinate the inducible expression of multiple genes collectively in response to specific hormone signals.

One important class of membrane protein receptors has intrinsic tyrosine kinase activity. The ligands of these receptors include growth factors and cytokines, both of which regulate cell growth. Important to this class of receptors are the *signal transducers and activators of transcription (STATs)*. STATs are transcription factors that reside in the cytoplasm in an inactive form. The binding of cytokines to membrane-bound receptors leads to phosphorylation of the receptor by activation of the receptor tyrosine kinase activity. This provides a binding site for the STAT proteins. The bound STAT proteins are phosphorylated on tyrosine residues and undergo dimerization prior to migration to the nucleus. There they act as TFs by binding to specific DNA sequences upstream of the TATA sequence.

3.4.2 *EUKARYOTIC REPRESSORS* [41]
Gene expression in eukaryotic cells is regulated by repressors as well as by activators. Repressors bind to specific DNA sequences and inhibit transcription through a variety of mechansims. In some instances the repressors simply interfere with the binding of other transcription factors to DNA. Other repressors have been shown to compete with activators in binding to specific

regulatory sequences. As a result, their binding to a promoter or enhancer blocks the binding of the activator, thereby inhibiting transcription. Other repressors contain specific functional domains, called repression domains, that inhibit transcription through protein–protein interactions.

The regulation of transcription by repressors as well as by activators extends the repertoire of mechanisms that control the expression of eukaryotic genes. One important role of repressors is the inhibition of expression of tissue-specific genes in appropriate cell types. Other repressors play key roles in the control of cell proliferation and differentiation in response to growth factors as well as hormones. Such intricate control is especially important when considering the coordination required for maintaining the vertical crypt-villus and horizontal jejunoileocolonic axis of the gut.

3.5 Post-transcriptional Processing and the Regulation of Eukaryotic Gene Expression [42–57]

The human genome contains coding information for approximately 100,000 different RNA molecules. However, within a single cell different genes are expressed at different times through a process known as *differential gene expression*. Differential gene expression occurs in response to signals that occur during cell development, proliferation and differentiation. The orderly, programmed expression of every gene thereby plays a central role in cellular and whole-organ homeostasis. Thus, it is not surprising that cells have evolved elaborate mechanisms that specifically control gene expression for particular genes. The pivotal step in all cells for the regulation of gene expression is at the level of transcription. The complex task of regulating gene expression in the many differentiated cell types in higher eukaryotes is a reflection of the combined actions of a diverse array of transcriptional regulatory proteins.

While the cellular events associated with the regulation of transcription represent the predominant step in the regulation of eukaryotic gene expression, additional levels of control include the following: (1) controlling the processing of mRNA by determining which exons present in the initial mRNA transcript are retained in the mature and fully functional mRNA; control mechanisms include either the alternative splicing of exons or the differential polyadenylation of the initial mRNA transcript; and (2) controlling the stability or the rate of degradation of the mature mRNA transcript. As well, the packaging of DNA into chromatin and its modification by methylation add further dimensions to the control of eukaryotic gene expression.

3.5.1 *RNA PROCESSING* [47]

The majority of newly synthesized RNAs are subsequently modified in a variety of ways to be converted to their functional forms. The regulation of the

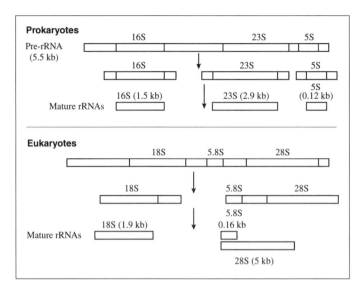

Figure 13. The processing of ribosomal RNAs. Prokaryotic cells contain three RNAs (16S, 23S and 5S) that are formed through cleavage of a pre-rRNA transcript. Eukaryotic cells contain four RNAs. One of these (5S rRNA) is transcribed from a separate gene; the other three (18S, 28S and 5.8S) are derived from a common pre-rRNA. Following cleavage, the 5.8S rRNA (which is unique to eukaryotes) becomes hydrogen-bonded 28S rRNA.

processing of RNA adds an additional level of control in eukaryotic gene expression.

RNA polymerase I is devoted to the transcription of rRNAs in the nucleolus. The processing of the 45S initial transcript, pre-rRNA, involves methylation of the RNA as well as ribonuclease-mediated cleavage of segments of the initial transcript to yield the 28S, 18S and 5.8S rRNAs (Figure 13).

The 5S tRNA is transcribed from a separate gene by RNA polymerase III, and the large precursor (pre-tRNA) undergoes cleavage and methylation. The processing of the 3′ end of tRNA involves the addition of a CCA terminus, such that all tRNAs have the sequence CCA at the 3′ end. This sequence is the site of an amino acid attachment to the tRNA during protein synthesis.

In eukaryotic cells, the mRNA synthesized in the nucleus by RNA polymerase II is exported to the cytoplasm before it can be used as a template for protein synthesis. The initial products of transcription in eukaryotic cells (pre-mRNAs) are extensively modified prior to export from the nucleus. The processing of eukaryotic mRNAs is illustrated in Figure 14. This processing involves the modification of both ends of the mRNA, as well as the removal of introns from its mid portion. The 5′ end of pre-mRNA is modified by the

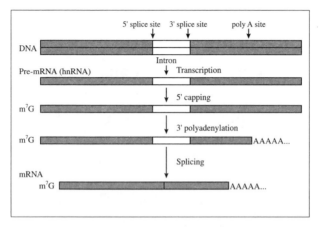

Figure 14. The processing of eukaryotic messenger RNAs. The processing of mRNA involves modification at the 5' end by capping with 7-methylguanosine (m⁷G), modification at the 3' end by polyadenylation, and removal of introns by splicing. The 5' Cap is formed by the addition of a GTP in reverse orientation to the 5' end of the mRNA, forming a 5'-to-5' linkage. The added G is then methylated at the N-7 position, and the methyl groups are added to the riboses of the first one or two nucleotides in the mRNA.

addition of a *7-methylguanosine (m⁷G) Cap*. The 5' Cap has several putative functions, including (1) protecting the RNA from 5'-to-3' exonuclease degradation; (2) facilitating transport to the cytoplasm; (3) facilitating RNA splicing; and (4) assisting in the alignment of mRNAs on the ribosomes during translation.

The 3' end of most eukaryotic mRNAs is modified by a processing reaction called *polyadenylation*. The signal for polyadenylation is the hexanucleotide sequence AAUAAA. This AAUAAA sequence is recognized by a protein complex that cleaves the RNA chain 15 to 30 nucleotides farther downstream. Subsequently, a poly A polymerase adds a poly A tail of approximately 200 nucleotides to the transcript. The initiation of polyadenylation heralds termination of transcription by RNA polymerase. The poly A tails have been envisaged to have several potential functions, including (1) facilitating transport of mRNA molecules to the cytoplasm; (2) stabilizing mRNAs in order to prevent degradation; and (3) facilitating translation by enhancing the recognition of the mRNA by the translational machinery.

Untranslated regions (UTRs) are found at both the 5' and 3' ends of the mRNA. UTRs represent sequences in the exons that remain in the mRNA but are not translated into protein. The 5' and 3' UTRs contain signals that are necessary for the processing of the RNA and subsequent translation into protein.

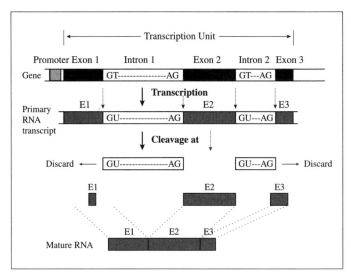

Figure 15. Splicing of primary RNA transcripts. RNA splicing involves endonucleolytic cleavage, removal of intronic RNA segments and splicing of exonic RNA segments.

3.5.2 *SPLICING MECHANISMS* [46, 49, 50]

Most genes contain multiple introns, which account for about 10 times more pre-mRNA sequences than do the exons. Thus, the most striking modification of the pre-mRNAs involves the removal of introns by a process known as *splicing*. Splicing involves endonucleolytic cleavage and removal of intronic RNA, and end-to-end ligation (i.e., splicing) of exonic RNA segments (Figure 15). The mechanism of RNA splicing is critically dependent on the *GT-AG rule*: introns start with GT and end with AG. The sequences adjacent to the GT and AG dinucleotides are highly conserved, and an additional conserved sequence situated just before the terminal AG at the end of the intron is the so-called *branch site*. The splicing mechanism is depicted in Figure 19 (Section 3.5.7), and involves the following steps: (1) cleavage at the 5′ splice junction; (2) joining of the 5′ end of the intron to an A within the intron (i.e., branch site) to form a lariat-shaped structure; and (3) cleavage at the 3′ splice site leading to the release of the lariat-like intronic RNA, and splicing of the exonic RNA segments. Splicing occurs in large complexes called *spliceosomes*. The RNA components of the spliceosomes are *small nuclear RNAs (snRNAs)*. These snRNAs range in size from approximately 50 to 200 nucleotides and are complexed with protein molecules to form *small nuclear ribonucleoprotein particles (snRNPs)*. SnRNPs play an important role in the splicing process. The snRNA part of the snRNP carries out the "intellectual task" of recognizing the splice and branch sites of the larger RNA molecule. In contrast, the protein part of the snRNP does the "manual labor" of cutting and reattaching the RNA molecule.

The central role that splicing plays in the processing of pre-mRNA affords another mechanism for regulation of gene expression by the control of the activity of the cellular splicing machinery. Since most pre-mRNAs contain multiple introns, different mRNAs can be produced from the same gene by different combinations of the 5' and 3' splice sites. The possibility of joining exons in various combinations provides a novel mechanism for the control of gene expression through the generation of multiple mRNAs (and thus multiple proteins) from the same pre-mRNA. This process is termed *alternative splicing*, and occurs frequently in genes of higher eukaryotes. Alternative splicing affords an important mechanism for the tissue-specific and developmental regulation of eukaryotic gene expression. In the case of transcriptional regulatory proteins, alternative splicing of pre-mRNAs yields products with dramatically different functions (e.g., the ability to act as either activators or repressors of transcription). An important variation of the theme of splicing is a phenomenon known as *trans-splicing*, where exons originating from two separate transcripts are ligated together. The biological significance of trans-splicing remains to be elucidated.

3.5.3 *EXON SELECTION DURING SPLICING* [51–53]

An additional level of control of gene expression occurs through the process of *exon splicing* during the processing of the pre-mRNA. The cell determines which exons present in the pre-mRNA are conserved in the final mRNA. This allows for the production of more than one protein from the same gene. For example, the same gene encodes calcitonin and the calcitonin gene–related peptide (CGRP). These proteins differ with respect to their amino acid sequence, function and tissue localization. The synthesis of these different proteins using the same genetic information occurs by a combination of alternative polyadenylation and differential exon selection. This is illustrated in Figure 16.

3.5.4 *RNA EDITING* [54, 55]

The protein-coding sequences of some RNAs are altered by RNA-processing events other than splicing. The best-characterized example is the editing of the mRNA for apolipoprotein B, where tissue-specific RNA editing gives rise to two different forms of apolipoprotein B (Figure 17). Apo B100 is synthesized in the liver by translation of the unedited mRNA, whereas a smaller protein specific to the intestine, apo B48, is synthesized as a result of translation of an

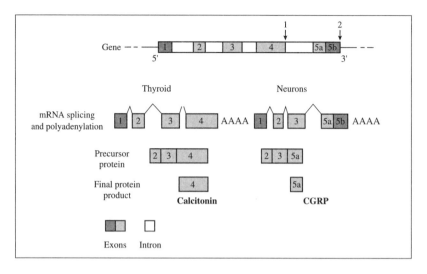

Figure 16.   The role of exon selection in the production of two proteins from the same gene. The calcitonin gene contains two polyadenylation signals and six exons (1, 2, 3, 4, 5a, 5b). In the thyroid, the upstream polyadenylation signal (arrow 1) is recognized, and this results in cleavage and polyadenylation of the mRNA at the 3′ end of exon 4, to produce a precursor mRNA containing exons 1, 2, 3 and 4. These four exons are spliced together, forming the mature mRNA, which codes for the calcitonin precursor peptide. This peptide is processed to yield calcitonin that contains amino acid sequence information only from exon 4. In neurons, the downstream polyadenylation signal (arrow 2) is recognized, resulting in cleavage and polyadenylation of the mRNA at the 3′ end of exon 5b to form a precursor mRNA containing exons 1, 2, 3, 4, 5a and 5b. During the splicing process, exon 4 is deleted, and the mature mRNA contains exons 1, 2, 3, 5a and 5b, which code for the calcitonin gene–related peptide (CGRP). The final processing gives CGRP, which contains the amino acid information that is found in exon 5a.

edited mRNA where a C in a single codon has been changed to a U. This nucleotide substitution alters the codon for glutamine (CAA) in the unedited mRNA to a translation termination codon (UAA) in the edited mRNA. This results in the synthesis of the shorter apo B protein. This tissue-specific editing of apo B results in the expression of structurally and functionally different proteins in the liver and intestine. The full-length apo B100 produced by the liver transports lipids of the circulation, whereas apo B48 mediates the absorption of dietary lipids by the small intestine.

3.5.5 RNA DEGRADATION [44, 45, 48]
The final aspect of the processing of an RNA molecule is its eventual degradation. The intracellular level of any particular RNA species reflects a balance between synthesis and degradation. In this way the rate at which particular

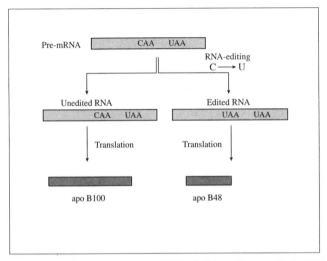

Figure 17. The editing of apolipoprotein B mRNA. In the human liver, unedited mRNA is translated to yield a 4,536-amino-acid protein called apo B100. In the human intestine, however, the mRNA is edited by a base modification that changes a specific C to a U. This modification changes the codon for a glutamine (CAA) to a termination codon (UAA), resulting in the synthesis of a shorter protein (apo B48, consisting of only 2,152 amino acids).

RNAs are degraded constitutes another potential level at which gene expression can be controlled. In eukaryotic cells different mRNAs are degraded at different rates, and this allows for the differential regulation of eukaryotic gene expression.

The degradation of most mRNAs is initiated by the trimming of the poly A tail. This is followed by the removal of the 5′ Cap and degradation of the RNA by nucleases. The mRNA half-life varies from 30 minutes to about 24 hours. The mRNAs with short half-lives usually encode for regulatory proteins. These mRNAs often contain specific AU-rich sequences situated near the 3′ end, which appear to signal rapid degradation by promoting deadenylation at the 3′ poly A tail.

The stability of some mRNAs can be regulated in response to extracellular signals. For example, the level of abundance of the mRNA encoding the transferrin receptor, a cell-surface protein involved in iron uptake, is regulated by the availability of iron (Figure 18). This occurs by modulation of the stability of the transferrin-receptor mRNA. When iron is replete, the transferrin-receptor mRNA is rapidly degraded by specific nuclease cleavage that occurs at a sequence near the 3′ end. When the supply of iron is rate-limiting, the transferrin-receptor mRNA is stabilized, and this leads to an increased synthesis of

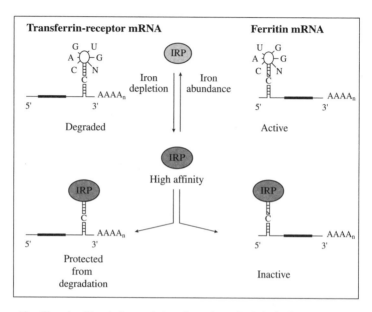

Figure 18. The role of iron in the regulation of protein synthesis in the liver. A stem-loop structure is located at the 3′ end of the transferrin-receptor mRNA. Additional structures located at the 3′ end include the iron-response element, which binds an iron regulatory protein (IRP) when the cell is depleted of iron. The binding of the IRP to the 3′ end of the transferrin-receptor mRNA protects the mRNA from degradation and results in an increase in the level of the transferrin-receptor mRNA and a corresponding increase in the level of the transferrin-receptor protein. At the 5′ end of the ferritin mRNA molecule is a stem-loop structure that binds IRP when iron is depleted in the cell. Binding of the IRP at the 5′ end of the ferritin mRNA inhibits the translation of this mRNA and results in a decreased level of ferritin protein. When iron levels are abundant, the ferritin mRNA no longer binds IRP and actively translates ferritin protein. At the same time, iron abundance inhibits IRP from binding to the 3′ end of the transferrin-receptor mRNA, and the mRNA is degraded. This results in a reduction of the level of transferrin-receptor protein.

transferrin receptor. Thus, more iron is transported into the cell. The regulation of the transferrin receptor is mediated by a protein that binds to specific sequences, called the iron-responsive element (IRE), which is located near the 3′ end of the transferrin-receptor mRNA. Binding protects the transferrin mRNA from cleavage and is controlled by the levels of intracellular iron.

3.5.6 PROMOTER SELECTION [56, 57]
The presence of more than one promoter within a particular gene can result in different amounts of the same gene product being produced in different tissues. Furthermore, tissue-specific availability of certain transcription factors

also contributes to this process. For example, the α-amylase gene contains two promoter sites that control the expression of this gene in a tissue-specific manner. Salivary gland cells have very high levels of α-amylase, whereas hepatocytes have very low levels. The relative difference in amounts of α-amylase is controlled at the transcriptional level. In salivary gland cells, the first promoter site, located just 5' to the first exon of the α-amylase gene, determines the start of transcription as well as the rate of gene transcription. This is a strong promoter, because it has the ability to transcribe the gene at a high transcriptional rate. By contrast, in hepatocytes the available transcription factors do not recognize the first strong promoter of the gene, and divert the RNA polymerase II to the second and weaker promoter located just 5' to the second exon of the α-amylase gene. This results in the same α-amylase protein being transcribed, albeit at lower levels. When the pre-mRNA is later spliced to form the mature mRNA, this 5' untranslated exon in each cell type is spliced to the first exon containing the amino acid sequence information. The final result is that the mature mRNA in hepatocytes differs from that which is found in salivary gland cells with respect to the 5' untranslated sequence only (the amino acid coding regions are identical).

3.5.7 ALTERNATIVE POLYADENYLATION SITES [43]

The differential production of the membrane form and the secreted form of immunoglobulin M (IgM) depends on the structure of the heavy-chain component of the antibody molecule. The membrane form of IgM contains a heavy chain with a carboxy terminal amino acid sequence rich in hydrophobic amino acids that facilitate its interaction and binding to the cell membrane. In contrast, the secreted form of the antibody contains a heavy chain devoid of this carboxy terminal amino acid sequence, and is unable to bind to the plasma membrane.

By using alternative polyadenylation signals within the gene, the precise type of heavy-chain mRNA is determined during B-cell development (Figure 19). When the mRNA encoding the membrane form of the heavy chain is produced, a polyadenylation signal present at the distal 3' end of the message determines the site of cleavage and polyadenylation of the mRNA. After polyadenylation of the mRNA occurs, splicing of all of the exons follows, including the 3' exon, which codes for the hydrophobic amino acid sequence located at the carboxy terminal end of the membrane-bound form of the heavy chain. This yields the mature mRNA. Translation of this particular mRNA produces a form of the heavy chain that has a hydrophobic tail and is found in the membrane-bound form of IgM. In contrast, in the cells in which the secreted form of the IgM molecule is produced, a second polyadenylation signal, which is recognized by the cell-specific polyadenylation system of mature B

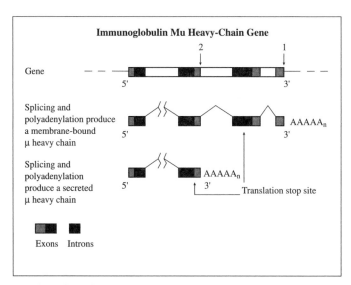

Figure 19.   Alternative polyadenylation in the immunoglogulin μ heavy chain gene. Only some of the exons of the μ heavy chain gene are represented. In cells in which the membrane-bound form of the antibody is produced, a polyadenylation signal present at the distal 3′ end of the mRNA (indicated by arrow 1) determines the site of cleavage and polyadenylation of the mRNA. During the splicing process of this mRNA, all the exons, including the 3′ exon coding for the hydrophobic amino acids found at the carboxy terminal end of the membrane-bound form of the μ heavy chain, are spliced together to produce the mature mRNA. In cells in which the secreted form of the antibody is produced, the upstream polyadenylation signal (arrow 2) is recognized and determines the site of cleavage and polyadenylation of the mRNA found in mature B cells. The mRNA produced after splicing is lacking the exons located 3′ to this polyadenylation signal. This results in the production of a μ heavy chain devoid of a hydrophobic tail, which is thus secreted.

cells, is located further upstream of the distal 3′ polyadenylation signal. In these cells, the cleavage and polyadenylation of the mRNA occurs at this second site, and the exons located 3′ to this site are no longer present in the mRNA produced. Following polyadenylation, the remaining exons are spliced together to yield an mRNA that encodes a heavy chain that is lacking the hydrophobic tail. Translation of this mRNA produces the heavy chain found in the secreted form of IgM.

3.6 DNA Methylation and the Control of Transcription [42]

Not only is methylation important in DNA synthesis and repair, but it also represents another general mechanism associated with the control of eukaryotic gene transcription. Cytosine residues in eukaryotic DNA are modified by the addition of methyl groups. DNA is methylated specifically at the Cs that precede Gs (*CpG dinucleotides*). Methylation is correlated with reduced transcriptional activity of several genes. Distinct patterns of methylation are seen in different tissues. The DNA of inactive genes is more heavily methylated, as compared to the DNA of genes that are actively transcribed. Moreover, some genes contain high frequencies of CpG dinucleotides in the region of their promoters. Transcription of these genes is repressed by methylation through the action of a protein that binds specifically to methylated DNA and inhibits transcription.

4. PROTEIN SYNTHESIS AND POST-TRANSLATIONAL PROCESSING IN EUKARYOTIC CELLS

4.1 Translation of mRNA [58–63]

The tRNAs serve as carriers and adapters for the alignment of each of the 20 amino acids with their corresponding codons on the mRNA template. tRNAs consist of 70 to 80 nucleotides, with a characteristic "clover leaf" configuration that results from complementary base pairing between regions of the molecule. The tRNAs possess unique identifying sequences that allow the correct amino acid to be attached and aligned with the appropriate codon in the mRNA. All tRNAs have the sequence CCA at the 3' end where free amino acids covalently attach to the ribose of the terminal adenosine residue. Recognition of the mRNA template occurs through interaction with an *anticodon loop*, located at the other end of the tRNA, which binds to the appropriate codon through complementary base pairing. The attachment of amino acids to specific tRNAs is mediated by *aminoacyl tRNA synthetases*. The three-base sequence on the anticodon loop is complementary to a specific codon found in the mRNA. For example, if the codon in the mRNA is GGC, it is recognized by the anticodon of the tRNA as CCG.

While there are 61 codons specifying amino acids, there are fewer than 61 tRNA molecules. Thus, some of the tRNA molecules are able to recognize more than one codon; this phenomenon is called *wobble*. Wobble effects are found with the third base of the codon.

4.2 The Steps in Protein Synthesis

Particles consisting of RNA and protein, known as *ribosomes*, are located in the cytoplasm and serve as the site of protein synthesis. The principal components of the protein synthesis machinery include mRNA, tRNAs, amino acids and ribosomes.

Each ribosome is composed of two subunits, the 40S (or small subunit) and 60S (or large subunit). The size of the entire particle is 80S. The 40S subunit is made up of the 18S rRNA and 30 different proteins. The 60S subunit is

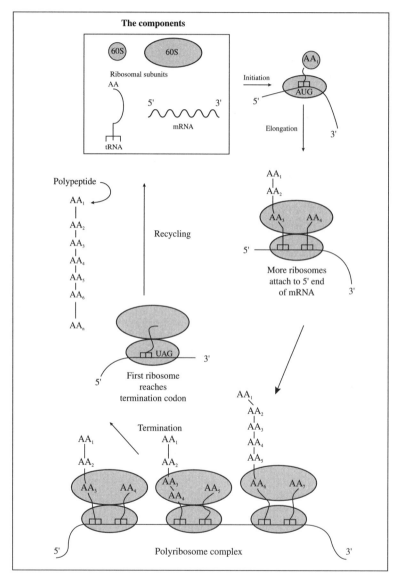

Figure 20.   Overview of translation. Translation involves three stages. Initiation occurs when the ribosomal subunits and charged tRNA associate with an mRNA molecule to form the initiation complex. Elongation occurs when additional tRNA molecules bring additional amino acids to the mRNA, where they are added in a stepwise fashion to the growing polypeptide chain. Termination occurs when a stop codon appears in the mRNA, and the completed polypeptide is released from the ribosome.

made up of the 5S, the 5.8S and the 28S rRNA as well as 50 different protein species. Ribosomal proteins are imported to the nucleolus from the cytoplasm, and begin to assemble on pre-rRNA prior to its cleavage. As the pre-rRNA is processed, additional ribosomal proteins and the 5S rRNA assemble to form pre-ribosomal particles. The pre-ribosomal particles are exported from the nucleus to the cytoplasm, yielding the 40S and 60S ribosomal subunits.

The ribosome physically moves down the mRNA in the 5'-to-3' direction, with the sequential addition of amino acids from tRNAs to form the nascent polypeptide. Amino acids are attached to tRNA by a process called *charging,* which is mediated by *aminoacyl tRNA synthetases.* For each of the 20 amino acids, there are 20 different aminoacyl tRNA synthetases. When the protein is completed, it is released along with the ribosome and tRNA molecules, which are free to begin the cycle again.

Protein synthesis comprises three specific steps: *initiation, elongation* and *termination.* Each of these steps involves specific proteins, and the energy for this process is derived from either ATP or GTP. These steps are illustrated in Figure 20.

4.2.1 INITIATION OF TRANSLATION

In eukaryotes, the initiation of protein synthesis involves approximately 10 different proteins (Figure 21). The initiation factors eIF3 and eIF1A bind to the 40S ribosomal subunit. The initiation factor eIF2 binds to GTP to form a complex that binds a tRNA charged with initiator methionine. The 5' Cap of the mRNA is recognized by eIF4, which brings the mRNA to the ribosome. The eIF2-Met-tRNA-GTP complex subsequently interacts with the 40S subunit at the 5' end of the mRNA. After binding to the 5' end of the message, the 40S subunit with the eIF2-Met-tRNA-GTP complex moves down the mRNA. This process is known as *scanning.* Scanning continues until the complex reaches the first AUG (i.e., the initiator codon) on the mRNA. Then, the 60S ribosomal subunit binds to the complex to form the final ribosomal structure. This process requires GTP as an energy source. The formation of this final structure signals the completion of the initiation step. eIF2 and GDP are released from the complex and are able to reinitiate the cycle. When the initiator codon (AUG) is located, eIF5 triggers the hydrolysis of GTP bound to eIF2, followed by the release of eIF2 (complexed to GDP) and other initiation factors. The 60S ribosomal subunit then joins the 40S complex to form the 80S initiation complex.

4.2.2 PEPTIDE ELONGATION

The various steps involved in the elongation phase of protein synthesis are illustrated in Figure 22. The ribosome has three sites for tRNA binding desig-

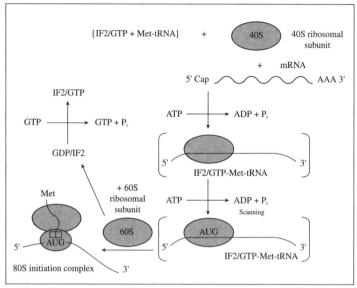

Figure 21. Initiation of protein synthesis. The initiation factor 2 (IF2) complex with GTP binds to a tRNA charged with methionine (Met). This complex interacts with the small 40S ribosomal subunit at the 5′ end of an mRNA molecule. After binding to the 5′ end of the mRNA, the 40S subunit scans the mRNA until it reaches the first AUG codon. At this point, the 60S ribosomal subunit binds to the complex to form the final initiation complex.

nated the P (peptidyl), A (aminoacyl) and E (exit) sites. The initiator Met-tRNA is bound at the P site. The first step in elongation is the binding of the next aminoacyl tRNA to the A site by pairing with the second codon on the mRNA. The aminoacyl tRNA is escorted to the ribosome by an *elongation factor* (eEF1α), which is complexed to GTP. The GTP is hydrolyzed to GDP after the correct aminoacyl tRNA is inserted into the A site of the ribosome, and the elongation factor bound to GDP is released.

Once the eEF1α has left the ribosome, the peptide bond is formed between the initiator met-tRNA at the P site and the second aminoacyl tRNA at the A site. This reaction is catalyzed by the large ribosomal subunit. The result is the transfer of methionine to the aminoacyl tRNA at the A site of the ribosome, forming a peptidyl tRNA at this position and leaving the uncharged initiator tRNA at the P site. The next step in elongation is translocation, which requires the elongation factor eEF2, and is again coupled to the hydrolysis of GTP. During translocation, the ribosome moves 3 nucleotides along the mRNA, positioning the next codon in an empty A site. This step translocates the peptidyl tRNA from the A site to the P site, and the uncharged tRNA from the P

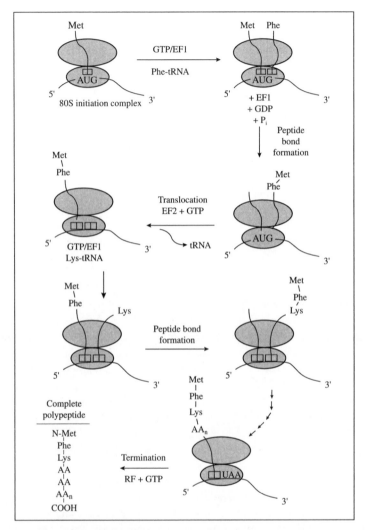

Figure 22. Elongation and termination of protein synthesis. Protein synthesis is initiated by the binding of methionine (Met)-tRNA to the AUG codon in mRNA bound to the ribosome. A second aminoacyl-tRNA interacts with the elongation factor 1 (EF1) and GTP followed by the binding of this complex to the second codon on the mRNA. In the presence of peptidyl transferase, a peptide bond is formed between methionine and phenylalanine (Phe). Subsequently, in the presence of GTP, EF2, and an enzyme known as translocase, the ribosome translocates one codon along the tRNA in the 5'-to-3' direction. This is followed by the release of the uncharged tRNA and the exposure of a new codon. The next aminoacyl-tRNA binds, and the cycle is repeated until a termination codon is encountered. In the presence of release factor (RF), the completed peptide is released from the ribosome.

site to the E site. The ribosome is then left with a peptidyl tRNA at the P site, and an empty A site. The binding of a new aminoacyl tRNA to the A site then causes the release of the uncharged tRNA from the E site. This leaves the ribosome ready for the next amino acid in the growing polypeptide chain.

4.2.3 TERMINATION OF TRANSLATION

Elongation of the polypeptide chain continues until a termination codon (stop or terminator codon) is translocated into the A site of the ribosome. The *release factor (eRF)* recognizes all three termination codons. The eRF binds to a termination codon at the A site and stimulates the hydrolysis of the bond between the tRNA and the polypeptide chain at the P site. This results in the release of the completed polypeptide from the ribosome.

The mRNAs are usually translated by a series of ribosomes, spaced at intervals of about 100 to 200 nucleotides. The group of ribosomes bound to an mRNA molecule is called a *polyribosome (polysome)*, and each ribosome within the group functions independently to synthesize a separate polypeptide chain.

4.3 **Regulation of Translation** [58–63]

Although transcription is the primary level at which gene expression is controlled, the translation of mRNA represents an additional regulatory control point in eukaryotic cells. One of the best examples of translational regulation in eukaryotic cells is the cellular mechanisms associated with the regulation of ferritin synthesis. The translation of ferritin mRNA is regulated by the supply of iron (Figure 18). More ferritin is synthesized when iron is abundant, and this regulation is mediated by a protein that binds to the iron-responsive element (IRE) in the 5′ untranslated region of ferritin mRNA. In the presence of iron, the repressor no longer binds to the IRE, and ferritin translation is able to proceed.

The regulation of ferritin translation by iron is similar to the regulation of the stability of transferrin receptor mRNA, which is regulated by protein binding to an IRE in the mRNA's 3′ untranslated region. The same protein binds to the IREs of both the ferritin and the transferrin receptor mRNAs. However, the consequences of the binding of this protein to the two IREs are quite different (Figure 18). The protein bound to the transferrin receptor IRE protects the mRNA from degradation, rather than inhibiting its translation. These distinct effects probably result from the different locations of the IRE in the two mRNAs. Thus, binding of the same regulatory protein to different sites on mRNA molecules can have distinct effects on gene expression, in one case inhibiting translation, and in the other case, stabilizing the mRNA to increase protein synthesis. In the case of the ferritin mRNA, the IRE blocks translation

by interfering with 5' Cap recognition and binding of the 40S ribosomal subunit. This protein binding to the same sequence in the 3' UTR of transferrin
receptor mRNA protects the mRNA from nuclease degradation and prolongs
its half-life.

4.4 Post-translational Processing of Proteins [64–72, 79, 82–84, 87]

Newly synthesized polypeptides are subsequently folded into three-dimensional structures. In many instances, multiple polypeptide chains are assembled into a functional complex. Many proteins undergo further modifications,
which include the covalent attachment of carbohydrates and lipids that are
critical for determining the function and correct localization of proteins within the cell.

Earlier studies suggested that protein folding is a self-assembly process
determined primarily by its amino acid sequence. However, more recent studies have shown that the proper folding of proteins is mediated by the activities of a group of proteins called *molecular chaperones*. Chaperones catalyze
protein folding by assisting the self-assembly process: the folded conformation of a protein is determined solely by its amino acid sequence. Chaperones
bind to and stabilize partially folded polypeptides. In the absence of chaperones, unfolded or incompletely folded polypeptides are unstable within the
cell and aggregate into insoluble complexes. Some chaperones bind to nascent
polypeptides that are still being translated on ribosomes. This prevents incorrect folding of the amino terminal region of the polypeptide before the synthesis of the chain is terminated. This interaction is important for proteins in
which the carboxy terminal region is required for correct folding of the amino
terminus. Other classes of chaperones stabilize unfolded polypeptide chains
during their intracellular transport to organelles such as the mitochondria.
Finally, chaperones are also involved in the assembly of proteins that consist
of multiple polypeptide chains.

Many of the molecular chaperones were originally identified as *heat-shock
proteins (Hsp)*, a group of proteins that are expressed in cells that have been
subjected to increased temperature or other forms of environmental stress.
The heat-shock proteins appear to stabilize and facilitate the refolding of proteins that have been partially denatured as a result of exposure to increased
temperature. However, many heat-shock proteins are expressed under normal
growth conditions. They function as molecular chaperones required for
polypeptide folding and transport under normal conditions, as well as under
conditions of environmental stress. Members of the Hsp-70 family stabilize
unfolded polypeptide chains during translation as well as during intracellular
transport to subcellular compartments such as the endoplasmic reticulum and
mitochondria. These proteins bind to short segments of seven or eight amino

acid residues of unfolded polypeptides and maintain the polypeptide chain in an unfolded conformation, thereby preventing aggregation. Proteins in the Hsp-60 family facilitate the folding of proteins into their native conformations. In several instances, members of the Hsp-70 and Hsp-60 families act together in a sequential fashion, and may therefore represent a general pathway of protein folding.

In addition to molecular chaperones, cells contain enzymes that catalyze protein folding by breaking and reforming covalent bonds. The formation of disulfide bonds between cysteine residues is an important step in the stabilization of the folded structures of many protein species. In this regard, *protein disulfide isomerase (PDI)* catalyzes the breakage and reunion of these bonds. Disulfide bonds are usually restricted to secreted proteins and some membrane proteins. In eukaryotic cells, disulfide bonds form in the endoplasmic reticulum where the activity of PDI is correlated with the level of protein secretion. Another example of an enzyme that plays a pivotal role in protein folding is *peptidyl-prolyl-isomerase,* which catalyzes the isomerization of peptide bonds that involve proline residues.

Proteolysis is a critical step in the maturation of many proteins. A simple example of proteolysis is the removal of the initiator methionine residue from the amino terminus of many polypeptides after the growing polypeptide chain leaves the ribosome. As well, proteolytic modification of the amino terminus plays a central role in the translocation of many proteins across the membranes. This includes the translocation of secreted proteins as well as proteins destined for targeting to the plasma membrane, lysosomes and mitochondria of eukaryotic cells.

Active enzymes and hormones are formed via proteolytic processing of larger precursors. For example, insulin is synthesized as a large precursor polypeptide (pre-proinsulin) containing an amino terminal sequence that targets the polypeptide chain to the endoplasmic reticulum (ER). Proinsulin is formed through the removal of the signal sequence during transfer to the ER. Proinsulin is subsequently converted to insulin, which consists of two chains held together by disulfide bonds, by proteolytic removal of an internal peptide.

The levels of proteins within cells reflect a balance between synthesis and degradation. The differential rates of protein degradation represent an important aspect of cell regulation. Rapidly degraded proteins function primarily as regulatory molecules, such as transcription factors. The rapid turnover of these proteins is necessary to allow their levels to respond quickly to external stimuli. Two major pathways mediate protein degradation: the ubiquitin-proteasome pathway and lysosomal proteolysis. The major pathway for selective protein degradation employs *ubiquitin* as a marker that targets cytoplasmic and nuclear proteins for rapid degradation. Ubiquitin is a 76-amino-acid polypeptide that attaches to the amino group of lysine residues. The ubiquinated proteins are recognized and degraded by a multi-subunit protease complex called *proteasome*. Ubiquitin is subsequently released and recycled. The other major pathway for protein degradation involves the transport of proteins to lysosomes, where they are taken up and degraded by proteases.

4.5 The Cellular Compartmentalization of Protein Sorting and Intracellular Transport [70, 77–79, 95]

Eukaryotic cells are distinct from prokaryotic cells by the presence of membrane-delimited compartments wherein specific cellular activities occur. The sorting and targeting of proteins to their appropriate destinations such as the plasma membrane, the endoplasmic reticulum or the Golgi complex are key features in the maintenance of these specific cellular activities.

Proteins destined for the endoplasmic reticulum, the Golgi appartatus, lysomes, the plasma membrane, and cellular secretion are synthesized on ribosomes that are bound to the ER membrane. Nascent polypeptide chains are transported from the cytoplasm into the ER, where protein folding and further processing occur prior to transport to the Golgi apparatus via ER-derived vesicles. In the Golgi appartatus, proteins are further processed and sorted for transport to the plasma membrane or to lysosomes, or export from the cell as secretory proteins. The various cellular compartments associated with protein sorting and transport are depicted in Figure 23.

Proteins synthesized on free ribosomes either remain in the cytoplasm or are transported to the nucleus, mitochondria or peroxisomes. Proteins destined for transport to the nucleus are responsible for important aspects of genome structure and function. These include histones, DNA and RNA polymerases, transcription factors and splicing factors. These proteins are targeted to the nucleus by specific *nuclear localization signals* that direct their transport through the *nuclear pore complex*. The first nuclear localization signal characterized was that of the SV40 viral T antigen. The amino acid sequence Pro-Lys-Lys-Lys-Arg-Lys-Val is necessary for the nuclear transport of the T antigen and other types of cytoplasmic proteins. Proteins are transported through the nuclear pore complex, a process mediated by the action of a nuclear receptor called *importin*.

4.5.1 *PROTEIN TARGETING TO THE ENDOPLASMIC RETICULUM* [70, 77–79, 85–87, 89, 90, 92, 95]

Ribosomes that participate in the synthesis of proteins that are ultimately destined for secretion are targeted to the ER. This targeting is directed by the amino acid sequence of the newly synthesized polypeptide chain, rather than by the intrinsic properties of the ribosome. A *signal sequence* spans about 20

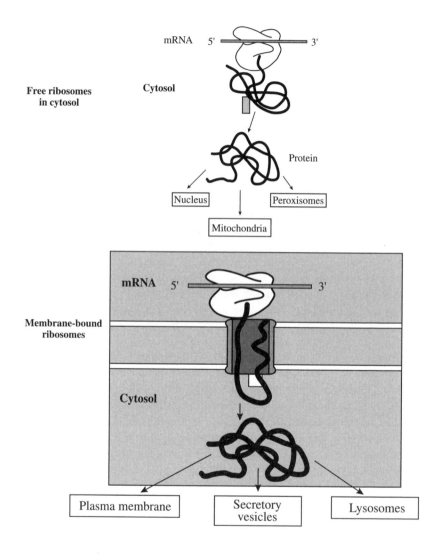

Figure 23.   Overview of protein sorting. Proteins synthesized on free ribosomes either remain in the cytoplasm or are transported to the nucleus, mitochondria, chloroplasts or peroxisomes. By contrast, proteins synthesized on membrane-bound ribosomes are subsequently translocated into the ER while their translation is in progress. They may be either retained within the ER or transported to the Golgi apparatus and, from there, to lysosomes or to the plasma membrane, or secreted outside the cell within secretory vesicles.

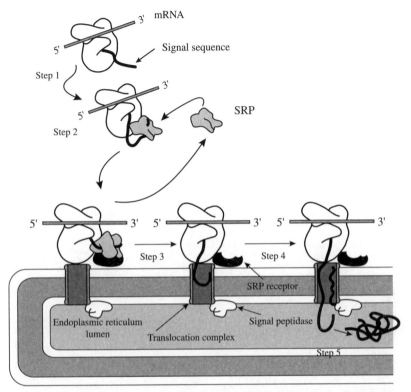

Figure 24. The targeting of secretory proteins to the ER. Step 1: As the signal sequence emerges from the ribosome, it is subsequently recognized and bound by the signal-recognition particle (SRP). Step 2: The SRP escorts the complex to the ER membrane, where it binds to the SRP receptor. Step 3: The SRP is subsequently released, the ribosome binds to a membrane translocation complex, and the signal sequence is inserted into a membrane channel. Step 4: Translation resumes, and the growing peptide chain is translocated across the ER membrane. Step 5: A signal peptidase catalyzes the cleavage of the signal sequence, and this releases the polypeptide into the ER lumen.

amino acids, including a stretch of hydrophobic residues, and is located at the amino terminus of the polypeptide chain. As they emerge from the ribosome, signal sequences are recognized and bound by a *signal-recognition particle (SRP),* which consists of six polypeptides and a small cytoplasmic RNA. The binding of the SRP inhibits translation and targets the complex (polypeptide chain, SRP, ribosome) to the rough ER. This is mediated by binding to the SRP receptor on the ER membrane. Binding to the receptor releases the SRP from the ribosome and the signal sequence of the polypeptide chain.

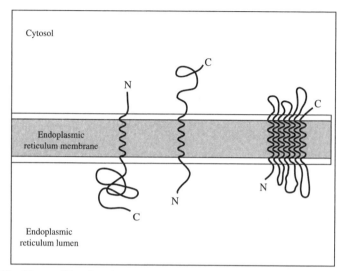

Figure 25.   The possible orientations of membrane proteins. Integral membrane proteins span the membrane via α-helical regions of 20 to 25 hydrophobic amino acids, which can be inserted in a variety of orientations. The proteins at left and center each span the membrane only once, but they differ in whether the amino (N) or carboxy (C) terminus is on the cytoplasmic side. On the right is an example of a protein that has multiple membrane-spanning regions.

The ribosome subsequently binds to the *protein translocation complex* of the ER membrane, and the signal sequence is inserted into an ER membrane channel. Translation resumes, and the growing polypeptide chain is translocated across the membrane into the ER lumen. The signal sequence is cleaved by the action of *signal peptidase*, and the polypeptide is liberated into the ER lumen. The sec-61 complex comprises three membrane-spanning proteins and is the principal component of the ER protein-conducting channel in mammalian cells. The targeting of secretory proteins to the ER is illustrated in Figure 24.

Proteins destined for incorporation into the plasma membrane, ER membranes, Golgi or lysosomes are inserted initially into the ER membrane, instead of being liberated into the ER lumen. These proteins then proceed to their final destination along the secretory pathway: ER → Golgi → plasma membrane or lysosomes. The proteins are transported along this pathway as membrane constituents, which differentiates the process from that of secretory proteins. These integral membrane proteins are embedded in the plasma membrane by hydrophobic regions that span the phospholipid bilayer of the membrane. The orientation of proteins inserted into the ER, Golgi, lysosomal and plasma membranes is established as the polypeptide chain is inserted into

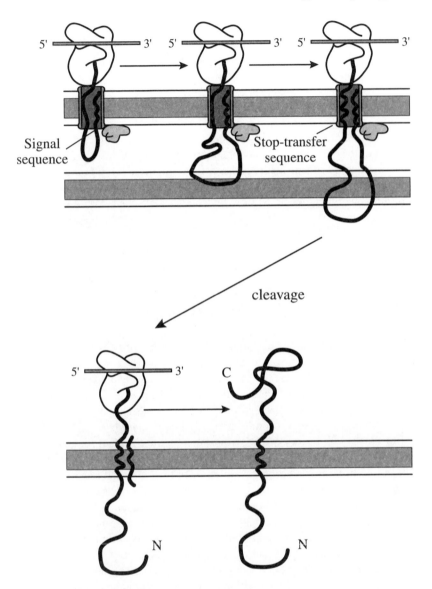

Figure 26. The insertion of a membrane protein with a cleavable signal sequence and a single stop-transfer sequence. The signal sequence is cleaved as the poplypeptide chain is exposed within the ER lumen. However, translocation of the polypeptide chain across the membrane is halted by a stop-transfer sequence that anchors the protein to the membrane. The ribosome is released from the membrane, and continued translation results in a membrane-spanning protein with its C terminus on the cytoplasmic side.

the ER. The ER lumen is topologically equivalent to the exterior of the cell membrane, such that the domains of plasma membrane proteins that are exposed at the level of the cell surface correspond to the regions of polypeptide chains that are translocated into the ER.

A variety of orientations of membrane proteins are found in eukaryotic cells. Transmembrane proteins are observed with either the carboxy or amino termini exposed to the cytosol (Figure 25). Other proteins have multiple membrane-spanning regions called *α-helical regions,* which consist of 20 to 25 hydrophobic amino acids. Some integral membrane proteins span the plasma membrane only once, while others have multiple membrane-spanning regions. As well, some proteins are oriented in the membrane with their amino terminus on the cytoplasmic side, and others have their carboxy terminus exposed to the cytoplasm. Two additional features of membrane proteins have been discovered, which play a key role in determining the orientation of membrane proteins: the *stop-transfer sequence* and the *internal signal sequence.* The consequences of these sequences in determining membrane protein orientation are illustrated in Figures 26–28.

4.5.2 *PROTEIN PROCESSING IN THE ENDOPLASMIC RETICULUM* [66–68, 72, 87, 91]

A variety of modifications to polypeptides at the level of ER include folding and assembly, as well as covalent modifications.

The proteolytic cleavage of the internal signal sequence takes place as the polypeptide chain is translocated across the ER membrane. The translocation occurs while translation is still in progress, and molecular chaperones facilitate the folding of the polypeptide chains. The *binding protein (BiP)* is a member of the Hsp-70 Family of chaperones that mediate protein folding and the assembly of multi-subunit proteins within the lumen of the ER (Figure 29). The correctly assembled proteins are released from BiP and are available for export to the Golgi apparatus. By contrast, abnormally folded or improperly assembled proteins remain bound to BiP and are retained within the ER, where they are subsequently degraded. Disulfide bond formation represents an important aspect of protein folding and assembly within the ER. This process is facilitated by the enzyme *disulfide isomerase,* which is located within the lumen of the ER.

Some proteins are anchored within the plasma membrane by *glycosylphosphatidylinositol (GPI)* anchors, which are assembled in the ER membrane. The GPI anchors are added immediately after completion of protein synthesis to the carboxy terminus of some proteins, which are subsequently transported to the cell surface via the secretory pathway. Their orientation within the ER dictates that GPI anchor proteins reside outside the cell.

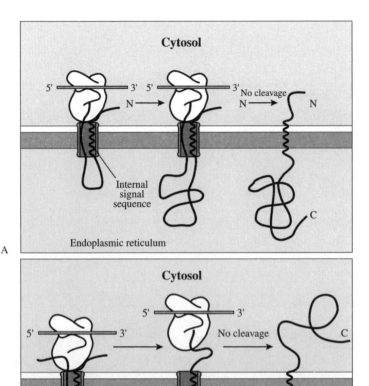

Figure 27. The insertion of membrane proteins with an internal non-cleavable signal sequence. Internal non-cleavable signal sequences result in the insertion of polypeptide chains in either orientation in the ER membrane.

A. The signal sequence directs insertion of a polypeptide such that its N terminus is exposed on the cytoplasmic side. The remainder of the polypeptide is translocated into the ER as translation proceeds. The signal sequence is not cleaved, so it acts as a membrane-spanning sequence that anchors the protein to the membrane with its C terminus within the ER lumen.

B. Other internal signal sequences are oriented to direct the transfer of the N terminal portion of the polypeptide across the membrane. Continued translation results in a protein that spans the ER membrane with its N terminus in the lumen and its C terminus in the cytoplasm. This orientation is the same as that resulting from insertion of a protein that contains a cleavable signal sequence followed by a stop-transfer sequence.

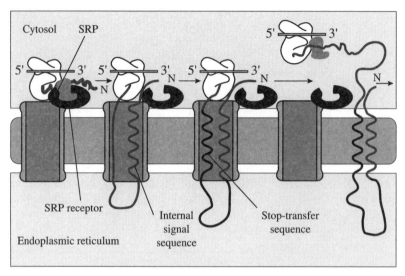

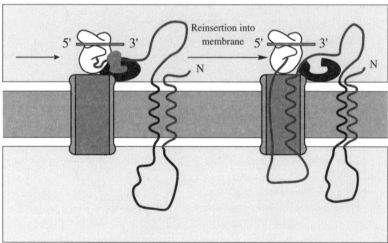

Figure 28.   Insertion of a protein that spans the membrane multiple times. In this example, the internal signal sequence results in insertion of the polypeptide chain with its N terminus on the cytoplasmic side of the membrane. A stop-transfer sequence then causes the polypeptide chain to form a loop within the ER lumen, and translation continues in the cytoplasm. A second internal signal sequence triggers reinsertion of a polypeptide chain into the ER membrane, forming a loop within the cytoplasm. This process can occur many times and results in the insertion of proteins with multiple membrane-spanning regions.

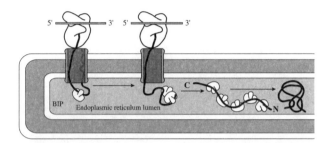

Figure 29.   Protein folding in the ER. The molecular chaperone BiP binds to polypeptide chains as they cross the ER membrane and facilitates protein folding and assembly within the ER lumen.

4.5.3 *TRANSPORT OF PROTEINS FROM THE ENDOPLASMIC RETICULUM* [70, 71, 78, 79, 88, 94, 95]

Proteins travel along the secretory pathway in transport vesicles derived from the ER. These proteins subsequently fuse with the membrane of the Golgi apparatus. The subsequent steps in the secretory pathway involve vesicular transport between the different Golgi compartments, and from the Golgi to the plasma membrane or lysosomes. The Golgi apparatus consists of a series of membrane-delimited cisternae and associated vesicles. Proteins derived from the ER enter the Golgi at the cis-face and exit the Golgi from its trans-face. Proteins marked for residence within the ER are recognized by the Golgi and are returned to the ER. Other proteins are carried by transport vesicles to the trans-Golgi network where the final stages of protein modification are completed prior to their being targeted to lysosomes and to the plasma membrane.

Most proteins travel from the ER to the Golgi. However, some proteins particular to the functioning of the ER must be retained within that organelle (e.g., BiP, signal peptidase, protein disulfide isomerase). Targeting sequences specifically designate proteins destined for retention in the ER or transport to the Golgi (Figure 30). The proteins that are retained in the ER lumen contain the targeting sequence KDEL (single-letter amino acid code; Lys-Asp-Glu-Leu) at their carboxy terminus. The retention of certain transmembrane proteins within the ER is dictated by the carboxy terminal sequence KKXX. Soluble ER proteins are packaged into vesicles and are transported into the Golgi where they are subsequently retrieved and returned to the ER via a recycling pathway. Thus, proteins bearing the KDEL and KKXX sequences bind to

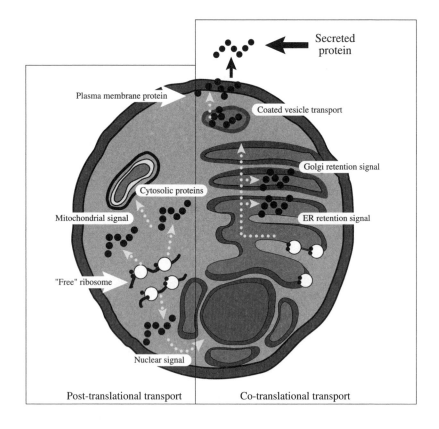

Figure 30. Proteins that are localized post-translationally are released into the cytoplasm after synthesis on "free ribosomes." Some have signals for targeting to the nucleus or mitochondria. Proteins that are localized co-translationally associate with the ER membrane during synthesis so that their ribosomes are "membrane-bound." The proteins pass into the ER, travel to the Golgi and then to the plasma membrane, unless they possess the signals that cause retention in one of the compartments along the pathway. They may also be directed to other organelles, such as lysosomes. Transport along this pathway occurs by way of secretory vesicles.

specific recycling receptors in the Golgi membrane and are selectively transported back to the ER (Figure 31). Proteins destined for transport from the ER are selectively packaged into transport vesicles targeted to the Golgi apparatus. Thus, protein export from the ER is controlled not only by retention/retrieval signals, but also by targeting signals that mediate the selective transport to the Golgi.

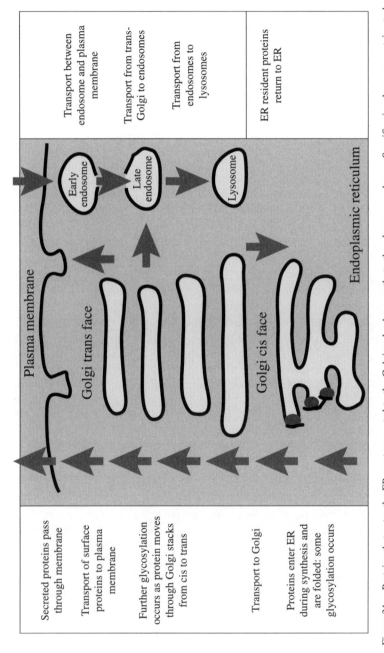

Figure 31. Proteins that enter the ER are transported to the Golgi and subsequently to the plasma membrane. Specific signals cause proteins to be returned from the Golgi to the ER, to be retained within the Golgi, to be retained in the plasma membrane, or to be transported to endosomes and lysosomes. Proteins may be transported between the plasma membrane and endosomes.

4.5.4 *PROTEIN GLYCOSYLATION* [71, 78, 85, 94]

Protein glycosylation takes place on specific asparagine residues (N-linked glycosylation) while a translation is taking place. The oligosaccharide is synthesized on a *dolichol carrier* anchored to the ER membrane. The membrane-bound enzyme oligosaccharyl transferase transfers the oligosaccharide unit to acceptor asparagine residues in the consensus sequence (Asn)-X-Ser/Thr. Thereafter, three glucose residues and one mannose residue are trimmed while the protein is still within the ER. The sequence of steps associated with protein glycosylation in the ER is illustrated in Figure 32.

The N-linked oligosaccharides are processed within the Golgi complex in an ordered sequence of reactions. The first modification is the removal of three additional mannose residues. This occurs on proteins destined for secretion or for targeting to the *plasma membrane*. This is followed by the sequential addition of an N-acetylglucosamine residue, the removal of two more mannoses, and the addition of fucose as well as two more N-acetylglucosamines. Finally, three sialic acid residues and three galactose moieties are added; these reactions occur at the level of the trans-Golgi network. The processing of the N-linked oligosaccharide of *lysosomal* proteins differs from that of secretory and plasma membrane proteins. The proteins destined for incorporation into lysosomes are modified by mannose phosphorylation, followed by the removal of the N-acetylglucosamine group, leaving mannose 6-phosphate residues on the N-linked oligosaccharide. These phosphorylated mannose residues are specifically recognized by the mannose 6-phosphate receptor in the trans-Golgi that directs the trafficking of these proteins to lysosomes. Proteins can also be modified by the addition of carbohydrates to the side chains of serine and threonine residues within specific sequences of amino acids (O-linked glycosylation). The serine or threonine is usually linked directly to N-acetylgalactosamine to which other sugars can be subsequently added.

4.5.5 *PROTEIN SORTING AND TRANSPORT FROM THE GOLGI APPARATUS* [78, 79, 93, 95]

Proteins are transported from the Golgi apparatus to their ultimate destinations via the secretory pathways. This involves sorting the proteins into different kinds of transport vesicles that bud from the trans-Golgi network and deliver their contents to the appropriate cellular addresses. In the absence of specific targeting signals, proteins are delivered to plasma membranes by *bulk flow*. This transports proteins in a nonselective fashion from the ER to the Golgi and ultimately to the cell surface. This bulk flow pathway accounts for the incorporation of new proteins and lipids into the plasma membrane as well as for the continuous secretion of certain proteins from the cell.

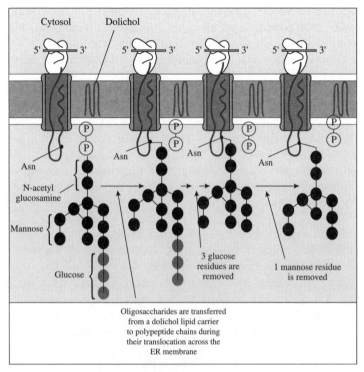

Figure 32. The sequential process of protein glycosylation in the ER.

The bulk flow pathway leads to continuous, unregulated protein secretion. In contrast, in some cell types, a distinct, regulated secretory pathway exists in which specific proteins are secreted in response to particular stimuli. Examples of regulated secretion include the release of hormones and neurotransmitters, and the release of digestive enzymes from the pancreatic acinar cells. These proteins are packaged into specialized secretory vesicles, which store their contents until specific signals direct their fusion with the plasma membrane. The sorting of proteins into the regulated secretory pathway involves the recognition of signal patches shared by multiple proteins that enter this pathway.

Proteins that function within the Golgi complex must be retained within that organelle. Retention of Golgi membrane proteins is based on the trans-membrane domains of those particular proteins. Golgi membrane proteins have short trans-membrane α-helices of about 15 amino acids, which contribute to the retention of these proteins within the Golgi complex. As well, signals in the cytoplasmic tails of some Golgi proteins mediate the retrieval of these proteins from subsequent compartments along the secretory pathway.

The plasma membrane of polarized epithelial cells, such as the enterocyte, is divided into apical and basolateral domains. Each domain contains compartment-specific proteins related to the unique functions of each domain. In some types of epithelia, membrane proteins are sorted at the level of the trans-Golgi network for *selective transport* to the domains of the plasma membrane. The GPI anchor is one signal that directs proteins to the apical membrane domain.

A specific receptor in the trans-Golgi network recognizes mannose 6-phosphate residues. The resulting complexes comprise the receptor plus lysosomal enzyme, and are packaged into transport vesicles destined for lysosomes.

4.5.6 *VESICULAR TRANSPORT* [73–76, 80, 81, 96–98]

The first step in vesicular transport is the formation of a vesicle by a process of "budding" from the membrane. The cytoplasmic surfaces of these transport vesicles are coated with proteins. Three types of coated vesicles that participate in vesicular transport have been characterized. *Clathrin-coated* vesicles are responsible for the uptake of molecules from the plasma membrane by endocytosis, as well as the transport of molecules from the trans-Golgi network to lysosomes (Figure 33). The two remaining types of coated vesicles that arise from the ER and Golgi complex are called *non-clathrin-coated* or *COP-coated* vesicles. COP-I-coated vesicles arise from the Golgi apparatus, whereas COP-II-coated vesicles bud from the ER. The COP-II-coated vesicles transport material from the ER to the Golgi, whereas COP-I-coated vesicles mediate transport between Golgi stacks, recycling from the Golgi to the ER, and possibly other transport processes.

The binding of clathrin to membranes is mediated by *adaptins*. These adaptins are responsible for the assembly of clathrin-coated vesicles at the plasma membrane and at the trans-Golgi network, as well as being responsible for selecting specific molecules to be incorporated into the vesicles.

Distinct protein complexes comprise the coats of COP-I- and COP-II-coated vesicles. The components of the COP-I coat interact with the KKXX motif that is responsible for the retrieval of ER proteins from the Golgi apparatus, and is consistent with the role for COP-I-coated vesicles in recycling from the Golgi to the ER. The budding of clathrin-coated and COP-I-coated vesicles from the trans-Golgi network requires the activity of a GTP-binding protein called *ARF (ADP-ribosylation factor)* (Figure 34). ARF is related to Ras proteins, which function as oncogenes in human cancers. ARF bound to GTP

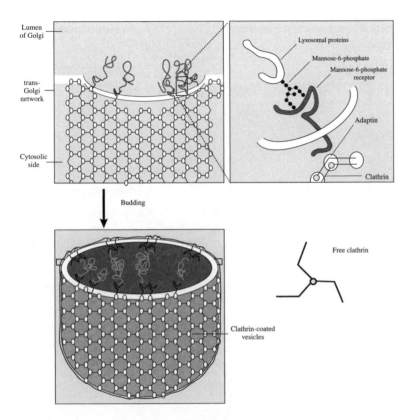

Figure 33. The incorporation of lysosomal proteins into clathrin-coated vesicles. Proteins targeted for delivery to lysosomes are marked by mannose-6-phosphates, which bind to mannose-6-phosphate receptors in the trans-Golgi network. The mannose-6-phosphate receptors span the Golgi membrane and function as binding sites for cytoplasmic adaptins, which in turn bind clathrin. Clathrins comprise three protein chains that associate with each other to form a lattice structure that distorts the membrane and promotes vesicle budding.

associates with the Golgi membranes and is required for the binding of either COP-I-coat components or clathrin adaptins.

Several other Ras-related GTP-binding proteins have also been characterized in the secretory process. These include more than 30 Ras-related proteins (termed Rab proteins) that are implicated in vesicular transport in eukaryotic cells.

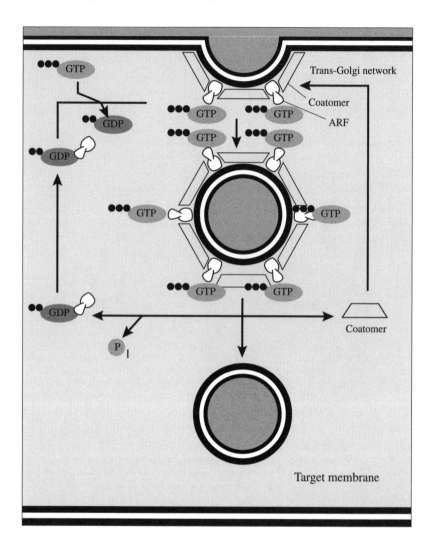

Figure 34. The role of ARF (ADP ribosylation factor) in the formation of COP-coated vesicles. ARF alternates between GTP-bound and GDP-bound states. When bound to GTP, ARF associates with the membrane of the trans-Golgi network and promotes the binding of COP-coat protein (coatomer). This leads to the budding of vesicles. The hydrolysis of the bound GDP then converts ARF to the GDP-bound state. This leads to the disassembly of the vesicle coat prior to fusion with the target membrane. The GDP-bound ARF is subsequently reconverted to the GTP-bound state. This is mediated by the action of a Golgi membrane protein that promotes a GDP–GTP exchange process. This leads to another cycle of coatomer assembly.

Two types of events characterize fusion of the vesicle with its target. First, the transport vesicles recognize the correct target membrane. Second, the vesicle and target membranes fuse, thus delivering the contents of the vesicle to the target organelle. Recognition between the vesicle and its target is mediated by interactions between unique pairs of transmembrane proteins. In contrast, fusion between the vesicle and target membranes arises from the action of general fusion proteins.

Biochemical analyses of reconstituted vesicular transport systems from mammalian cells have defined two classes of proteins involved in vesicle fusion: NSF and SNAPs. NSF (N-ethylmaleimide-sensitive fusion) is a soluble cytoplasmic protein that binds to membranes with other proteins called SNAPs (soluble NSF attachment proteins). NSF and SNAPs bind to families of specific membrane receptors called SNAP receptors or SNAREs. According to the SNARE hypothesis, interactions between specific vesicle SNAREs (v-SNAREs) and target SNAREs (t-SNAREs) membranes dictate the specificity of the vesicle fusion. Following specific vesicle–target interaction, the SNARE complex recruits NSF and SNAPs, resulting in the fusion of the vesicle and target membranes. For example, transport from the ER to the Golgi requires SNAREs that are located on both the vesicle and target membranes. These interactions are additionally regulated by the Rab GTP-binding proteins that are essential for vesicle transport. The SNARE hypothesis provides a central framework for understanding the molecular mechanisms of vesicle docking and fusion.

The major functions of lysosomes relate to the digestion of material taken up from outside the cell by *endocytosis*. Lysosomes are formed by the fusion of transport vesicles arising from the trans-Golgi network with endosomes, which contain the molecules taken up by endocytosis at the level of the plasma membrane. Acid hydrolyases are targeted to lysosomes by mannose 6-phosphate residues, which are recognized by mannose 6-phosphate receptors in the trans-Golgi network and packaged into clathrin-coated vesicles. After removal of the clathrin coat, these transport vesicles fuse with endosomes, and the acidic internal pH results in dissociation of the hydrolyases from the mannose 6-phosphate receptor. The hydolyases are thus released into the lumen of the endosome. The endosome then matures into a lysosome as it acquires a full compliment of acid hydrolyases that digest the molecules taken up by endocytosis.

4.6 Conclusion: Cystic Fibrosis as a Paradigm of Mutations Leading to Alterations in Transciptional and Post-transcriptional Processing of an Integral Membrane Transport Protein [99–101]

The largest family of membrane transport proteins consists of the *ABC transporters*, so designated because they contain a basic structural unit characterized by six transmembrane domains followed by a highly conserved *ATP binding cassette*. One of the most important members of the ABC family of transporters is the gene responsible for cystic fibrosis. This gene encodes a protein, the *cystic fibrosis transmembrane regulator (CFTR)*, which functions as a Cl⁻ channel in epithelial cells.

Cystic fibrosis (CF) is the most common (1 in 2,500 newborns) lethal recessive genetic disease of Caucasians. The fundamental physiological abnormality in CF is characterized by failure of cyclic adenosine monophosphate (cAMP) regulation of chloride transport across epithelial cell membranes. The CFTR maps to chromosome 7 and comprises 27 exons (i.e., 230 kb of DNA) that encode a glycosylated protein containing 1,480 amino acids with a molecular mass of 170 kilodaltons. The CFTR gene product has two transmembrane domains, each containing six membrane-spanning segments, two nucleotide-binding domains (NBD) and a regulatory (R) domain (Figure 35). The hydolysis of ATP occurs at the NBD sites, while the R domains play an inhibitory role in keeping the Cl⁻ channel closed. The closed state of the Cl⁻ channel arises through the dephosphorylation of the R domain.

The CFTR is restricted to the apical membrane domain of epithelial cells, where it functions as a cAMP-dependent channel that allows the selective transport of chloride ions across the epithelial cell membrane. The binding of ATP leads to the gating of the Cl⁻ channel. As well, the CFTR is regulated by phosphorylation, which is accomplished by the action of a cAMP-dependent protein kinase A (PKA). The phosphorylation of the R domain results in a conformational change that leads to the opening of the chloride channel. The phosphorylated R domain plays a stimulatory role by enhancing the interaction of NBDs with ATP. The binding of ATP by the NBDs and its subsequent hydrolysis control the opening and closing of the chloride channel. The activated CFTR conducts Cl⁻ out of the epithelial cell and functions as a regulatory switch that allows cAMP to inhibit Na⁺ absorption through Na⁺ channels, and stimulate Cl⁻ secretion through channels distinct from the CFTR.

Chloride conductance at the apical membrane domain is dramatically reduced in CF. This is explained on the basis of quantitative or qualitative alterations in the CFTR, such that the clinical phenotype of CF patients is characterized by the inability of epithelial cells to transport or secrete chloride. The specific deletion of 3 bp in exon 10 results in the loss of a phenylalanine residue at position 508 within one of the ATP-binding domains of the CFTR protein (ΔF508). This particular mutation is associated with 70% of the mutant alleles in CF. More than 800 additional mutations within the CF gene comprise the remaining 30% of the mutant alleles in CF.

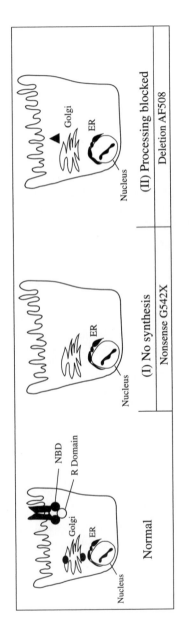

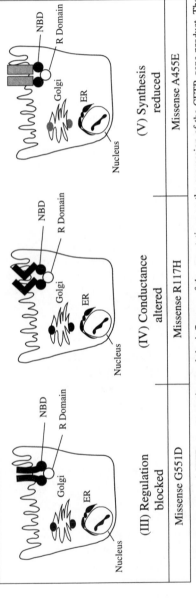

Figure 35. The five classes of CFTR gene mutations and the influence of these mutations on the expression of the CFTR gene product. The CFTR comprises a nucleotide-binding domain (NBD) and regulatory (R) domain.

The ΔF508 mutation, for example, results in defective post-translational processing and intracellular trafficking of the CFTR such that it does not reach the apical membrane domain. Other mutations in the CFTR reduce its function in CF patients by a variety of mechanisms that act at one or several points in the flow of DNA to RNA to protein. Five classes of CFTR mutations have been described, and the molecular consequences of these different classes of mutations are illustrated in Figure 35. However, the various classes of CFTR mutations are not mutually exclusive. For example, in the ΔF508 CF mutation the deletion of phenylalanine leads to misprocessing of the CFTR but also failure of the CFTR protein to respond normally to activation signals.

In summary, mutations in the CFTR gene lead to alterations in transcription, post-transcriptional processing, translation and post-translational processing of the CFTR membrane protein along the secretory pathway. Importantly, the various types of CFTR mutations underscore the importance of each of these critical steps in the regulation of CFTR gene expression.

ABBREVIATIONS

DNA	Deoxyribonucleic acid
A	Adenine
G	Guanine
C	Cytosine
T	Thymine
U	Uracil
RNA	Ribonucleic acid
mRNA	Messenger RNA
tRNA	Transfer RNA
rRNA	Ribosomal RNA
hnRNA	Heterogenous nuclear RNA
snRNA	Small nuclear RNA
UTR	Untranslated regions
SINEs	Short interspersed nuclear elements
LINEs	Long interspersed nuclear elements
G phase	Gap phase
S phase	Synthetic phase
M phase	Mitotic phase
Cdk	Cyclin-dependent kinases
CKI	Cyclin-dependent kinase inhibitors
INK	Inhibitor of Cdk
KIP	Kinase inhibitory protein

REFERENCES

General References

1. Lodish H, Baltimore D, Berk A, Zipursky SL, Matsudaira P, Darnell J. Molecular cell biology. 3d ed. New York: WH Freeman, 1995.
2. Alberts B, Bray D, Johnson A, et al. Essential cell biology – an introduction to the molecular biology of the cell. New York: Garland, 1998.
3. Cooper GM. The cell – a molecular approach. Washington, DC: ASM, 1997.
4. Lewin B. Genes VI. New York: Oxford UP, 1997.
5. Glick BR, Pasternak JL. Molecular biotechnology – principles and applications of recombinant DNA. 2d ed. Washington, DC: ASM, 1998.
6. Alberts B, Bray D, Lewis J, Raff M, Roberts K, Watson JD. Molecular biology of the cell. 3d ed. New York: Garland, 1994.
7. Jameson JL. Principles of molecular medicine. New Jersey: Humana, 1998.
8. Strachan T, Read AP. Human molecular genetics. New York: Wiley-Liss, 1996.

The Cell Cycle

9. Hartwell LH, Kastan MB. Checkpoints: controls that ensure the order of cell cycle events. Science 1989; 246:629–634.
10. Murray AW. Creative blocks: cell-cycle checkpoints and feedback controls. Nature 1992; 359:599–604.
11. Norbury C, Nurse P. Animal cell cycles and their control. Ann Rev Biochem 1992; 61:441–470.
12. Morgan DO. Principles of CDK regulation. Nature 1995; 374:131–134.
13. Levine AJ. The tumor suppressor genes. Ann Rev Biochem 1993; 623–651.

DNA Replication

14. Blackburn EH. Telomerases. Ann Rev Biochem 1992; 61:113-129.
15. Diller JD, Raghuraman MK. Eukaryotic replication origins: control in space in time. Trends Biochem Sci 1994; 19:320–325.
16. Heintz NH, Dailey L, Held P, Heintz N. Eukaryotic replication origins as promoters of bidirectional DNA synthesis. Trends Genet 1992; 8:376-381.
17. Kelman Z, O'Donnell M. DNA polymerse III holoenzyme: structure and function of a chromosomal replicating machine. Ann Rev Biochem 1995; 64:171–200.
18. Roca J. The mechanism of DNA topoisomerases. Trends Biochem Sci 1995; 20:156–160.
19. Zakian VA. Telomeres: beginning to understand the end. Science 1995; 270:1601–1607.

Mutations and DNA Repair

20. Kolodner RD. Mismatch repair: mechanisms and relationships to cancer susceptibility. Trends Biochem Sci 1995; 20:397–401.
21. Leach FSE. Mutations of *mutS* homology in hereditary nonpolyosis colorectal cancer. Cell 1993; 75:1215–1225.
22. Modrich P. Mismatch repair, genetic stability, and cancer. Science 1994; 266:1959–1960.

23. Sancar A. Mechanisms of DNA excision repair. Science 1994; 266:1954–1956.
24. Seeberg E, Eide L, Bjoras M. The base excision repair pathway. Trends Biochem Sci 1995; 20:391–397.
25. Tanaka K, Wood RD. Xeroderma pigmentosum and nucleotide excision repair of DNA. Trends Biochem Sci 1994; 19:83–86.
26. Davis MM. T cell receptor gene diversity and selection. Ann Rev Biochem 1990; 59:475–496.

Eukaryotic Gene Transcription
27. Buratowski S. Mechanisms of gene activation. Science 1995; 270:1773–1774.
28. Grunstein M. Histones as regulators of genes. Sci Amer 1992; 267(4):68–74B.
29. Paranjape SM, Kamakaka, RT, Kadonaga, JT. Role of chromatin structure in the regulation of transcription by RNA polymerase II. Ann Rev Biochem 1994; 63:265–297.
30. Tjian R. Molecular machines that control genes. Sci Amer 1995; 272(2): 54–61.
31. Tjian R, Maniatis T. Transcriptional activation: a complex puzzle with few easy pieces. Cell 1994; 77:5–8.
32. Goodrich JA, Cutler G, Tjian R. Contacts in context: promoter specificity and macromolecular interactions in transcription. Cell 1996; 84:825–830.
33. Beato M, Herrlich P, Schutz G. Steroid hormone receptors: many actors in search of a plot. Cell 1995; 83:851–857.
34. Gehring WJ, Qian YQ, Billeter M, et al. Homeodomain-DNA recognition. Cell 1994; 78:211–223.
35. Maniatis T, Goodbourn S, Fischer JA. Regulation of inducible and tissue-specific gene expression. Science 1987; 236:1237–1244.
36. Pabo CO, Sauer RT. Transcriptional regulation in mammalian cells by sequence-specific DNA binding proteins. Ann Rev Biochem 1992; 61:1053–1095.

Eukaryotic RNA Polymerases and Basal Transcription Factors
37. Buratowski S. The basics of basal transcription by RNA polymerase II. Cell 1994; 77:1–3.
38. Conaway RC, Conaway JC. General initiation factors for RNA polymerase II. Ann Rev Biochem 1993; 62:161–190.
39. Young RA. RNA polymerase II. Ann Rev Biochem 1991; 60:689–715.
40. Zawel L, Reinberg D. Common themes in assembly and function of eukaryotic transcription complexes. Ann Rev Biochem 1995; 64:533–561.
41. Hanna-Rose W, Hansen U. Active repression mechanisms of eukaryotic transcription repressors. Trends Genet 1996; 12:229–234.

Post-transcriptional Processing of RNA
42. Bird A. The essentials of DNA methylation. Cell 1992; 70:5–8.
43. Staudt LM, Lenardo MJ. Immunoglobulin gene transcription. Ann Rev Immunol 1991; 9:373–398.
44. Beelman CA, Parker R. Degradation of mRNA in eukaryotes. Cell 1995; 81:179–183.
45. Foulkes NS, Sassone-Corsi P. More is better: activators and repressors from the same gene. Cell 1992; 68:411–414.

46. Green MR. Biochemical mechanisms of constitutive and regulated pre-mRNA splicing. Ann Rev Cell Biol 1991; 7:559–599.
47. Keller W. No end yet to messenger RNA 3' processing! Cell 1995; 81:829–832.
48. Klausner RD, Rouault TA, Harford JB. Regulating the fate of mRNA: the control of cellular iron metabolism. Cell 1993; 72:19–28.
49. Maniatis T. Mechanisms of alternative pre-mRNA splicing. Science 1991; 251:33–34.
50. McKeown M. Alternative mRNA splicing. Ann Rev Cell Biol 1992; 8:133–155.
51. Bennett MM, Amara SG. Molecular mechanisms of cell-specific and regulated expression of the calcitonin/alpha-CGRP and beta-CGRP genes. Ann NY Acad Sci 1992; 657:36–49.
52. Zandberg H, Moen TC, Baas PD. Cooperation of 5' and 3' processing sites as well as intron and exon sequences in calcitonin exon recognition. Nucleic Acid Research 1995; 23(2):248–255.
53. Lou H, Cote GJ, Gagel RF. The calcitonin exon and its flanking intronic sequences are sufficient for the regulation of human calcitonin/calcitonin gene-related peptide alternative RNA splicing. Mol Endocrinol 1994; 8(12); 1618–1626.
54. Chan L. Apolipoprotein B messenger RNA editing; and update. Biochimie 1995; 77(1–2): 75–78.
55. Chan L, Chang BH, Nakamuta M, Li WH, Smith LC. Apobec-1 and apolipoprotein B mRNA editing. Biochim Biophys Acta 1997; 1345(1): 11–26.
56. Schibler U, Hagenbuchle O, Wellauer PK, Pittet AC. Two promoters of different strengths control the transcription of the mouse alpha-amylase gene Amy-1a in the parotid gland and the liver. Cell 1983; 33: 501–508.
57. Sierra F, Pittet AC, Schibler U. Different tissue-specific expression of the amylase gene Amy-1 in mice and rats. Mol Cell Biol 1986; 6(11):4067–4076.

Translation of mRNA
58. Hershey JWB. Translation control in mammalian cells. Ann Rev Biochem 1991; 60:717–755.
59. Klausner RD, Rouault TA, Harford JB. Regulating the fate of mRNA: the control of cellular iron metabolism. Cell 1993; 72:19–28.
60. Kozak M. Regulation of translation in eukaryotic systems. Ann Rev Cell Biol 1992; 8:187–225.
61. Merrick WC. Mechanism and regulation of eukaryotic protein synthesis. Microbiol Rev 1992; 56:291–315.
62. Noller HF. Ribosomal RNA and translation. Ann Rev Biochem 1991; 60:191–227.
63. Rhoads RE. Regulation of eukaryotic protein synthesis by initiation factors. J Biol Chem 1993; 268:3017–3020.

Protein Folding and Processing
64. Casey PJ. Protein lipidation in cell signaling. Science 1995; 268:221–225.
65. Clarke S. Protein isoprenylation and methylation at carboxy-terminal cysteine residues. Ann Rev Biochem 1992; 61:355–386.
66. Dalbey RE, von Heijne G. Signal peptidases in prokaryotes and eukaryotes – a new protease family. Trends Biochem Sci 1992; 17:474–478.

67. Englund PT. The structure and biosynthesis of glycolsyl phosphatidylinositol protein anchors. Ann Rev Biochem 1993; 62:121–138.
68. Freedman RB, Hirst TR, Tuite MF. Protein disulphide isomerase: building bridges in protein folding. Trends Biochem Sci 1994; 19:331–336.
69. Gething M-J, Sambrook J. Protein folding in the cell. Nature 1992; 355: 33–45.
70. Gierasch LM. Signal sequences. Biochemistry 1989; 28:923–930.
71. Hart GW, Haltiwanger RS, Holt GD, Kelly WG. Glycosylation in the nucleus and cytoplasm. Ann Rev Biochem 1989; 58:841–874.
72. Hartl FU. Molecular chaperones in cellular protein folding. Nature 1996; 381:571–580.

Protein Sorting and Transport
73. Fischer von Mallard GB, Stahl CL, Sudhof TC, Jahn R. Rab proteins in regulated exocytosis. Trends Biochem Sci 1994; 19:164–168.
74. Mellman I. Protein mediators of membrane fusion. Cell 1995; 82:869–872.
75. Novick P, Brennwald P. Friends and family: the role of Rab GTPases in vesicular traffic. Cell 1993; 75:597–601.
76. Pelham HRB. About turn for the COPs? Cell 1994; 79:1125–1127.
77. Pryer NK, Wuestehube LJ, Schekman R. Vesicle-mediated protein sorting. Ann Rev Biochem 1992; 61:471–516.
78. Rothman JE. Mechanisms of intracellular protein transport. Nature 1994; 372:55–62.
79. Rothman JE, Wieland FT. Protein sorting by transport vesicles. Science 272: 227–234, 1996.
80. Schekman R, Orci L. Coat proteins and vesicle budding. Science 1996; 271:1526–1533.
81. Whiteheart SW, Kubalek EW. SNAPs and NSF: general members of the fusion apparatus. Trends Cell Biol 1995; 5:64–68.

Protein Degradation
82. Ciechanover A. The ubiquitin-proteasome proteolytic pathway. Cell 1994; 79:13–21.
83. Dice JF. Peptide sequences that target cytosolic proteins for lysosomal proteolysis. Trends Biochem Sci 1990; 15:305–309.
84. Goldberg AL. Functions of the proteasome: the lysis at the end of the tunnel. Science 1995; 268:522–523.

The Endoplasmic Reticulum
85. Abeijon C. Hirschberg CB. Topography of gylcosylation reactions in the endoplasmic reticulum. Trends Biochem Sci 1992; 17:32–36.
86. Gilmore R. Protein translocation across the endoplasmic reticulum: a tunnel with toll booths at entry and exit. Cell 1993; 75:589–592.
87. Hendrick JP, Hartl FU. Molecular chaperone functions of heat-shock proteins. Ann Rev Biochem 1993; 62:349–384.
88. Hurtley SM. Golgi localization signals. Trends Biochem Sci 1992; 17:2–3.
89. Rapaport TA. Transport of proteins across the endoplasmic reticulum membrane. Science 1992; 258:931–936.
90. Sanders SL, Schekman R. Polypeptide translocation across the endoplasmic reticulum membrane. J Biol Chem 1992; 267:13791–13794.

91. Udenfriend S, Kodukula K. How glycosylphosphatidylinositol anchored membrane proteins are made. Ann Rev Biochem 1995; 64:563–591.
92. Walter P, Johnson AE. Signal sequence recognition and protein targeting to the endoplasmic reticulum membrane. Ann Rec Cell Biol 1994; 10:87–119.

The Golgi Apparatus
93. Burgess TL, Kelly RB. Constitutive and regulated secretion of proteins. Ann Rev Cell Biol 1998; 3:243–293.
94. Machamer CE. Targeting and retention of Golgi membrane proteins. Curr Opin Cell Biol 1993; 5:606–612.
95. Pelham HRB, Munro S. Sorting of membrane proteins in the secretory pathway. Cell 1993; 75:603–605.

Lysosomes
96. Dunn WA, Jr. Autophagy and related mechanisms of lysosome-mediated protein degradation. Trends Cell Biol 1991; 266:21327–21330.
97. Kornfeld S. Structure and function of the mannose 6-phosphate/insulinlike growth factor II receptors. Ann Rev Biochem 1992; 61:307–330.
98. Kornfeld S, Mellman I. The biogenesis of lysosomes. Ann Rev Cell Biol 1989; 5:483–525.

Cystic Fibrosis
99. Collins FS. Cystic fibrosis: molecular biology and therapeutic implications. Science 1992; 256: 774–779.
100. Zielenski J, Tsui LC. Cystic fibrosis: genotypic and phenotypic variations. Ann Rev Genet 1995; 29:777–807.
101. Davis PB, Drumm M, Konstan MW. Cystic fibrosis. Am J Respir Crit Care Med 1996; 154:1229–1256.

ACKNOWLEDGMENTS

This work was supported by operating grants from the Medical Research Council of Canada and the Crohn's and Colitis Foundation of Canada. Dr. Gary E. Wild is a senior clinician scientist of the Fonds de la recherche en santé du Québec. Dr. Wild wishes to extend his appreciation to Drs. David Fromson, John Southin, Howard Bussey and Bruce Brandhorst of the McGill Biology Department. Their tireless efforts in the area of undergraduate science education fostered a sense of inquiry and collegiality that guided a cohort of students through the early recombinant DNA era.

List of Contributors

ADAMS, P., London Health Sciences Centre - University Campus, 339 Windermere Rd., P.O. Box 5339, London, ON N6A 5A5. Tel: (519) 663-3513 Fax: (519) 663-3232 E-mail: padams@julian.uwo.ca

ARCHAMBAULT, A., Hôpital Maisonneuve-Rosemont, 5415, boulevard de l'Assomption, Montréal, QC H1T 2M4. Tel: (514) 252-3822 Fax : (514) 252-1452.

BAIN, V.G., University of Alberta, 2E3.27 W.M.C., 8440-112th St., Edmonton, AB T6G 2B7. Tel: (780) 407-7238 Fax: (780) 439-1922 E-mail: vince.bain@ualberta.ca

BARKUN, A.N.G., Director, Division of Gastroenterology, McGill University Health Centre, Montreal General Hospital Site, 1650 Cedar Avenue, Room D7.148, Montréal, QC H3G 1A4. Tel: (514) 934-8233 Fax: (514) 934-8375 E-mail: alan.barkun@muhc.mcgill.ca

BECK, I.T., Gastrointestinal Diseases Research Unit, Queen's University, Hotel Dieu Hospital, 166 Brock St., Kingston, ON K7L 5G2. Tel: (613) 544-0225 or 544-3400 ext. 2289 Fax: (613) 544-3114 E-mail: becki@hdh.kari.net

BURNSTEIN, M., St. Michael's Hospital, 38 Shuter St., Suite 504, Toronto, ON M5B 1A6. Tel: (416) 864-6050 Fax: (416) 864-5668 E-mail: burnsteinm@smh.toronto.on.ca

BURSEY, R.F., Memorial University of Newfoundland, Faculty of Medicine, Health Sciences Centre, 300 Prince Philip Dr., St. John's, NF A1B 3V6. Tel: (709) 737-6960 Fax: (709) 737-3605 E-mail: fbursey@morgan.ucs.mun.ca

BUTZNER, J.D., University of Calgary, Health Sciences Centre, 3330 Hospital Dr. NW, Calgary, AB T2N 4N1. Tel: (403) 220-4561 Fax: (403) 283-3028 E-mail: butzner@ucalgary.ca

CHAMPION, M.C., Division of Gastroenterology, The Ottawa Hospital - Civic Campus, 1053 Carling Ave., Ottawa, ON K1Y 4E9. Tel: (613) 761-4674 Fax: (613) 761-5269 E-mail: mchampion@civich.ottawa.on.ca

FARDY, J.M., Memorial University of Newfoundland, Faculty of Medicine, Health Sciences Centre, 300 Prince Philip Dr., St. John's, NF A1B 3V6. Tel: (709) 737-7064 Fax: (709) 737-3605 E-mail: jfardy@morgan.ucs.mun.ca

FARIA, J., Division of Gastroenterology, McGill University Health Centre, 1650 Cedar Ave., Montreal, QC H3G 1A4. Tel: (514) 934-8308 Fax: (514) 934-8411.

FEAGAN, B.G., University of Western Ontario, Faculty of Medicine, London Health Sciences Centre, University Campus, P.O. Box 5339, London, ON N6A 5A5. Tel: (519) 663-3589 Fax: 519-663-3807 E-mail: feagan@lctrg.com

FEDORAK, R.N., University of Alberta, 519 Newton Research Building, 11315-87 Ave., Edmonton, AB T6G 2C2. Tel: (780) 407-6941 Fax: (780) 407-3744 E-mail: richard.fedorak@ualberta.ca

FREEMAN, H.J., UBC Hospital, Acute Care Unit, Room F-137, 2211 Wesbrook, Vancouver, BC V6T 2B5. Tel: (604) 822-7216 Fax: (604) 822-7236.

GILLIES, R.R., (formerly) The Ottawa Hospital - Civic Campus, 1053 Carling Ave., Ottawa, ON K1Y 4E9. Tel: (613) 761-4603 or (613) 729-8926 (home) Fax: (613) 761-5269.

GIRGRAH, N., The Toronto Hospital, General Division, 200 Elizabeth St.,10 NU - 146, Toronto ON, M5G 2C4. Tel: (416) 340-5221 Fax (416) 340-3492 E-mail: nigel.girgrah@uhn.on.ca

GRÉGOIRE, S., The Ottawa Hospital - General Campus, 311 McArthur Rd., Suite 203, Vanier, ON K1L 6P1. Tel: (613) 744-8180 Fax: (613) 744-7982 E-mail: daniel.foucaud@sympatico.ca

HABAL, F., The Toronto Hospital, General Division, 200 Elizabeth St., EN9-229, Toronto, ON M5G 2C4. Tel: (416) 340-5023 Fax: (416) 595-5251 E-mail: flavio.habal@utoronto.ca

HEATHCOTE, J., University Health Network, The Toronto Hospital, Western Division, 399 Bathurst Street, 6B Fell Wing - 172, Toronto ON M5T 2S8 Tel: (416) 603-5914 Fax: (416) 603-9195 E-mail: jennyheathcote@earthlink.net

HILSDEN, R.J., Department of Community Health Sciences, University of Calgary, Health Sciences Centre, 3330 Hospital Dr. NW, Calgary, AB T2N 4N1. Tel: (403) 220-6536 Fax: (403) 270-7287 E-mail: rhilsden@ucalgary.ca

HUNT, R.H., McMaster University Medical Centre, 1200 Main St. W, Room 4W8, Hamilton, ON L8N 3Z5. Tel: (905) 521-2100 ext. 76404 Fax: (905) 521-5072 E-mail: huntr@fhs.mcmaster.ca

HURLBUT, D.J., Department of Pathology, Queen's University, Kingston General Hospital, 76 Stuart St., Kingston, ON K7L 2V7. Tel: (613) 549-6666 ext. 6035 Fax: (613) 548-6076 E-mail: hurlbut@cliff.path.queensu.ca

LEE, S.S., Dept. of Medicine, University of Calgary, Health Sciences Centre, 3330 Hospital Dr. NW, Calgary, AB T2N 4N1. Tel: (403) 220-3245 Fax: (403) 270-0995 E-mail: samlee@ucalgary.ca

LEMOYNE, M., Hôpital Saint-Luc, 1058, rue Saint-Denis, Montréal, QC H2X 3J4. Tel: (514) 281-2121 Fax: (514) 281-6135.

LEVY, G.A., The Toronto Hospital, General Division, 621 University Ave., NU10-116, Toronto, ON M5G 2C4. Tel: (416) 340-5166 Fax: (416) 340-3378 E-mail: fg12@msn.com

LILLY, L.B., The Toronto Hospital, General Division, 621 University Ave., NU10-162, Toronto, ON M5G 2C4. Tel: (416) 340-4629 Fax: (416) 340-3492 E-mail: les.lilly@uhn.on.ca

MA, M., University of Alberta, 2E1.04 W.M.C., 8440 -112th St., Edmonton, AB T6G 2R7. Tel: (780) 407-7485 Fax: (780) 439-1922 E-mail: mang.ma@ualberta.ca

MacDONALD, P.H., Hotel Dieu Hospital, 166 Brock St., Kingston, ON K7L 5G2. Tel: (613) 544-3400 ext. 2424 Fax: (613) 546-4854 E-mail: phm@post.queensu.ca

MacINTOSH, D.G., Queen Elizabeth II Health Sciences Centre - Victoria General Site, Room 927, Centennial Wing, 1278 Tower Rd., Halifax, NS B3H 2Y9. Tel: (902) 473-3620 Fax: (902) 473-4406 E-mail: dgmacint@is.dal.ca

MACHIDA, H., Alberta Children's Hospital, 1820 Richmond Rd. SW, Calgary, AB T2T 5C7.

MALKAN, G., Consultant Hepatologist, Bombay Hospital and Medical Research Centre, Marine Lines, Mumbai, India.

MARTIN, S.R., Service de gastro-entérologie et nutrition, Hôpital Sainte-Justine, Université de Montréal, 3175, Côte Sainte-Catherine, Montréal, QC H3T 1C5. Tel: (514) 345-4626 Fax: (514) 345-4999. E-mail: martinst@magellan.umontreal.ca

MAY, G.R., University of Calgary, Health Sciences Centre, Room 701, 3330 Hospital Dr. NW, Calgary, AB T2N 4N1. Tel: (403) 220-4557 Fax: (403) 220-8747 E-mail: gmay@ucalgary.ca

MAYRAND, S., GI Division, Montreal General Hospital, D7120 - 1650, av Cedar, Montréal, QC H3G 1A4. Tel: (514) 934-8308 or 514-934-8233 Fax: (514) 934-8375 E-mail: serge.mayrand@muhc.mcgill.ca

MERCER, C.D., Dept. of Surgery, Hotel Dieu Hospital, 166 Brock St., Kingston, ON K7L 5G2. Tel: (613) 544-3400, ext. 2474 Fax: (613) 546-4854 E-mail: mercerd@HDH.KARI.NET

MORRISON, D.J., Developmental Paediatrics, Alberta Children's Hospital, 1820 Richmond Rd. SW, Calgary, AB T2T 5C7. Tel: (403) 229-7821 Fax: (403) 229-7649 E-mail: diane.morrison@crha-health.ab.ca

PAPALIA, P., Division of Gastroenterology, McGill University Health Centre, 1650 Cedar Ave., Montreal, QC H3G 1A4. Tel: (514) 934-8308 Fax: (514) 934-8411.

PARÉ, P., Hôtel-Dieu de Québec, 11, Côte du Palais, 7th Floor, Québec, QC G1R 2J6. Tel: (418) 691-5252 Fax: (418) 691-5348 E-mail: Medecine.PHDQ@dechuq.ulaval.ca

PARSONS, H.G., Paediatric Gastroenterology and Nutrition, Faculty of Medicine, University of Calgary, Health Sciences Centre, 3330 Hospital Dr. NW, Calgary, AB T2N 4N1. Tel: (403) 220-7496 Fax: (403) 283-3028 E-mail: hparsons@ucalgary.ca

PATEL, D.G., Division of Gastroenterology, The Ottawa Hospital - Civic Campus, 1053 Carling Ave., Ottawa, ON K1Y 4E9. Tel: (613) 761-4501 Fax: (613) 761-5269 E-mail: dpatel@civich.ottawa.on.ca

PATERSON, W.G., GI Division, Hotel Dieu Hospital, 166 Brock St., Kingston, ON K7L 5G2. Tel: (613) 544-3310 ext. 2332 or 3376 Fax: (613) 544-3114 E-mail: patersow@hdh.kari.net

ROPELESKI, M.J., Division of Gastroenterology, McGill University Health Centre, 1650 Cedar Ave., Montreal, QC H3G 1A4. Tel: (514) 934-8308 Fax: (514) 934-8411.

SALENA, B.J., McMaster University Medical Centre, 1200 Main St. W, Room 4W8, Hamilton, ON L8N 3Z5. Tel: (905) 521-2100 ext. 76782 Fax: (905) 521-4958 E-mail: salenab@fhs.csu.McMaster.ca

SCHREIBER, R.A., British Columbia's Children's Hospital, 4480 Oak St., Room D611, Vancouver, BC V6H 3V4. Tel: (604) 875-2332 Fax: (604) 875-3244 E-mail: rschreiber@cw.bc.ca

SCOTT, R.B., Paediatric Gastroenterology and Nutrition, Faculty of Medicine, University of Calgary. Alberta Children's Hospital, 1820 Richmond Rd. SW, Calgary, AB T2T 5C7. Tel: (403) 229-7802 Fax: (403) 229-7665 E-mail: Brent.Scott@CRHA-Health.ab.ca

SCULLY, L.J., Division of Gastroenterology, GI Unit A1, The Ottawa Hospital - Civic Campus, 1053 Carling Avenue, Ottawa, ON K1Y 4E9.

Tel: (613) 761-4830 Fax: (613) 761-5269.
E-mail: dthompson@ottawahospital.on.ca

SEKAR, A.S.C., Division of Gastroenterology, The Ottawa Hospital -
Civic Campus, 306-1081 Carling Avenue, Ottawa, ON K1Y 4G2.
Tel: (613) 729-3179 Fax: (613) 729-1026.

SHAFFER, E.A., Professor and Head, Department of Medicine, University
of Calgary and Head, Regional Department of Medicine, Calgary Regional Health Authority, Foothills Hospital, 1403-29 St. NW, Room C210,
Calgary, AB T2N 2T9. Tel: (403) 670-1500 Fax: (403) 670-1095
E-mail: eldon.shaffer@crha-health.ab.ca

SIDOROV, J.J., Victoria Medical Building, 307-1669 Victoria St.,
Prince George, BC V2L 2L5. Tel: (250) 564-2182 Fax: (250) 964-6110
E-mail: jsng@telus.net

SIMON, J.B., Division of Gastroenterology, Queen's University,
Hotel Dieu Hospital, 166 Brock St., Kingston, ON K7L 5G2.
Tel: (613) 544-3310 ext. 2483 Fax: (613) 544-3114
E-mail: simonj@post.queensu.ca

STEINBRECHER, U.P., Professor of Medicine and Head, UBC Division
of Gastroenterology, Vancouver Hospital & Health Sciences Centre,
Willow Chest Centre, 100 - 2647 Willow St., Vancouver, BC V5Z 3P1.
Tel: (604) 875-5862 or 875-5244 Fax : (604) 875-5447
E-mail: usteinbr@interchange.ubc.ca

THOMPSON, W. G., Emeritus Professor of Medicine, University of
Ottawa, 7 Nesbitt Street, Ottawa, ON K2H 8C4. Tel: (613) 761-4147
Fax: (613) 761-5269 E-mail: wgthompson@compuserve.com

THOMSON, A.B.R., University of Alberta, 519 Newton Research Building,
11315-87 Ave., Edmonton, AB T6G 2C2. Tel: (780) 407-6490
Fax: (780) 407-7964 E-mail: alan.thomson@ualberta.ca

TOMALTY, D. , Department of Diagnostic Radiology, Queen's University,
c/o Imaging Services, Kingston General Hospital, 76 Stuart Street,
Kingston, ON K7L 2V7. Tel: (613) 548-2301 Fax: (613) 548-2412
E-mail: RDT1@post.queensu.ca

TURNBULL, G.K., Queen Elizabeth II Health Sciences Centre - Victoria
General Hospital Site, 1278 Tower Rd., Room 927, Halifax, NS
B3H 2Y9. Tel: (902) 473-3620 Fax: (902) 473-4406
E-mail: turnbull@is.dal.ca

VANNER, S.J., Hotel Dieu Hospital, 166 Brock St., Kingston, ON
K7L 5G2. Tel: (613) 544-3310 ext. 2473 Fax: (613) 544-3114
E-mail: vanners@hdh.kari.net

WATTERS, J.M., The Ottawa Hospital - Civic Campus, 737 Parkdale

Avenue, Room 208, Ottawa, ON K1Y 1J8 Tel: (613) 761-4780
Fax: (613) 761-4698 E-mail: jwatters@lri.ca

WHITTAKER, J.S., 550 - 1144 Burrard St., Vancouver, BC V6Z 2A5.
Tel: (604) 683-6393 Fax: (604) 681-2421.
E-mail: whitaker@interchange.ubc.ca

WILD, G.E., Montreal General Hospital, 1650 Cedar Ave., Montreal, QC
H3G 1A4. Tel: (514) 934-8308 Fax: (514) 934-8411
E-mail: gwild@is.mgh.mcgill.ca

WITHERS, G., (formerly) Dept. of Paediatrics, University of Calgary,
Health Sciences Centre, 3330 Hospital Drive NW, Calgary, AB T2N 4N1.
(currently) 28 Ardross Cres., Mount Lawley West, Australia 6050.

WONG, F., The Toronto Hospital, General Division, 200 Elizabeth St.,
Toronto, ON M5G 2C4. Tel: (416) 340-3834 Fax: (416) 340-5019
E-mail: florence.wong@utoronto.ca

WOROBETZ, L.J., Dept. of Gastroenterology, Royal University Hospital,
University of Saskatchewan, 103 Hospital Dr., Saskatoon, SK S7N 0W8.
Tel: (306) 966-7964 Fax: (306) 966-7996
E-mail: worobetz@sk.sympatico.ca

ZAMORA, S.A., Hôpital des Enfants, 6, rue Willy-Donze, Geneva,
Switzerland. Tel: 41 22 382 45 16 Fax: 41 22 382 45 04
E-mail: Samuel.Zamora@HCUGE.CH

Index

The bold letter **t** or **f** following a page reference indicates that the information appears on that page only in a table or figure, respectively.